your church a house of healing

MICHAEL GEMIGNANI

Foreword by Keith Miller

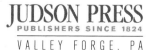

JUDSON PRESS
PUBLISHERS SINCE 1824
VALLEY FORGE, PA

Making Your Church a House of Healing
© 2008 by Judson Press, Valley Forge, PA 19482-0851
All rights reserved.

The author and Judson Press have made every effort to trace the ownership of all quotes. In the event of a question arising from the use of a quote, we regret any error made and will be pleased to make the necessary correction in future printings and editions of this book.

Bible quotations in this volume, unless otherwise noted, are taken from *Holy Bible, New International Version*®. NIV®. Copyright © 1973, 1978, 1984 by International Bible Society. Used by permission of Zondervan. All rights reserved.

Library of Congress Cataloging-in-Publication Data
Gemignani, Michael C.
Making your church a house of healing / Michael Gemignani. — 1st ed.
    p. cm.
ISBN 978-0-8170-1530-5 (pbk. : alk. paper) 1. Spiritual healing. 2. Church work with the sick. 3. Pastoral medicine. I. Title.
BT732.5.G46   2008
    234'.131—dc22

                                                                    2008005894

Printed on recycled paper in the U.S.A.
First Edition, 2008.

*To Nancy McCann and
the Glory Bound Singers
of the Daughters of the King,
in recognition of their glorious music
and deep commitment to the Lord.*

CONTENTS

FOREWORD

Making Your Church a House of Healing is a remarkable book. Rarely does a brilliant intellectual come up with a deceptively simple and user-friendly theological insight that can transform life in a local congregation. Michael Gemignani has done that.*

At a time when many churches are crying out for an authentically Christian focus and practical structures to implement this focus, Michael's perceptive definition of Christ's purpose for his church—based on solid biblical and psychological foundations—is a bright light in what can seem to be a swirling darkness of confusion, controversy, and division engulfing the Christian community today.

The author sees Jesus' vision for the church primarily as a place for specifically diagnosing and treating "spiritual illnesses." Furthermore, he perceives that spiritual healing is inherent in the "life-in-community" described and inaugurated by Jesus. This kind of community life can be a remedy for all kinds of dis-ease revealed in the symptoms of physical and emotional illnesses and abuse, which often results from marginalization of individuals and races separated by social and economic pressures. These and other casualties of the self-centered competitive culture of the world—and sometimes churches—are examples of "spiritual illness." From this recognition of our current brokenness, the author leads us to see how the local church can become a safe place—a house of healing in which all kinds of people (including present parishioners) can discover, or recover, their spiritual balance, freedom, and courage. We are transformed in a culture of Christ's caring love and healing among other people whose lives are also being healed.

Michael Gemignani is a wise and honest pioneer. He is clear about how this can be a rewarding and fulfilling adventure. He is equally direct in pointing out and describing the fact that life will not be easy or trouble free. In this volume, the reader will find clear descriptions of what a congregation will likely face, suggestions from actual case histories, and personal illustrations of methods used to deal with all kinds of resistance and change.

This is not another scheme to attract more people to your local congregation. But when the church becomes a house of healing, I predict that the transformation in progress in the lives of the members will attract all the new "patients" you would wish for.

As members each begin their journey of seeing the nature of their own personal needs—and of receiving help in terms of God's healing, they are asked only to learn how to pass on specific aspects of the *same healing and loving acceptance* they have already received. The sharing of these discoveries can be seen in day-sized, achievable goals.

I am happy to recommend this honest and insightful book and the man who wrote it because both are realistic and Christ-centered guides for congregations and individuals looking for a new and exciting adventure with God in real-life terms.

Keith Miller, Author
The Taste of New Wine,
The Edge of Adventure (with Bruce Larson),
A Hunger for Healing, and
What to Do with the Rest of Your Life:
Awakening and Achieving Your Unspoken Dreams

An Additional Word about the Author

Michael Gemignani is a secret treasure for the church. I suspect that most people who know him have little or no idea of the breadth and depth of the education and experience that have prepared him uniquely to write this book. In a world obsessed with mathematical evidence and the need for scientific and intellectual prowess, Michael's humility about his background is a significant qualification for writing this particular book. Additional qualifications are that he has earned an MS and PhD in mathematics from Notre Dame University as well as a law degree (Juris Doctorate, *summa cum laude*) from Indiana University Law School. His career includes teaching at St. Mary's College, South Bend, SUNY Buffalo, and Smith College. Michael was professor and chair of mathematical sciences at Indiana University; dean of arts and sciences at the University of Maine, Orono; and senior vice-president for academic affairs and provost at the University of Houston in Clear Lake. He has written fourteen books in the fields of law, computer science, mathematics, and spiritual development, and he has completed many articles and lectureships—including being national lecturer for the Association for Computer Machinery. Michael has also written the music and lyrics for numerous hymns. These experiences in the mainstream of the world's culture plus his theological training and experience as an ordained minister combine to give the author an unusual perspective regarding ministry in a congregation interfacing contemporary culture.

The Reverend Dr. Gemignani founded the Brazosport Medical Center to provide health care for an underserved population and the spiritual director training program for the largest Episcopal Diocese in the US. During many of the years he was accomplishing these things in the "real world," the author has been—and still is—a parish priest in the Episcopal Church, learning how to live out the concepts he has now described in *The Church as a House of Healing*.

KM

PREFACE

The central thesis of this book is that Jesus Christ established the church primarily to be an instrument of spiritual healing. Each local church, as an embodiment of the church, should, therefore, have spiritual healing as the focus of its ministry.

These simple statements lead at once to many complex questions. What is spiritual healing? Why is it so important? If our church wants to become deeply involved in spiritual healing, how should it go about it? What are some of the obstacles we are likely to encounter and how might we overcome them? This book was written to try to address each of these questions.

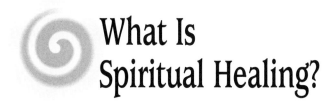 # What Is Spiritual Healing?

The church universal was established by Christ first and foremost as an instrument of spiritual healing. If one considers spiritual disease as the inability of human beings to come into a right relationship with God on their own, then becoming a member of the church, the body of Christ, is a cure for our inherent estrangement from God. If one considers spiritual disease as the human inability to become ever more Christlike, to be drawn ever deeper into the life of God, then Christ has cured that disease by sending the Holy Spirit, the Sanctifier, to his church, that Spirit through which we may become holy by becoming more and more like God. If spiritual disease is our innate inability to see God as God is, then Christ offers the cure for that disease because, although now we see but a poor reflection in a mirror, through Christ we may come to see God face to face and know as we are known (1 Corinthians 13:12).

It is true, of course, that all true spiritual cures come through Christ and the Holy Spirit, but both Christ and the Holy Spirit act in, and through, the church, the body of all faithful believers, the organic extension of God's presence in the world, of which Jesus Christ is the Head and the Holy Spirit is the vital element or soul.

Spiritual healing consists of growing ever more into the life of God through Jesus Christ by the power of Holy Spirit. Athanasius, a bishop in the early church and a great theologian, stated that God became a human being so that human beings could become God. No, we do not become God as God is God, or even as Jesus is God. We remain finite creatures, but we are privileged, graced by God, to share in God's own life through our sharing in life of Christ, and thus to gain a fullness, a blessedness, a life that transcends any merely natural life, however happy and fulfilled that natural life may be.

Spiritual healing and love

As we are healed spiritually, we become more highly conformed to God. Though our minds may still suffer from the turmoil of the human condition, our wills become more and more attuned to the will of God. We not only love God in a more profound way by choosing as we believe God wants us to choose. In loving God more, we find that God's love pours out from us on to our neighbors. As we become more like God, we love more like God loves. God's love embraces the entire human race. We seek to love others with the same love with which Christ first loved us.

If we find ourselves becoming proud that we are being healed, then we may be sure that our healing is false. True healing comes about only through the power of the Holy Spirit, not because we have the ability ourselves to make it happen. As we come to know God more, we recognize our own weakness, our own nothingness in comparison with the infinite power and grandeur of God. We may rejoice in our weakness, for it magnifies the power of God. "'My grace is sufficient for you, for my [God's] power is made perfect in weakness.' Therefore I will boast all the more gladly about my weaknesses, so that Christ's power may rest on me" (2 Corinthians 12:9).

And if we find ourselves being healed, then our most ardent desire is that others be healed as well. We recognize that if God has had such mercy on us, then others are even more deserving of

God's mercy. We pray that the whole world will be aflame with the love of God.

Spiritual healing and physical healing

The essence of spiritual healing is growing into God's divine life. It therefore seems paradoxical that our natural lives all too often engage in a process of decline as we grow older. But even the young can become seriously ill, blind, crippled, or in acute physical pain. Doesn't spiritual health imply physical health as well? A substantial portion of Jesus' ministry consisted of healing physical ailments, giving sight to the blind and restoring bodily wholeness to the crippled and lame. Should the church not be about physical healing as well as spiritual healing?

Of course, the church should seek to alleviate all manner of human suffering. The church should be a prophetic voice for social justice, work to clothe the naked and feed the hungry, compassionately tend to the sick and the dying, and work for physical healing through its prayers and ministries. Jesus himself ordered his disciples to go forth and heal the sick (Matthew 10:5-8; Luke 9:1-2). What's more, Jesus stated that whatever act of kindness we do for the least of his brothers and sisters, we do for him (Matthew 25:40).

Nevertheless, the disciples went forth not primarily to heal physical ailments but to preach that the kingdom of God was close at hand. We might say that their mission was to announce that spiritual healing was at hand, and their physical cures were signs that they spoke the truth. Our earthly life will rarely be free of physical pain and suffering, but spiritual healing draws us into a new dimension of living where even physical illness can be a source of grace. In any event, no matter how healthy we may be throughout our earthly lives, our earthly lives will one day end. We will all die even if we have no illness whatever until the moment our hearts stop forever. If we are healed spiritually, we will not fear death or even bodily illness, for our true life resides in the eternal love and glory of God.

The local congregation and spiritual healing

A congregation, as the local embodiment of the church universal, should be an instrument of the broader church, an instrument of Christ himself, for the spiritual healing of its members. Spiritual healing is almost always something that does not happen instantly but, rather, is progressive as the Holy Spirit continues the work of transformation. Local churches should challenge their members to be open to the Spirit's power—that is, to be open to spiritual healing. They should be places where Christians are supported and encouraged in spiritual healing and where the many gifts God has given the church to assist Christians in their healing are freely available. For healing is not one of many programs of the church and the local congregation. It is the central mission of the church and should be the central mission of every congregation, even though the mission may be realized in different ways in different churches.

Perhaps one of the reasons for the decline in some denominations is that they have lost sight of their healing mission. Spiritual healing is nothing less than growth into God, coming to an intimacy with God that is possible only through Christ by the power of the Spirit. This quest engages a person at the deepest levels of his or her life. It recognizes that each human, knowingly or unconsciously, yearns for the knowledge of God. As Augustine said, "O Lord, thou hast made us for thyself, and our hearts are restless until they rest in thee." Spiritual healing involves coming to an open acknowledgment that our hearts were made for God and then seeking after God with all our hearts until God finds us. If a church does not teach and actively engage in this spiritual healing, it is little wonder if its flock wanders off.

This book is intended to be a practical primer in spiritual healing for churches. Healing is always a work in progress. Studying the principles set forth in this book is a beginning, but, for all of us, it is but the beginning of a journey that lasts an eternity.

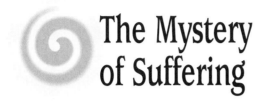 # The Mystery of Suffering

Any religion that does not address the problem of human suffering is unlikely to attract many followers. For suffering is a central concern for virtually every human being who has reached the age of reason, either because of the individual's own pain or because he or she is exposed, often graphically, to the pain of others. All of the world's great religions address suffering as part of their core message.

The church and a local church must address suffering

Christianity itself, however, is not of one voice in addressing "the problem of pain," to use the title of one of the great modern apologist C. S. Lewis's books. Some Christians state that the first human beings, Adam and Eve, lived in an earthly paradise without any unhappiness or discomfort until their violating God's will resulted in their being cast out of paradise into a world of strife and suffering. In other words, suffering came about because humanity deserved to suffer because of the sin of their first parents.

But many good Christians do not take the story of Adam and Eve literally. For them, suffering can be a result of our own bad decisions. Someone who uses illegal drugs may shorten his or her life or be forced into a degrading life of crime to satisfy his or her addiction. Someone who overindulges in eating runs the risk of Type II diabetes and high blood pressure.

Suffering can also come from the biological and physical laws of nature that govern our bodies and our environment. Gravity requires that when a wing falls off an airplane in flight, the plane will crash, killing all on board. Unthinking bacteria use a human host for their survival, thus threatening, in some cases, the survival of their host. Genetic defects can cause premature death as well as tragic physical deformities.

Many Christians believe that Jesus suffered primarily to pay the penalty due for our sins, but others believe that Jesus suffered to show his solidarity with suffering humanity. Jesus showed the lengths to which God was willing to go to prove his love for us and to demonstrate that his Son shared fully in the human condition.

Nevertheless, suffering remains a great mystery. I do not intend to try to solve that mystery in these pages. I do intend to discuss the response a church can make toward suffering, both the pain of its own members and the pain in the community and world around it. And just as a religion that does not provide a response to suffering will not attract many members, the Christian church that cannot provide a response to suffering will be incomplete, if not altogether inadequate, in carrying out the ministry of the One whose name it bears.

For suffering is real and it is all too present among us. My experience as an Episcopal priest of more than thirty years leads me to believe that there is more suffering and pain, even among those who outwardly appear to be happy and content, than most people are willing to reveal. And the daily news reminds us that even if we consider ourselves to be well off, there are millions, if not billions, of others around the world caught in the web of war, disease, and famine.

Healing is an integral part of Jesus' ministry

Whatever the cause may be of suffering and pain, Jesus' foremost ministries were healing the sick, restoring sight to be blind, casting out demons, and bringing strength and wholeness to withered limbs. Never once did Jesus tell someone he or she deserved to suffer. Nor is there any account in the Gospels where he ultimately refused a request to heal. "I have come that they may have life, and that they may have it more abundantly" (John 10:10) was his message. Jesus expressly confirmed that he was the Messiah in his reply to messengers sent by John to Baptist by declaring: "Go back and report to John what you hear and see: The blind receive sight, the lame walk, those who have leprosy are cured, the deaf hear, the dead are raised, and the good news is preached to the poor" (Matthew 11:4-5, echoing Isaiah 35:5-6).

One might try to argue that Jesus healed just to prove that he was the Messiah. He wanted to establish his credentials, and miracles were the surest way to reveal his power and prove the truth of his message. But except for the instance just mentioned when Jesus replied to a question posed by John the Baptist, Jesus does not seem eager to promote himself through his miracles. There are even instances when he tells those for whom he performed a miracle not to tell anyone about it. (See, for example, Luke 8:56.) Had he wished to prove his divine standing through miracles, there are certainly other acts of power, such as striking his enemies dead when they came to arrest him, that would have been more convincing to the authorities than his healing the sick.

The point is that it was an integral part of Jesus' message and ministry to engage in healing. And he gave authority to his disciples to heal in his name when he sent them forth to preach the Kingdom of God. If it was integral to Jesus' ministry to heal, then it is integral to the church's ministry to heal, and if the church universal, then healing is also integral to the local embodiment of the church. The church can be a more effective witness for Christ as a house of healing. As suffering may, alas, be integral to the human condition, so healing is integral to the mission of the church. Spiritual healing is the primary mission of the church.

Physical suffering is not essentially evil

Suffering and pain are not essentially evil. Jesus suffered, but his suffering led to our healing. We might prefer that Jesus not have suffered, but he did suffer as have many of the great heroes and heroines of faith throughout history. Paul rejoiced that he was able to suffer for Christ. His suffering for the Lord was a source of joy for him because of the spiritual benefits it brought him (see Romans 5:3).

Pain, too, can be beneficial. Without pain, we might not realize that we burned our hand or stepped on a nail, and, thus, the initial injury might lead to more serious consequences. It is "senseless" pain, pain that seems to have no purpose and that cannot be relieved, that wears us down and brings about meaningless suffering. How we view our trials and tribulations determines, to a large extent, how much and what kind of suffering they cause. Obviously, one purpose of a church is to provide its members' lives with meaning and to enable them to interpret their trials in the context of Christ's love and redemptive acts. We will be exploring how to help make this happen in later chapters.

But this is hardly the entire purpose of the church. Even when we are suffering for and with Christ, we are still suffering. My first wife died of cancer at age forty-seven. Her dying was a deeply spiritual experience for the two of us. At that time, the support of hospice and my church was of immeasurable value for us both. But there was still suffering in her dying for me, for her, and for our children, not to mention those who loved us.

The grief that flows from the death of a beloved spouse is no less grief because our faith tells us that the spouse now enjoys a broader life in heaven. The fear that comes from the diagnosis of a terminal illness or the realization that a loved one has Alzheimer's is no less fear because Christ loves us. Even Jesus was afraid as he faced his Passion, and even he felt abandoned by God as he hung on the cross. Our spiritual life in Christ is bound to our earthly flesh; just as Christ's divine nature was indivisibly bound with his fully human nature. We do not cease being human by becoming a new creation in Christ.

Neither is a man or woman made spiritually or physically whole by virtue of seminary training or ordination. Pastors can be dysfunctional and, instead of being sources of healing for their congregations, they can spread spiritual dis-ease. Likewise, congregations can suffer illness even with the holiest of pastors. Jesus' hand-picked apostles suffered one major defection. All the rest fled when Jesus was arrested and hid for fear of their lives after his death on the cross. I will address the issue of pastoral and congregational dysfunctions later in this book.

The church must help us with our pain

Thus, the church must not only provide us a Christian framework within which to view all aspects of our lives—our sorrows as well as our joys—but it must address the pain and anguish we will feel even if our faith is deep and solid. The church must not merely provide a context of faith, but it must also serve to dress our wounds and comfort us when we are afflicted, and, if possible, to bring us to health. And if physical health is not possible, then the church must help us to grow whole spiritually.

Our spiritual health is tied in large part to our knowledge of God. We begin as "baby Christians" (see 1 Corinthians 3:1-2), and grow to maturity in Christ by the transforming power of the Holy Spirit. We can initially be spiritually healthy babes in Christ, but we cannot remain babes forever and remain spiritually healthy, any more than a human infant who fails to thrive and grow will remain healthy. Thus, part of our healing consists in our continuing to grow toward spiritual maturity, a process that cannot be completed in this life. It is the role of the church to assist and support in this growth, to challenge us to grow spiritually, and to provide an environment in which spiritual growth can take place.

With the help of God and the church, we can come to recognize the presence of God's love in our lives even in the depths of adversity, even if that presence is grasped only in the darkness of faith. We can seek to conform our wills as much as possible to what we discern as God's will in our regard. We can seek to live as we believe Christ would live in our particular circumstances, ever mindful that, though we are not Christ, yet we live in Christ and Christ lives in us. We can seek to serve God in every word and deed, recognizing we will fail, but trying nonetheless. We should try to be able to say with Paul, "I have been crucified with Christ and I no longer live, but Christ lives in me. The life I live in the body, I live by faith in the Son of God, who loved me and gave himself for me" (Galatians 2:20), or again, "So whether you eat or drink or whatever you do, do it all for the glory of God" (1 Corinthians 10:31).

In this attitude—in this striving to become what God calls us to become, other Christs—is spiritual health on earth.

And just as few, if any, human beings enjoy total health of mind and body, so few, if any, Christians, enjoy total spiritual health in this life. But the church should be a powerful instrument of God in moving us toward this spiritual health. For in this spiritual health is peace. In this spiritual health is the ability to endure physical and emotional suffering. In this spiritual health is the assurance that God is with us, the assurance that God loves us, the assurance that we are one with God as much as we can be on this earth.

Can I be spiritually healthy yet physically ill?

History provides many examples of spiritually healthy Christians who suffered painful physical ailments. Paul complains about a "thorn in his flesh, a messenger of Satan." Although we are not sure what this ailment was, it must have troubled Paul deeply since he prayed several times that God would cure him of it. Yet no cure came; rather God told Paul, "My grace is sufficient for you, for my power is made perfect in weakness" (2 Corinthians 12:9).

John of the Cross, Teresa of Avila, Francis of Assisi, and Therese of Lisieux, all of whom were great saints and mystics, suffered terrible physical trials, and this list could be extended indefinitely. Mother Teresa of Calcutta, a source of comfort to innumerable poor in the streets of India, endured terrible emotional and psychological torments. Henri Nouwen, a renowned contemporary spiritual author, suffered a nervous breakdown and was several times in need of psychiatric counseling. Physical and, yes, mental, ailments are part of the human condition. I personally believe that even those whom we recognize as spiritual giants had periods of intense pain. Nor can any of us avoid death indefinitely no matter how skilled the physicians are that attend us. Jesus himself wept at the tomb of Lazarus (John 11:25), sweat blood in his agony in the Garden of Gethsemane (Luke 22:44), and cried aloud on the cross asking why God had abandoned him (Matthew 27:46).

Unfortunately, there are those who believe that a physical illness is a punishment for sin. We have seen this in our own day when some Christians claim that AIDS is God's penalty for homosexual conduct. Even Jesus' own disciples, on seeing a man born blind, asked Jesus, "Rabbi, who sinned, this man or his parents, that he was born blind?" (John 9:2). Jesus, however, would have none of this blame game, stating that neither the man nor his parents sinned. Elsewhere in the Gospels, Jesus teaches that the fact that someone suffers misfortune is no indication that that person is more sinful than others (see Luke 13:1-5).

There are also Christians who think that if someone prays for the healing of a physical or mental illness and it is not cured, the effect of the prayers is being blocked by insufficient faith or some secret sin. Although certain passages of the Gospels appear to teach that if you ask for something with sufficient faith you will get it, such an interpretation is contradicted over and over again in such cases as Paul's where God did not provide a physical cure when one was sought by a person of faith.

Pushed to its logical limits, the idea that God must grant us whatever we want if we ask for it with sufficient faith implies that we can bend God to our own wills. This way of thinking attempts to make God our servant rather than we being servants of God. This view reduces faith and prayer to little more than magic. Jesus taught we must seek first the kingdom of God, and all things will be added on that are necessary for us (Matthew 6:33). If we are earnestly seeking the kingdom, God can transform even adversity into a source of grace. "And we know that in all things God works for the good of those who love him, who have been called according to his purpose" (Romans 8:28-29).

Even though suffering and spiritual health are not incompatible, we do know that God can, and sometimes does, cure physical illness. Let us look at some accounts of healing in Scripture to see what we might learn from them.

CHAPTER 3

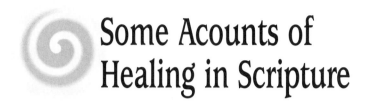

Some Acounts of Healing in Scripture

The Old Testament contains few examples of healing. God in the Old Testament tends to be supremely other; Yahweh's horizons are broad, generally embracing the Hebrews as a whole rather than expressing compassion toward, or even interest in, ordinary citizens. Yet even in the Old Testament there are notable and dramatic glimpses of the more personal and immanent God who is revealed most powerfully in the New Testament through Jesus.

Raising two dead sons of widows

I want to call attention to one such example and use that story to highlight the difference between this Old Testament healing and similar healings in the New Testament. The account is found in 1 Kings 17.

The prophet Elijah was staying with a widow in Sidon during a great famine. Elijah and the widow and her son were miraculously fed from a jug of oil and jar of flour that never became empty. While Elijah was staying at their house, the widow's son died and she complained loudly to Elijah: "What do you have against me, man of God? Did you come to remind me of my sin and kill my son?" (1 Kings 17:18).

Elijah took the child to the upper room he was using as his bedroom and laid the boy on his bed. "Then he cried out to the LORD, 'O LORD my God, have you brought tragedy also upon this widow I am staying with, by causing her son to die?' Then he stretched himself out on the boy three times and cried to the LORD, 'O LORD my God, let this boy's life return to him!' The LORD heard Elijah's cry, and the boy's life returned to him, and he lived." (1 Kings 17:19-22)

Now contrast this restoring life to a dead son with Jesus' resurrecting the dead son of another widow:

> As he approached the town gate, a dead person was being carried out—the only son of his mother, and she was a widow. And a large crowd from the town was with her. When the Lord saw her, his heart went out to her and he said, "Don't cry." Then he went up and touched the coffin, and those carrying it stood still. He said, "Young man, I say to you, get up!" The dead man sat up and began to talk, and Jesus gave him back to his mother (Luke 7:12-15).

Note that Elijah cries out to the Lord and provides a justification why his prayer should be answered. It is basically for Elijah's sake that God raises the widow's son, that is, so the widow will not blame Elijah, her guest, for her misfortune. Even so, Elijah has to stretch himself on the boy three times before the boy's life is restored.

Jesus heals out of compassion. No one will think less of him if he fails to raise the widow's son, but "his heart went out to her." Jesus does not throw himself on the boy or cry out loud to God. He simply touches the coffin and issues a command: "Young man, I say to you, get up!" Jesus knows his own power, which is nothing less than the power of God.

What conclusions might we draw by contrasting these two healings? Elijah's miracle is, in a sense, self-serving. Jesus' miracle is gratuitous, done out of concern for the widow who lost her only son. Elijah calls on God to act because he does not want the widow to think ill of himself or God. Jesus simply issues a personal command. With Elijah, God is remote. With Jesus, God and God's healing are present among us.

Jesus is filled with compassion for those who suffer. He did not have to raise the widow's son. Jesus was, in some sense, putting himself at risk by performing so public and so dramatic a miracle. He took that risk out of love. Healing and being healed has its risks, as we shall see later.

Other examples of healing in the New Testament

The instances of healing in the New Testament are too numerous to catalog here. The examples below are intended to highlight specific issues related to healing. The first example deals with ten lepers (Luke 17:12-16). In sum, ten lepers cried out to Jesus to take pity on them and cure their dread disease, a disease which made them outcasts and beggars. Nine of the lepers were Jews and the tenth was a Samaritan. Pious Jews considered Samaritans to be heretics and unclean even if they did not suffer from leprosy. Jesus told all ten to show themselves to the priests as required by Jewish law, so that the priests might certify they were no longer leprous and were thus free to reenter society.

All ten lepers were cleansed of their leprosy. Nine went straight to the temple priests, as the Law required and as Jesus had instructed them. But the tenth leper, when he realized that he was no longer leprous, immediately turned around, went back to Jesus, threw himself at Jesus' feet, and offered heartfelt thanks for his cure.

We do not know what happened to the other lepers or even to the tenth leper after he returned to thank Jesus. We may assume that they all remained cured of their dread disease. But the one we admire most is the one who returned to thank Jesus. His thankfulness opened the way for a deeper healing, a spiritual healing, rather than just a cure for his leprosy. Ten were cured, but we might say that only one was healed at a level deeper than the physical. The lesson here is that physical cures do not necessarily lead to spiritual healing.

We observe, too, that the leper who returned was the Samaritan, the one with whom devout Jews would normally never associate. It would have done him no good to go to the Jewish priests because they considered all Samaritans unclean. Just as their common affliction had brought Jews and the Samaritan into a community of shared suffering, so their physical cure destroyed that community and left the Samaritan again an outcast. The Samaritan was more open to running back to Jesus to thank him because he knew he would not be welcome in the temple. Those who believe in their own righteousness will have a harder time finding their way to Jesus. We must recognize ourselves as spiritually ill before we can recognize our need for spiritually healing.

Another of Jesus' healings involved a paralytic who lay by the pool of Bethesda in Jerusalem. The Jews believed that when the waters of the pool were stirred, the first one who entered the pool would then be cured. Thus, many ill and disabled people were brought to the pool in the hope that they might be cured, including the paralytic who had lain by the pool for thirty-eight years. Jesus, seeing the man and knowing he had been paralyzed a long time, asked him if he wanted to be healed. The man did not answer Jesus' question, but stated that others had always been able to get into the pool ahead of him. Jesus then ordered the man to pick up the mat on which he lay and walk. The paralytic found himself cured (John 5:1-9).

Note that neither Jesus' restoring the widow's son to life nor the cure of the paralytic at the pool involved faith on the part of the one who was healed. The paralytic did not even know that it was Jesus to whom he was talking. Neither the widow nor the paralytic asked Jesus to perform a miracle, but Jesus, out of compassion for the suffering, performed a miracle anyway. We thus learn that Jesus can heal even when we do not ask for healing, even when we don't believe that he can heal or that we can be healed, even when we do not know that it is Jesus who offers healing in the first place.

But why did Jesus ask the paralytic what at first hearing seems to be a strange question: "Do you want to get well?" We ourselves might think that if we had been the paralytic, we would have responded enthusiastically, "Of course I want to get well." But perhaps the paralytic subconsciously was afraid of being healed. As we shall see, there are responsibilities that come with being physically healed, and there are also responsibilities in being spiritually healed. Did the paralytic fear, as he reasonably might have, that his life might be harder without his handicap than with it? No longer crippled, he could no longer beg. And what kind of a job could he expect with a résumé that only listed lying by the pool of Bethesda for thirty-eight years? We should not be judgmental if the paralytic might have thought twice about how to answer Jesus' question.

But Jesus does not ask only the paralytic whether he wants to be healed. He asks all of us that same question. He asks it of dysfunctional pastors and dis-eased congregations. Jesus healed the paralytic, even though the paralytic did not expressly ask to be healed. Rarely will Jesus heal unless someone truly wants to be healed, unless someone consents to be healed. If we do not think of ourselves as spiritually ill, then we will not think of ourselves as needing spiritual healing. If Jesus were to ask if we want to be healed, we would simply tell him that we are not ill. Denial is a form of spiritual dis-ease. We are all sinners, and we all fall short of the glory of God (Romans 3:23). This applies not only to humans but to human institutions, including churches.

Consider now another account of a healing, the story of the blind beggar, Bartimaeus. Jesus, along with his disciples and a large crowd, was leaving Jericho. Bartimaeus heard the commotion and was told that Jesus was passing by. Immediately, Bartimaeus cried out as loudly as he could, "Jesus, Son of David, have mercy on me!" Some of those close by told him to be quiet, but he cried out all the more, "Jesus, Son of David, have mercy on me!" Jesus heard his cries and ordered the man to be brought to him. Now those who had wanted to silence Bartimaeus told him, "Cheer up! . . . He's calling you," and they brought him to Jesus. Jesus asked the blind man what he wanted, and Bartimaeus asked for his sight. Jesus gave the man his sight saying, "Your faith has healed you." Bartimaeus then followed Jesus along the road (Mark 10:46-52).

Surely the faith of the blind beggar is evident. He calls out to Jesus despite efforts by others to silence him. Why would they have wanted to silence someone crying out to Jesus for mercy? Perhaps for the same reason some are embarrassed by someone praying too loudly in church or expressing their faith in ways that seem out of character with what is considered appropriate in a "proper" congregation.

Nevertheless, Jesus calls the man and those who tried to silence him now offer him encouragement. "Cheer up! On your feet! He's calling you." Then Jesus asks him a question we all would rejoice to hear from the Savior's lips: "What do you want me to do for you?"

We might all profitably reflect on how we ourselves would answer this question. Might our answer be, "Lord, please let me be completely healed according to your will"? Blind Bartimaeus asks for his sight, and Jesus tells him that his faith has healed him. Jesus gives no command, nor does he take some other action such as touching the blind man's eyes. Bartimaeus may well have been given spiritual sight as well because we hear that he then followed Jesus along the road.

Unlike the paralytic at the pool, Bartimaeus knows what he wants and has faith that Jesus can provide it. Unlike the paralytic who does not even know it is Jesus who healed him and who fails to seek him out afterwards, Bartimaeus becomes a follower of Jesus.

God speaks to us through Scripture, and if the primary purpose of the church is spiritual healing, then God must speak to us about spiritual healing in the Scriptures. It is stories such as those presented here that should cause us to reflect on what Scripture is saying to us about healing. Even though their accounts primarily concern physical healing, we depend even more on Jesus for our spiritual healing. But these biblical accounts do not speak just to us as individuals. They speak also to the church universal and to local churches.

What must a church believe
if it is to be a house of healing?

If a church is to be a house of healing, 1) it—that is, the members of the body of Christ in that place—must want their church to be a house of healing. Involvement in the healing ministry must be intentional, not accidental. 2) They must believe that Christ can exercise his healing ministry with them as his instruments. 3) The church must not believe, or act as if, there should be no suffering among its members.[1] Let us examine each of these points more carefully.

First, the congregation must believe—truly believe—that spiritual healing is not merely important but central to its mission. If the church is satisfied the way it is, this is a sign that it does not want to grow spiritually. Just as spiritual healing for individuals involves spiritual growth, so the mission of spiritual healing requires constant attention and openness to the transforming power of the Holy Spirit. As healing for an individual is a process, so, too, the continuing mission of healing for a church is a process, not a fixed point at which the church stagnates.

Second, a church must be convinced that true spiritual healing comes only through Jesus Christ and the power of the Holy Spirit. I do not mean to imply that a church sits back and waits for the Spirit to act. But if a church places its faith in youth programs or Bible studies or anything other than Christ and the Spirit, it is building its house on sand. Church programs and even the Bible are only instruments through which God can heal if we are open to healing. But no church should ever mistake the means for the end.

Third, the church that believes that a "true" Christian is always joyful and that anyone who prays for a physical cure with sufficient faith will be cured fails to understand the gospel. Even Jesus himself had moments of suffering and grief. Yes, faith can bring greater peace, but it will not end suffering. Moreover, I have known powerful prayer warriors, whose devotion and faith were beyond question, who prayed for the healing of a sick Christian but the person prayed for was not cured physically. To accuse those who pray of a lack of faith or the sick person of a secret sin that blocks healing is worse than cruel. It is dis-eased theology of the worst kind.

What must a church do to become a house of healing?

Once a church is committed to, and believes in, the healing ministry, then it can progress to asking itself how best to carry out that ministry. I will offer a number of suggestions toward this end later on. I provide a brief summary now.

A church must provide a Christian framework—a context of faith, hope, and love grounded in Christ—that helps shape its members' lives. The church should provide meaning for its members, a meaning embracing the new life that we have in Jesus Christ, God's unfailing love, and our exalted status as children of God and heirs of heaven. The church must then challenge and assist all its members to grow toward spiritual maturity within this framework using the gifts God has given the church for this purpose. What programs the church implements to focus on a framework of faith and to challenge its members to grow will vary from church to church. Churches may use Bible studies, small group spiritual development, a series of teachings on healing, and a host of other means to achieve these purposes. We will talk about some of these programs later. Again, the programs are not as important as the spirit in which they are offered and the spirit that participants bring to them.

A church must keep in mind that spiritual depth and deep faith do not imply that a Christian will not suffer. Jesus himself suffered, as most surely his mother and his disciples did, when he was arrested and crucified. The church must never deny the reality of suffering—be it mental, spiritual, or physical—or assume that suffering is God's way of punishing a lack of faith or a secret sin. The church must be a source of comfort for the afflicted.

Tragically, however, many of those who suffer have not found comfort or understanding in their churches. As a spiritual director, I have talked with individuals who have had powerful spiritual experiences that drew them nearer to God that they dared not discuss with their pastor. Or, worse, they had tried to discuss their experience with a minister and felt put down. I have personally known instances where someone who sought solace through a church was rebuffed because he or she did not fit the pattern with which the members were comfortable. I would like to be able to say that I myself never have been wounded by representatives of the church, but it would not be true. If a church is to be a house of healing it must not sweep such matters under the rug but confront them openly and honestly. Later we will explore ways in which churches and pastors can engage in positive and constructive self-evaluation to assist in their own spiritual healing and to make them better instruments of spiritual healing for others.

In the coming chapters we will develop a number of the themes introduced in this chapter and explore ways in which a church might move toward becoming a more effective house of healing.

Note

1. There are proponents of the "prosperity gospel" who preach that the sign of a true Christian is perpetual joy and freedom from anxiety and that illness and suffering represents sin or insufficient faith. They believe that true Christians will enjoy good health and prosperity in this life as well as the next.

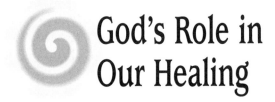# God's Role in Our Healing

An example from a pastor

Rev. Dr. Ralph Heller has been involved in the ministry of healing for more than thirty years. He has served both as a paramedic—as an active volunteer on a rescue squad—and pastor of a Sharon Lutheran Church in Greensboro, North Carolina, which bills itself as "A Healing Community in Christ."

Pastor Heller states that "one of the aspects of the healing ministry is that we can never say with absolute certainty a 'miracle' took place." There are incidents where God seems to have intervened, but there is no scientific or objective proof that such intervention occurred. I will let Pastor Heller describe in his own words three events from his ministry experience:

> Many years ago my mother-in-law was diagnosed with congestive heart failure. At a family reunion I had the family gather around her and I anointed her with oil and we laid hands on her and prayed. Later her physicians found her much improved. Another time I prayed for a lady at the altar rail of my church who was to have back surgery the next day. At the hospital they did a preoperative exam, including x-rays, and told her she didn't need the

surgery after all. Some therapy, yes, but not surgery. Another incident involved an elderly gentleman in my church who collapsed right during my sermon! I could have sworn he was dead—no chest movement, no breathing. We all gathered around, anointed, prayed, etc., and he revived. An ambulance squad took him to the hospital for treatment, [and] he lived on for a few more years. (He died at the age of ninety-eight!) In all of these instances and many others, I am always forced to ask the question, "What if I (or we) had *not* prayed?" And the corollary, "Was the recovery due to prayer and the intervention of God in response to that prayer?" I must honestly say, "I don't know."

Pastor Heller teaches that Jesus directs us to heal the sick. We do what we are supposed to do and leave the rest to God.

Note that in two of the cases Pastor Heller relates, the illness was abated, but it was not completely cured. Was the partial cure a sign of partial faith? Of course not! But we should know that cures can be partial, even in a response to prayer. Cures can take time, and sometimes they are incomplete. This is particularly true of spiritual cures because we can, and should, continue to grow into spiritual healing throughout our lives on earth, and, in the belief of many, into eternity as well. No finite being can ever exhaust the knowledge of an infinite God. That a dramatic and complete cure does not occur instantly does not mean a cure is not taking place.

Does God always heal?

Pastor Heller's accounts relate primarily to physical healing. Physical healing does not always take place in response to even the most fervent prayer offered in profound faith. But I said before, and I will repeat it because it is central to the healing ministry of the church: God wants all human beings to be healed spiritually. God will heal all human beings who continue to pray for spiritual healing and are open to the transformation that God will work in them to bring about spiritual healing.

But why doesn't God heal physically as well as spiritually? Didn't Jesus give sight to the blind, cleanse the leper, and cause the lame to walk? Isn't Jesus still present with his church so that the church can cure physical ills in Jesus' name?

There is ample evidence that in some instances God does indeed effect physical cures. Many churches can provide accounts of miraculous physical healings. Many persons claim to have been physically healed at famous shrines such as Lourdes. Such healings are attested to by the vast numbers of crutches and other supportive devices that line the walls at these shrines, discarded there when a man who had been lame found himself able to walk and when a woman immobilized by arthritis suddenly found that she could move freely and without pain.

But one can also observe that many who visit a holy place in the hope of a physical cure are not cured. There are probably more who come to Lourdes on crutches and leave on crutches than those who have been able to throw their crutches away.

We must never forget either that God often heals through natural means: through the amazing capacity of the diseased body to heal itself, through the skill and knowledge of medical science, through the compassion of caregivers, and through the indomitable spirit of a patient who works tirelessly to regain her health. Truly miraculous healings due to the direct intervention of God in situations where medicine has proved powerless are extraordinary and rare. God acting in nature through human agents happens all the time.

I have also seen situations where I could not in good conscience pray for a physical cure, but, rather, prayed that God would heal the patient and his or her family according to his loving will. We do not know in advance all the effects that will follow from getting what we think we need. All too many people who have suddenly found themselves rich beyond their imaginations, such as when winning a lottery megajackpot, find their seeming good fortune brings only tragedy in its wake.

Jesus told us to seek first the kingdom of heaven rather than riches and good health (e.g., Matthew 6:33). Jesus also promised that if we knock, the door to the kingdom will be opened for us (Matthew 7:7). It is the kingdom of heaven, spiritual healing, that we must seek above all. For what does it profit us if we are in excellent physical health and can enjoy all that this world has to offer if we thereby lose sight of what truly matters. "What good is it for a man to gain the whole world, and yet lose or forfeit his very self?" (Luke 9:25).

God, in God's immeasurable love for us, gives us the gifts we need, not those we think we need.

Only God can heal us spiritually

Whereas physical and mental cures usually come about through skilled medical intervention or the natural defenses of the human body, God, and God alone, can bring about spiritual healing. Why?

In the previous chapter we looked at two kinds of spiritual healing. The first is fulfilled only in heaven when we experience God directly. We see God face to face and know God as God knows us in an intimacy of love we cannot even begin to imagine now. "However, as it is written: 'No eye has seen, no ear has heard, no mind has conceived what God has prepared for those who love him'—but God has revealed it to us by his Spirit" (1 Corinthians 2:9-10). It is only through the Holy Spirit that the knowledge of God—rather than knowledge about God—comes to us.

But in this life, we can still strive for that spiritual health, which consists of conforming our wills to God's will, our lives to the life of Christ in us. Spiritual growth consists of letting God take ever greater control of our lives.

We have no natural ability to come to know God directly. This knowledge comes only as a free gift of God. Nor do we have the natural ability to grow ever more into the life of God. It is only through Christ that we are born into the life of God, and it is only through the Holy Spirit, the Sanctifier, that this life develops toward full maturity.

Thus, spiritual healing is substantively different from physical or mental healing. Whereas the latter healing generally takes place through such natural causes as medicines, physical therapy, or surgery, spiritual healing only takes place through the action of God. Spiritual healing is always miraculous. It can be neither explained nor effected by natural means. It rests ultimately on the greatest miracle in history, the Incarnation, when God took on the nature of one of his creatures. As God took on a human nature in Jesus Christ, so humans, through Christ, can share in the divine nature.

All this is fine in theory, but it must be played out in real lives. That God wants me to grow into a more godly life does not provide me with a concrete blueprint to make it happen, nor does this abstract truth tell me how I can best cooperate with the Holy Spirit so that the Spirit can transform me more fully into Christ as only the Spirit can. Thus, in order for a church to become a house of spiritual healing, it must keep two principles in mind:

First, it must develop concrete and practicable means to assist members to discern how the Spirit is at work in their lives and how they might best respond to, and cooperate with, the Spirit's action. Second, it must respect the individual differences of its members. The Spirit acts differently in different people. There is no "one size fits all" in spiritual growth, nor is there any checklist so that once we tick off all of the tasks on it we can say we have reached spiritual maturity.

This is often a difficult lesson for pastors to learn and practice since the pastor must be willing to subordinate personal preference to how the Spirit is leading someone. But, at the same time, the pastor must have sufficient wisdom and discernment to judge whether someone's promptings truly flow from the Spirit. If lacking these gifts, then the pastor must have the humility to rely on trusted advisors who do have them. Those who might support pastors in their efforts to bring healing in themselves and others include, for example, therapists, family counselors, physicians, and spiritual directors.

Fortunately, God has also given the church gifts that both ordained and lay ministers can use as aids for discernment and spiritual growth, and, of course, for spiritual healing. We now will consider some of these gifts.

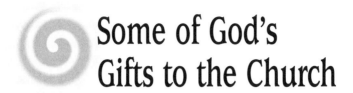 # Some of God's Gifts to the Church

The gift of Scripture

Scripture can be studied in a variety of ways and used for a variety of purposes, but because this is a book about healing with an emphasis on spiritual healing, we will look at how Scripture can be used as an instrument for spiritual healing.

The Bible, of course, is more than just another book. It is the inspired Word of God. Whether you read the Bible "literally" or "contextually," what I hope all readers affirm is that the Bible is a gift that God has given the church to assist her members to grow spiritually. The mere reading of the Bible with an open mind and heart directs thoughts toward God.

What are some practical techniques for using the Bible for spiritual healing?

We can express our true feelings to God using Scripture

First, spiritual healing requires openness with God. God knows our hearts better than we ourselves know them, so it does not help us to try to hide our feelings from God. If we are angry at God—and who has not been at some time—it is better to tell God we are angry and why. Releasing our feelings to God is healing and shows that God is more than an abstract idea to us. God is a person to whom we can relate at the deepest levels of our feelings.

Perhaps you do not believe this. You may feel that being honest with God is presumptuous, arrogant, or even childish. After all, if God knows us all as we are, there is no need to tell God about how we feel, so why now acknowledge our feelings openly to God?

Perhaps you think Christians should constantly be praising God and thanking God for all the blessings God has showered on us even when we are mad as hell and suffering intensely over the death of a loved one, the loss of a job, or a fire that destroyed everything we own. If so, you are doing yourself and God an injustice. You are being dishonest with God and repressing genuine human feelings that will ultimately find some way to express themselves.

If spiritual health is the knowledge of God and God is all truth, then the knowledge of God implies knowledge of ourselves as well. We will know God as God knows us, and in our knowledge of God, we will know ourselves as God knows us, that is, as we really are, warts and all. And we also know that God loves us as we are. We do not have to achieve perfection to enjoy God's love.

What has all of this to do with Scripture as an instrument of spiritual healing? In Scripture we find expressed the full range of human emotions. If we are afraid to tell God how we feel, we can turn to Scripture to speak for us. We can channel our feelings through Scripture to God. The Psalms, in particular, span the full range and depth of human feelings.

Are you angry with God? Do you feel abandoned by God in your hour of need? Consider the opening verses of Psalm 69:

> Save me, O God, for the waters have come up to my neck. I sink in the miry depths, where there is no foothold. I have come into the deep waters; the floods engulf me. I am worn out calling for help; my throat is parched. My eyes fail, looking for my God. (Psalm 69:1-3)

Are you contrite and sad because you have sinned? Consider Psalm 130:

Out of the depths I cry to you, O LORD; O Lord, hear my voice. Let your ears be attentive to my cry for mercy. If you, O LORD, kept a record of sins, O Lord, who could stand? But with you there is forgiveness; therefore you are feared. (Psalm 130:1-4)

Are you thankful for an answered prayer? Consider Psalm 116:

I love the LORD, for he heard my voice; he heard my cry for mercy. Because he turned his ear to me, I will call on him as long as I live. The cords of death entangled me, the anguish of the grave came upon me; I was overcome by trouble and sorrow. Then I called on the name of the LORD: "O LORD, save me!" The LORD is gracious and righteous; our God is full of compassion. The LORD protects the simplehearted; when I was in great need, he saved me. (Psalm 116:1-6)

I could go on at great length giving examples of how the Psalms enable us to express every human emotion. They enable us to pour out our hearts honestly and openly to God and, in such honesty and openness, to enable God to work more powerfully in and through us.

The book of Psalms isn't the only Scripture we can draw on to encourage us to express the full range of human emotions when we talk to God. In fact, the biblical models for candor in prayer can liberate us to go beyond the words of Scripture and speak to God in our own words. Scripture should open us to a more complete, honest, and healing relationship with God, relating to God as we are and not as we imagine others think we ought to be.

Scripture allows God to speak to us

I have taught that if someone reads the phone book every day with the specific intention of opening him or herself to the transforming power of the Holy Spirit, he or she will be transformed. If we want God to heal us, God will heal us. That is the fundamental premise of this book. But it is also a fundamental premise of the New Testament.

And if this is true with the phone book, then how much more does reading Scripture with the intention of opening ourselves to God's power, God's Word, God's Holy Spirit, transform us?

Here I am not proposing reading the Bible with concordance and commentary close by. Instead, I am suggesting reading the Bible as a prayer, beginning with a petition to God such as the following:

> Lord, I want more than anything else to love you with all my heart, mind, soul, and strength; to make my will your will; to make my life your life. As I read this, your holy Word, I pray that as you inspired your holy men and women who wrote this sacred book to hear with the ears of their heart what you wanted them to say, so inspire the ears of my heart that I may hear you speak to me. Let what I read, by the power of your Holy Spirit, be as healing oil for my body and soul to make me more completely yours through your Son, Jesus Christ, who with you and the Holy Spirit are God, now and forever. Amen.

We then read a passage of Scripture slowly and reflectively, not asking ourselves whether the translation is accurate or what God was trying to tell the people to whom the words of the passage were originally directed, but what God is trying to tell us now. Perhaps what we will hear has nothing to do directly with the passage being read. Perhaps we will hear nothing at all. But we will be present to God in a special way that God will honor.

The power of the Incarnation

Sometimes when my wife does not feel well—she has two painful autoimmune diseases—she asks me to sit by her and hold her hand. She tells me that this always helps her feel better. Humans are "embodied" creatures, and it is through our bodies that we relate to one another, through touch, speech, sight, or simply presence. Simply being bodily present to someone can be a source of comfort. I am using my body, the empathy expressed through my touch, to try to bring healing to my wife.

As is the case with my wife, our bodies also can be sources of pain, crosses to be shouldered. Even for my wife, however, the body can be a source of pleasure and joy, as when our grandchildren visit. For better or worse, we are stuck with our bodies. They are an integral part of how God created us. As a kindly doctor once remarked when I complained about some flaws in my own body, "We must play with the cards we are dealt, not the ones we would prefer to have."

But our bodies are not just crosses to bear, an affliction we must tolerate until we are able to shed our bodies in death and live as pure spirits. Our bodies must participate in our spiritual healing, and, because we believe in the resurrection of the body, they will share in our spiritual healing as well. If we have any doubt of this basic truth, we should remember that God also took on a human body, and he rose from the dead, not as a ghost, but as an embodied, glorified human being.

If nothing else, the Incarnation teaches us that God understands our pain because God shared it through the Son. God understands our human limitations because God once had a body like we do, with all of its limitations except sin. Jesus himself ministered through his body. His words brought us knowledge about God. His touch and words cured many. By his suffering, we are healed. By his life, we are brought into the life of God, bodies and all.

The Incarnation healed the breach between God and creation and made all things new. The Incarnation made spiritual healing possible. The Incarnation now works in and through us to complete the work that Christ began, to restore all creation to its creator in Christ by the power of the Holy Spirit.

As we share in the divine life of Christ through our incorporation into his body, the church, so our bodies share in the work of Christ here on earth. But we are not *just* members of the body of Christ. We are *the* body of Christ on earth, his hands and feet, eyes and ears, workers to bring about the kingdom, and, therefore, "physicians" to help bring about healing. That may be why my wife is comforted by my holding her hand. I have no magic pow-ers, but Christ's love joins with my love to bring her some relief. Christ acts through my body to lessen the pain in her body.

Through healthcare professionals, human bodies help heal wounded human bodies. Similarly through pastoral care, minis-ters use their embodied faculties to help bring spiritual healing.

It is tempting to neglect our bodies rather than see them as instruments of healing. Too often our bodies are in need of heal-ing and seem as much a hindrance to ministry as a help. How can we heal others when we ourselves are in need of healing? But our own need of healing should bring compassion for others in simi-lar need. Through serving as an instrument of healing, we our-selves are sometimes healed.

We ought not to think about just our bodies. Our minds, too, are valuable in our healing and in our serving as instruments of healing. Jesus not only cured the sick, he taught about the king-dom of God. His miracles attested to the truth of his teaching. Our spiritual healing is growth into truth, not truth as we would like it to be, but truth in God who is the fullness of truth and as found in the Son of God who is the Way, the Truth, and the Life (see John 14:6).

Mental and emotional dis-eases can often be more painful than bodily diseases. Can someone be mentally ill and spiritually well at the same time? There is a fine line between sanity and sanctity. I am convinced that some of the great saints had their feet on both sides of that line during much of their lives.[1]

The power of the Holy Spirit

We are spiritually healthy to the extent that we have become what God wills us to be, other Christs. As Christ's perfection con-sisted in his lifelong faithfulness to the will of his Father, so our perfection consists of being faithful in love to the will of Christ according to our circumstances. We are to grow into the life of God in Christ so that Christ lives in and through us. This growth into the life of God in Christ comes about through the action of the Holy Spirit.

Consider the disciples in the upper room after Jesus had ascended into heaven. Although they had found their hope and faith restored by the resurrection, Jesus was no longer with them. They were there according to his command waiting for the coming of something, but they did not know what. But he had promised them a Counselor who would guide them into all truth.

We all, of course, know what happened, but we must also remember that the disciples did not know what would happen. They would, not unreasonably, still have been afraid of the Jewish and Roman authorities, and, although they had been given the Great Commission before Jesus' ascension, they had no idea how to carry it out and were probably afraid of what would happen to them if they tried to do so.

We might say that the disciples, prior to receiving the Holy Spirit, were in a state of dis-ease. They were anxious because they did not know what the future held. They were fearful because they thought the authorities might come to arrest them at any moment. They were stressed because they had been told to wait for something but they did not understand what, or who, it was they were waiting for or how long they would have to wait. They lacked understanding of their mission and, in all probability, the courage to carry it out had they understood it. Once they received the Holy Spirit, their dis-ease was cured and they burst from the upper room to proclaim the gospel, for most of them at the cost of their lives.

Pentecost teaches us forcefully about the power of the Holy Spirit to transform lives and to shape us as God wants us shaped.

If we need additional evidence of the healing power of the Holy Spirit, we learn from Paul in 1 Corinthians 9 that healing is a gift of the Holy Spirit. And if our true healing is to consist in the vision of God as God is, then that healing also comes from the Spirit (1 Corinthians 2:9-10). And because our bodies are temples of the Holy Spirit (1 Corinthians 6:19), we are made holy by no less than the presence of God in us. Healing comes about by our letting that presence grow until it fully controls our lives and God lives in and through us as perfectly as is possible on earth.

It is through the Holy Spirit that we gain spiritual healing, and it also through the Holy Spirit that both we and our churches become instruments of healing. For the individual to become an instrument of healing and for a church to become a house of healing does not happen automatically. It requires intentional choices, an open heart, and hard work. We will return to this theme when we consider specific strategies to help individuals and churches in their ministries of spiritual healing.

Note

1. The noted spiritual writer and Roman Catholic priest Henri Nouwen gave up a career in academia to live and work with the mentally handicapped living in the L'Arche community in Toronto. Nouwen wrote of Adam, a severely mentally impaired young man whom Nouwen called his friend, teacher, and guide. Nouwen died of a heart attack in 1996.

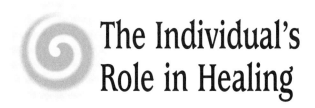

CHAPTER 6

The Individual's Role in Healing

In this chapter we explore some issues that individuals face that may impede their spiritual healing. In Chapter 14, we will discuss ways in which these hindrances may be addressed.

Do you want to be healed?

We looked at the paralytic at the pool of Bethesda in chapter 3. We now revisit this story and examine it more closely. Imagine a man whose legs were paralyzed for more than thirty-eight years. What caused this paralysis? Perhaps his mother accidentally dropped him when he was an infant. Perhaps he had some genetic defect or a disease like polio. But we are not told why he is lame. Rather, we see him, as Jesus did, lying by the pool of Bethesda for some thirty-eight years. Each day he is brought to the same location by friends or relatives to lie there begging for handouts until dusk when he is carried back to his house.

It is hard for me, someone who is in relatively good health with the freedom to go where I please, to imagine the indignity this beggar felt, even if his paralyzed limbs no longer suffered pain. Did he soil his clothes attending to the calls of nature he must have had while lying all day by the pool? Did he harbor resentment at the able-bodied people who dropped coins into his outstretched hand?

And why was he lying there by the pool? The Gospel of John tells us of the belief that when the waters of Bethesda were stirred, it was an angel who roiled the pool and the first person who went into the pool after the waters were stirred would be healed of his or her illness (John 5:1-14).

One day Jesus saw this man lying there and was told that the man "had been in this condition for a long time." Jesus asks the man a question, "Do you want to get well?" What an odd question. The man had been coming to the pool for thirty-eight years so that he could, at some point, be the first into the pool when the angel roiled the waters and thus be healed. We might have expected the man to blurt out, "What a dumb question! Would I have been here day after day in this miserable situation if I did not want to get well?" But he does not answer Jesus' question; rather, he gives an excuse why he has not yet been made well: "'Sir,' the invalid replied, 'I have no one to help me into the pool when the water is stirred. While I am trying to get in, someone else goes down ahead of me'" (John 5:7).

We ourselves might think of a number of questions to ask the man: "Why don't you have someone position you closer to the edge of the pool?" "Couldn't you have one of your relatives stay with you during the day so you will have someone to help you into the pool?" "If you have been unsuccessful in being the first into the pool for thirty-eight years, why don't you simply give up and stay home so at least you won't have to lie here in the heat of the day?"

Jesus does not ask any more questions. We are not told if the man had enough faith to be healed. In fact, he probably had no faith at all in Jesus because he had no idea that it was Jesus speaking to him (see John 5:13). Jesus simply told the man, "Pick up your mat and walk."

Oddly, the man obeyed. I say oddly because if I had been in his situation for such a long time and some stranger told me to hop out of bed and walk across the room, I would have thought the stranger was crazy. Yet the man somehow sensed that feeling had returned to his legs and something had changed. So he tried to rise from his mat and was startled to find that he could stand up. And then he picked up his mat and left. We are not told that he thanked Jesus. We are told that he still had no idea who cured him. He did not find that it was Jesus until later when people began to ask him about his miraculous healing.

The question that Jesus asked the paralyzed man is one that he asks us as well: Do you want to be healed? Do you really want to be healed, or are you merely saying that you want to be healed? Or is that you want some aspects of your life to change for the better but not others that would force you to radically reexamine your priorities?

Obstacles to being healed

There may be benefits to being sick

A tale is told of three men seated in a diner when Jesus enters. Jesus goes up to one of the men and asks, "What illness do you have, my son?" The man says that he has a painful slipped disk in his back. Jesus touches his back and says, "Be healed." The man breaks into a broad smile and declares that the pain in his back vanished as soon as Jesus touched him. Jesus goes to the second man and asks him what illness he has. This man replies that his eyesight is failing and there is nothing the doctors can do to save his sight. Jesus touches his eyes and says, "Be healed," and the man cries out that the blurriness in his vision has gone away and he can see clearly again. Jesus walks toward the third man, but the man backs away, shouting, "Get away from me! I'm on disability."

One reason that someone may not want to be healed is that she thinks that being healed will cause her to lose some benefit. The person may not even be aware of the benefit or the fear of losing it; both may be subconscious. This may well have been the case with the paralyzed man at the pool of Bethesda. For true healing is a life-changing experience, and many people do not really want their lives to change.

One reason people resist change is summarized in this old adage: Better the devil you know than the devil you don't know. True healing consists of letting God take ever greater control of our lives. Ultimately, we must belong entirely to God and all that is not God in us has either been converted or burned away in the purifying flame of the Holy Spirit, or we decide that we prefer our own desires to God's desires for us. We, in effect, make ourselves our own gods.

The riskiest prayer people can pray is to ask God to teach them to love God with all their hearts and souls and minds and strength, to let them belong completely to God, and if there is something they are trying to withhold that God will seize it from them by force, if necessary. If someone prays in this way and is open to having it answered, God will answer it. And the person will find that his or her life belongs totally to God and no longer to himself or herself. Christians might say that this is what they want, but most are consciously or subconsciously afraid of opening themselves completely to God, of letting themselves be swept up in the transforming power of the Holy Spirit. They do not want to take the risk of God answering this prayer. When answering this prayer, God asks us to yield total control of our lives. Can we blame those who do not want to take the risk? Look at what happened to Jesus and many of his closest disciples.

Psychologists use the term "secondary gain." Someone who is in pain, like the man at the pool, may not like the pain, but they like some of the benefits that the pain brings with it. I'm not talking about a kind of masochistic pleasure. Certainly, it could not have been comfortable for the man to lie there day after day, depending on the charity of others for food and drink. It must have been demeaning to be carried every day by friends to the same spot and left there while the friends went off to work.

It might well have been that the man could never find a way to get to the pool first. It might be that he had no one to help him into the pool. It might be that the "devil he knew," the demeaning life style of a crippled beggar, was preferable to the devil he did not know. What was he to do if he could walk? He had no skills and he was, for his time, already an old man.

And the lifestyle brought secondary gain. He knew he could live with his situation as a beggar. He did not have the responsibilities that healthy men had. He did not have to work for a living. Others would take care of him. He had a ready excuse why he could not get married, start a family, assume those duties that were so important for men in his society but at which the cripple might have feared he would fail if he undertook them. He may not have understood the notion of secondary gain, but when Jesus asked him if he wanted to be healed, an alarm may have gone off in the back of his mind. *Do I want to make the adjustments I will have to make once I can walk? Do I really want to be healed?* Secondary gain can be a powerful obstacle to healing.

Thus, one role of the church as a house of healing is to challenge members not to be complacent where they are, but to provide them a vision of where they might be. A church should help anyone whose situation resembles that of the paralyzed man to envision a better life and to challenge him or her to seek it. Secondary gain is an obstacle to healing, but churches should compassionately and prayerfully assist their members in every way possible to identify, and, with the help of God, overcome any obstacle to spiritual growth.

Sin

We usually think of sin as deliberate disobedience of God's will. But if we accept the premise that we must be open to God's transforming grace and cooperate with God to become all God wants us to be, then a more useful definition of sin is any obstacle that hinders God's action in us. Obviously, turning our backs on God is sin in this sense, but sin in this broader sense can be far more subtle than this.

Consider prayer, for example. No Christian would argue that prayer is sinful, but it can become an obstacle to spiritual progress. Prayer can become the symptom of a spiritual illness. How?

I may find one particular method of prayer especially helpful in the sense that it creates strong feelings of closeness to God or joy that God loves me. But there is a danger that my special prayer method that gives me so much satisfaction will become an end in itself. I may slip into praying for the warm emotions it brings me rather than because I want to be more available to God. And if God is trying to lead me to another form of prayer, or perhaps away from my prayer time to an active ministry, I may resist. Even worse, if the positive feedback I get from my prayer should cease, I may give up praying altogether, or even stop caring about God because God is not giving me the emotional satisfaction I previously enjoyed.

Sin was a relevant concept for Jesus, and it is a relevant concept in our day if for no other reason than it can prevent our realizing the potential that God has given us through Jesus Christ and the Holy Spirit. Sin should perhaps even be studied as part of a church's healing ministry. I will provide some suggestions in this regard in the next chapter.

Failure to forgive and to accept forgiveness

Forgiveness is a central theme in the New Testament. Even if someone should offend us again and again, but continue to seek forgiveness, Jesus tells us to continue to forgive (Matthew 18:21-22).

Someone once said that deliberately harboring anger against someone is like drinking poison and hoping your enemy will die. We cannot help it if we are upset and even angry because someone injured us in some way. We often cannot control our emotions, but we can usually control how we act in response to our emotions. A business owner may be angry because his partner embezzled company funds. He may seek justice in the court system. But he should not pray that God will wreak vengeance on the thief, much less take justice into his own hands and murder the partner. Better yet, he can pray for the partner's spiritual welfare, that God will touch his heart and let him realize and repent of the damage he has caused. He can pray for the embezzler's family and pray that he himself will be healed of his anger and any desire for revenge.

I had the privilege of being the spiritual advisor of a Beginning Experience team. Beginning Experience is a ministry for those who have lost a spouse through divorce, separation, or death. The ministry, through a well-designed weekend retreat, assists participants in working toward closure on their loss. Naturally, many of those who take part in such a weekend are deeply grieving and many, particularly those involved in a divorce, are exceedingly angry as well. Yet even those who have been abandoned by a spouse who deserted them to go to a new partner are encouraged to forgive. They cannot forget, but they can forgive by praying for their former spouse and by continuing to pray for the errant spouse they eventually find they have forgiven him or her and found greater peace themselves.

As important as forgiving another is being able to forgive oneself. An important part of a Beginning Experience retreat is the rite of reconciliation. In this ritual, participants have an opportunity to lay before God their sins for which they are sorry and be assured of God's forgiveness. After assuring the participants that God has put away their sins, I always ask each whether he or she forgives himself or herself. Many people cling to the guilt associated with past sins, confessing them again and again, seemingly unable to forgive themselves even though their faith and a representative of the church has assured them that God has forgiven them. Ironically, much of what these grieving individuals confess is not sinful because it is involuntary, such as the anger they feel toward an unfaithful spouse.

We all sin. We all fall short of the glory of God (Romans 3:23). We all make mistakes. We all are subject to human weaknesses, emotions over which we have little control, all the foibles and missteps that are part of the human condition. Yet God loves us and offers us complete forgiveness of those sins of which we repent if we but ask for forgiveness in the name of Jesus. The inability to accept that forgiveness and move on is often a powerful obstacle to spiritual growth. It is in every sense a spiritual dis-ease that needs healing. The church can assist in that healing by continuing to teach that God does indeed forgive and that if God can forgive us, we must be willing to forgive ourselves and others. If God puts aside our sins so that we can grow more fully into his divine life, we must not frustrate God's purpose by clinging to what is no longer there.

Indifference

If the good news of Jesus Christ is true, if Jesus Christ is indeed the Son of God and the Way, the Truth, and the Life, then this is the most important information ever provided the human race. It is more important than all of the scientific knowledge accumulated over the ages. It is more interesting than all of the fiction written from the dawn of time. And yet research seems to show that there is little difference between the way Christians and non-Christians live their lives. The gospel is all too often stripped of its life-transforming power when we fail to understand its implications or are indifferent to those implications.

If most humans were told there was a vast treasure buried somewhere in their backyards, they would immediately begin digging to find it. If most humans were told that they had a life-threatening illness, they would immediately search the Internet and seek out the best treatments for a possible cure. But when the gospel tells them that Jesus is the way to God and that through him they can grow into the life of God and come to know God directly even as God knows them, they fail to take action. This failure is a spiritual dis-ease since it is essential that we cooperate with God in God's transforming work, even if it is God who is doing the heavy lifting.

A church must, therefore, do all it can to impress on its people the importance of the Good News and to assist them in understanding its implications for their lives. The gospel is not just to be studied; it is to be lived. Consider carefully Jesus' statement in Matthew: "Everyone who hears these words of mine and does not put them into practice is like a foolish man who built his house on sand. The rain came down, the streams rose, and the winds blew and beat against that house, and it fell with a great crash" (Matthew 7:26-27).

Failure to live the gospel fully is not necessarily spiritually fatal any more than chronic arthritis necessarily prevents someone from living a reasonably full life. But indifference, like arthritis, can be debilitating, and it is an obstacle to God's transforming grace. Therefore it is a dis-ease that calls for a cure.

Responsibilities that come with being healed

We might wonder what emotions the man at the pool of Bethesda felt once he found he could walk. He could walk, but where was he going? Back to whatever home he had away from the pool itself? To the temple to give thanks to God? To look for a job at whatever passed for an employment agency in those days? What skills could he offer anyone? His résumé could state only that he lay by the pool of Bethesda for much of his life. One thing we can say with certainty. Once he could walk, the man's life was fundamentally changed. We can say the same thing about spiritual healing.

The fact that the man was no longer paralyzed meant that he had new responsibilities that he may not have wanted. He could no longer beg for alms. He could no longer shirk the responsibilities that his society and the Jewish law laid on the shoulders of able-bodied men. He might have even incurred the suspicion of his friends who may have wondered if he had been feigning his illness.

What of the others that Jesus healed of physical infirmities? Some thanked him. Some even followed him. Many simply went on their way cured of whatever ailed them. Newfound health, however, did bring new responsibilities or brought a return to old ones. What are our responsibilities if we are spiritually healed?

First, we must remember that spiritual healing is a process that is rarely, if ever, completed in this life. It is a growing more and more into the life of God, becoming ever more Christlike, until we no longer live, but Christ lives in us (see Galatians 2:20). It is a process of our wills conforming to God's will in our circumstances, of God taking ever greater control of our lives. Thus, the responsibilities we assume are those associated with God's will in our regard.

All too often Christians want to choose their ministries, determine what it is they will do in the service of God, and then ask God's help in doing it. If we allow God to take control of our lives, then we may find that God has other plans for us. Instead of our teaching Sunday school, God may want us to establish a soup kitchen. Instead of our entering the ministry, God may want us to witness to his love in a secular workplace.

Being healed involves turning more and more control of our lives over to God, to let God direct our paths, to seek the choices God would have us make rather than the choices we would make for ourselves. We become ever more aware of our responsibility to God and, through God, our responsibility to the rest of humanity and all of God's creation. We begin to understand and echo Paul's cry, "I have been crucified with Christ and I no longer live, but Christ lives in me" (Galatians 2:20).

We would be naive to think that everyone wants the responsibility that comes with spiritual healing. To some it appears like the ultimate loss of freedom, the inability to control one's own life ceded to an unseen God. We must be convinced, however, that true freedom is found only in God for it is only in God that we realize our full potential as human beings. Until we belong entirely to God we are chained to those things that are not God, things that may satisfy temporarily but can never bring lasting happiness. We may gain the whole world and still have nothing if we do not have God.

> "For whoever wants to save his life will lose it, but whoever loses his life for me and for the gospel will save it. What good is it for a man to gain the whole world, yet forfeit his soul?" (Mark 8:35-36)

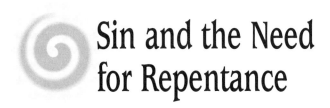

CHAPTER 7

Sin and the Need for Repentance

Spiritual healing involves a complete turning around of our lives, a true conversion. No longer do our lives belong to us, but they belong to God. In repentance, we turn away from what God does not want of us toward what God does want of us. We become open to what God wants us to be rather than what we ourselves would naturally prefer to be.

Conversion of life

Because spiritual healing is a transformation that only God can bring about in us, sin in its broadest sense is any obstacle we place in the way of that transformation, any hindrance to God's working in us. Repentance involves the sincere desire to have all those obstacles removed, even those of which we may not be aware, particularly those that only God can break down. Forgiveness in its broadest sense is the removal of those obstacles to our spiritual healing.

Repentance need not be accompanied by wails of grief and cries to God for mercy. Repentance does involve a decision that we freely choose God above all us. We truly, in the depths of our hearts, want to be spiritually whole. In this regard churches might plan services of repentance coupled with assurance of forgiveness through Christ. Reflections on sin can also help identify obstacles to God's work in us that must yet be removed.

Rituals of repentance and forgiveness

Many participants in a Beginning Experience weekend, described in the previous chapter, have experienced enormous relief and joy at the assurance that God had forgiven those sins for which they were sorry. They had a chance to lay their sins, real or imagined, before God and were told, entirely in keeping with the promises of Christ, that their sins were taken away. As a sign that God had taken away their sins, they were offered the opportunity to write the sins on a piece of paper (which no one else saw), and these papers were burned as an offering to the Lord.

All Christians believe in God's forgiveness of sin through Jesus Christ. A ritual in which people can lift up their sins to the Lord and receive formal assurance that God has taken away those sins and no longer holds the penitents responsible can be a source of immense healing. Participants should be reminded, of course, that if God forgives them, they need to forgive others and themselves as well.

Joy at being forgiven should not stem from no longer fearing God's punishment for transgressions but from the realization that God is working with us to remove obstacles to our growing into God's own life. Rituals of repentance and forgiveness should inspire participants to recognize their need for God's help in spiritual transformation and inspire them to be more open to God's ardent desire to draw all human beings to himself. Forgiveness is least of all remitting any punishment that sin may deserve. It must be a challenge to make us want to be free of any barrier that can separate us from God. It is not a magic wand to remove fear, but a motivation to embrace that love that casts out fear.

A practical exercise to make people more sensitive to sin

Because sin is an obstacle to our spiritual healing, churches should instruct their members in the basics of sin, not holding out the threat of hell, but teaching that sin is a spiritual dis-ease that needs to be healed. Below are short descriptions of the Seven Deadly Sins which often considered as the foundation for all sin. Following each summary are questions that church members can reflect on. A study of the Seven Deadly Sins and reflecting on how these effects our lives can be a salutary exercise for any congregation. I will take a more modern approach to these sins while using the traditional names to try to illustrate that these sins are still very much with us, though perhaps in contemporary guises.

Anger

The emotion of anger in itself is not sinful. Emotions are a natural part of our human makeup. It is only when we allow anger to lead us into a desire for vengeance or to hatred for God or another human being that anger becomes sinful. When anger is given free rein, it can result in prejudice and persecution against those whom one blames for one's problems. Both reason and anger cannot simultaneously be in control of a person or a church. Anger can divide congregations and result in unjust actions against the clergy and others alike. A church is guilty of anger when real or imagined slights bring about attempts to exclude, or drive out, those at whom anger is directed.

Two questions for self-examination:

1. Review those times when someone has hurt you. Ask yourself, Have I made any special efforts to pray for those who have hurt me or to reconcile with someone from whom I have become alienated when reconciliation was a genuine possibility?

2. If I have ever wanted some evil to befall someone because of the harm that person caused me, I will now pray for that person that God may bless him or her and that God may remove all anger from my heart toward him or her.

Envy

Envy is a violation of the command that we shall not covet what is our neighbor's. Envy involves an untamed desire to have something that someone else has. I do not sin if I simply admire my neighbor's house or car and would like to have a car or a home like my neighbor has. Envy creeps in when I hope that my neighbor will suffer some misfortune that will deprive her of the goods I covet, or when I am willing to steal from my neighbor if I think I could get away with it. Envy can lead to hatred of my neighbor because he has something I want and cannot have. Envy can lead to sorrow and frustration because I cannot get what I want. A church can be guilty of envy when it demeans the reputation of another church because that church is seen as more successful.

Two questions for self-examination:

1. How would I feel if a neighbor had a stroke of good fortune at the same time I suffered some misfortune?

2. If I have been in a situation where someone got a promotion or recognition that I thought I deserved instead, how have I handled it? In what way could I have handled it that is more in keeping with what I believe God wants of me?

Gluttony

Traditionally, the sin of gluttony involved eating or drinking in excess. We can expand this sin to include any form of overindulgent consumption. Someone who works so hard that he or she has no time for family or friends is guilty of a form of gluttony. So is someone who has far more goods than he or she could ever reasonably enjoy. So is a nation that uses far more of the world's resources than is necessary for its population's welfare. So is a church that is more concerned about displaying its worldly success than in healing its members.

Two questions for self-examination:

1. What worldly thing can I not get enough of? How is my desire for this thing interfering with my search for God or my

obligations toward others? What can I do to overcome this inordinate desire?

2. How might I alter my lifestyle or habits to be a better steward of the earth's natural resources?

Greed

Traditionally, greed was a desire for excessive wealth or material goods. A greedy individual is generally willing to use almost any means to gain a material advantage, even betraying others. Thus, someone who is willing to lie to a business partner so that she can receive more than her fair share of the partnership's income is guilty of greed. So is someone who has more than he needs, yet will not contribute to charities or those in need.

By extension, greed is an inordinate desire for any worldly possessions, even abstract possessions like honors and offices. Rather than seeking the kingdom of God, the greedy person wants to accumulate the things the world values. Both the wealthy and the poor can be greedy if their heart's desire is great wealth, even if they never achieve it. A church can be greedy by measuring its success in the numbers of members it can attract or the income it generates rather than in the spiritual healing that takes place there.

Two questions for self-examination:

1. What would I be unwilling to give up if giving up that something would remove some obstacle to my spiritual healing? Pray that God will give me the grace to overcome my attachment to this obstacle.

2. When have I deceived someone or lied to gain a personal advantage? What is the worldly advantage or good that I want more than anything else? Would I be willing to compromise my morals to get it? Why or why not?

Lust

Generally, people associate lust with illicit sexual activity. Thus, to lust after someone connotes a desire to have sex with the object of desire. Lust, as opposed to the genuine love found in a healthy marriage, wants to use another human being for one's own pleasure. The other person is not truly loved but is an "object," a toy as it were, for the pleasure and amusement of the one who lusts. The feelings and well-being of the other person are of little or no concern.

Let us expand the notion of lust. Lust occurs when a person desires to use another person for his or her benefit without regard to the welfare of that person. "If you can help me sign a lucrative contract, I will wine and dine you. Otherwise, you are no use to me." "I care about you only for what you can do for me, not for what you are in yourself or in the eyes of God."

Through lust we place ourselves at the center of the universe. We make ourselves our own gods. Even a church can be guilty of lust when it seeks new members simply to add to its numbers or to gain more income but refuses to share leadership and ministry with the newcomers.

Two questions for self-examination:

1. When have I cared about someone only so long as I believed that person could do something for me? What steps might I take to make sure that this pattern does not recur?

2. How might I try to see Christ in each person I meet, even someone I do not naturally like?

Pride

Pride is generally considered to be the foundation of all sin because it was the sin of Satan who wanted to be accorded greater dignity than he merited. Milton's classic formulation of Satan's motto is "Better to reign in hell than to serve [God] in heaven."[1] Pride is deeming ourselves better and more deserving than we are, and, therefore, valuing others less, particularly those who do not give us the praise and honors that we are sure we deserve. A proud person thinks that God "owes" her or him a reward for being so good. The proud person exalts him or herself in the eyes of God, and even wants to play the role of God in relation to others. Churches can be guilty of pride if they deem that only they are worthy of God's favors, only their members are going to heaven, or only they have the fullness of the truth.

Two questions for self-examination:

1. When I learn that someone I thought had high morals had been exposed as having committed some sin or crime what are my feelings? I will imagine myself in that person's situation and recognize that I too might have fallen.

2. Imagine that someone who is obviously a "street person" comes into a service at my church. How do I feel toward that person? How do I extend myself to greet that individual as a child of God and brother or sister of Christ?

Sloth

If we take sloth, as some have, to be an insufficient love of God, then we are all guilty of this sin. I will define sloth as willfully avoiding seeking the kingdom of God. The slothful person might declare that when he is older he will devote more time to spiritual growth, but not just yet. The slothful person is aware that she is supposed to love God with all her heart and mind and soul and strength, but that seems just too difficult for her. Let those who have a special call attempt it, but she is content to be an "average" Christian. Churches are slothful when they do not challenge their members to continuing spiritual growth and when they do not reach out to others to carry on the work of Christ and spread the kingdom of God.

Two questions for self-examination:

1. What do I do each and every day that is for God and not merely for myself?

2. What special effort do I put forth to make sure that I keep the Sabbath holy? What special effort do I put out to live Christ in my workplace or home?

Note

1. This classic quote is paraphrased from John Milton's epic poem, *Paradise Lost*, book 1, line 263.

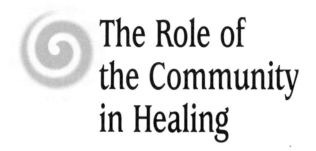

CHAPTER 8

The Role of the Community in Healing

All Christians are one in Christ

All members of the church are bound by their common membership in the body of Christ. This membership is essentially different, however, from membership in a club. The members of a club, while dedicated to the purposes of the club, remain distinct individuals. Their common bond is external to each individual. Members may devote part of their time to the club, but their lives are their own.

Membership in the body of Christ, however, implies an organic unity. Members share a common life in Christ in the same way that an organ of a human body shares in the life of that body. If the organ is ill, the body is ill. If the organ cannot function properly, the whole body suffers.

Jesus himself expresses this organic unity of the members of his Body with himself by comparing himself to a vine and the members to branches (see John 15:5 and following). If the branches are separated from the vine, they not only cannot bear fruit but will wither and die. Paul develops this doctrine in his epistles. Here is an example: "Just as each of us has one body with many members, and these members do not all have the same function, so in Christ we who are many form one body, and each member belongs to all the others" (Romans 12:4-5).

But Paul points out those who belong to Christ do not merely form a unity. Each member of the body of Christ has some particular function to perform. No Christian should want to carry out any function in the body of Christ other than the one to which God calls him or her. Instead the Christian should recognize that God's desire in his or her regard is important for the welfare of the whole. Thus, there should be no envy concerning the roles others are assigned because each member is essential and all must function as God intends so that the whole Body can be healthy (see 1 Corinthians 12:12-27).

To summarize, all Christians are incorporated into Christ and share his life. All Christians are members of that organic whole which is the body of Christ. Each member has his or her role to play in that body in the same way that each organ of a human body has a role to play. If the member, or the human organ, is ill, then the whole body is ill. "If one part suffers, every part suffers with it" (1 Corinthians 12:26). These truths have significant implications for spiritual healing.

Implications for spiritual healing

If the community is diseased, it may contribute to its members' disease

If a civic community fails to carry out some function necessary to the welfare of its members, then the members will suffer. If a city, for example, cannot provide clean water, the citizens who drink the water may very likely contract serious illnesses. Similarly, if a church cannot carry out some function necessary for the spiritual health of its members, then it may not serve as an effective house of healing. Even worse, the church may itself serve as a source of spiritual dis-ease.

We have all heard of tragic situations where a minister betrays the trust placed in him and disgraces his office. In most such cases, the congregation itself is wounded. A church should be a place in which members are able to trust the leadership and one another because they are able to see Christ in one another. Likewise the leaders should recognize that they are servants of God who must teach about Christ more by example than by words. Patients must trust a doctor if they are to take her advice. Passengers must trust the pilot if they are to fly. If members of the church cannot trust one another or their leadership, the church will be an environment is which genuine healing will be difficult. Indeed, members may be deceived into thinking they are being healed when, in reality, their pathologies are deepening. One only has to think of Jim Jones and Jonestown to know this can be the case.[1]

I will have more to say about the health of the church as a community later, but now I simply underscore Paul's point about the unity of the body of Christ of which the church is a local realization. If the members are ill, the body suffers, but if the body is ill, the members also suffer.

We each have our own role to play in the church

There are a number of churches that have too many cooks in their kitchen—with everyone jostling to lead and too few wanting to follow. Conversely, there are churches where the members are happy to let the pastor or a handful of members do almost all that needs to be done. The commonly quoted statistic tends to be regrettably true, that 20 percent of a congregation does 80 percent of the work of the church. Neither of these situations is healthy. If some members are doing all the work, then either some members are being deprived of the opportunity to engage in ministry, or too many members are unwilling to engage in ministry. Likewise, if everyone wants to lead, dissension is almost sure to follow and some of the vital work that no one wants to do because it is not "important" will not get done.

A healthy church should enable each of its members to identify the ministries to which God may be calling them and to respond to an authentic call, be that ministry hospitality, teaching, administration, or any other ministry vital to the church. Likewise, members should try to discern prayerfully what role or roles the Lord is calling them to play and then to respond faithfully without regard to whether it is the service they originally had in mind.

Some churches administer spiritual gifts inventory tests to members. There are a number of these tests available on the Internet. They vary in the questions asked and in what they consider to be gifts. The success of these tests can depend heavily on the honest answers of those who take them. I do not mean to imply that anyone deliberately lies, but we each suffer from some illusions as to what we truly prefer and what we are good at. Even if they are not infallible, such tests may stimulate members to think about what ministries they are called to exercise. The leadership of the church should provide appropriate training and oversight as well as periodic evaluation to enable members to improve their performance, or, in some cases, to recognize that they are not well suited to the tasks they are performing.

This may seem unduly idealistic since no one likes to be criticized and each of us would like to choose the areas in which we will serve. Churches have a hard enough time recruiting volunteers for all the work that needs to, or can, be done, and they are unwilling to risk offending someone who wants to engage in a particular activity by turning them away.

But we do not heal through being dishonest. God is a God of truth, not of illusions. We may fool ourselves, but God knows us as we are. And the doctrine of the body of Christ indicates that there are appropriate roles for every member of the body, and that someone serving in the role or roles to which he or she is called by God best insures the health of the church universal and the local church. Allowing someone to think he or she is a good teacher, for example, when, in reality, he or she is ignorant of the subject matter or fails to present it clearly does a disservice both to that individual and those who are being taught. A pastor may protest that "Sam was the only one willing to teach the high school youth," but if Sam does not work well with young people—even if he thinks this is his strong suit—several bad outcomes will occur that will contribute to the dis-ease of the church. First, others may hesitate to volunteer to teach the high school youth because Sam is already doing it. Second, the high school youth will not be "fed" appropriately. And third, Sam will not learn from the experience either. He will continue to foster his illusion that he interacts well with youth.

Never let me suggest it is easy for a church to create a program to enable its members to serve in those areas to which God may call them and to assist all members to see their strengths and weaknesses honestly. But I do suggest that such a program is important for the overall health of the church and for the spiritual health of its members. No one grows spiritually by avoiding what God calls them to do and to become. And while illusions are sometimes vital for our psychological well-being, those illusions that tell us we are capable of a role for which we are not suited can cause dis-ease both for ourselves and for the church.

Spiritually ill members can cause the church to be ill

Churches, it has been truly noted, are hospitals for sinners. No one who comes to church is perfect. Each of us has spiritual diseases that need healing, and we hope that God will use our church as an instrument in our healing. However, just as someone with a contagious disease can infect others, those with "contagious" spiritual dis-eases can make a church ill. How does this happen?

I personally have served in a number of churches in three Episcopal dioceses, many times as a "visiting firefighter" to try to extinguish the flames of a troubled situation. Sometimes a well-meaning diocesan officer would tell me to watch out for certain members because they were the troublemakers, the ones who created the problems from which the church suffered and which I was supposed to help fix. These have, of course, been the first people I have sought out, not to warn them to behave, but to hear their concerns and their stories. All too often, I found that the church was to blame for their pain. They were not causing problems because they were troublemakers at heart but because they felt, usually with good reason, that the congregation or its leadership did not listen to their genuine concerns. They felt the church had written them off without trying to understand what they were trying to say. In other words, they did not believe that the church loved or respected them. When someone feels alienated from the church, the pastor or senior leadership would do well to listen carefully and without judgment to what that person has to say. A pastor must try to determine, with an open mind, if these members are troubled because the church itself is troubled and is the cause of their spiritual affliction.

But we all know there are those who, for whatever reason, have not been ill-treated by the church but are a source of dis-ease within the congregation. Often these folks need professional help that the church is not qualified to give, but they act out their issues within the congregation by spreading rumors, insisting that the pastor never does anything right, getting themselves elected to the lay governing board and then paralyzing its work with their endless diatribes, scheming to replace the current "inadequate" pastor with another pastor they will also soon deem inadequate as well. The litany of problems caused by troubled troublemakers is almost as varied as are the troubled members themselves. Like a diseased organ can bring discomfort to the entire body, so these people bring discomfort to the entire church. What is a pastor supposed to do?

Ideally, of course, the church would heal the troublemaker and thus heal itself. But this is not always possible. Many church members feel that listening to Hannah or old Tom is just part of the cross they bear, even if Hannah and Tom are obstructing the work of the church, making members uncomfortable and discouraging visitors from joining.

There are a number of books on how to resolve conflict in the church, and this is not intended to be one of them,[2] but I have found that the healthier a congregation is, the fewer are the real troublemakers, and the few there are become isolated and ignored. Generally, for a troublemaker to cause trouble, he or she must have someone who will take his complaints seriously. To put it differently, a troublemaker wants to engage in games consistent with her pathology. It takes more than one to play such a game. If no one wants to play, the troublemaker becomes frustrated and often moves to another church where he might get a more sympathetic hearing—mumbling, of course, about how uncharitable and uncompassionate his previous church was. If almost all of the church members are engaged in healthy ministries in which they are encouraged, and if members see the church deeply involved in the work of the Lord, then they will have little time for gossip and gamesmanship.

Central to a healthy congregation is love—love of the members for one another and love of the pastor for the congregation. Love toward a troublemaker involves accepting him or her as a child of God, but it does not involve becoming a player in the troublemaker's games. The chief "lover" of the church and its members, of course, must be the pastor who is the representation or reminder of Christ in the community whether he or she wants to be or not. A healthy church starts with a healthy pastor, and their people know that a healthy pastor not only loves the Lord but loves them in the Lord. If the people do not sense this, the church has an illness that must be addressed. A wise old bishop once remarked to me, "If the people know you love them, you can get away with anything, but if they sense you do not love them, you can't get away with anything."

Churches are organic bodies like human bodies

Paul depicts the church as a body, with members that must carry out their intended functions for the health of the whole. It reminds us that a church, a microcosm of the church universal itself, is a body whose health depends on the well-being of its congregants, its bodily members. Whether we like it or not, we are all in this together, and what each of us does affects the other members either positively or negatively. The church, universally and locally, is an inherently social organism. There can be no such being as a Christian who acts entirely by himself or herself.

One may conjure up the image of the desert mother or father living alone in a cave, waging a spiritual battle totally apart from civilization. But the image is misleading. The hermit is as much a part of the body of Christ as the member of a large church. What the hermit does, or does not do, affects the Body, even if those effects are not immediately visible.

Even cloistered monasteries serve as a powerful symbol of lives dedicated to prayer and the transience of material goods. But the desert hermits soon found support in one another and formed communities, and those with reputations of particular wisdom and holiness soon attracted followers. Members of monasteries interact with one another in more intimate ways than do members of most churches. How they live out Christ to one another creates an atmosphere in which spiritual growth abounds or in which spiritual growth is stifled.

The social nature of the Church and the church was intended by Christ. We need each other to grow spiritually. And just as some may bring spiritual dis-ease to the church, so others may bring spiritual healing. But how the church deals with its most spiritual dis-eased members largely determines whether it is a house of healing or a house of pain.

Notes

1. Jim Jones founded the Peoples Temple in San Francisco but in 1977 founded a colony with 900 of his followers in Guyana when his church came under investigation by the IRS. An investigation into the group's activities and a visit to the colony by Congressman Jim Ryan in 1978 led to a deadly attack on the congressman's party and mass suicide by Jones' followers.

2. I have listed a few such books in Appendix B.

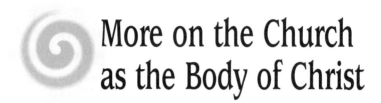

CHAPTER 9

More on the Church as the Body of Christ

Members, one yet individual

So important is the concept of the church as the body of Christ, and the church as a local realization of that body, that is worthwhile spending additional time reflecting on its implications. We must, however, still distinguish between the church as an organic whole and the church as a community of individuals. In one sense, all of the members of a church are one in Christ, bound together by the life of Christ. Nowhere is this expressed more powerfully than at the Communion table, where the entire church family gathers in unity at the banquet of the Lord.

But even when they recognize Christ in one another, the members are still separate human beings. They each have their own personalities, strengths and weaknesses, degrees of faith, and so on. Thus, the body of Christ on earth and the local congregation suffer from the same potential diseases of any human institution. The effect of these diseases may even be magnified within a church because the members are expected to love one another in Christ and put up with one another's failings since we all fall short of the glory of God (Romans 3:23). But the fact remains that some failings and some people are hard to tolerate.

In such a situation we might ask who it is that needs healing. Perhaps the person who is hard to tolerate needs healing. But many saints have been hard to tolerate because they rightly and courageously stood against the values of their societies. The leadership must listen to the "troublemaker" to discern whether God is trying to teach them through this difficult person.

But a person whom many find abrasive and irritating may simply be abrasive and irritating. Gentleness and constructive counseling may cause the individual to moderate his or her behavior. The troublesome person may yet remain troublesome. Our greatest challenges to charity and compassion can come from those we find it hard to get along with. Thus, those members who cannot act compassionately toward those who chronically annoy them are themselves in need of healing. Christ is present even in the person who most displeases us.

And perhaps those who stand idly by, who could help the situation but choose not to do so, are also in need of healing. One strategy to help us deal with someone we dislike is to ignore that person. In some instances that may be the only viable strategy, but only after other approaches to try to relate to the annoying individual fail, or are reasonably deemed to be futile. Remember that we may well have to embrace in heaven those whom we could not abide on earth.

It was into an imperfect world filled with problems caused by human beings being human beings that Jesus came. God became a human being knowing what he was getting into but coming nonetheless. God, therefore, is fully aware from his Son's own experience of what it means to be human.

> For we do not have a high priest who is unable to sympathize with our weaknesses, but we have one who has been tempted in every way, just as we are—yet was without sin. Let us then approach the throne of grace with confidence, so that we may receive mercy and find grace to help us in our time of need. (Hebrews 4:15-16)

Jesus felt loneliness, rejection, sorrow and other negative human feelings, but he likewise experienced the joys of being human through his powerful positive relationships with others. Think, for example, of the incident in which a woman poured ointment on his feet and wiped them dry with her hair (Luke 7:36-38). This, John tells us, is Mary, the sister of Lazarus whom Jesus raised from the dead (John 11:2). How healing this tender show of love must have been for Jesus, particularly when he had been treated so coldly by the Pharisee whose dinner guest he was. The bonds between Mary and Jesus were deep. Mary was one of the few disciples who stayed by him at his crucifixion and who wanted to care for his body after his death. She was rewarded by being the first to witness his resurrection.

Human experiences, both good and bad, in the church

Members of a congregation will suffer the same problems as other humans, but they can also enjoy the same healing experiences as well. Let us look at several of the common human experiences, both negative and positive, and see how these might be experienced by individuals in a church and by the church as a whole. We will also explore in greater depth later how the negative experiences can be lessened or overcome so that healing can take place at the individual and congregational level, and how the positive experiences can be reinforced to foster greater opportunities for spiritual growth.

Alienation

I remember visiting a church some years ago that gave me a colored ribbon to wear to identify me as a visitor. The ribbon was clearly visible, but I felt invisible. I went to the coffee hour following the service and stood quietly, expecting someone to notice my ribbon and welcome me. No one came forward. After a reasonable time of being ignored, I left, saddened that this church had intentionally instituted a method to mark someone as a visitor but failed to welcome a visitor thus marked. They thus doubled a visitor's sense of alienation. It would have been less hurtful if I was not singled out and ignored. But to single me out in a special way and then ignore me made me feel particularly unwelcome.

I wish I could say this is the only such incident I have had in visiting other churches. Instead, it is the rule. Yes, once I had identified myself as a priest, I was accepted, but I was not accepted as a stranger. Too often, when I was not "one of the group," I was treated like an alien and because I was treated like one, I felt like one.

The human body has defense mechanisms against invaders like viruses and bacteria that the immune system recognizes as foreign to the body. All too many churches have defense mechanisms as well to exclude those who are "not like us" or who have not been invited by a current member. Although a good immune system is important for the health of the human body, it can cause spiritual illness for a church.

A healthy church should be a welcoming place. If members feel good about their church, if their church is a house of healing, then they should want to share the healing they are receiving with the entire world, and, certainly, with those who take the trouble to visit. A healthy church feels good about itself and knows that it has much to offer potential members. Members are joyful and excited and anxious to lavish the abundant love and healing they feel on others, knowing that it is not theirs to hoard, but theirs to give away. This is one of the signs of a healthy congregation. What are some others?

Health-giving relationships

Becoming a member of a church necessarily puts us in relationship with others. Relationships can be neutral, constructive, or destructive, but relationships with others in a healing community should always be constructive. The relationships themselves should be instruments of spiritual healing. How is this so?

First, there are others who genuinely care about us, who love us in Christ. Thus, when I am physically ill I have someone to visit me and perform useful services for me both to alleviate my discomfort and to ease my anxiety.

I was spiritual director of a woman who lived alone and was dying of cancer and able to do very little for herself. But women at her church took it on themselves to make sure that she always had a companion, that her house was clean, and that she was fed and cared for. She was able to stay at home and died there. But this care provided by her companions in Christ was what made this possible. She died a most holy death, and I am sure that those who attended to her needs were inspired by her own love and example. Her relating to them was as important as their relating to her.

Second, within the church we can see that others are struggling with many of the same problems with which we struggle. We can be inspired by examples of courage, and we can give of ourselves to help those who need encouragement. Through the example of others, we can be inspired and learn, and through our giving to others, we can be strengthened and grow in the Lord. I have often learned a great deal from the example that others set in their relationship with God. But this is certainly to be expected. Young children learn from the example of their parents. In the secular world, we learn much of our behavior (both good and bad) as well by following the example of others. But examples in a healthy church should be infused with the grace of God and based on the example given to us by Christ. Christlike examples should help us to become more spiritually healthy. Almost everyone who has made a commitment to seek Christ at a deeper level has been inspired to do so by someone else. We should be especially grateful to those who have been a holy inspiration to us. We might well pause in a moment of prayerful reflection and gratitude for those who have been such inspirations in our own lives.

Third, Jesus said that where two or three are gathered in his name, he is in the midst of them (Matthew 18:20). Jesus is with each church in a special way. The members can count on his presence if they are willing to do so. There might even be regular reminders in sermons, banners, or prayers that Jesus is present to his people in church. For example, a hanging in front of the altar could read, "We are all one in Christ at this table." A banner near the door to the church could quote Paul, "In Christ, we who are many form one body and each member belongs to all the others." A Sunday school class could be assigned to produce pictures to represent the unity of Christians with one another in Christ.

Fourth, the members can pray for one another. The knowledge that others are praying for us can itself be healing, but the prayer itself often brings special graces as well. Perhaps it does not bring the physical healing we might be seeking, but it can bring peace that enables us to endure our physical suffering with patience and to offer it as a prayer to God. When we pray for others, we ourselves benefit because we are directing our hearts and minds to God and allowing God to transform us by the power of the Holy Spirit. A church that truly is a house of prayer will also be a house of healing. Most churches have prayer chains to enlist immediate prayers for critical needs and prayer lists for continuing needs. Often a church will have prayer teams to pray at, or before or after, services for those who feel the need for prayer. Healing prayer teams are discussed at length in chapter 15.

Special healing services should also be a part of any church's worship that aspires to be a house of healing. But the services must be conducted in a way that is likely to lead to healing rather than to increased guilt or feelings of spiritual inadequacy. We will explore this theme at greater length later on and include a sample healing service in appendix A.

Finally, there is often consolation is just having others around—simply in companionship. No one likes to be alone all the time. No one likes to feel isolated as I did standing at the coffee hour with my colored ribbon and no one paying the least attention to me, or visiting other churches and feeling alone even though I was in a crowd. Belonging to a caring, healing congregation is like belonging to a healthy family where each of the members love and care for one another. There are few better satisfactions than walking into a group of people and feeling that you belong and are welcome. If strangers feel this way about your church, you are well along in being a house of healing.

Health-giving harmony

I love music and have a musical background. But one need not be a trained musician to appreciate the elegance and beauty of choral voices singing in harmony. Nor need one be much of a musician at all to recognize how poorly selected music or music poorly performed can detract from an otherwise well-conducted service. There is power in harmony.

A church that promotes healing seeks harmony in its members without demanding subservience or forcing members to think and act in lockstep. In fact, to require everyone to think and act alike contradicts Paul's statements that the body of Christ has many members and each has its proper role to play. Perhaps one member's role is to play the gadfly, to challenge tradition and "facts" that may prevent the congregation from being more open to the Holy Spirit.

But if harmony is not thinking alike, then what is it?

Some will insist that it consists of a common agreement on a core set of beliefs, traditions, values, or goals. If this is the case, then the question becomes what beliefs, traditions, values, or goals are contained in the "core." What must every member of the community say or do to be in harmony with all of the other members? Can an atheist, for example, join a Christian church because he has many friends there and enjoys the social activities the church sponsors?

This issue is more than theoretical. I have given quizzes to congregations in such a way that the respondents remained anonymous and, thus, did not feel constrained in their answers. These quizzes present general Christian and specific denominational statements—for example, "Jesus Christ physically rose from the dead," or "The head of the church has the authority to pronounce its doctrine." Respondents are asked to give a score to each statement with one meaning they completely disagree and ten meaning they completely agree. The only statement that has gotten an average of ten is "Jesus Christ is Lord and Savior." If you think all of your members think alike, you might try giving a quiz of your own, but make sure it is carried out anonymously. And even if every member agrees say that there is life after death, I can assure you that there are as many different descriptions of that life as there are members.

Compounding the problem of basing harmony on common beliefs and practices is the fact that the central truths of Christianity, such as the Incarnation—God becoming human—soar far beyond the natural powers of our understanding. They are mysteries, not because they are false, but because we cannot grasp them using our natural intellectual powers. Moreover, even members of churches whose members strongly agree on a common set of beliefs and practices can fight like cats and dogs over issues of control, the quality of the pastor's sermons, or even the color to use for painting the ladies room. In what then does harmony lie?

How we live and practice Christianity is conveyed, not as much in what we say, but in multidimensional symbols. How we live our lives is a symbol of what Christianity means to us. If our actions are divisive, arrogant, and controlling, we send a strong message that this is how we interpret the gospel and how Christ would act in our shoes. The symbols of our faith are also contained in our manner of worship. Worship can be healing, or it can be a source of spiritual illness. What are the symbols we use in worship? Are the symbols able to bring worshipers in contact with the reality that underlies the symbols? I suggest that it is through its worship and through the behavior of its members that a church builds either harmony or dissension, heals or serves as a pathogen. The worship, by bringing members in contact with the symbols of their faith and, hopefully, with a deeper experience of God and God's love for us, should strengthen and teach its members to lead lives that are also symbols of the Good News.

It is in worship and the symbols therein, including the preaching of the gospel, that harmony will be found or lost; the members brought together or divided, inspired to live the Good News or left with a sense that church is a burdensome duty rather than a spiritual aid. For the symbols to be most helpful, however, the members must have an appreciation for why the symbols are present. We use symbols to represent the unseen and unintelligible realities of our faith. The symbols confer power, not in themselves, but because they make present in a special way the timeless realities they represent.

We will close this chapter by suggesting powerful symbols that can promote spiritual healing and ways in which they can be incorporated into the worship of a church. These symbols are more than signs of faith. They are balms that can promote spiritual healing and, in some cases, physical healing as well.

Symbols of faith and spiritual healing

Symbols from the Epistle of James

A passage from James has been used as the basis for many healing rituals and services.

> Is any one of you sick? He should call the elders of the church to pray over him and anoint him with oil in the name of the Lord. And the prayer offered in faith will make the sick person well; the Lord will raise him up. If he has sinned, he will be forgiven. Therefore confess your sins to each other and pray for each other so that you may be healed. The prayer of a righteous man is powerful and effective. (James 5:14-16)

Anointing with oil was used in a variety of ways in both the Old and New Testament as well as in society at large. Oil was used by athletes to make their skin smoother and more supple and to reduce perspiration. Oil was used for cleansing. It was also used to consecrate certain persons or locations as sacred (see, for example, Genesis 28:18).[1] Oil was used in the coronation of kings, and still is used in this way today, such as in the coronation of the kings and queens of England. Oil also symbolizes the pouring out of the Holy Spirit, and it is not uncommon today to talk of someone being anointed by the Spirit with special gifts. Thus, oil has been, and still is, used in many rituals.

The prayers used at the laying on of hands and anointing, and the prayer following the anointing are instructive as to the meaning of what for some denominations is considered a sacrament. The Episcopal *Book of Common Prayer* is not copyrighted (although its supplements are); therefore any denomination is free to use these time-honored prayers if it finds them appropriate. Some prayers for healing found in the *Book of Common Prayer* have been included in appendix A.

We used the prayers from that historic volume at our healing service at St. Paul's, a congregation I served for some sixteen years, but your church might prefer prayers from your own tradition or your church might want to write its own prayers. We incorporated our healing service into our Sunday worship, but other churches I know of have their healing services or prayers for healing during the week or apart from the Sunday services.

Entire services can be constructed around the theme of healing, but symbols of healing must be an important component of such services. Of course, words are symbols, but they are immensely enhanced if accompanied by other appropriate symbols. Laying on hands, if it conveys no other meaning, tells the recipient that the minister is one in Christ with him or her. The touch expresses the human connection between two members of the body of Christ, but it also expresses Christ himself reaching out to that person.

Symbols of forgiveness and fellowship

The prayer following the administration of the laying on of hands and anointing speaks of forgiveness. The message of forgiveness is central to Christianity; hence it too should be expressed in symbols. Forgiveness is essential to spiritual healing, forgiveness of our sins by God through Christ, and our forgiveness of others for real or imagined injuries.

James states that we ought to confess our sins to one another and pray for one another that we might be healed. Forgiveness comes through Christ, but we can assure penitents that Christ has forgiven them for those sins for which they are sorry. I remarked earlier about what joy participants in a Beginning Experience weekend often felt once they had confessed their sins and been assured that God had put away their sins.

Some denominations may be skittish about having a penitent confess his or her sins, even to a minister, because they believe that the sinner should confess his sins to Jesus and receive forgiveness from him rather than from a human intermediary. Moreover, many penitents are ashamed and afraid to tell another human being how they have sinned, particularly if the sin involves deeply personal activities.

The ceremony can be tailored to a denomination's traditions and beliefs. But all Christian denominations, so far as I know, believe that sinners who repent are forgiven for their sins by God because of the saving work of Jesus Christ. So all the penitents will be reminded that God will continue to forgive and forgive again if they sin and sin again so long as they are sorry and try their best to sin no more.

Some denominations place a heavy emphasis on sin, our human corruption in the eyes of God, and God's anger at our continuing transgressions. I respectfully suggest that this emphasis does not promote spiritual healing any more than reminding someone with cancer how painful and fatal the disease can be. Jesus came so we could be healed, not scared out of our wits. He raised the dignity of human nature by taking that nature on himself. As I noted before, Jesus saved his harshest comments for those who thought they were righteous, and he was merciful and forgiving toward those who knew they were sinners. Fear may work in some rare cases as a means of getting someone to "accept Jesus" as "fire insurance," but do we really want to present the gospel in that way? It is love to which God calls us. "There is no fear in love. But perfect love drives out fear, because fear has to do with punishment. The one who fears is not made perfect in love" (1 John 4:18). Those who have been spiritually healed are not afraid of God.

Common meals

Yet another symbol of fellowship in Christ is sharing a common meal. At more informal and intimate celebrations of the Lord's Supper, I allow participants to administer Communion to one another as a symbol of how, though being fed by Christ, we must feed one another in Christ. In giving Communion to another person, it is hard to harbor a grudge or not see Jesus in that person.

But a meal need not be Communion to symbolize unity. Pitchins or covered dish suppers at the church, or smaller groups gathered at homes, can be reminders of unity in Christ. The food that is shared should be a sign of a deeper sharing. Indeed, small groups sharing a meal at home can often turn into groups in which participants share their lives and support one another in Christ at a deeper level.

Whenever a symbol is used, there must be continuing reminders of the meaning of that symbol. A meal can easily become just a meal with friends if teaching about its symbolism does not take place and if prayers are not said that remind those present at a meal that the meal is a sign of something that is more than a meal. The more skeptical may say that teachings and reminders may not make much difference in the underlying attitudes that people have toward one another; the symbolism will mainly be ignored. But if the reminders, prayers and teaching are consistent and continuing, many will "get it."

The exchange of the peace

"Greet one another with a holy kiss" (Romans 16:16). More controversial than meals is the exchange of the peace, the greeting with a "holy kiss" as Paul puts it. In an age that is rightly sensitive to sexual misconduct, all Christians, particularly pastors, must pay close attention to personal boundaries.

Even so, touching, and even hugging, if done appropriately, can help build community and convey warmth and acceptance within a church. The exchange of the peace can also be used as a sign of reconciliation and forgiveness.

Jesus touched people often in the act of healing them. Through appropriate touching we establish a connection with someone that mere words cannot accomplish. When I visit someone who is seriously ill, I often hold that person's hand while praying for him or her so that the patient better senses my presence and my concern. I, thus, become more available to the patient. Both the sense of touch and sense of hearing are involved, which reinforces my prayer.

The exchange of the peace, like the other rituals mentioned above, should be a symbol of a deeper reality. Through it members can not only express their reaching out to one another in Christ but their integral unity in Christ. Through words alone, we remain separate. In touching, there is a more profound sense of connection. Through the words we use in the exchange of the peace, we also express our prayer for the spiritual welfare of the one we greet.

Note

1. In the ordination of Roman Catholic priests, the fingers which are to handle the consecrated elements in Communion are also anointed with oil.

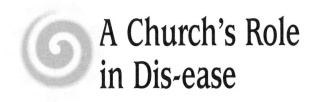

CHAPTER 10

A Church's Role in Dis-ease

Even a hospital can be a dangerous place

A common cliché is "The church is a hospital for sinners." Statements often become clichés because people recognize they concisely express a truth, and such is the case with this statement. The church should be a hospital for sinners, a house of healing for our spiritual dis-eases, a place where we not only receive forgiveness for our sins through Jesus Christ, but a community in which, and through which, the Holy Spirit can act to renew us and transform us into what God calls us to be, other Christs.

But hospitals can be dangerous places. Hospital staff can make mistakes that aggravate existing illnesses. Patients can contract new illnesses despite a hospital's best efforts to contain infection or isolate communicable diseases. Although most patients are discharged from a hospital in better health than when they were admitted, some few experience complications that worsen their conditions and that may even prove fatal.

The church as a hospital for sinners must confront the possibility that it is harming some members more than it is helping them. If a church cannot bring itself to face this possibility, then it may not recognize when it is contributing to its members' dis-eases, nor will it take steps to reform itself to make itself a better house of healing.

There are two principle carriers of spiritual dis-ease for a con-gregation. The first is the congregation itself. The second is the pastoral leadership. Rarely, however, is either the congregation or the pastoral leadership a carrier without the complicity—explicit or implicit—of the other. Let us consider some ways in which con-gregations and pastors can be dysfunctional.

Congregational dysfunctions

Because congregations are composed of human beings, they are subject to all of the faults and failings of the human condition. Moreover, there are faults that humans will commit in a crowd that they are not likely to commit as individuals. Examples might include hiding behind the "will of the people" or claiming that "everyone was doing it," to absolve oneself of inappropriate behavior. Let us consider some sources of spiritual dis-ease that may be present in a congregation. Those issues I present below by no means exhaust the faults of which a congregation may be guilty. We will identify certain faults now, but we will return to them later when I suggest ways to try to overcome them.

Exclusivity

A congregation that is exclusive will be reluctant to reach out to bring others in, or, if others do start to attend the church, the con-gregation will not make them feel wanted or welcome. Of course, few congregations would post "No Trespassing" signs on their doors or go out of their way to offend visitors. Exclusivity will show itself in more subtle ways. For example, does your church:

- have a member of the congregation sit with visitors to help guide them through the service and accompany them to the social time following the service?

- have a lay person contact visitors within twenty-four hours after their visit to tell them how much their visit was appreciated and to invite them back?
- have a visitor welcome and orientation dinner each month as well as a program to inform newcomers about your denomination and your church?
- involve newcomers as quickly as possible in the work and ministry of the church?
- welcome new members who have shown fidelity in attendance to share in the leadership of church programs?

What has this to do with the church as a house of healing? Aren't we talking rather about outreach and stewardship? Yes, but healthy outreach and healthy stewardship are both necessary for a healthy church. A church that is too turned in on itself, that fails to take steps like those listed above, is like someone who isolates himself from other people. That person will be deprived of new ideas and may, at worst, become narcissistic. Jesus commanded his disciples to go into all nations, not remain together in Jerusalem. A church, like any living organism, must either thrive or die. The church that retreats within itself and fails to entertain new ideas, or that will not train and engage new members in leadership, will ultimately wither away. Members of a congregation that does not actively seek growth both numerically and spiritually will themselves stagnate spiritually and risk losing whatever understanding of the message of the gospel they may have had.

Inflexibility

Related to, but different from, exclusivity is inflexibility. Here is an example of a congregation that will die because of its inflexibility. A church I knew of personally (the name and denomination will not be mentioned to protect the guilty) was asked by its area executive head to work closely with a church of another denomination only blocks away. The two denominations involved were in full communion and could share their ministers with one another. The church that was asked to work with the sister church refused, even though the average age of its members was in the sixties and they had no hope of obtaining even a part-time minister. The congregation decided that they were only interested in their own church, and when the last member died, their church would close. No doubt, that is exactly what will happen. The members were inflexible to the point of being willing to see their church die rather than partner with another church with similar theological views.

One sees this same phenomenon in the South where there may be multiple Southern Baptist Convention congregations in the same small town—none of which can support themselves—yet there is no interest among these churches in forming a cooperative venture that could be viable. Why? Because members are not willing to give up "their" congregation.

Many Christians consider inflexibility a virtue, meaning that they are unwilling to compromise on doctrine or Scripture. They point out that many Christians have been willing to suffer death rather than renounce their faith. And they are correct. In those matters that are truly central to the gospel and a life of faith, one cannot compromise. The gospel is not to be watered down, even if it means fewer members in the pews.

But, all too often, inflexibility extends to matters that have little to do with faith. One cannot argue, for example, that tastes in music have changed through the ages. If a congregation claims that they will not tolerate any hymn written after 1750, they are depriving themselves of some excellent hymns; moreover, they are pushing away those who want more contemporary, though tasteful, music. A congregation that insists that anyone who wants to be part of their services must hug other participants at the exchange of the peace will drive out those who find even a handshake difficult. Instead, we might take Augustine's famous advice: "In essentials, unity, in non-essentials diversity, in all things charity."

As has oft been said, the cry of "We've always done it this way before" can be the death knell for a church. Human beings adapt and change regularly in their daily lives. A couple who tries to live exactly as they did before their new baby came will wind up frustrated and unhappy. Changes in life bring changes in the way we do things. Once again, we must realize that a church is a living organism, a body in Christ in the Body of Christ. The members of the church are members of this body. The organism must be adaptable to thrive.

Although exclusivity and inflexibility often look much alike in the behaviors they inspire, they are not the same dis-ease. An exclusive congregation can still be open to different viewpoints among its members—that is, it is not inherently inflexible—but it can be completely indifferent to the ideas of outsiders. Inflexibility will generally not entertain new ideas, no matter where they come from. In an inflexible church, members do not listen to those whose viewpoints differ from the status quo, hence there is little dialogue or openness. A member who feels he or she is not heard by the church will often leave it or simply fade into the background. In either case, that person has been treated with disrespect by his or her brothers and sisters in Christ—a spiritual dis-ease indeed.

Just as exclusivity can bring spiritual stagnation, so too can inflexibility. Each church needs to be able to ask itself: Yes, this is the way we've acted until now, but is there a way we should act now that is more in harmony with the gospel and in accord with our desire to support our members in their spiritual growth? An unwillingness to ask this question and answer it openly and honestly is a sign of spiritual dis-ease in a church.

Control issues

Denominations often differ in the way decisions are made both at the denominational level and in their local churches. A church itself may even be independent of any denomination. Such a church might stand alone, having been established by a self-ordained individual, who usually exercises tight control over its members. In some denominations members are given wide latitude and encouragement for independent thought and forming their own consciences.

Churches that more strictly monitor their members' beliefs and behaviors generally adhere to the principle that the way to salvation is narrow and the temptations to stray many. Therefore it is necessary to keep members on the right path lest they deviate from it and are lost.

Churches that encourage more independent thought and action among their members would argue that God treats each person as an individual and there is no "one size fits all" in the spiritual life. We cannot bind the Holy Spirit, and since God gave humans minds to think, they should use them to discern how and where God is leading them. These Christians feel that blind obedience to any authority is a perversion of their God-given freedom and human reason.

Other Christians feel more comfortable when they are told what to believe and how to live. They want strong guidance from their spiritual leaders since they feel obedience to such guidance gives them greater certainty that they are pleasing God and living correctly. They sacrifice their own wills to the will of their superiors because, whether the superior is right or wrong, obedience is never wrong. God will bless their fidelity in following the instructions of their church's lawful authority.

Thus, individual Christians will choose the mode of polity that they find comfortable. Nevertheless, tight control by a pastor can sometimes stifle spiritual growth, just as excessive freedom can. Both dis-eased control and dis-eased freedom can lead to a dis-eased congregation and dis-eased individuals.

Pastors must always remember that they are servants of Jesus Christ and are to be as Christ to their flock. Jesus said, "Come to me, all you who are weary and burdened, and I will give you rest. Take my yoke upon you and learn from me, for I am gentle and humble in heart, and you will find rest for your souls. For my yoke is easy and my burden is light" (Matthew 11:28-30).

When a pastor presumes to speak exclusively for God to the congregation, instead of recognizing in the mirror a person with all the weaknesses of a human being called to a special ministry of service, then tyranny may replace servant leadership. This control is based on fear rather than love and example. Moreover, pastors who believe that only they are right must logically conclude that everyone else is wrong. Thus, there is no room for discussion or listening sympathetically to the ideas of others.

Christians who are controlled by a human pastor cannot be guided by the Holy Spirit if the Holy Spirit should be so bold as to disagree with the pastor. Demanding that a Christian submit absolutely to human authority, even human authority that claims to speak with the voice of God, necessarily binds the Spirit. Christians and churches who blindly subject themselves to such authority risk spiritual stagnation, pride ("We are the only ones saved"), exclusivity, and inflexibility.

We must not assume, however, that only pastors can be guilty of control issues. Most pastors know of congregations where a small number of members insist on their right to control the church and the pastor is reduced to little more than a chaplain to the real decision makers. This situation too is dis-eased. It is simply another group, rather than the pastor, that is raising the control issue.

At the opposite extreme, churches and denominations that refuse to set boundaries for those who wish to call themselves members likewise are a source of spiritual dis-ease. Increasingly, individuals are attending churches just because they feel comfortable there rather than because they agree with those churches' teachings or even know what those teachings are.

One may argue about what someone must believe to be a Christian, but surveys seem to indicate that a fair number of churchgoers think that the most important element of Christianity is obeying the Ten Commandments and living a good life. No doubt many churchgoers believe that Jesus was a great prophet who taught people how they ought to behave, but they do not think that Jesus was fully divine in any unique sense. And, yet, without the Incarnation—Jesus is both fully divine and fully human—Jesus has little more claim to our allegiance than Muhammad or Buddha or John the Baptist.

Just as healthy human beings set boundaries to protect their integrity, so too must a healthy church set boundaries to protect its integrity. A healthy church must state openly and clearly what it believes and what its mission is. Without such statements, a church will be more a social club than a house of healing. For, as noted earlier, genuine healing only comes about through continuing growth into the life of God through Jesus Christ by the power of the Holy Spirit. God can still act in those who do not believe in Jesus Christ or the Holy Spirit. But a church, at least, should promote healing through its active and open promotion of Jesus Christ as the Way, the Truth, and the Life, and the Holy Spirit as Sanctifier. Different denominations may stress different aspects of the reality that is Christ and the Spirit, have different polities and even different views of how best to worship, but no denomination, in my opinion, can call itself Christian unless it is founded on Jesus Christ as the Incarnate God. A church that has no foundation in Christ is dis-eased, and any healing that takes place in its members happens in spite of it rather than because of its ministry.

Other issues that lead to a dis-eased congregation

I have passed over the more glaring issues of violations of pastoral trust, perhaps through misuse of authority, perhaps through embezzlement, perhaps through sexual misconduct. Whenever a congregation has been wounded by pastoral misconduct, it stands in need of healing. A congregation that tries to bury its past trauma will continue to suffer from it. In some way the past trauma will bubble up and manifest itself in dysfunction and in congregational disease.

Generally, it is the denominational executive who must recognize that the church needs healing and who intervenes, perhaps by providing a skilled interim minister, to guide the church through a period of coming to grips with its past and moving beyond it. Unfortunately, from what I have seen over my more than thirty years in the ministry, all too often this is not what happens. The dis-eased congregation is allowed to call another pastor who may not even be briefed on the trauma the church has suffered. The church is not given a chance to heal, and the wound continues to fester, often creating animosity among the members and toward the new pastor, who is unaware of the true root cause of the dysfunctions being displayed.

Thus, denominational executives themselves must be sensitive to dis-eases in congregations under their charge. If the judicatory as pastor to pastors is itself dis-eased, that dis-ease will filter down through the churches, or a healthy church may simply isolate itself from the executive to keep from getting infected.

The church as an unsafe place

A dis-eased congregation is one that is handicapped in one or more ways in its efforts to assist its members to grow into spiritual maturity. This does not mean, of course, that many members do not continue to grow spiritually. The Spirit is able to work even in the most adverse of circumstances. Moreover, just as there is no such thing as a perfect human being (except Jesus), there is no such thing as a perfect congregation. A church is made up of imperfect human beings and is bound to reflect those imperfections in imperfections of its own. In sum, a church can be dis-eased but still be a house of healing in spite of its faults if its members can still be supported in their spiritual growth and if the church is a safe place to be.

The most obvious manner in which a church can be unsafe is if the leadership demeans members and so lessens their self-esteem. This occurs if the members are constantly berated for their alleged sinful behavior and warned of God's anger toward them, or if the leadership has assumed such absolute control over the members that they are, in effect, letting the pastor, rather than God, control their lives.

Another way that a church can be unsafe is if the confidences of its members are not respected. A secret revealed, even inadvertently, can mean a church member both lost to the congregation and deeply offended. Churches must be places in which members can tell their stories with the assurance that they will be respected and not judged. I know of specific cases from my work in spiritual development where a member did not dare reveal her deepest religious experiences to her pastor for fear of being perceived as crazy. Worse was the case where she did dare to reveal such experiences and was demeaned.

Extending the metaphor of church as hospital for sinners, we know that hospitals today try to assure patients that their situations will not be revealed without their consent. The same must be true in churches. Those involved in compassion ministries, pastoral leadership, small groups, or other programs in which confidences might be shared must be given clear instructions concerning confidentiality.[1]

All too often sharing takes place in a church only at a superficial level, the depth of sharing being even less than one might find at a cocktail party. In some sense, the extent to which members are willing to open themselves to the pastor and other members so as to seek spiritual guidance, prayers, and support is a measure of the health of the congregation. A church that functions only at the level of small talk is not much of a church at all. And yet, to create an environment where members are encouraged to share at a deeper level and have developed the trust to do so is hard work. It is not something that comes naturally. It comes only supernaturally when members trust the Holy Spirit and sense the Holy Spirit is operating in and through others in the church.

Sometimes members believe they are safe when, in reality, they are not safe at all. If members are taught that their salvation is completely assured only so long as they remain completely obedient to their pastor, then they are substituting the pastor, a fallible human being, for God.[2]

Still, human beings yearn for certainty. We want to believe that we are doing whatever is necessary to gain entry into heaven and avoid the pains of hell. But a church that stresses the rewards of heaven and the pains of hell is dis-eased. The promise of a reward or the threat of punishment to control what members do and believe guarantees a low level of spiritual development, a stagnation of the spiritual life in its early childhood. Christians are to grow into a more perfect love of God and neighbor, and perfect love casts out fear (see 1 John 4:18). Indeed, perfect love is founded neither on hope of reward nor fear of punishment but on an absolute desire to possess God as the source and meaning of all that is good. A church in which members are held in bondage to fear or are deliberately infantilized is not a spiritually safe place.

A failure to acknowledge healing as a principal mission of the church

Many devout Christians believe that the primary mission of the church, a mission subordinate to all other missions, is to bring people to Christ. Once someone has been brought to Christ, that person can then be trained as a disciple who will bring others to Christ. The most important function of the church is to offer salvation, and, since salvation only comes through faith in Jesus Christ, the church must concentrate on bringing people to faith in Christ and then enabling them to bring others to faith in Christ. If someone is not saved, little else matters, so the church's emphasis must be on saving souls.

Whether a church should be primarily interested in making converts to Christ or making saints of its members is a serious question. Evangelicals, among others, will stress bringing souls to Christ. They will argue that if the house is on fire, you must concentrate on getting its occupants to safety, not work on the interior decorating. Once someone is saved, they will be completely happy in heaven later on. Having that person worry about spiritual growth on earth might lead inevitably to works righteousness.

But the New Testament is clear that being "saved," becoming a new person in Christ, is but the first step toward spiritual growth. "Brothers, I could not address you as spiritual but as worldly—mere infants in Christ. I gave you milk, not solid food, for you were not yet ready for it. Indeed, you are still not ready" (1 Corinthians 3:1-3). Even after Jesus rose from the dead, his disciples still did not understand his message, but they continued to meditate on it and grow into it throughout their ministries. We are called to achieve the fullness of Christ (see Ephesians 4:13), and Paul indicates this is a process, not something that has already taken place.

Concerning works righteousness, no saint has argued that he or she grew ever more into the love and service of God through his or her own efforts. Rather the saint became more holy by opening him or herself to the work that only God could do. A premise that underlies this book is that God wants to draw us more and more into God's own life through Jesus Christ (who made it possible) by the power of the Holy Spirit (who accomplishes it if we will let the Spirit work in us). Works righteousness implies that we can bootstrap our way to holiness, that by appropriate works and spiritual exercises, we can come to see God face to face, to know God as God knows us, to love God with God's own love. This is bad theology in every Christian denomination since it implies there is no need for either Christ or the Holy Spirit.

But, in reality, there is no conflict between bringing people into the life of Christ and growing in the life of Christ. Those who grow in the life of Christ are more likely to be successful in attracting others to Christ since they will serve as better windows to Christ's love and glory. And since they will love more fully with the love of God, they will want even more to bring others to God in accordance with the desire of God's love.

Some may be led to profess faith in Christ as "fire insurance," but most people I know are turned off by threats of hell if they do not accept Christ in the way that some well-meaning evangelists demand. People are generally more attracted to a merciful and loving God than a harsh, punitive God.

Those who love the Lord with all their hearts and souls and minds and strength (see Matthew 22:37) will want more than anything else to do what they believe the Lord wants them to do. If they have experienced the love of God, they will want others to experience it as well, not because others will go to hell if they do not claim to love God, but because the love of God brings spiritual riches beyond any riches that the earth can give. The knowledge of God is of greater worth than any human knowledge. Human knowledge is useful in this life, but the knowledge of God not only gives meaning to our current lives on earth but is the foundation of our eternal life.

Notes

1. Would that the matter were as simple as not revealing to "outsiders" information received in a pastoral relationship. In most states, only an ordained minister receives confidences as privileged, that is, he or she cannot be made to reveal such confidences in a trial. Some states require anyone, even an ordained minister, who learns about abuse of a child to reveal that information to law enforcement or risk prosecution. Then, of course, there is the case where someone threatens, or hints at, harm to himself or another. These situations illustrate that it generally insufficient just to tell someone to keep certain information in confidence. More extensive training and discussion is called for, even if a trainee may never encounter a problem.

2. Recall the Jonestown tragedy referenced in footnote one of chapter 8.

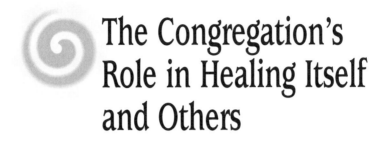

CHAPTER 11

The Congregation's Role in Healing Itself and Others

Now that we have looked at some of ways in which both individuals and churches may need spiritual healing, we look at some of the steps that can be taken to facilitate such healing.

Acknowledging the dis-ease in self and others

Someone who is ill and refuses to admit he or she is ill may still get better. The human body has amazing mechanisms to heal itself. Of course, that person may also die, because dis-eases that are ignored can, in some cases, prove fatal. So it is with congregations and with individual Christians.

But acknowledging dis-ease is easier said than done. First, what someone else may see as a dis-ease in me, I may see as a virtue. I may, for example, be absolutely adamant that a certain style of hymns must be used in worship. All other forms of music profane the service and do not instill the proper attitude of reverence. Of course, I am wrong, and others find my unyielding demands annoying and neurotic, but they go along with me because I am the pastor and they do not want to cause dissension . . . or they leave and go to another church that has music more to their liking.

In the example above, there are two dis-eases. The first is my unwillingness to honor any opinion other than my own. The second dis-ease is that the congregation enables my dis-ease instead of calling me to account. Because I am the pastor, any "intervention" concerning my neurotic behavior must be done with special care. But pastors have dis-eases too, and their dis-eases can infect their congregation with dis-ease, so it does not help me or the church to gloss over my irrational behavior.

But I, of course, think my behavior is entirely rational; in fact, I am sure that I am acting in the best spiritual interests of the members of my church. Christians who suffer from spiritual maladies may not realize that they are dis-eased and are causing dis-ease in others. Denial is one of the basic spiritual illnesses.

A church that has had a serious breach of trust by a pastor has to confront that tragedy if its wounds are to heal. I know one church where the congregation spent more than a year under the guidance of a loving and skilled pastor dealing with and healing the wounds it suffered from an alcoholic minister. I know of another church, however, where the denominational executive accused the church of a lack of compassion toward an alcoholic pastor. The church wanted to get rid of the pastor after he had been to rehabilitation twice and relapsed after returning each time. That church had to recover not only from the harm caused by the dis-eased pastor but from the lack of support and understanding shown it by those who should have cared most about its well-being.

In sum, acknowledging a dis-ease, whether it is in an individual or in the congregation, is usually an essential prerequisite to healing. But what steps can a church take to help it identify congregational or pastoral dysfunctions and to help members identify those areas in which they need healing without doing more harm than healing?

Means to identify spiritual dis-eases

Whatever methods the church employs to identify and seek healing for spiritual illnesses must not be worse than the illnesses themselves; that is, they ought to facilitate healing rather than produce wounded feelings or bring about angry recriminations. A church, however, should be a place where members do want to be healed, and they should think of their church as a house of healing. If healing is to take place, then the dis-eases that need to be healed must be brought to light. Moreover, Christians must think of dis-eases as illnesses that need healing rather than crimes that need to be punished. Here, then, are some practical mechanisms that may help in this regard.

Annual evaluations of the leadership

Every leader needs to be accountable. Because a pastor serves his or her members, the members have the right and obligation to evaluate the pastor on a periodic basis. A credible and helpful evaluation needs to be carried out against a background of clearly delineated goals, expectations, skills, and characteristics that pastors might reasonably be expected to have. Moreover, not all skills and characteristics are equally important for a given pastor. If someone was hired as a youth minister, then an inability to relate to young people may be fatal to his or her ministry, but the ability to relate well with youth may well be of far less importance for the senior pastor.

Although a congregation may expect its pastor to be a Jack or Jill of all trades, such an expectation is unreasonable. Some seminaries may not offer training in carrying out a stewardship campaign. Someone who is not a skilled musician on entering seminary is unlikely to graduate as a skilled musician. Some ministers are good at preaching and others are good at pastoral visits, but few, if any, ministers are good at everything. A congregation should spell out those areas in which it wants its pastor to be especially skilled and concentrate on those.

The CREDO Program of the Episcopal Church offers priests an opportunity to do an extensive self-review in several areas of their lives, including ministry, spirituality, finances, and health.[1] As part of the preparation for a CREDO eight-day retreat, a priest rates himself in numerous areas and subareas of skills related to his or her ministry. Each area receives not only the priest's estimate of how well she is doing, but also her estimate of the overall importance of that area to her ministry. The priest gives the same evaluation instrument to not fewer than six nor more than ten persons who are to rate the priest in the same way. The evaluators also have the opportunity to make comments that will be shared with the priest.

At the CREDO retreat the priest is given the joint evaluations: her own and the composite of the ratings by others. Thus, a priest can see whether his self-assessment concerning quality and importance in each area is consistent with how others see him in those areas. If there are areas where the priest's and the evaluators' scores as to skill or importance are substantially different, particularly if the priest has an exalted opinion of her skill or an off-base idea of how important an area is to those she works with, then this is a warning to rethink those areas.

The purpose of the CREDO evaluation is not to embarrass priests or to determine whether they ought to be dismissed from their positions. The evaluation provides greater self-understanding and helps the priest see herself as others see her. It provides guidance on those areas considered important that might need improvement and those areas that are relatively unimportant that do not merit a high level of attention. If the comments contain a consistent message—for example, Pastor Sam works too hard and does not look out for his health—then the priest needs to take that message to heart too. Since the priest is the one to choose his evaluators, he might expect the marks to be higher than if evaluators were chosen at random, which is why signs of weakness need to be taken particularly seriously.

I believe the CREDO model is a good model for any church to use in evaluating its clergy. Each church can design its own instrument consistent with its polity, doctrine, and priorities. The minister might also help in designing the instrument, but neutral parties should review the evaluation instrument to make sure that it is not biased toward or against the minister. Rather, it must represent a balanced and reasonable catalog of areas that should be reviewed. Each area is to be graded not only on how well the minister performs in that area, but how important that area actually is in the work of the church.

What has all of this to do with healing? A great deal. The evaluation, if well designed, should detect areas in which healing needs to take place or even areas in which the minister may contribute to dis-ease among the members. Christians are often afraid of criticizing others because they do not want to seem judgmental and do not want to cause hard feelings. We are not to be judgmental, nor are we to hurt another without good cause. But Paul exhorts us to speak the truth in love when it is necessary for the good of the church.

> Then we will no longer be infants, tossed back and forth by the waves, and blown here and there by every wind of teaching and by the cunning and craftiness of men in their deceitful scheming. Instead, speaking the truth in love, we will in all things grow up into him who is the Head, that is, Christ. From him the whole body, joined and held together by every supporting ligament, grows and builds itself up in love, as each part does its work. (Ephesians 4:14-16)

There is no falsehood in God. Even if Christians are in denial, God is not. Any evaluation, whether of clergy or layperson, should never be carried out in a spirit of meanness. Instead, in an attitude of love, it should help bring about spiritual growth in the one being evaluated and help that individual carry out as well as possible the work to which God has called him or her.

It should go without saying that evaluations should commend individuals for their strengths and the work they are doing well to help them build on those strengths and to be encouraged in their work. If a pastor is unwilling to be evaluated, then the lay authorities of the congregation should counsel with the pastor to discover the reasons for his resistance and convince the pastor that an evaluation will benefit both him and the congregation. Perhaps the pastor is uncomfortable with the design of the evaluation instrument or how the evaluation will be conducted. Mutual discussions may find compromises to make the pastor more comfortable with the evaluation instrument and methodology.

"'Come now, let us reason together,' says the LORD" (Isaiah 1:18). Charity, coupled with reason and a loving spirit, can heal many of the dis-eases of a pastor and a congregation. But if healing is to take place, then whatever dis-eases need healing must be brought to light. As noted earlier, dis-eases that are denied or ignored can sometimes prove fatal.

Small groups

People need a safe place to share their stories and to receive positive, nonjudgmental support. In my years as a priest and active spiritual director, I have learned the following:

- When people are given a setting in which they feel safe in telling their stories, what is most important in their lives, their joys and their trials, their deepest spiritual experiences and longing, then surprising and wonderful things can happen. We begin to see that those we thought we knew, we knew only at a superficial level. But by learning more about someone's spiritual struggles and how God is acting in his or her life, we see Christ more clearly in that person and develop bonds in Christ through prayer and mutual encouragement.

- One of the most serious dis-eases a member of a church can suffer from is to feel that he or she is not loved or respected. Tragically, this feeling is often founded in the way the member is treated by the pastor or other members, sometimes because the member is a newcomer in a closed, exclusive congregation or because he or she simply does not look or act like "one of us." It may be that the excluded member is shy and hard to approach, but instead of reaching out to that person in Christ, or to Christ in that person, the congregation finds it easier to just ignore him or her. In situations where I was about to take over a congregation, I found that some of those I was told would be troublemakers were those who had just felt neglected and unloved. Once they were no longer excluded, they became some of the hardest workers and most faithful supporters of the church.

Many church small groups function more at the social than the spiritual level. They are good at providing fellowship and a chance to gather with friends. Sometimes they also provide mutual support. Some seniors groups, for example, form networks of care, and members regularly check on one another to see if someone needs assistance or is having special health problems. Fellowship and the concern of others can affect healing because they demonstrate that others value someone's friendship, care about how someone is doing, and are willing to offer help if needed.

But churches should be more than social clubs and mutual-aid groups. Churches exist because God demonstrated love for us through the Incarnation and the cross. Churches, as I cannot stress strongly enough, need to be places where members are supported, encouraged, and challenged to grow ever more into the life of God through Jesus Christ by the power of the Holy Spirit. They are not to be just clubs to make Christians comfortable until they can collect their eternal rewards. Churches must provide the tools by which members can discern how God is acting in their lives and then be uplifted to respond faithfully to God's action. If such discernment is to take place, there must be opportunities for members to share the deepest longing of their hearts and their personal encounters with God. I believe that this interaction can best take place in small groups.

Small groups can suffer from the same dis-eases as the congregation can, however, and may well be more apt to contract such dis-eases such as exclusivity, elitism, and isolation. They may also wind up opposing the broader church if they become cliques for politicking or personal agendas. Despite the risks, small groups can be an important instrument to aid Christians in spiritual healing. There are books that help structure small groups to help members grow spiritually. See, for example, my book *To Know God: Small Group Experiences in Spiritual Formation*, also published by Judson Press.

Prayer partnering, prayer lists, and prayer teams

Churches should be houses of healing, but they must also be houses of prayer. What is prayer? It is intentionally directing our body, mind, soul, and strength to God in faith, hope, and love. Prayer can take many forms. It can, for example, be verbal, a service activity, or simply "being" there for God in silence. All too often, Christians think of prayer as being only verbal. We are talking to God. But we must also listen for God's response. We must actively serve in ways that we believe God calls us to serve. Sometimes, we must just be silent and enjoy the embrace of God's love.

The customary form of prayer in churches is worship, but outreach in service to the community is also prayer if it is carried out for the love of God. Even though there are activities where the church as a whole prays, there are also steps a church can take to enable its members to support one another in prayer. One common method is prayer lists. Persons seeking prayers for some intention place that intention on a prayer list. Prayer for those intentions, asking God to hear and answer them, occurs during worship, and such prayer may also be lifted up by groups within the church with a special ministry of prayer. Some churches also have e-mail or telephone prayer chains for special prayer needs that are more immediate, such as when someone enters the hospital.

Church members should also pray for one another. One way of bringing about such prayer is to form prayer partnerships, where two members agree to pray for one another on a regular basis. Prayer partners can meet together on a periodic basis to pray for one another in person and to support one another in their walk together. Prayer partnerships can allow members to get to know at least one other member's story and to share their own story as well.

A church can also train healing prayer teams. This is such an important topic that I have devoted a later chapter to a discussion of it.

93

Compassion ministries

There are a church organizations, some denominational and some ecumenical, devoted to the compassion ministry for those who have suffered some special grief or loss, or who are suffering from a serious illness. Beginning Experience, for example, reaches out to those who have lost a spouse through divorce, separation, or death. The Stephen Ministry tries to provide compassionate ears to those who need them. Some churches and denominations have special programs, such as food banks, devoted to feeding the needy. Many churches have assistance funds to help the poor with rent, utilities, and health care. Many denominations have special programs to help the needy on a more global scale such as the American Baptist Churches One Great Hour of Sharing offering or Episcopal Church's Presiding Bishop's Fund for World Relief. I know of at least two churches that helped start medical clinics in their communities to serve the poor and medically underserved. The list of ways in which churches and denominations are trying to bring healing to their communities and the world, and, thus, assist their own spiritual healing through doing the work of Christ, can be extended almost indefinitely. A partial list of such programs is found in appendix B.

Having an organization to help people in times of trouble or stress can be a valuable assistance in healing both for those served and those serving. Knowing that others care and love them in Christ can be a powerful balm for the afflicted.

Nevertheless, members of compassion groups must recognize their limitations. Only licensed professionals are competent to carry out psychotherapy. Group members should be trained sufficiently to recognize potential psychological pathologies as well as to observe appropriate boundaries in any situation they might encounter. They should be able to consult an appropriate professional for advice as needed and have a list of resources to which persons might be referred if that seems warranted.

Although programs that bring together a number of people and resources to minister collectively to one another and the community are valuable instruments of healing, often a one-on-one relationship is important for an individual's spiritual growth. We discuss such relationships in the next chapter.

Note

1. I am familiar with this program because I am an Episcopal priest and been a participant at a CREDO retreat. Perhaps your own denomination has its own program to assist clergy in a constructive evaluation. A well-known ecumenical program is the Centers for Career Development and Ministry. Its offices are in Oakland, California (708-343-6268); Columbus, Ohio (614-442-8822); Kansas City, Kansas (913-621-6348); and Dedham, Massachusetts (781-329-2100).

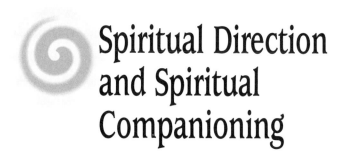

CHAPTER 12

Spiritual Direction and Spiritual Companioning

Soul friends

There is a Celtic tradition of an *anam kara*, a soul friend. A soul friend is someone to whom a Christian can unburden his or her heart and know that the soul friend will respond honestly, compassionately, and in Christian love. At times, the soul friend will simply listen quietly and prayerfully to the Christian. At the heart of the *anam kara* relationship is trust: trust that the soul friend will not reveal to others what the Christian tells her, trust that the soul friend will not be judgmental, trust that the soul friend will pray with and for the Christian.

Having a fellow Christian of deep faith to talk to about our own deepest spiritual experiences and longings, our joys and sorrows, is a great treasure. In such a relationship there is shared prayer and a partnership in faith that helps the Christian better explore how God is acting in his or her life and what God might be asking that person to do. Human to human, Christian to Christian, pilgrims together on the journey.

Having a soul friend is much like belonging to a small spiritual-development group, but it is also quite different as well. In a small group, all participants are equal and all are expected to share their spiritual walk together. In a soul-friend relationship, the soul friend is more a sounding board for the Christian and may share his or her own spiritual experiences as part of the soul-friend relationship. Whereas in a group, the emphasis is on all participants equally, with a soul friend it is the person being companioned who remains the focus, even though two Christians may be soul friends to each other.

Because sharing occurs at such a deep level, the emotional ties can be strong, and therefore, the temptation to turn the soul friend relationship into a more personal one may arise. The same temptation may arise in spiritual direction (discussed below), in a pastoral relationship, or in any relationship, for that matter, where sharing is profoundly personal and emotions run deep.

When I was in a religious community quite a few years ago, we were discouraged from having what were called "particular friendships" for fear that closer relationships with one person would detract from our ability to relate to others in the community and might even lead eventually to immoral behavior. Though, of course, the dangers were there, in my mind, an even greater danger lay in not having someone to confide in and with whom to share the deepest spiritual movements of one's heart. Not being permitted a soul friend could lead to human isolation and a stagnation of spiritual growth.

In all human relationships there are potential dangers of various kinds. Yet, it is usually through and in others that Christ works in us. We must accept the possible dangers and pray not to fall victim to them if we are to enjoy the benefits of having a soul friend.

Spouses, pastors, and prayer partners as soul friends

If someone wants a soul friend, it would seem that the most reasonable candidates would be a spouse, pastor, or prayer partner. Sometimes developing a soul friend relationship with one of these works out, but more often, in my opinion, it does not.

Although a pastor may be spiritually strong and knowledge-able, as well as an excellent teacher, he or she is still an authority figure and therefore is not someone to whom a church member may want to open his or her heart. Moreover, pastors may want to instruct, while a Christian may simply want someone who will listen. A person seeking a spiritual friend may also be afraid that deep sharing with his pastor may cause the pastor to think less of him. For better or worse, a pastor stands in a different relationship to members of a church than members do to one another. The pastor's role as teacher and leader will frequently prevent the pastor from being considered a soul friend.

A prayer partner may or may not make a good soul friend. There are many people with whom I pray but with whom I would be uncomfortable sharing my deepest spiritual experiences. The "chemistry" is simply not there, or I may be afraid that they would not respond to what I might say in a way that I would find help-ful. For example, someone might want to use my sharing with them as an opportunity to pour out his own problems on me. This might enable me to minister to him, which could in itself be a good thing, but he is not then serving as my soul friend.

Even a spouse may not be a suitable soul friend. Such is the case with my own wife. Even though she is my best friend, she is not particularly interested in my spiritual endeavors, and I do not intend to force them on her. It is somewhat rare, in my experience, that a husband and wife can truly serve one another as soul friends as well as mates, but it can and does happen.

Spiritual direction

Spiritual direction is a traditional term for a form of spiritual "companioning." The term, however, is becoming increasingly unpopular with many directors, because a good spiritual director does not direct, that is, tell a directee what he or she must do. Therefore, some directors prefer to call themselves spiritual mentors. I will, nevertheless, continue to use the more traditional term.

A spiritual director works with a directee to help the directee clarify how God is acting in her life and how she might faithfully respond to God's action. Although a spiritual director will pray with and for a directee, the director's role is different from that of a spiritual friend.

A spiritual friend is primarily a sounding board, but may ask questions and offer advice. A spiritual director is expressly expected to ask questions to help the directee discern God's movement in his life and how to respond to that movement. The director may offer advice, such as recommending a prayer technique suited to the directee's temperament or suggesting a book to give the directee more training in an area of interest, but the director leaves decisions to the directee.

In other words, a spiritual director is more than someone who listens in a compassionate manner to what the directee might say. A director tries to draw the directee out, provide specific suggestions concerning prayer or training, and even give the directee assignments to help her make the most of the direction relationship. A director, for example, may ask a directee to write down special insights and experiences as soon as possible after they occur so these instances can be brought to the next session of direction. Or the director may ask the directee to try a particular prayer method and report at the next session on his experience with it.

In spiritual companioning, there is more or less an equality between the participants; little special training or expertise is expected on the part of the soul friend. But in spiritual direction the directee is in a subordinate relationship to the director, even if the director tries to pretend otherwise, and the director is presumed to have special knowledge or experience that goes beyond that expected of a spiritual companion.

Although I do a good deal of spiritual direction and also am a recipient of spiritual direction myself, I always tell a potential directee that the first two sessions are simply getting to know one another and determining if the chemistry of the relationship seems right to both of us. If there does not seem to be a good match, then it is easier to part company without hard feelings if only two sessions have taken place. What I primarily look for in potential directees is a sincere desire to grow spiritually. I am not particularly interested in their theological knowledge or even what denomination they belong to. They must be willing to be open to the power and the promptings of the Holy Spirit—who is the real spiritual director—and I am there as an instrument to try to help them clarify what the Holy Spirit is doing in them.

Just as spiritual companioning has potential pitfalls, one must beware of possible dangers in spiritual direction.

Possible pitfalls in the path of spiritual direction

Lack of an appropriate background to do direction

St. Teresa of Avila, a sixteenth-century Carmelite mystic, one of the greatest teachers of spiritual theology in the west, thought that a spiritual director must have three attributes: 1) common sense, 2) a sound theological background, and 3) experience in the spiritual life. Someone who tries to be a spiritual director who is not herself widely experienced in the spiritual life and has merely read books about spirituality is like someone who tries to pilot an airplane after reading a flight manual. It may work out, but I would not board the aircraft.

Thus, a spiritual director should have adequate training and experience to carry out his or her ministry. But since there is a certain prestige that comes with being a spiritual director and there are no universally recognized credentials to become one, there are some who claim to be spiritual directors who have neither the call nor the background to be directors.

Neither the ministry of spiritual direction, nor spiritual companioning, can be carried out without the special help of the Holy Spirit. Both are calls. Usually, someone discovers a call to spiritual direction because people start coming to him or her and asking the kinds of questions involved in direction. Even being ordained does not necessarily make someone a good spiritual director for some of the same reasons it may prevent a pastor from being a suitable spiritual companion. Some of the best directors I know are laypersons.

But all of the directors I know whom I trust to do direction have either been through a reputable training program or have had other experience, such as a number of years in a religious community. These qualifications provide them with the additional tools a director should have above and beyond those needed by a spiritual companion. Nevertheless, one question someone should ask a potential director is, "What background do you have to do spiritual direction?" If no seemingly satisfactory answer is forthcoming, then the candidate for direction might better look elsewhere.

Unfortunately, even some who can cite credentials for being a director are not necessarily good directors. There are probably hundreds of programs in the United States purporting to train spiritual directors, with more programs seeming to come online every day.[1] Some of these programs run for three years, with most of training taking place in classrooms and coupled with internships in which a student does direction under the supervision of an experienced director. In some of them, most of the work is done at home or online with no supervised practice before the would-be director is turned loose on the world. Because there are no governing boards or widely recognized certification examinations for directors, all any program can provide one of its graduates is a certificate of completion. And even some directors who have been through more rigorous training programs may have flaws that compromise their work as directors.[2]

Inappropriate attitudes toward direction

"If it worked for me, it will work for you." "God speaks to you through me." If a director says anything that sounds like these statements, run in the opposite direction. A director must be flexible because the Holy Spirit treats every individual as, well, an individual. Inflexibility in a director often indicates a lack of adequate training or experience since the director can only imagine one way to spiritual growth.

Likewise, the director who requires a directee to obey his demands is serving his own interests, not those of the directee or of the Spirit. A director is to be an instrument of the Holy Spirit, not *be* the Holy Spirit. A good director leaves all decisions to the directee. This does not mean that a director cannot point the directee toward resources that she thinks might be helpful. A director may also legitimately ask a directee to carry out practices, such as writing down experiences or trying some form of prayer, that are designed to help make the direction sessions more profitable and offer help in the discernment process. But a director cannot, and should not, try to command obedience. On the other hand, if a director believes that the directee is simply ignoring whatever the director says, and therefore gaining little from the relationship, the director might terminate the relationship.

A spiritual director must always respect the appropriate boundaries of spiritual direction. Spiritual direction is not psychotherapy, family counseling, or even pastoral counseling.[3] The purpose of spiritual direction is to help a directee discern how God is acting in that individual's life. Direction can continue indefinitely so long as both director and directee feel comfortable with the relationship. If a director identifies an issue that lies outside of direction, then he or she should refer the directee to an appropriate professional and may even make continuation of direction contingent on the directee's seeking needed help.[4] A director who tries to deal with issues outside his or her competence is inviting trouble.

Because the direction relationship is not one of equality, unlike the relationship in spiritual companioning, directors must be particularly sensitive never to abuse their power. The directee is placing great trust in the director, and that trust must never be abused. If a directee is concerned that the relationship is developing in an unhealthy manner, he or she should terminate it immediately.

Issues for churches related to spiritual direction

A number of churches have added spiritual directors to their staffs or allowed trained volunteers to do spiritual direction under the church's auspices. Inasmuch as there are no recognized certification requirements for spiritual directors, such sponsorship of direction may pose insurance issues. Denominational malpractice insurance may cover only ordained persons, paid staff, or licensed professionals, or the denomination or church might not even have such insurance.

And since direction is such a highly personal experience and demands confidentiality if it is to be successful, spiritual directors cannot report to the pastor concerning their sessions, except in a manner that preserves confidences, which makes it difficult for pastors to oversee the direction taking place in their churches.

Placing spiritual directors on staff, whether paid or volunteer, raises issues that each denomination and church must address according to its particular circumstances. While taking such precautions is always prudent, I personally know of no director who has ever been sued for malpractice. It is difficult to see how a director can be sued for malpractice if there are no standards of practice to begin with. Please note, however, even though a director may not be liable for malpractice as a director, the director, and, hence the sponsoring church, may be liable for boundary violations or attempted practice in an area in which the director is not qualified or licensed.

Notes

1. I provide a partial list of training programs for spiritual directors in appendix B.

2. In better programs, students are evaluated carefully before being admitted to training and are evaluated each year concerning their progress toward becoming competent directors. Likewise, in those programs with internships, the supervisor will try to help the student work out issues that might interfere with being a good director.

3. Pastoral counseling involves helping people resolve moral questions or life issues such as preparation for marriage or deciding whether to study for the ordained ministry. Once the issue in question has been resolved—the person has formed his conscience on the moral issue, the marriage has taken place, or she reached a firm decision concerning a call to the ordained ministry—pastoral counseling on that matter is complete.

Pastoral counseling is not psychotherapy, and it is not spiritual direction. Psychotherapy addresses mental pathologies that are sufficiently serious as to interfere with someone's ability to function normally in society or to enjoy life at a level considered satisfactory by the patient. Once the patient has reached a point where he or she is able to function or live at a level she considers acceptable, the treatment is complete. Psychotherapy may have little or nothing to do with moral issues or religion of any persuasion. Spiritual direction, on the other hand, is an ongoing relationship the purpose of which is to support someone in her spiritual walk. Although a direction relationship may end for any of a number of reasons, our spiritual growth is never complete in this life.

Pastoral counseling can be part of the healing process by helping Christians resolve questions that they find troubling in ways that bring them greater assurance and peace. It can also help them reach important life decisions and prepare them for various new roles.

4. An important component of respectable training in spiritual direction is clarifying the limits of direction and helping the student recognize conditions that require the intervention of a qualified professional. A director should have a list of professionals to whom he or she can refer.

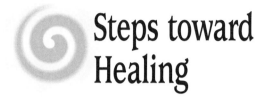 Steps toward
Healing

In previous chapters we looked at some of the issues that potentially hinder healing—individual healing as well as congregational healing. In this chapter I address some of the means by which those issues might be resolved.

Education concerning, and commitment to, the importance of healing

As already noted, unless the senior pastor is committed to the healing ministry, there is little chance it will take root in a congregation even if the lay leadership would like to see it happen. And even after a pastor is convinced that his or her church must become a house of healing, much work still needs to take place.

First, the pastor must have a clear rationale why the healing ministry is foundational to what a church does and be able to articulate that rationale to both the lay leadership and the congregation. The pastor must recognize and be able to get others to recognize that healing is more than a physical cure or "being saved." Christian healing involves a *continuing* transformation of lives through Jesus Christ by the power of the Holy Spirit as God draws people deeper and deeper into God's own life. People are dying to self by the power of God so that Christ can live in them.

This is a powerful message and one that some people do not want to hear. It threatens their control over their lives, and they sense that if they take their healing seriously, God may make demands on them that they may not want to obey. But if the church is unwilling to challenge Christians to grow into spiritual maturity, then who will? It may well be that churches' unwillingness to challenge their members has resulted in loss of those who found that they are not being spiritually fed. They unwittingly might have caused some Christians to seek spiritual healing and growth in non-Christian religions and New Age spiritual practices that demand more of them.

Once the pastor is convinced, the lay leadership must be educated, or, if the church is small, then the congregation can be educated as a whole. Before I instituted the laying on of hands and anointing for healing as part of our first Sunday services at my local church, I gave a series of sermons setting out the theology of healing. In these sermons I tried to give the congregation a sense of the meaning and importance of the healing service. Bringing the lay leadership and the congregation to recognize the importance of healing can proceed rapidly or slowly, depending on how well disposed everyone is already to the ministry of healing.

Once the ordained and lay leadership and the congregation have become convinced of the importance of healing, then the ministry of healing must be incorporated into the church's mission statement so that the church's programs, worship, and teaching are evaluated, at least in part, according to how well they serve to make the church a house of healing.[1]

In sum, education and commitment concerning healing are essential to a church's becoming a house of healing. This education and commitment must be embraced by the ordained and lay leadership if it is to succeed. The church's denomination might also produce educational and training materials to assist a congregation in developing its ministry of spiritual healing.

Even if a church is convinced it wants to be a house of healing, issues might arise (discussed in earlier chapters) that hinder a church from fulfilling its healing mission. We now revisit these potential obstacles and suggest ways to address them.

Overcoming congregational obstacles to the healing ministry

Three particular obstacles to a congregation's healing ministry were noted in chapter 10. The first step in removing an obstacle is to recognize that it exists. Thus, removing an obstacle involves acknowledging its presence and then identifying what needs to be done to get rid of it.

Addressing exclusivity

Have you ever visited a new church and surveyed those present? Does it seem that everyone present is from the same social class or economic level? The great majority of churches of any denomination that I have visited have consisted of people sharing similar characteristics.

It is a stereotype, but not without foundation, that the Episcopal Church is one of the most white, most educated, and most affluent in any community. Even my largely blue-collar, working-class parish was considered to be the "rich church" by many of my minister colleagues, even though most of them had some members who had substantially more money than any of mine did.

Examine your own congregation with an open mind. Are there certain types of people you assume would not want to come to your church? If so, your church may be unintentionally exclusive. How can a church be less exclusive? First, go out of your way to invite some of these people you think would not fit in to visit.

Second, the church might require further education. Are there members of your church who resent someone from another ethnic or racial background attending services? Preach that Christ came for all human beings and that all should be welcome in any house of God, particularly a church that intends to be a house of healing. What might need healing more than stereotyping and prejudice?

Other steps to heal exclusivity

Most congregations, I believe, do not start out trying to be exclusive. Members invite their friends, who are generally like themselves. A particular style of service develops that appeals to those who attend but that may not be appealing to visitors looking for a church. Visitors are expected to accommodate themselves to what the existing congregation wants; after all, a church cannot offer a service that appeals to everyone, and those who actually come to services are those whose preferences have to be considered first. If visitors find the service pleasing, we will welcome them, but, if not, they would probably be happier at a church where they find the service more to their liking. This argument seems compelling, but there are still steps that a church can take to reach out to those who are not "like us."

Because a visitor is likely to be confused by the service if he is not already familiar with a church's or denomination's style of worship, someone from the congregation might sit with the visitor to help guide him through the service, for example, showing him what books are being used and where hymns are found. The church might also provide every visitor with a flyer or pamphlet containing a brief explanation of their service.

A member should invite the visitor to the social hour following the service, introduce her to others, and offer to answer any questions she might have about the church or the service. And, of course, also invite the visitor to return. A follow-up phone call or short visit by a lay member of the church (research shows that visitors are more favorably impressed when lay persons follow up than when the clergy do so) may also help to prove that the church is genuinely interested in the visitor. A church member could even offer to give the visitor a ride to church the following Sunday or take the visitor—and family, of course—out to lunch after the service.

Addressing inflexibility

The old cliché tells us that the seven last words of a church are, "But we've always done it this way." Often there are good reasons to do something a certain way. Change for change's sake is not a solution to any problem. And just as there must be reasons for keeping something unchanged that are understood and can be articulated, so too a proposed change should have a compelling rationale to give to those who might oppose the change. A change can even be introduced as an experiment that will be evaluated after a certain length of time, usually two or three months, to see if it is making a positive difference.

If someone has a proposal for a change, the leadership should always listen respectfully with an open mind. Whatever decision the leadership reaches, it needs to be defensible and explained to those affected by it. Each year, the congregation should evaluate its strengths and weaknesses and seek positive changes to make itself more effective, particularly as a house of healing.

Generally, the worship, programs, and decisions of the congregation should be judged against their stated mission statement, goals, and objectives. If some proposal or program does not contribute to implementing the church's priorities, then it should be pruned. Too often a church will institute a program simply because someone is interested in it and willing to do it. Unless the implementation, however, is in accord with the way the church defines itself, then the church may end up with set of programs with little coherent theme and no clear direction.

Here are some short rules that should help a church avoid inflexibility.

- If the rationale for a practice cannot be clearly explained to someone unfamiliar with the church in terms that a reasonable person would accept, that practice probably should be eliminated or changed in favor of a practice that can be so explained.

- If a practice is not consonant with the church's mission, goals, or objectives, or worse, draws resources away from them, then it probably should be discontinued.

- At least every year or two, a church should do an open-minded examination of its mission, goals, and objectives to see if they are still relevant and if the church is acting in accordance with them.

- If someone who *is* seeking a church does not choose to join your congregation, then rather than simply letting that visitor go, make a call or send a letter to ask why he or she chose another church. The reason may be simply that the visitor wanted a Baptist service and your church was Episcopal, but the individual may also have insights that might lead to changes in the way the church deals with visitors.

Addressing control issues of the congregation

I have encountered a number of churches where newer members are simply not considered for a position of leadership until they have "paid their dues." I even heard of one church near a prestigious university that allegedly would not elect anyone to their leadership board unless that person had at least one doctorate. In some churches, members of the lay board are elected but the elections are tightly controlled and only the "right" people are candidates. And in other churches, essentially no checks and balances are put in place against absolute control by the minister. None of these are healthy situations because they exclude from leadership those who might be fine leaders and bring new ideas, and these members might ultimately leave the church in frustration.

One might reasonably expect that someone must have some level of knowledge about a church and its polity before he or she can become a leader there. Even when a church does make needed changes, it generally must do so in a fashion that is transparent, is in accordance with the polity of the denomination, and invites participation from all members. But newer members must be trained for leadership, not merely left to languish until their time has come. They need to be given some responsibilities as soon as possible to tie them more closely to the church and to enhance their learning process. If someone feels no ownership in an organization, his or her participation and continued membership is at best doubtful.

Members should be helped to recognize their spiritual gifts and given opportunities and encouragement to exercise them. Constructive mentoring by a more experienced and senior member may also assist the new member to take more and more responsibility and grow into senior leadership. Persons offering to start and lead programs that are consonant with the mission, goals, and objectives should be allowed to do so whenever possible.

Control issues can be addressed by considering everyone, new and old, a potential leader whose opinions are heard and respected, even when they are not implemented.

Addressing control issues of the pastor

Pastors, of course, can also have control issues. All pastors must recognize that they are servants of God, not replacements for God. And as servants of God, they serve the people of God. Though they are responsible for leadership, it is servant leadership that supports and challenges church members to grow spiritually.

A good reality check on the pastor's effectiveness, including the manner in which he or she exercises authority, is the evaluation process described in chapter 11. If a pastor is unwilling to be evaluated by, or consider advice from, the members of the congregation with an open mind and heart, then denominational intervention may be needed to mediate the situation, and, in all probability, remove the pastor. Although this is a measure of last resort, a denomination, and the pastor, must recognize that the church exists to carry out the work of Christ and to assist its members in their spiritual healing. If the pastor is an impediment to spiritual healing and will not reform, then he or she must be removed for the good of the church. How denominations deal with problem pastors and with problem congregations is, of course, a matter of denominational polity.

Note

1. Some training programs for the healing ministry are referenced in appendix B.

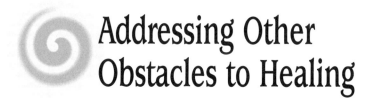

CHAPTER 14

Addressing Other Obstacles to Healing

In chapter 6 we pointed out some hindrances to healing that apply primarily to individuals. We revisit each of these now and suggest means to address these hindrances.

Addressing not wanting to be healed

A church must teach the value of spiritual healing. Yes, true healing involves sacrifices and giving up control of one's life to God, and this message is definitely threatening to many Christians who are quite satisfied just to have been saved. No one can be forced to cooperate with the Holy Spirit. To help someone overcome the attraction of secondary gain, the alternative—healing—must be made even more appealing than the benefits that come from remaining ill. This is largely a matter of education, prayer, and modeling the benefits of spiritual health. A spiritually sick person (and we are all spiritually sick to a greater or lesser degree) must come to see that spiritual healing will bring authentic peace rather than the false "safety" of the status quo.

But to know God is the one thing that can keep us happy for all eternity. To know and love God as fully as we can, we must become as much like God as we can through Jesus Christ by the power of the Holy Spirit. Ultimately, we must either belong totally to God, loving God with the totality of our being, or decide to be our own gods and separate ourselves from God. That is, we must choose to go to hell. God does not send people to hell. Rather, they choose to embrace a false idea of freedom by refusing to yield themselves entirely to God.

But one cannot be persuaded to love for fear of hell. Indeed, to many, the idea of maintaining control of their existence without having to yield control to God may seem attractive. Yet we are finite creatures, so no matter what pleasures we may gain from satisfying our every personal desire will eventually lead to disillusionment and pain. It is only in knowing the Truth that true freedom is found. "You shall know the truth and the truth shall set you free" (John 8:32). Healing is growing into the Truth that is God alone.

It is ironic that anyone would choose partial truth or partial goodness or partial beauty, not recognizing that they thereby pass up the fullness of Truth and Goodness and Beauty of which the partial objects are but a pale reflection. True healing involves a passionate desire to have the fullness of Truth, Love, Beauty, and Goodness, all of which is found in God alone. How odd that people would choose the counterfeit coin over genuine gold. Churches must challenge their members to choose the genuine, not the counterfeit.

Addressing an inability to forgive

What does it mean to forgive? Perhaps the clearest sign that we have forgiven someone is our no longer wanting to see the offending party suffer any harm for what he or she has done; that is, we have no desire to seek vengeance for the wrong done to us. This does not mean that we do not remember the wrong, since memories, as well as the emotions we feel on remembering the wrong, are often outside of our control. I might understandably experience fear, anger, and resentment toward someone who has robbed

113

and beaten me. But I can choose to pray that God will turn the robber's heart and lead him to repentance and a better life, or I can choose to pray that God will strike the robber with some dread disease in repayment for the pain he has caused me. I may still cooperate with the state in identifying, arresting, prosecuting, and imprisoning the robber. But I do so, not to extract vengeance, but to protect others whom the robber might harm in the future and in the hopes that the robber might be rehabilitated and become a law-abiding and productive citizen.

I have often observed difficulties in forgiving, primarily in my work in Beginning Experience, where a woman who had been abandoned by her husband, often for another woman, found it difficult to forgive what the ex-spouse had done to her. The feeling of loss, betrayal, humiliation, loneliness, and fear of the future were such that we might not expect that she would forgive someone who had wounded her so grievously. And, yet, this is what Christ expects of us. Even more, it is what must happen before real healing can take place. So long as the desire for revenge rages inside someone, it is a cancer that eats at the soul and is a serious obstacle to healing.

In addition to teaching the need to forgive others so we ourselves can be healed, we who have been wounded should be encouraged to pray for that person who wounded us. In keeping with Jesus' injunction to forgive as we have been forgiven, we can ask God to cause that wounder to see the pain caused by his or her actions and be led to repent. The prayer can include requests that God give peace both to we who are injured and to those who have caused the injuries. I genuinely believe that if we can sustain this prayer for at least two weeks, we will find peace and will also have shown that we have truly forgiven the one who hurt us.

Addressing sin

Sin is more than deliberate disobedience of what we believe God wants of us. Sin is any obstacle that interferes with God's working in us. In this general sense, we may not even be aware of many of our sins, our hindrances to God's transforming power. But God is aware of these hidden sins and can work to remove them if we are open to God's doing so. The removal of obstacles to full healing is forgiveness of sin in its broadest and deepest sense.

Consider the paralytic whose friends lowered him through the roof of the house because they could not reach Jesus through the large crowd that surrounded him. Once the man was placed at Jesus' feet, Jesus told him, "Take heart, son; your sins are forgiven" (Matthew 9:2). When the Pharisees present criticized Jesus for presuming to forgive sins, Jesus asked them if it was easier to forgive sins or to cure the man of his paralysis. The implication was that it was harder to forgive sins—to heal someone spiritually—than to heal someone physically. It is more difficult to remove the obstacles to God's grace working in us than it is to cure our bodily ills. Yet Jesus was able to forgive the paralytic's sins and to prove his power to forgive sins by then healing the man of his paralysis.

Jesus can and will forgive sin if we want to be forgiven. Jesus will remove the obstacles that stand between us and a more complete love of God if we will allow him to do so. But we must recognize our need for spiritual healing and want to be healed spiritually. We must accept the fact that there are barriers between us and a deeper life in God that only God can remove.

The study of the Seven Deadly Sins as outlined at the end of chapter 7 might help make church members more aware of the most basic sins and how these can enter their lives in subtle ways. Beyond greater sensitivity to the basic sins and self-examination to determine how these sins are influencing our relationship with God, there must be repentance, a genuine desire to change and, with God's help, drive these sins from our lives. Members can then be assured of forgiveness once they have repented. They must also be taught, as Jesus taught, that even if someone relapses into sin, God will forgive again and again so long as the sinner repents again and again.

Once someone has confronted the most basic sins, then he or she must move on to more subtle occasions of sin. Such sins, or obstacles, can include such things as preferring the feelings we obtain from prayer to the object of our prayer (making prayer an end in itself rather than a means to open ourselves to God) or an unwillingness to forgive someone we think has wronged us. Perhaps only God is aware of what sins still have to be forgiven so that we can belong completely to God. But our minds and hearts must be open to cooperating with the power of God in removing those sins. We might pray regularly as follows:

> Lord, I want more than anything else to love you with all my heart and soul and strength. Only you can purify my love to make me yours alone. Do whatever is necessary to make me totally yours. I offer you my life, my mind, my will, all that I have and am for you to do with as you will in your immeasurable love for me and your desire to make me what you would have me become. Remove all obstacles between me and you that I may be yours completely now and forever. Amen.

I am certain God will honor our desire and continue to draw us ever more deeply into his own divine life, even if we do not sense the progress God is making.

Addressing indifference

It is the role of a church not merely to provide support in healing but to challenge its members toward healing. Without appropriate teachings and examples, most members will not understand what spiritual healing consists of and will, therefore, not be much interested in it. Indeed, surveys seems to reveal that, although the vast majority of US citizens consider themselves to be Christians, they are remarkably uninformed about the content of Christianity—many cannot name even one of the four gospels. Moreover, many, if not most, of those who claim the name of Christian believe that Christianity primarily involves leading a moral life.

But if Christianity is nothing more than being good, following the Golden Rule, and keeping the Ten Commandments, then it is has little to do with Jesus Christ and the Holy Spirit. In such a view there is no need for Christ and the Holy Spirit at all. This is, of course, totally inconsistent with traditional Christianity where Jesus is the Way, the Life, and the Truth and the Holy Spirit provides Christians with many gifts to aid in their sanctification. If the moral life is the sum and substance of Christianity, then spiritual healing is nothing more than becoming more moral, not becoming more holy or growing ever more deeply into the life of God.

Thus, it is imperative that churches have sound teaching on spiritual healing and not lapse into letting members think that healing consists in feeling good, becoming wealthy, achieving one's earthly desires, or just leading a good life. Pastors may question how many members truly want to hear this message or will accept it, but that does not make it less true. Christianity must not water down its exciting and critically important message just to allow people to follow their own inclinations under the guise of leading a Christian life.

But teaching about genuine spiritual healing will not be effective unless the church supports its members in seeking true spiritual healing. To tell members what their goal is and not provide aids to achieve that goal is worse than useless. Members will see what they want and seek it elsewhere if they see that their church is not helping them get it. In earlier chapters I have suggested various aids that a church can implement to assist members toward spiritual healing.

Assistance from healing services and rituals

Ritual is a fundamental, perhaps a defining, element of religion. If healing is to take place in a church, then the rituals of that church must incorporate healing. As I described in chapter 1, one church I pastored incorporated laying on of hands and anointing for healing in their services on the first Sunday of each month. Thus, members were reminded of the healing function of the church on a continuing basis.

Some churches have healing prayer teams. Such teams are discussed in the next chapter. Rituals, however, need to be explained in order to have their greatest effect, which means that teaching about healing and the structure of the healing ritual generally must precede the use of the ritual. Some denominations propose a form for a healing service. The Episcopal Church includes a public service of healing in its *Book of Occasional Services*. I include a sample healing service in appendix A. Any church might design its own service in keeping with its polity and doctrine. The greater the involvement of members in designing the service, the more likely will be both understanding and participation once the service is implemented.

If a church is using small groups, then time for healing prayer can be incorporated into the group meetings, or each group could discuss and design a ritual for healing that it might employ periodically. Some churches have organizations devoted to promoting the healing ministry, the international Order of St. Luke the Physician being perhaps the foremost.

I personally believe that the laying on of hands and anointing should be central to a healing service since these actions are scripturally sound and have been practiced since ancient times. They also provide a personal contact for those conducting the ritual. Touch can be healing. Be aware, though, of the cautions set out in the chapter on healing prayer teams. If someone does not want to be touched, his or her wishes must be respected. All touching, obviously, must be done respectfully and appropriately without invading a person's boundaries.

In addition to rituals that deal directly with healing, there are rituals that deal less directly with healing. A rite of reconciliation wherein someone is assured of God's forgiveness of sins, a bereavement service to help someone come to closure with a loss, or simply lending a compassionate ear to someone suffering depression or going through a crisis can be deeply healing. I include sample rituals of reconciliation in appendix A.

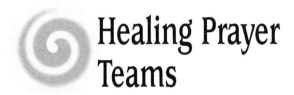

CHAPTER 15

Healing Prayer Teams

A substantial number of churches with which I am familiar have healing prayer teams. Some teams function during Sunday services, some after services, and some during the week in connection with, or apart from, a formal service. For example, part of each meeting of a chapter of the Order of St. Luke the Physician, an ecumenical organization dedicated to the Christian healing ministry, is devoted to praying for those requesting prayers for healing.

Members of both the Order of St. Luke and the Order of the Daughters of the King (a devotional community of women in the liturgical tradition) create lists of prayer intentions, primarily for healing, for which they pray on a regular basis.

There are, of course, other organized forms that healing prayers can take, including those offered by television evangelists, by hospital chaplains, and lay persons doing sick calls, but we will focus in this chapter on healing prayer teams.

My experience at St. Paul's revisited

At St. Paul's Episcopal Church in Freeport, Texas, where I pastored for sixteen years, we incorporated the laying on of hands and anointing for healing in both services on the first Sunday of each month. When I first initiated this practice, only a year or two after I arrived at St. Paul's, I gave a series of teaching sermons on healing and then told the congregation that we would incorporate the laying on of hands and anointing on a trial basis. I stressed that no one should feel any embarrassment at not coming forward. But the first time we offered the rite of healing, almost everyone came forward.

I expected that fewer people would come up after the novelty wore off, but almost everyone continued to come forward on each first Sunday. There were no dramatic physical healings—although I was told that some physical healings occurred—but I think that members kept coming forward again and again because they craved spiritual healing and they sensed the power of the Holy Spirit in this sacrament. Indeed, the presence of the Holy Spirit was often almost palpable. Although I was previously devoted to the healing ministry, the experience at St. Paul's convinced me anew of the deep desire Christians have for spiritual wholeness and their faith that God will heal if we allow God to do so.

Most experiences with healing rituals or the use of prayer teams are positive and uplifting for those who participate, but prayer teams must also be carefully trained and be accountable to the pastor in their ministries because the exercise of this ministry does have potential pitfalls.

Potential pitfalls for prayer teams

Healing prayer teams, like medical doctors, should adhere to the sound Hippocratic dictum, "First, do no harm." How can I suggest that a team's prayers can do harm? Are prayers ever harmful?

Prayers, as such, are not harmful any more than a knife is harmful in itself. But the knife can be used to good or bad effect, and the manner in which a prayer team approaches its work can also have a good or bad effect. If a team accuses a petitioner of sinful behavior or blames him or her for a failure to be healed, the petitioner will go away feeling even worse than before and may wind up leaving the church. It is not the prayer team's role to accuse or judge. Nor is the session with the prayer team an opportunity for confession as with a priest in a confessional. In almost all denominations, there are opportunities for some form of confession and absolution, but a session with a healing prayer team should not be one of them.

Those who come forward for prayers for healing are often vulnerable as well. Some seek healing prayers only in fear and desperation, perhaps as a last resort after private prayer and medical science have failed to bring relief. One prayer team member related that someone had presented himself to the prayer team trembling in fear and embarrassment, someone who was vulnerable indeed. Those who are vulnerable, particularly those who are suffering, are in need of protection and especially sensitive treatment. First, the healing prayer team must not harm such persons.

In the remainder of this chapter we will first consider boundary issues, which may be physical or psychological, then theological issues related to healing prayers, and finally, miscellaneous other issues related to this topic.

Boundary issues

Almost all pastors are aware that boundary issues are one of their most important considerations in dealing with others. Every human being sets boundaries around himself or herself. We set boundaries, for example, concerning how close another person can come to us without making us uncomfortable. Such boundaries are often cultural. Someone from a culture with a high population density may feel perfectly fine if someone talks to him inches from his face, but others may be uneasy if someone is less than two feet away.

And not all boundaries are physical. Almost everyone has some secret about himself or herself that he or she does not want others to know. Thus, someone who tries to pry the secret out is encroaching too closely on a psychological boundary rather than a physical one. Whether the boundaries are physical or psychological, boundaries must be respected by anyone engaged in healing prayer.

Physical boundaries

Some people like to be hugged; others find being hugged by any-one but a close friend or relative to be unduly intrusive. Even those who are willing to be hugged as a sign of Christian affection would take offense at contact that was inordinately familiar or protracted. "Yes, of course," you might counter, "but the people at my church have more sense than that. They would not engage in conduct that someone could take to be too forward."

Perhaps. But different people have different boundaries. Some want to be hugged. Others do not even want to be touched. The danger may be particularly subtle in healing prayer since someone from the prayer team may wish to place his or her hand on the part of the body that needs healing. So how does one discern what is appropriate? One asks.

Sometimes the person seeking prayers may be well known to the prayer team, and they are aware that holding hands or plac-ing hands on the head will not cause offense. Nonetheless, if there is any doubt whatsoever, perhaps hesitancy evidenced by the body language of the petitioner, a member of the team should ask, "Do you mind if we hold hands," or "Do you mind if I place my hands on your head?" Particular caution should be exercised if a portion of the body other than hand or head is to be touched.

The sensitivity associated with touching suggests that a prayer team should consist of at least two individuals, preferably includ-ing both a man and a woman. If the petitioner seems uncomfort-able with being touched, then the team members can simply extend their hands over the petitioner without actual contact. The effectiveness of prayer does not depend on touching or even, nec-essarily, physical proximity. If the petitioner chooses not to be touched, then he or she should not be made to feel uncomfortable or that he or she is are thereby showing less faith. Even if the team believes that the petitioner's physical boundaries are unreasonably restrictive, they must still be respected.

Too large a prayer team may also be intimidating to a peti-tioner. Two or three members is adequate.

Psychological boundaries

The psychological boundaries of a petitioner may be less obvious than physical boundaries, but they exist, and they are just as important as, if not more important than, physical boundaries. Moreover, whereas physical boundaries deal primarily with some form of physical contact, psychological boundaries come in several varieties.

Many people are unwilling to reveal a great deal about their problems. The common social convention in responding to the question "How are you?" is to say "Fine" or "Good," even if life is neither fine nor good. The implicit assumption is that the person asking the question is just being polite and has no real interest in hearing a litany of complaints. But also, the respondent may not want the questioner to know all that is going wrong in his or her life.

We may assume that members of prayer teams want to know why the petitioner is coming to them so that their prayer may be more specifically directed. But the petitioner may not want to reveal his problem for reasons good or bad and may not even be sure what the problem is other than feeling apprehension or discomfort. Prayer teams must allow petitioners this privacy. Thus, a member of the team may ask, "Is there something specific for which you want us to pray, or would you like general prayers for healing?" The team must not interrogate the petitioner concerning why he or she is coming to them. God knows why the petitioner is seeking prayers, and the prayer team does not need to know in order to ask God's healing.

Example 1 (inappropriate questioning):

Team Member: Is there anything specific you would like us to pray for?
Petitioner: No, I just feel the need for someone to pray for me.
Team Member: We prefer to pray for some specific intention. Prayer works better that way.
Petitioner: I would prefer you just pray for me without having to say more.

Team Member: You shouldn't be embarrassed to tell us what is wrong. After all, God knows all about you.

Example 2 (appropriate questioning):

Team Member: Is there anything specific you would like us to pray for?
Petitioner: No, I just feel the need for someone to pray for me.
Team Member: That's fine. We will ask God to heal you in whatever way God knows you need to be healed.

As noted earlier, prayer teams must not be accusatory or judgmental, blaming the petitioner for her illness or for harboring some secret sin that prevents a cure. The fact that the petitioner is coming forward for prayer is itself a sign of faith that should be respected and honored. Judgmental attitudes and blaming the victim are serious violations of psychological boundaries.

Petitioners also have every right to expect that whatever they do say to the prayer team, or even that they came forward for prayers, will be held in confidence not to be revealed to anyone without their express permission. If someone tells the team something that the pastor should know, such as that he or she is entering the hospital for a serious operation, the team might ask if it is all right to tell the pastor.

There are situations in which either the law or the urgency of the matter require that some revelation be reported, such as when someone is having suicidal thoughts or confesses to abusing a child. Fortunately, such incidents are exceedingly rare, but when they do occur, they raise serious questions of balancing privacy against the need to protect the petitioner or others as well as complying with the law. Prayer teams are not subject to the shield of the confessional, nor do they generally have the immunity that pastors do from having to testify in court. There are no easy answers in such matters; but even though a prayer team might never encounter the issue, they must still know how they will react if they do. If it appears that a petitioner is about to use the session with the team to confess sinful behavior, I strongly recommend that he or she should be told immediately and expressly that confessional issues should be taken to the pastor.

Because prayer teams often operate in the open in full view of the congregation, thought should be given to allowing petitioners to come to the team in private. Some people are embarrassed to seek healing prayer openly since it will lead others to ask what is wrong with them, or they may just not want to be seen having others pray for them. This does not represent a lack of faith; it is just another psychological boundary that, rational or irrational, must be taken into account when doing healing ministry.

In my view, after the team has prayed for a petitioner, they should not interrogate the petitioner about whether he has been healed or whether she feels better following the prayer. Neither should they continue to press on with their prayer until something tangible or obvious happens.

Example 3 (inappropriate questioning):

Team Member: Has something happened yet?

Petitioner: Not yet. Maybe we could stop now.

Team Member: No, we can't stop. God will think we don't have enough faith to keep trying. When we keep praying long enough something always happens.

The team member may be correct in saying that something eventually happens. After a petitioner is worn down, he or she will say almost anything to get away from the prayer team, even telling the team that he or she feels much better though it is a lie.

Example 4 (appropriate questioning):

Team Member: Do you feel any better now?

Petitioner: Not yet. Maybe we could stop now.

Team Member: All right. Sometimes healing takes place in God's good time, not ours. We will keep you in our prayers, and God bless you.

Here are some other issues related to healing prayer teams.

Theological issues

Before a team prays for petitioners, it should have a theologically sound view of what healing involves, how God answers prayers, and how God acts in the lives of individuals. Earlier, I spoke about what true healing means to me. The deepest healing, as I have tried to make clear before, is being made whole in God, becoming united to God in Christ through the power of the Holy Spirit as fully as any creature can be united to God. Eternal life is not found in physical health or wealth but in spiritual health. Our treasure should be in heaven, as Jesus himself told us (see Luke 12:33-34).

Because God loves us and is wiser than any of, or all of, us, God knows better than we what we need to become whole in God. And because God loves us "more than all we can ask or imagine" (Ephesians 3:20), God is constantly acting in our lives to bring us to wholeness whether we are aware of that action or not. Prayer teams are instruments of God's love whereby the love and mercy of God should shine forth to those who feel a need for healing. The experience with the prayer team should bring reassurance that God is present even at times when it seems that God has completely abandoned us.

When I served as spiritual advisor for our diocesan Episcopal Beginning Experience team, we also incorporated the laying on of hands and anointing as part of our weekends. This practice, along with the Rite of Reconciliation, seemed to bring immense comfort to many participants. Many of them had come to the weekend grieving deeply over the loss of a spouse but found a deep source of healing and restored peace through the ministry of the team and the healing rituals we offered. Although the team did not call itself a healing prayer team, that is what it was, as are many of the teams involved in compassion ministries.

Forms of prayer for healing to avoid

There are two forms of prayer that I believe should never be employed by prayer teams.

Healing as an exorcism

My own experience, and, more important, that of many spiritual directors and persons I trust involved in the healing ministry, is that true diabolical possession is extremely rare. Diabolical obsessions are less rare, but still should not be assumed to be the primary source of a petitioner's dis-ease.

Although accounts of demons taking control of a person's body occur in the New Testament, and Jesus himself was tempted by Satan, most of our "demons" are part of our own human makeup. Physical and mental illnesses, addictions, and other problems found all too often in members of the human family almost always have natural causes such as bacteria and biochemistry and are not brought on by evil spirits. Consequently, to "demonize" all dis-ease and treat healing prayer as an exorcism is psychologically offensive to many Christians as well as being poorly grounded in both science and theology.

Example 5 (inappropriate prayer):

Team Member: God, drive out now from Nancy the demon of cancer. Satan, you have allowed the evil spirit cancer to enter into Nancy. In Jesus' name we now cast out this demon. Go, cancer, into the eternal darkness from whence you came. Go out now and do not enter this woman again. In Jesus' name we pray, Amen.

Yes, there are people who pray for healing this way, and, if you are one of them, you are no doubt offended by what I've said. But consider the harm that can come from such a prayer. First, it tells the petitioner that she has been possessed by an evil spirit rather than having a well-defined medical illness. This, in turn, implies that she has been guilty of some sin that has allowed a demon to enter her. And if the prayer of exorcism fails and the cancer remains, it further implies that God is unwilling or unable to cast out the demon of cancer, so she must be giving it a willing home.

Name it and claim it

A form of prayer I find almost as theologically offensive as exorcisms for healing is what is often called "name it and claim it." Here is an example of such prayer.

Example 6 (inappropriate prayer):

Team Member: Lord, you have promised to give us whatever we ask for in your name. So now we thank you that, because we asked for it, you have cured Nancy of her cancer. Yes, Lord, thank you that Nancy's cancer has vanished. You have taken it away. Nancy, go to your doctor and tell her that the Lord has healed you. The Lord has given you healing just as you asked for.

Some may object that to pray otherwise than thanking God for what God has already given us is to doubt that God will answer our prayer. Yet to assume that God must answer any request we make—even a request agreed on by several Christians—is to make God our servant, a magical genie who must grant our wishes when we rub our Aladdin's lamp of prayer in the correct manner. In an extreme example of this magical thinking, a woman once told me that if she prayed in faith for the death of her enemies, God would kill them—hardly a thought in keeping with Jesus' message of forgiveness.

Moreover, if God does not grant the desired favor, then who is to blame? We cannot blame God without the risk of sounding blasphemous, so we must blame the petitioner. He is unwilling to accept the gift that God wants to give, or is guilty of some sin that stands in God's way. Neither view is likely to prove helpful to the petitioner, even if these views absolve the team members from responsibility for the "failure."

Prayer, however, is never a failure. I have taught, and will continue to teach, that continued prayer for healing will bring healing, though not necessarily in the manner in which we expect. Is it a greater miracle that a woman dying of cancer and in great pain and fear be cured of the cancer or that she find peace knowing with certainty that she is surrounded by God's love and is safe in God's hands? Those who doubt the efficacy of healing prayer will say that the former is more a sign of God's power than the latter, and that the latter is merely a cop-out to try to excuse God's failure to effect a cure. But we are all going to die sometime. Even the most devout and consistent prayer does not change this reality. Shall we pray then that we live forever on earth, and would this be a Christian prayer? Is not the goal of our lives in Christ to live forever in God, to see God face to face and know God as God knows us? Life in God is a greater miracle and favor than anything earthly that God can grant us. And yet if the woman with cancer were given the choice between a physical cure and a spiritual healing, which would she choose? Which would you choose?

Still other issues

Gifts of the Spirit

Yet another potentially controversial issue is "gifts of the Spirit." The number of such gifts is an oft-debated question, but certainly among the gifts mentioned in the letters of Paul are faith, healing, speaking in tongues, interpretation of tongues, and prophecy (1 Corinthians 12:7-11). An essential characteristic of the gifts of the Spirit is that they are not given arbitrarily, nor does anyone have a right to claim a gift. Even if someone receives a gift of the Spirit, it is not a sign of personal holiness. For the gifts are given solely at the discretion of the Holy Spirit (1 Corinthians 12:11). Such gifts as are given are given for the common good, not the personal welfare of the one to whom they are given (1 Corinthians 12:7). Thus, a gift of the Spirit is given to a particular person at a particular time and place for a particular purpose, a purpose related to building up the body of Christ at that time and place.

But all Christians are supposed to have faith, and all Christians should be engaged in the work of healing. How are the gifts of faith and healing different from "ordinary" faith and a desire for healing for oneself and for others? Given the nature of a gift, a particular Christian may receive certainty from the Spirit to trust the Lord in a particular venture for the welfare of the church (gift of faith), or a Christian may receive a special call to be God's instrument in effecting a special healing (gift of healing).

How do we know whether someone has received a gift? By their fruits you will know them. Gifts of the Spirit bear good fruit and help build up the Body. Nevertheless, even if someone believes he or she has received a special gift of the Spirit, it is still wise to ask the Lord's protection from error and to seek discernment from trusted devout friends and advisers.

Likewise, if a team member believes he has received a "word from the Lord" (prophecy) about the petitioner, I advise that he keep it to himself until discernment of its authenticity can be conducted. This latter point can be strongly disputed since the Lord may want the petitioner to hear the prophecy then and there if it is a true prophecy.

The problem, as always, is whether it is true and what harm it might do to the petitioner if it is false. Some prophecies may be at best harmless, or may even be helpful, even if they later turn out to be formed from the team member's own imagination. Here are some examples:

Example 7 (inappropriate):

Team member: Sally, the Lord has told me that when you wake up tomorrow you will be completely healed and you can stop taking your medicines then.

Example 8 (inappropriate):

Team member: Sally, the Lord has told me that you are living with a man to whom you are not married and that you will not be healed until you leave this sinful relationship.

Example 9 (possibly helpful, even if not a true prophecy):

Team member: The Lord told me to commend you on your faith for coming forward for prayer. Keep praying. The Lord hears you.

Example 10 (possibly helpful, even if not a true prophecy)

Team member: The Lord told me that the team should keep praying for your healing, and I can promise you that we will obey the Lord in this matter. Thank you for letting us pray for you.

Some may object that I myself am being blasphemous by suggesting team members refrain from exercising what may be true gifts of the Holy Spirit. For example, if a team member feels inspired to tell the petitioner to leave a sinful relationship, why should he be prevented from doing so?

It is not my, nor anyone else's, place to interfere with the work of the Lord. But we must be as certain as we can be that it is the work of the Lord. False prophets did great damage in the Old Testament, and they can also do great damage today. It is better, in my view, to err on the side of caution than to rush to judgment. Remember: "First, do no harm."

Anointing and sacramental language

Some denominations embrace the concept of a sacrament that, according to the catechism definition, is an outward sign instituted by Christ that confers inward grace.[1] Anointing is frequently mentioned in the Old Testament, but more for setting persons apart for special offices than for healing. Anointing for healing conducted by the apostles is mentioned in Matthew 6:13. Sacramental language for anointing is used by Episcopalians, Roman Catholics, and others in the liturgical tradition.

Is anointing as a ritual permitted in a particular denomination or church and, if so, may laypersons carry out this ritual? This is a matter that each church must decide in accordance with its own polity.

Note

1. The Episcopal *Book of Common Prayer* in response to the question, "What are the sacraments?" responds, "The sacraments are outward and visible signs of inward and spiritual grace, given by Christ as sure and certain means by which we receive grace." The Roman Catholic *Baltimore Catechism* states, "A Sacrament is an outward sign instituted by Christ to give grace."

Conclusion

Appendix A provides examples of prayers and rituals that might be used for healing. Appendix B lists some additional resources to assist churches in their healing ministries. Obviously, neither of these appendices is meant to be exhaustive. Appendix A may inspire a pastor or congregation to design its own healing rituals. Each of the possible resources in appendix B will lead toward additional possible resources.

Hopefully, this book has brought the reader to a deeper appreciation of the central role of spiritual healing in the ministry of the church and has provided some practical suggestions in identifying and removing obstacles to healing and in implementing ways to make a church a more effective house of healing. Please pray for my complete healing as I pray also for yours.

I close with a prayer from the *Book of Common Prayer*:

The Almighty Lord, who is a strong tower to all who put their trust in him, to whom all things in heaven, on earth, and under the earth bow and obey: Be now and ever more [our] defense and make [us] know and feel that the only Name under heaven given for health and salvation is the Name of our Lord Jesus Christ, Amen.
COME, LORD JESUS, MAKE US WHOLE.

APPENDIX A

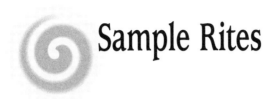 # Sample Rites

In this appendix we present sample prayers and rites that might be used in the healing ministry. This are intended as examples only. Churches are encouraged to develop their own prayers and rites in accordance with their particular doctrine, polity, and character. Books that may help in the design of such services include Brad Berglund's *Reinventing Sunday* and *Reinventing Worship*, both published by Judson Press. There are a number of books that contain collections of prayers, though they are not limited to prayers for healing. Examples of this genre are *The Doubleday Prayer Collection*, Mary Batchelor (compiler), and *The Oxford Book of Prayer*, George Appleton (compiler). Most denominations, of course, also have their own compilations of services and prayers.

A sample healing service

Some of the prayers have been taken, or adapted, from prayers found in the Episcopal *Book of Common Prayer*. Where this is the case, I have place the notation (BCP) after the prayer.

Hymn

Celebrant: We come together in the name of our Lord and Savior Jesus Christ, recognizing our need for forgiveness and for healing. He has given us assurance that where two or three are gathered together in his name, he will be among them. Let us pause silently for a moment to recognize his presence here with us.

Silence

Celebrant: The Lord be with you.
People: And also with you.
Celebrant: Let us pray.
The Celebrant says this or some other appropriate Collect
> O God, the source of all health: So fill our hearts with faith in your love, that with calm expectancy we may make room for your power to possess us, and gracefully accept your healing; through Jesus Christ our Lord. Amen. (BCP)

The Readings
Romans 8:31–9:1

[31] What, then, shall we say in response to this? If God is for us, who can be against us? [32] He who did not spare his own Son, but gave him up for us all—how will he not also, along with him, graciously give us all things? [33] Who will bring any charge against those whom God has chosen? It is God who justifies. [34] Who is he that condemns? Christ Jesus, who died—more than that, who was raised to life—is at the right hand of God and is also interceding for us. [35] Who shall separate us from the love of Christ? Shall trouble or hardship or persecution or famine or nakedness or danger or sword? [36] As it is written: "For your sake we face death all day long; we are considered as sheep to be slaughtered." [37] No, in all these things we are more than conquerors through him who loved us. [38] For I am convinced that neither death nor life, neither angels nor demons, neither the present nor the future, nor any powers, [39] neither height nor depth, nor anything else in all creation, will be able to separate us from the love of God that is in Christ Jesus our Lord.

Hymn

Mark 6:47-56
[47] When evening came, the boat was in the middle of the lake, and he was alone on land. [48] He saw the disciples straining at the oars,

because the wind was against them. About the fourth watch of the night he went out to them, walking on the lake. He was about to pass by them, [49] but when they saw him walking on the lake, they thought he was a ghost. They cried out, [50] because they all saw him and were terrified.

Immediately he spoke to them and said, "Take courage! It is I. Don't be afraid." [51] Then he climbed into the boat with them, and the wind died down. They were completely amazed, [52] for they had not understood about the loaves; their hearts were hardened.

[53] When they had crossed over, they landed at Gennesaret and anchored there. [54] As soon as they got out of the boat, people recognized Jesus. [55] They ran throughout that whole region and carried the sick on mats to wherever they heard he was. [56] And wherever he went-into villages, towns or countryside-they placed the sick in the marketplaces. They begged him to let them touch even the edge of his cloak, and all who touched him were healed.

Comments and discussion

Hymn

A Litany of Healing

The Celebrant introduces the Litany with this bidding
Let us pray.

A period of silence follows. Someone other than the Celebrant may lead the Litany.
Leader: Lord, you know all in us that yet requires healing.
Response: Heal us, merciful Lord.
Leader: Lord, you know how much our nation stands in need of healing.
Response: Heal our nation, merciful Lord.
Leader: Lord, you know how much our world stands in need of healing.
Response: Heal our world, merciful Lord.
Leader: Heal those who suffer because of injustice. Keep them strong in their faith.

Response: Heal those who suffer because of injustice, merciful Lord.

Leader: Heal those who are persecuted.

Response: Heal those who are persecuted, merciful Lord.

Leader: Heal those who are wounded by discrimination. Keep them strong in their faith.

Response: Heal those who are wounded by discrimination, merciful Lord.

Leader: Heal those who have been wounded by the violence of war.

Response: Heal those who have been wounded by the violence of war, merciful Lord.

Leader: Heal those who have been wounded by intolerance and ignorance.

Response: Heal those who have been wounded by intolerance and ignorance, merciful Lord.

Leader: Heal those who have been wounded because they are called aliens and are told that they are not worthy of compassion and justice.

Response: Heal those who are called aliens and excluded from compassion and justice, merciful Lord.

Leader: Heal those who stand in need of physical, mental, or spiritual healing whose names we now voice either aloud or in our hearts.

There is a pause to allow those present to name those for whom they wish healing.

The Celebrant concludes the litany with one of the following or some other suitable prayer:

Almighty God, giver of life and health: Send your blessing on all who are sick, and upon those who minister to them, that all weakness may be vanquished by the triumph of the risen Christ; who lives and reigns for ever and ever. Amen. (BCP)

Or this:

Heavenly Father, you have promised to hear what we ask in the Name of your Son: Accept and fulfill our petitions, we pray, not as we ask in our ignorance, nor as we deserve in our sinfulness, but as you know and love us in your Son Jesus Christ our Lord. Amen. (BCP)

Or this:

O Lord our God, accept the fervent prayers of your people; in the multitude of your mercies look with compassion upon us and all who turn to you for help; for you are gracious, O lover of souls, and to you we give glory, Father, Son, and Holy Spirit, now and for ever. Amen. (BCP)

A Confession of Sin follows, if it has not been said at the beginning of the service. See, also, the sample rite of penitence in this appendix.

The Celebrant: Let us confess our sins against God and against our neighbor.

Silence may be kept.

Celebrant and People:

Most merciful God, we confess that we have sinned against you in thought, word, and deed, by what we have done, and by what we have left undone. We have not loved you with our whole heart; we have not loved our neighbors as ourselves. We are truly sorry and we humbly repent. For the sake of your Son Jesus Christ, have mercy on us and forgive us; that we may delight in your will, and walk in your ways, to the glory of your Name. Amen. (BCP)

The Celebrant stands and says: Almighty God have mercy on you, forgive you all your sins through our Lord Jesus Christ, strengthen you in all goodness, and by the power of the Holy Spirit keep you in eternal life. Amen. (BCP) *Note: If it is deemed more appropriate, the Celebrant may substitute "us" for "you" in the prayer of absolution.*

Blessing of the oil

O Lord, holy Father, giver of health and salvation: Send your Holy Spirit to sanctify this oil; that, as your holy apostles anointed many that were sick and healed them, so may those who in faith and repentance receive this holy unction be made whole; through

Jesus Christ our Lord, who lives and reigns with you and the Holy Spirit, one God, for ever and ever. Amen. (BCP)

The Celebrant now invites those who wish to receive the laying on of hands (and anointing) to come forward.

The following anthem is sung or said:

Savior of the world, by your cross and precious blood you have redeemed us;

Save us, and help us, we humbly beseech you, O Lord. (BCP)

The Celebrant may say the following blessing over those who are about to come forward.

The Almighty Lord, who is a strong tower to all who put their trust in him, to whom all things in heaven, on earth, and under the earth bow and obey: Be now and evermore your defense, and make you know and feel that the only Name under heaven given for health and salvation is the Name of our Lord Jesus Christ. Amen. (BCP)

The Celebrant then lays hands on each person (and, having dipped a thumb in the oil of the sick, makes the sign of the cross on their foreheads), and says one of the following:

N., I lay my hands upon you [and anoint you with oil] in the Name of the Father, and of the Son, and of the Holy Spirit, beseeching our Lord Jesus Christ to sustain you with his presence, to drive away all sickness of body and spirit, and to give you that victory of life and peace which will enable you to serve him both now and evermore. Amen. (BCP)

Or this:

N., I lay my hands upon you [and anoint you with oil] in the Name of our Lord and Savior Jesus Christ, beseeching him to uphold you and fill you with grace, that you may know the healing power of his love. Amen. (BCP)

Or this:

N., I lay my hands upon you [and anoint you with oil] in the Name of the Father, and of the Son, and of the Holy Spirit. Amen. (BCP)

Or prayer may be offered for each person individually according to that person's need, with laying on of hands (and anointing). Lay persons with a gift of healing may join the celebrant in the laying on of hands. When the administration of the laying on of hands and anointing has been completed, the Celebrant prays as follows:

As you are outwardly anointed with this holy oil, so may our heavenly Father grant you the inward anointing of the Holy Spirit. Of his great mercy, may he forgive you your sins, release you from suffering, and restore you to wholeness and strength. May he deliver you from all evil, preserve you in all goodness, and bring you to everlasting life; through Jesus Christ our Lord. Amen. (BCP)

The service continues with the exchange of the Peace.

If there is not to be a Communion, the service concludes with the Lord's Prayer and the prayer and blessing given below.

If Communion is to be celebrated, the Liturgy continues with the Offertory.

In place of the usual postcommunion prayer (or, if there has not been a Communion, after the Lord's Prayer), the following prayer is said:

Lord, Jesus Christ, our great healer, we have come to you in faith asking that you make us whole. Heal us of our ills of mind and body, but most of all heal whatever might prevent us from growing evermore fully into your divine life. Make us yours, Lord, now and forever. Amen.

The Celebrant may pronounce a blessing such as the following:

The peace of God which passes all understanding fill your minds and hearts with the knowledge and love of God and of our Savior Jesus Christ. And may the blessing of God Almighty, Father, Son and Holy Spirit, be with you now and forever more. Amen. (BCP)

The people are then dismissed.

Hymn

A sample service of reconciliation

The following is one of the penitential rites found in the Episcopal *Book of Common Prayer*.

The Penitent begins, Bless me, for I have sinned.

The Priest says, The Lord be in your heart and upon your lips that you may truly and humbly confess your sins: In the Name of the Father, and of the Son, and of the Holy Spirit. Amen.

Penitent: I confess to Almighty God, to his Church, and to you, that I have sinned by my own fault in thought, word, and deed, in things done and left undone; especially _____ . For these and all other sins which I cannot now remember, I am truly sorry. I pray God to have mercy on me. I firmly intend amendment of life, and I humbly beg forgiveness of God and his Church, and ask you for counsel, direction, and absolution.

Here the Priest may offer counsel, direction, and comfort. The Priest then pronounces this absolution

Our Lord Jesus Christ, who has left power to his Church to absolve all sinners who truly repent and believe in him, of his great mercy forgive you all your offenses; and by his authority committed to me, I absolve you from all your sins: In the Name of the Father, and of the Son, and of the Holy Spirit. Amen.

Or this:

Our Lord Jesus Christ, who offered himself to be sacrificed for us to the Father, and who conferred power on his Church to forgive sins, absolve you through my ministry by the grace of the Holy Spirit, and restore you in the perfect peace of the Church. Amen.

Note: If either of these forms of forgiveness are not consonant with a denomination's doctrine, another form of a declaration of forgiveness might be used, e.g., Our Lord Jesus Christ, who offered himself to be sacrificed for us to the Father, forgives your sins by the grace of the Holy Spirit. Amen.

The Priest adds: The Lord has put away all your sins.

Penitent: Thanks be to God.

The Priest concludes: Go in peace, and pray for me, a sinner.

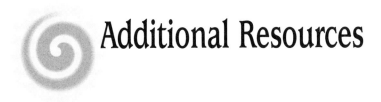 Additional Resources

This list of resources is not intended to be complete. Accessing the resources listed, however, will, in turn, lead to more resources on spiritual healing. These resources are listed alphabetically.

Alban Institute—The Alban Institute is involved in clergy and congregational development through publishing, leadership training, its magazine *Congregations*, research, and its various online activities. It is a rich source of information not only about clergy health and healing at the congregational level, but its website contains articles dealing with healing and links to other sites that might prove useful. Among the latter is www.congregationalresources. org/healingchurch/Resources.asp.

Its list of books include works on conflict resolution, clergy health and congregation health, and healing during clergy transitions or after a problem pastorate. The website for the Alban Institute can be found at www.alban.org. One of the many interesting articles available from Alban is Claudia Greer's "Becoming a Holy and Healing Church." Among the books on healing wounded congregations are David Lott's *Conflict Management in Congregations*; Denise Goodman's *Congregational Fitness: Healthy Practices for Layfolk*; and Jill Hudson's *Congregational Trauma:*

Caring, Coping, and Learning. A resource on evaluating ministries is David McMahill's *Completing the Circle: Reviewing Ministries in the Congregation*. Workshops are also available through Alban for leadership training; consultants are available to assist congregations in various ways.

Christian Healing Ministries—Francis and Judith MacNutt are prominent practitioners of the art of Christian healing. The center they founded in located near Jacksonville, Florida, and offers a number of workshops and conferences, including their well-known School of Healing Prayer. Their website is found at www.christianhealingmin.org.

Community of Hope—According to its website, "the mission of The Community of Hope is to create and sustain Christian communities of volunteer lay pastoral caregivers in the Episcopal Diocese of Texas, united in prayer, shaped by Benedictine spirituality, and equipped for and serving in pastoral care ministries." Learn more about the Community of Hope at www.slehc.org/AboutUs/Spirituality/COH.

Institute for Religion and Health—This Houston, Texas, based organization was initially involved in chaplaincy training, but it has morphed into an organization that "offers a wide range of programs that support healthcare provider wellness, promote compassionate healthcare, and provide a nurturing environment for collaborative education and research relevant to health, healing, and spirituality." It offers programs such as a Psychotherapy and Faith Conference, and a yearlong series on the meditation practices of various religions. It may be found on the Web at www.religionandhealth.org.

Order of St. Luke the Physician—According to its website, "The International Order of St. Luke the Physician is an ecumenical organization dedicated to the Christian healing ministry. Members meet together in local chapters to study Scripture, especially the biblical stories of the healing miracles, as well as other books on Christian healing. Members also engage in healing prayer, often with the laying-on of hands." The website for the Order of St. Luke is found at www.orderofstluke.org. The order has a bimonthly magazine, *Sharing*, that includes notices about healing retreats and workshops as well as accounts of healings.

Training materials for leadership in the healing ministry are available from the order. See the website for training for members and leaders in the OSL.

The order also has a recommended reading list of twenty-one titles, and prospective members must read at least three books on this list before they can be considered for full membership. Among the books on this list are Agnes Sanford's *The Healing Light* and Frances MacNutt's *Healing, The Prayer That Heals* and *The Power to Heal*. All of the books on the recommended list are available from the OSL Bookstore.

Although the OSL is an excellent resource, its members and its authors vary widely in their attitudes about healing, some of which I consider problematic, including "name it and claim it" or the health-and-wealth gospel.

The School of Pastoral Care, founded by the noted healer Agnes Sanford, has become a part of the Order of St. Luke that offers programs that used to be given under the separate auspices of the school, for example, a healing ministry training weekend.

Services for Healing—The *Episcopal Book of Occasional Services* contains a public service of healing on which the service in appendix A is modeled. A number of such services are available on the Internet. A Google search using "healing prayer services" brings up a listing containing hundreds of thousands of entries. There is a tremendous amount of New Age material that comes up in a search of a site like Amazon.com. Being on the best-seller list does not necessarily mean that a book is appropriate for the ministry of Christian healing.

Small Group Spiritual Development—Below are some books on the use of small groups as tools for spiritual formation:

- Gemignani, M., *To Know God: Small Group Experiences in Spiritual Formation*, Judson, 2002.
- Dougherty, R. M., *The Lived Experience of Group Spiritual Direction*, Shalem, 2006.

Spiritual Direction and Spiritual Companioning—There are perhaps several hundred programs in the United States that purport to train spiritual directors. Since there is no uniform certification, licensing, or accreditation of such programs, they vary in quality. Investigate carefully before signing up for such a program.

Spiritual direction is often offered through retreat houses; for example, in Houston, Texas, spiritual direction is available at the Ruah Center of the Villa de Matel and at the Cenacle Retreat House. Some books on the topic of spiritual direction and companioning are Guenther, Margaret, *Holy Listening: The Art of Spiritual Direction*, Cowley, 1992, and Leech, Kenneth, *Soul Friend*, Morehouse, 2001.

Spiritual Directors International—Spiritual Directors International, SDI, is by far the largest organization of spiritual directors. Anyone of any denomination who calls him or herself a spiritual director can join, so membership in SDI is not necessarily an indication that someone is a Christian spiritual director or is a competent director of any persuasion.

SDI has, however, put together a compendium of "enrichment, formation and training programs for spiritual directors" available on its website. See www.sdiworld.org/index.pl/northamerica enrichment.html. There are hundreds of listings for the United States, with a training program in almost every state. There are ten listed in my own state of Texas, including the International Association of Pastoral Counselors, Lebh Shomea House of Prayer, the Texas Annual Conference—United Methodist Church, Christian Renewal Center, the Episcopal Diocese of Texas, the

University of St. Thomas, the Cenacle Retreat House, the Center for Spiritual Growth and the Contemplative Life, HeartPaths Spirituality Centre—Dallas, and St. Peter upon the Water Spiritual Direction Center.

The SDI website also offers a list of "retreat centers with spiritual direction" at www.sdiworld.org/retreat_centers.html.

Stephen Ministry—Resources concerning the Stephen Ministry involve training and organizing lay people to provide one-to-one Christian care to hurting people in a congregation. More information about Stephen Ministry may be found at www.stephen ministries.org.

THE SMILE

GINNY VERE NICOLL

~

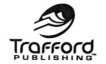

Trafford
PUBLISHING

*We at Trafford believe that it is the responsibility of us all, as both individuals
and corporations, to make choices that are environmentally and socially sound.
You, in turn, are supporting this responsible conduct each time you purchase a
Trafford book, or make use of our publishing services. To find out how you are
helping, please visit www.trafford.com/responsiblepublishing.html*

*Our mission is to efficiently provide the world's finest, most comprehensive
book publishing service, enabling every author to experience success.
To find out how to publish your book, your way, and have it available
worldwide, visit us online at www.trafford.com/10510*

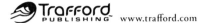 www.trafford.com

North America & international
toll-free: 1 888 232 4444 (USA & Canada)
phone: 250 383 6864 • fax: 250 383 6804 • email: info@trafford.com

The United Kingdom & Europe
phone: +44 (0)1865 722 113 • local rate: 0845 230 9601
facsimile: +44 (0)1865 722 868 • email: info.uk@trafford.com

10 9 8 7 6 5 4 3

ACKNOWLEDGEMENTS

A huge thank you to my two, brilliant, editors, for their endless work on my behalf: to my talented, graphic art designer daughter, for the beautiful cover and to my long suffering husband, family and friends, who have lived with all these extra 'people' in the house for so long!

To Tobie, for all the fun, help and encouragement from the very beginning: and, for my mother, watching from some far off place, high above, not forgetting Marmite and Treacle, my little four-legged companions.

How would I have managed without all the faith, love and support?

May you all be forever 'Smiling'.

~

THE SMILE

CHAPTER 1

Gianni Vivarini stood tense and still, aware of a deep, inexplicable unease. The nagging discomfort attacked his stomach in persistent, annoying waves. He stood on the beach, on his island, L'Isola Delfino, his beautiful home and wondered how it was possible to experience such disquiet in such a place?

A lone gull wheeled high above his head, its cries reaching him even after it disappeared through a veil of dawn mist, left behind from the receding night sky. Distracted, he took a long, restoring, breath of, fresh, salty air, then, stared out across the sea to the far horizon, considering the sky and his day ahead.

It was early, very early and so the movement in the distance to his right took him by surprise. Gianni recognized the woman; her figure a silhouette against the rapidly lightening sky, she was also turned to look, her pale hair touched by the rising sun. She had arrived late last night, beautiful and sad with very little luggage, surrounded by an aura of mystery and without a smile. He watched with interest. She bent down, perhaps tying a shoe lace or picking up a shell or smooth stone that caught her eye as it reflected in the early morning glow.

Gianni shifted his weight slightly, awkward with the familiar stiffness from the old wound in his leg. The sniper's bullet had lodged firm and true. Feeling conspicuous and conscious of invading the young person's privacy

I

he looked down at his own feet, big, reliable and familiar, friendly almost. He'd had them fifty odd years. He moved them apart, scrunching the sand as he took a more solid stance and straightened his back. With his hands in his pockets he could feel the knarled old knife in one and the roll of thin twine in the other. Comforting and normal, these tranquil days, he thought. He looked up again at the forlorn figure standing at the water's edge, one hand raised to shade her eyes from the glare, but she was, thankfully, still unaware of his presence. I'm intruding, he thought, looking away again, she needs to be alone.

He lingered a minute or two longer, watching the vivid ball of fire achieve its spectacular journey and ascend into an already azure sky. The whole surround was splashed vermillion, the retreating threads of cloud formations scattered and mismatched. A new day was born. Unsettled weather Gianni predicted as he glanced, now to the left, straining his eyes, searching for his brother's fishing boat and listening for the distant and reassuring beat of the throaty little engine.

Then he saw it: Dimitri's pride and joy the 'Amica', chugging home as regular as clockwork from around the next headland after completing its night's work. It was followed by a cloud of circling, shrieking, arguing gulls and a couple of the island's namesakes, the dolphins. They made a magical picture leaping and playing in the wake of the boat with the sea spray shimmering and sparkling, caught and coloured by the early rays of the sun. Dimitri, the shape of his body sharp against the dazzling light with one hand bent back to the helm, was also turned to watch.

Gianni looked around once more and studied the motionless form of the girl by the sea. He shivered, but with apprehension, for he was not cold. The goose pimples prickled the back of his neck and he shrugged deeper down into his coat. The Delfinos, as the island men were affectionately called, seldom felt cold for they were a tough breed, these third generation fishermen. 'We're just like the real dolphins,' Gianni would chuckle when the women remarked on his rolled up sleeves in wintertime, 'and warm blooded too', he would whisper as an aside to his wife if she happened to be there.

Gianni sighed, for his few minutes of solitude were up and it was time to get on with the innumerable practical matters planned for the day. He retraced his footsteps over the sand towards the little hidden path which wound its way up through the rocks to meet the edge of the rough field bordering his land. His eyes darkened with undefined worry. He was disturbed by the image of the young woman he'd just left, enveloped in sorrow and alone on the beach.

~

Gianni walked back through the vineyard more quickly than usual, his trained eye automatically checking the vines as he passed, while he pondered this new problem. He was anxious to hear his wife Giuseppina's thoughts on the subject and wondered what the two of them could do to help put the smile back on the lovely young woman's face. He was a kind man and he didn't like to see suffering in one so young. Why was she here all alone and so far from home? It wasn't the holiday season after all; it was, as yet, much too early for tourists on L'Isola Delfino.

~

Giuseppina was busy in her warm, fragrant, kitchen. She put the coffee on the hob to percolate while she prepared the pasta for the evening. This done she began on the bread, taking it from its usual resting place near the cooking range where, covered in a clean cloth, she'd set it to rise the night before. The aroma of the yeast filled her expectant nostrils, causing her to grunt with satisfaction as she looked at the size of this living thing that she had created. She loved the idea of the dough growing and expanding in the quiet dark place, while she slept. Now safe in her capable hands she kneaded, pummelled, pulled and shaped the loaf while she awaited her husband's return. The dough was warm, soft and pliable - a pleasurable job and conducive to thought. It was at such times, when her hands were busy, that she did her best thinking. Giuseppina, also, was worried about their English guest. She sensed an air of torment, vulnerability and heartache engulfing the sad girl, like a damp, all encompassing fog. She needed her mother concluded Giuseppina. Where was she? The poor thing was all over the place. Even

3

though their visitor was a stranger, Giusepinna, with a wealth of experience and a fondness for sorting out other peoples problems, wanted to gather up the young woman's shattered life and help her to set it straight again. It was in her nature to do these things.

Giusepinna was not accustomed to having unhappiness encroach on her family life, or for it to throw their daily routine into certain disarray. An easy mind was all important as far as Giuseppina was concerned. Trouble of any sort was not welcome and should be checked; otherwise it could spread quickly, far and wide, like a raging fire. The island was inhabited and protected by people with plenty to smile about, a happy, carefree bunch. Minor disputes or sad losses normal in the life span, yes, these were expected, dealt with and overcome. But the Delfino's gregarious love of life always resurfaced undaunted, with the help of family, friends and often with a large slice of Giuseppina's generosity and support.

She paused in her work, wiped her hands on her apron and tucked a loose strand of hair back behind her ear. Now she'd have flour on her face, which was pink with exertion and it wouldn't escape his notice. Her beloved Gianni never missed a thing. She'd only left their warm bed a couple of hours before and was still bathed in that warm afterglow of contentment. She looked down at her increasing figure and chuckled to herself. Not quite the same as when the bambinos were there, but at least it was still firm and he still seemed to take frequent delight in it.

She described herself nowadays as a 'comfortable' looking, forty-five year old woman, six years younger than her husband, neat, pink and plump! Her dark hair showed few telltale white streaks and was coiled tidily at the nape of her neck, held there with the same tortoise shell comb that Gianni had given her years before. Her mouth was habitually busy singing and her eyes shone just as they always had, with the sheer joy of living in the place and with the people she loved best.

Giuseppina glanced towards the stove, drawn by the noise and the pervasive smell of the strong rich coffee forcing its way up through the percolator.

It was ready. She looked out of the open window. Gianni was approaching, his head turned to one side checking the last of his vines as he walked up the path. He loved those bushes, the grapes and finally the wine. She sucked in her breath, shaking her head, an amused smile on her lips as she considered her husband: sound and solid as a rock physically, though a little more robust perhaps, but as upright and strong as ever. He was without doubt the best looking man in the whole of Italy, as she never ceased to tell their three girls, with his shock of thick, dark, unruly, hair and eyes full of humor. 'A film star' she would tell them. 'Your Papa could have been a film star, so just imagine all the women that your poor Mama would have had to fight off at the festival for films', she would add when, as young people do, they all collapsed in fits of giggles at the mere thought of their parents being feted at Cannes.

Giuseppina would prance up and down the kitchen with her hands on her hips, describing the pretended scene. The long dress, she'd say, would be in dazzling red silk, hugging her body tightly. It would swish and wrap its way seductively around her legs as she floated over the long, thick, carpet between rows of admiring fans. It would be slit high, just so high - she would tell her audience, indicating, - so as to allow her smooth passage while she made her grand entrance to the reception. Her husband would be there at her side bowing and waving to the imagined crowd.

Gianni would play his part until he'd had enough, then he'd turn to their rapt audience and becoming serious again, would wait for the noise to quieten. He'd tell them, almost reverently, that there was no film star born yet who could hold a candle to their mother as a young woman. The laughter would die and they would all nod in agreement, as they believed him. Giuseppina, silenced for once, would smile at her husband and kiss him tenderly, before getting back to cooking their meal. She would feel like a film star for the rest of the evening. What a lucky woman she was to command the enduring love of such a man.

~

But Gianni was concerned about something this early spring morning.

Giuseppina could tell by the hesitation in his walk. He was thinking, his mind in altogether another place and this time she knew the cause of his disquiet.

After living with her husband both through his active and secretive military life and later, after he'd seemingly left the army to help his father run things on Delfino island, Giuseppina had a sensitivity and an uncanny feel for the atmosphere surrounding people and places. In the early years of their marriage she had instinctively known when Gianni was about something difficult or dangerous. She'd seen it in his eyes when they said goodbye. On these occasions Gianni had always left the house unaware of his wife's perceptions. In those uncertain days she'd known how important it was for him to leave with an easy mind and so she had hidden her apprehensions well.

The island women had their own ideas about what had taken place on Delfino both during and after the last war. People of different nationalities had frequently arrived unexpectedly, even furtively and sometimes at dead of night, by boat or small plane. All had the same thing in common. They were shrouded in an air of secrecy. Allessandro, her father-in-law and the young Gianni had taken great trouble to see that the visitors had what they needed and were left undisturbed, with their privacy both well guarded and respected.

The islanders, fiercely loyal and above all desperate for a world at peace, absolutely trusted the judgement of both Allessandro and Gianni. They put their own lives on hold without question, whenever they were asked, doing whatever was required of them, in the certainty that it would be for the overall benefit of mankind. But whatever these guests were really up to on the island had never been a subject for discussion amongst the Delfino women, not even when their own men were present. This had been and still remained an unbroken rule. They had merely watched, waited and came to their own conclusions in silence. Gossip, centred around the endless small dramas and problems of their everyday lives, their very life's blood under normal circumstances, had no part in these events.

~

First things first, Giuseppina thought: Gianni's coffee and then she must give Alicia her breakfast in the sun. In Giuseppina's book, in order to recover from a bad state of affairs, whatever it was, you needed to eat and eat well! And a good dose of sunshine and sea air would do the poor girl the world of good too.

Gianni whistled as he passed the last of the vines. Bending down, he deftly tied up a branch that had come loose in the wind, with his large, but sensitive hands, giving Giuseppina the time she needed to make sure that his coffee was hot once she had seen or heard him coming. On this particular morning he really didn't think he wanted any coffee, but he'd have to have it or his wife would guess that something was up, that he was worried. She'd give him English tea instead, to settle his digestion. He hated the insipid drink, far preferring the strong black expresso coffee. But these days it affected his stomach, particularly when he was anxious.

He walked through the door, smiling. There she was, as usual, as if she didn't know after all this time. It was still their unspoken little joke together, the same every morning. The coffee was poured, ready and waiting.

"*Gioia mia,* how can you know I am here?"

"Come here, you silly man," she replied, as she pulled out the chair and put his own special mug on the table before him. She took his coat from him as he sat, then gave him a kiss, stepping back quickly, laughing, as he tried to grab her around her large waist.

"Enough! *Sei così pazza,* you have already had some of 'that' for breakfast! Now: what about our unhappy guest?" Giuseppina, asked quietly becoming serious again. "How can such a beautiful girl be so sad... perhaps it's a man?" she finished hopefully looking up at him as if in question.

"*Si, mia cara,* we must do something, but I think it's more than that," replied Gianni as he sipped his coffee carefully.

"I think so too. In fact, I have this feeling that it is something very much more than that," Giuseppina answered, patting her equally large chest and becoming thoughtful too. "Anyway she's too thin. She needs building up with good, nourishing, Italian food." she said returning to practical matters. "Now drink up and I will see to it." She bent to ruffle his hair affectionately. "She is not down yet."

"*Si si*, yes she is," said Gianni, as he turned to look out of the window to watch the lonely figure wending her way slowly back through the distant vines. "She's been out and about for some time already and up in the night several times too. I heard her."

"Poor girl!" muttered Giuseppina sadly, "but maybe that's just a woman's thing."

"I very much doubt it." answered Gianni getting up from his chair as he finished his coffee. He kissed the top of his wife's head and went out of the room to get on with his day. Giuseppina agreed with her husband. Yes, she thought, their guest's lovely face was bathed in undiluted misery, it was quite obviously very much more than just 'a woman's thing'.

★★★

CHAPTER 2

Alicia Spence was twenty-six, tall and angular, with genuinely blonde hair and startling aquamarine blue eyes. She was intelligent, with an enquiring mind, interested in everything, which she put to good use as a freelance travel journalist and writer. She dressed with an understated air of sophistication. Her natural charm drew both men and woman of all ages to her side and children suffered no adult threat of exclusion or patronization. She would talk and play with them at their own level with evident enjoyment.

Normally Alicia was a serene, happy person, but not today, nor for many days past, since it had happened.

Today was to have been the day; the day that she should have married Guy Hargreaves, an erudite young lawyer with a brilliant mind, good looking fit and funny. That was what had attracted Alicia most when they had first met: the constant fun and laughter which seemed to surround him and infect everybody else within range. He believed nothing to be out of reach. His life, mapped out ahead, had spelled success. Together they'd had everything, or so she had believed.

~

They'd met two years previously, over a bank holiday, at a week-end party given by mutual friends in Scotland. Alicia had thought she was going to be bored stiff, she had only gone to please her mother, in the first place. She was busy, with several articles to finish for her office, she was tired and in need of a break. The trip to Scotland, often grey and dismal in wintertime, was not what she would have planned from choice. It was a long way, an expensive journey and Alicia didn't even know the couple who owned the house very well. Their parents were friends of her mother, but against her better judgement, she had travelled north. There, fate had played its inevitable hand: little did Alicia guess what life had in store.

There was one conspicuously empty chair when they had all sat down to dinner on the Friday night, but just as the first course was put on the table the late arrival had walked in.

'Good timing', Guy announced surveying the room, then staring unashamedly at Alicia, as he caught and held her eyes, whilst greeting their host. Alicia's stomach lurched, her heart beat double time and she felt unable to speak. Her world turned upside down in one soul-stirring moment. The other guests glanced from one to the other with amusement as they recognized the symptoms and sensed the charged atmosphere. Alicia sat down again, very fast, saying to herself, 'this is ridiculous, it just doesn't happen this way'. But it did happen for them both, 'just like that'. Instead of being embarrassed, Guy took over the room. He soon had everyone laughing with him over his journey on the train, with a dreadful woman and her equally awful dog and then, without further ado, made them all move around so he could sit next to Alicia.

Guy had never left her side throughout the whole week-end, yet, whenever he tried to get Alicia alone, someone had disturbed them. They all went for a walk on the Sunday. He made her walk more slowly than the rest until they were well behind. Then he had grabbed her and pulled her behind a tree, kissing her until she could hardly stand. If it hadn't been for the others they would have made love then and there despite the cold, frosty weather. They couldn't wait to be on their own together. He had insisted that he'd fly back with her on the plane to London on the Monday night, wasting his own return train ticket. He had taken her out to dinner the following evening, after which they saw each other at least twice a week. It was as if they'd known each other always. From then on their relationship progressed and developed, enriched by an intense and spontaneous love life, which surpassed anything that either had experienced before.

Guy had soon persuaded Alicia to leave her own flat and move into his immaculate house in Fulham. They couldn't survive apart and were happier than either could have ever imagined. She loved the house, with the extra space it gave them and had immediately seen the potential for its unkempt and unloved garden. It hadn't remained so for long. Once Alicia went into action, the small piece of land was speedily transformed, much to Guy's amazement and admiration. He teased her mercilessly about her 'green fingers', saying that perhaps she should give up her hectic journalistic pursuits and go into horticulture instead.

Nonetheless, she hadn't sold her flat, rather renting it out to an American couple, just in case. Looking back now, she wondered if that decision had been in some way a premonition of what was to come.

~

Over and over again Alicia would reflect on the recent sequence of events, remembering as much detail as she could. What could possibly have happened? Where was he? Was he safe? Could he have been 'taken' for some reason? Was he alive? These last possibilities sent shivers racing down her spine. How could she not know? How could he have disappeared without trace and without a word? They were on the same wavelength. Nobody knew Guy as well as she did. He would face up to a problem, no matter how difficult. He always did. They discussed everything and had no secrets, until now. He would have told her, if he could; and there lies the rub thought Alicia, 'if he could'. What or who was stopping him?

There had seemed to be no cloud on their horizon. Alicia could swear that Guy was looking forward to their wedding as much as she was. She had scoured the house for a sign, any clue that something else was wrong, but that hadn't taken long, they didn't have many possessions. They both liked plenty of space. Guy's desk was tidy, with the bills and correspondence up to date. Everything was in order, as always. She had leapt on the post as soon as it had fallen through the door each morning, but had found nothing of interest and only disappointment followed.

A discreet search in Guy's office had not revealed anything either, except his immediate travel plans, cut short. His secretary and partners had, so far, showed little concern. Alicia realized they were at a loss as to what to say to her, they didn't know where he was themselves. So she had left quickly to avoid further embarrassment. She sensed, but with no real, reasonable, explanation that for the moment perhaps the whole world shouldn't be alerted to her belief in her own fears, as yet unfounded.

Alicia had telephoned friends, family and acquaintances, trade and business contacts at home and abroad, both past and present, everybody she could think of. She had literally spent hours on the telephone. This was difficult, as quite a few hadn't been invited to the wedding. Perhaps she had rather under-played things. She had taken such care not to spread alarm, just gently enquiring if they'd seen Guy recently as she was trying to pass on a message and had lost track of where he said he would be on his travels. Nothing. Nobody else had heard anything since the day before the flowers had arrived, when he had been to a scheduled meeting at his bank in Guernsey and gone on to lunch at a restaurant with a business associate. She had managed to trace his lunch companion who had merely said that Guy had been well and had been intending to continue to Paris that evening. She hadn't admitted that he'd disappeared or that she was worried and the man had politely wished them well for their wedding.

In spite of her carefully worded questions, Alicia could tell that some of their friends, sensing intrigue, thought she'd most likely just been dumped, albeit in a rather callous way. 'Let's face it', those that knew her well enough would say, 'these things do happen'. 'Not to me they don't', she'd mutter, after finishing the conversation more abruptly than she meant, hoping she hadn't been rude. Then her natural confidence would begin to dwindle. Perhaps they were right. She'd almost start to believe these faithless people with their glib comments and knowledgeable explanations, but not for long. After quietly reviewing the whole scenario, yet again, she returned to the same conclusion every time. Something extraordinary had to have happened.

Guy's last assignment abroad had seemed un-noteworthy. A short hop to the Channel Islands: from there to Paris and on to New York, before returning home in time for their wedding. Then they'd both made no commitments for a month, until after the honeymoon they had planned in the West Indies.

The last she had heard was the card on the box of freesia's flown in from Guernsey signed, 'For Ever and Always G.' Nothing odd, nothing untoward. He always managed to send her flowers en route. When she'd left the house for Italy the freesia's had remained limp and colourless in their vase. Alicia could not bring herself to throw out this last link.

She discovered that Guy's meetings in Paris and New York had been inexplicably cancelled by somebody unknown to those offices. At this point his text messages had also suddenly stopped. The last 'goodnight' text had come through the day before the flowers arrived. Her answer was never received. She continued to try his mobile, only to be told 'please hold, this call is being transferred', then, maddeningly, 'please try again later' and finally, 'I'm sorry, this number is no longer available', followed by an ongoing, eerie, silence. The line was dead.

Guy's elderly parents lived in Devon. They'd had a call from Guernsey the same day as her last text so they knew he was travelling. She hadn't wanted to worry them and had again played the whole thing down. As far as the rest of the world was concerned they had merely postponed their wedding for work reasons. At least she hadn't had to send all the presents back.

Alicia wracked her brains day and night. She was unable to sleep. How could someone go missing or just vanish without trace? The relevant authorities had said that the Channel Islands were one of the easiest places from which to disappear, with regular ferry sailings and scheduled flights, not to speak of the constant comings and goings of small private boats and planes. They hadn't been very helpful. She supposed it was because Guy was a so-called responsible adult rather than a wayward child and that they were too busy to deal with domestic problems. After two weeks the police had given up. She suspected that, finding no evidence of foul play or violence, they had decided Guy had probably planned the whole thing for some personal reason. They were not particularly sympathetic and made it quite clear that she was wasting their time and that 'time was money'.

She had gone home and waited - waited for something, anything, to happen. It had turned out to be the longest and worst week of her life. She couldn't eat. She felt anaemic, weary, thoroughly depressed and totally abandoned.

~

Alicia needed to talk to Julian. Julian Birchall was Guy's oldest friend. They had been in the army together as younger men and before that at the same school. She had rarely, if ever, heard either of them refer to their mutual military experiences. Alicia always thought this strange, as they talked about their shared adventures at school on many occasions. Perhaps that branch of the army had been some special unit, not to be discussed. She often wondered what their actual work had been. If ever she mentioned the subject they both neatly turned the conversation around, so neither she, nor Julian's girlfriend Adriana, ever bothered to pursue it. After all, it in no way encroached on their present day lives, or so they had thought.

Alicia wished that Julian had been at home in England. He might have some idea, or be able to throw some light on the matter, the two men were always talking. She needed his reassurance. Adriana, unaware of the full extent of Alicia's misgivings, had merely said that Julian was still in America on some job, but was also overdue in returning to his office. He was a war correspondent and Adriana was used to him being out of touch. Nevertheless she was obviously concerned for Alicia and promised to contact her if she heard anything.

Alicia considered the last few days she had spent with her fiancé. Work was normal. There were a couple of business dinners and an evening at the theatre with friends. It had been fun and they'd all laughed a lot: she remembered an especially light-hearted, late night. Nothing could have been wrong then, surely?

There had been one curious telephone call on Guy's mobile, in the middle of the night, before he left for the Channel Islands. He'd said it was a business man from the Far East, who had mistaken the time difference. Guy had definitely been uneasy after that call. He'd gone next door and Alicia heard his voice, lowered purposefully. The conversation had been short and intense, followed by a gap. Then she thought he'd made another call: she could tell from the murmurings and the slight noise as he punched in the numbers. He hadn't said anything more to her but she had the distinct feeling that it hadn't been a misdirected call and that he had responded to it. This was the only odd occurrence that Alicia could come up with. No doubt it could be easily explained by others, but for the moment she kept it to herself.

With Julian's absence there was only one person to whom Alicia told the whole story, with all her fears and worries and that was Guy's young first cousin, Nick Hargreaves. Nick worked in the Foreign and Commonwealth Office. 'Our man from the F.O', as Guy would insist on calling him. He was doing everything he possibly could to help her. Nick seemed to have all the contacts he needed at his fingertips and Alicia liked and trusted him. He'd been brilliant, using his Home Office contacts to help her with the Channel Islands' police, when she had finally become exasperated with them. Also, most importantly and to this she clung like a drowning person, he believed her when she said that under no circumstance would Guy have left, out of the blue and with no explanation, unless for some very serious and exceptionally dramatic reason.

Alicia's mother, Diana, was beside herself with worry and devastated by what had happened to her daughter, although she was clever enough not to show too much in Alicia's presence. It was without doubt the most bizarre of situations.

The final straw for Diana was when she found Alicia sitting one day in her bedroom at their home, literally staring at a blank wall. Her mother had decided to take control. She persuaded Alicia to go away for the period over the cancelled wedding.

'You'll end up making yourself ill with the worry of it all', Tony, her stepfather had commented tactlessly, just at the wrong moment. 'It depends how you define illness', Alicia had retorted with annoyance, jumping up and walking out of the room, realizing that he probably wanted to get rid of her as she was becoming a nuisance. She had never liked the man, found his behaviour overbearing and so avoided him whenever she could. She wondered why her mother had ever married him. Perhaps it had just been loneliness.

Alicia felt the usual wave of aggravation flooding over her just thinking about the wretched Tony. Guy disliked him even more than she did. Alicia used to giggle when Guy only just managed to hide his dislike and hold his tongue in her stepfather's presence. He did so only out of respect and politeness to Diana, of whom he was very fond.

Diana was typically calm and reassuring, dealing with the various wedding cancellations as if they were mere everyday occurrences and Alicia was constantly grateful to her mother for not badgering her with endless questions that she couldn't answer. It was a difficult time for them both. Diana adored her future son-in-law and was also at a complete loss herself as to what had caused Guy's mysterious disappearance.

★★★

CHAPTER 3

Diana Trefford-Spence, as she preferred to be called, was well aware of Alicia and Guy's dislike for her present husband. Alicia was correct in her assumption. Diana had married for the second time out of loneliness and had regretted it ever since. She was an attractive woman and with her first husband had led a busy, smart, life, always together, very social with frequent, international, travel. Diana could never have replaced Alicia's father, Peter, he was a wonderful man. Much respected and well liked: she missed him as much as ever. He and Guy would have had shared much in common and Guy would have become the son they were never able to have.

It was some years before Diana, only forty-five at the time of her husband's accident, recovered enough to show any interest in another man. She was just fifty when she finally married Tony, Major Anthony Trefford-Sharpe. He had one obnoxious, unmarried, son from a previous marriage, but luckily Diana and her daughter didn't see much of him as he lived in Australia.

It still hurt to remember the awfulness of Peter's untimely death. It had badly affected Alicia, who was at boarding school at that time. Diana went down to tell her as gently as she could. Her heart contracted even now at the memory of the distraught child in her arms beginning to absorb the shocking news that her father was gone.

A fine and experienced rider, he'd fallen from his horse whilst riding in the woods near their home in the Cotswolds. Nobody could work out quite what had happened but he'd been killed instantly and his favourite hunter had to be put down with a badly broken leg. The only living creature left who really knew the answer was the family dog, who had always gone everywhere with Peter. How she'd wished Max could have told them his own, sorry, story. He had stayed faithfully beside his master, keeping him company, until they were found and then wouldn't eat or come out of Peter's dressing room until finally persuaded by hunger.

It was her job, Diana told Alicia when she came home from school, to look after poor Max so that one day he might be happy again, as her father would wish. Alicia had been only just fifteen at the time and had taken this responsibility most seriously, ministering to Max's every need and determinedly insisting that he slept in her bed, but only after Diana had given the dog a much needed bath. Diana, Alicia and Max were a comfort to each other for the three weeks after the funeral.

After being sent back to her boarding school, Alicia had missed Diana and her little companion badly and had cried herself to sleep for many nights. Alicia's misery had not gone unnoticed at school and her friends and room mates became unsettled and upset for her too. Finally, coming to the conclusion that this state of affairs had been going on far too long, her headmistress had suggested that Diana visit the school for a chat. The outcome was a wonderful plan for them both to stay with her mother's sister in Venice.

This was the first of several visits and the beginning of Alicia's love affair with Italy, the Italians and their way of life, the architecture, their culture, the food and everything Italian. She was hypnotized by the wonder of Venice, absorbed every smallest detail and completely exhausted both Diana and her aunt Caro! When Alicia came down from university some years later with a first class honours degree in history of art, it was mainly because of the thorough, local, knowledge and understanding poured into her written thesis on Venice. Both Caro and Diana had been exceptionally proud.

Alicia's six months stay in Venice, as a grown woman, had been greatly enhanced by an enlightening love affair with an older Italian who, according to Caro, although not entirely suitable had certainly taught Alicia 'the things she needed to know'. He had adored her, treated her like a queen, was great company and impossibly flirtatious. The only difficulty had arisen when Alicia came to leave, but then as Caro told Diana, 'what man in his right mind would let a girl like Alicia go without a fight'.

~

Diana smiled at the thought of Alicia's conquest in Venice in her late teens, little knowing that, at that time, back in England she had been perfectly well aware of the affair and was kept well up to date at all times by her sister, who seemed to condone the liaison, which had somewhat soothed Diana's protective, motherly, instincts.

Diana felt immensely relieved that, for the moment, Alicia was away from England, living another life in her beloved Italy. She hoped she would go on to Venice soon, when she'd had enough peace and quiet on Delfino Island. Alicia could never be miserable for long in Caro's company.

Her heart went out to her daughter. What a weird and horrible predicament. Guy loved Alicia, she was certain of that, but where on earth was he? Diana could never believe ill of her future son-in-law, but at present she just didn't know what to make of it. She wished, beyond anything, that they could get to the bottom of it all. She must think how best to help; whom she could approach. There had to be someone, somewhere, who knew something and they must find out, wherever that might lead. Diana had a bad feeling about the whole situation and it left her chilled to the bone.

~

Alicia's office in London had been both supportive and considerate, enabling Alicia to take the time off to deal with the present crisis in her life. Her duties were being well covered by other members of the staff and in return she was asked merely to collect together any interesting material for the travel department and to check in once in a while. 'Take a sabbatical', she was told, 'you've earned it'.

'Brilliant, no real commitments, just what the doctor ordered'. Alicia could hear her mother's voice again. Diana hadn't wanted her to go away alone, but Alicia knew she'd be company for no one. She needed to recover by herself, she needed to be on her own and have the time to think it all out.

Diana had driven Alicia to Heathrow to catch her flight. The last thing her mother had said, during a tearful goodbye, was that no matter what the future held, she must always believe in the absolute certainty that Guy loved her completely. Something beyond the bounds of their own knowledge and understanding must have happened but Alicia should never give up hope. She must rest and try to get over the shock in order to be able to go forward again. Diana was as reassuring as anybody could be, given the circumstances, saying that she would try to do a little more research herself while Alicia was away, … 'but with the utmost discretion', Diana had added, winking at her daughter, conscious of Alicia's feelings towards her stepfather.

~

Her mother had originally heard of the Italian island of Delfino through friends who had all spent a day there, exploring, while on their holiday a year before. They had looked around the guesthouse after lunch in the restaurant and had been enchanted with both the location and Gianni Vivarini's family. They had intended to return there themselves one day and Diana, remembering the photos of the holiday, thought what an ideal place it would be for her daughter to recuperate.

Alicia wanted to hide and Diana was quite right, Delfino Island was perfect for her. She had been dealt a shattering blow which had deeply undermined her usual self-confidence. Alicia didn't wish to go anywhere she might run into somebody she knew and who might be aware of her unhappy situation. How could she explain what had occurred, when she had no idea and was in such turmoil herself?

Had she just been dumped, almost at the altar? No, never that, it just was not possible. There had to be some explanation, somewhere, as to what had happened to Guy. He would never have left her in this way. First and foremost Alicia knew she had to find out if he was alive. Her gut feeling told her that he was and that he could only have disappeared for some fundamental and unavoidable reason. For now, she needed time to recover and regain her strength so that she could think rationally before making a sensible plan of action. God willing, she would by then have had some news from either Julian or Nick or even from her mother.

★★★

CHAPTER 4

Alicia arrived at the guest house on Delfino in a state of utter disarray. Normally she loved being on the sea, but nothing was normal and she hadn't even enjoyed the boat trip across from the mainland. She felt as if she'd aged ten years and been through several hedges backwards. But, with a mammoth effort, or so it had seemed at the time, she managed to struggle up the stairs to her room, where she collapsed on the bed, in a heap, quite oblivious to her surroundings. Her hosts were kind and considerate and after seeing Alicia settled, left her to her own devices that first night.

It was late and Giuseppina, sensing Alicia's exhaustion perhaps, had put a tray of food, covered with a cloth, on the table in the window. Alicia ate thankfully, gulped down copious amounts of water and then sat for a while in a daze, considering whether or not she had the energy to attempt a shower. Yes, she would feel better if she did, she decided. She stripped off her crumpled clothes, leaving them in a pile on the floor. She was alone, they could stay there till the morning: there was no one to see, to tell her off or to tease.

An immense sense of relief flowed over her with the warm and cleansing water, drowning the prospect of more unshed tears. The shower was a comfort and she stood in its warm, steamy atmosphere for a long time. Falling into bed and finding a hot water bottle there before her, had to be the greatest luxury she could possibly have wished for at that precise moment. When I die, thought Alicia as she passed into oblivion, I hope that I'll have an old fashioned hot water bottle to hang on to.

~

The next morning Alicia woke early. It was her 'sad and bad' time these days, when she felt at her lowest ebb, so she got up, dressed in her tracksuit and trainers and went outside. She would go down to the beach and watch the sunrise, finding the path which she had noticed lit by the house lights, when she had arrived the night before. It wound its way towards the vineyard and Gianni had said it led to the sea.

Alicia took her coat from the peg by the door and crept out of the house, not wishing to disturb her hosts. It was still cool. She licked her lips and tasted the slight salt in the damp air. As she listened, she could hear the gentle rhythm of the sea, in the distance, as it caressed the sand, in and out, like a whisper slithering up the beach only to retreat, drawn incessantly back again. Alicia loved that nostalgic sound. She must find it. The soft scent of a rose reached her nostrils. She'd unwittingly brushed against it when putting on her coat. She bent to touch its perfect velvet petals, releasing more of its sweet, musky fragrance. Even in an unkind world, thought Alicia disconsolately, nature and natural beauty still managed to emerge triumphant, making a mockery of man's destructive efforts.

She walked down the well-worn path, past some chicken coops in which the birds were beginning to stir. The sickly, acrid, stench from the hen house invoked memories of collecting eggs as a child on her grandparents' farm. The smell was poignantly strong in the chill atmosphere. She walked on towards the vines. The sky was lightening all the time. She could just see the face of her watch: twenty past five. The sun would soon be on its way. The footpath was easy to follow, soon becoming a wider, rutted, track, running straight as a die between the bushes. The grapes were already well in leaf and beautifully tended, Alicia noticed, peering at them with interest. That must be Gianni's work. She had only just met the couple the night before but she had taken an instant liking to both of them. She would be safe here. The whole place had a good feel about it.

The path came to an abrupt halt by the end of the vineyard at the edge of a narrow, rough cut, field. The sound of the sea was much louder now: she was almost there. She felt her adrenalin pump with the excitement of this small achievement. Her eyes had become accustomed to the light and she could see the way better. Someone else walked this route and often, by the look of the flattened grass. It led through some rocks and finally onto the beach.

When Alicia walked onto the sand her heart lifted. A boost of energy surged through her body and hope lifted her spirits. Yes, indeed; she was going to be very fine here.

~

Alicia resolved to leave her unsettling thoughts and worries well alone until she felt of a calmer mind. Her first day fulfilled its dawn promise perfectly, so she decided to explore the whole island. The best thing was that it didn't matter how long it took, there were no time limits. She set out on this 'positive plan of action' with determination and interest, fuelled with the added bonus that she might also exhaust herself into sleeping properly again at night. Her mother's advice to do something constructive had not gone unheeded: so she'd take some paper and make notes for the office travel department on the way.

She soon came to know and love the island; it was unique. Delfino was quite small, only about seven miles in length and maybe three across, so she could bike the whole way round in a day and often did, taking one of Giuseppina's *ciabatta* sandwiches and a bottle of water in a small bag on her back.

The single road was little more than a track and as the islanders used tractors or bicycles, for the most part, it was unusually quiet. There were some who kept an old car on the mainland, in the port of Biri, for visiting family and friends off the island. One Italian family, Alicia thought, could quite likely populate an entire city. Everybody with whom she ever came in touch seemed to be some sort of relation to Gianni's family. When she mentioned this to him, he proudly told her, laughing, that the population of the whole island came to some sixty-nine people and every one was either a direct relation or had some particularly strong family connection.

The islanders were self-sufficient in most things. They grazed sheep, kept cows and goats and everybody had chickens! The eggs tasted quite different, laid by hens that were free, in the true sense of the word. Fish was plentiful, for most of the year, and even in the winter the sea was seldom dangerously rough for long, the main fishing waters being well protected by the natural lie of the land. The farmers made hay in the summer, harvested their fruit, olives and grapes in the autumn and spent the winter preparing for the next season. The elder women made lace or knitted so that there would be plenty to sell in the summer shops or in the weekly market. Everyone's income was in some way supplemented by the influx of summer tourists. All in all, the island's people earned enough income from the holiday makers to carry them through the winter months.

Rosato was the only village, with a picturesque little harbour, a restaurant and one shop. It was named, many years ago, after the island's special brand of sparkling rosé wine, or the other way around, nobody seemed to know which had come first. The shop was owned by Gianni's father Allessandro and his cherished wife, Ana Maria. Soon they would have been married fifty years.

The family gave the elderly couple willing help in the store, especially the little ones, who could always count on some little treat from the old lady. Ana Maria kept the shelves well stocked with all of the items she considered to be essential for both the men and women and particularly for the children, and she was still considered to be the best cook on the island. The fresh fruit and vegetables all came from the local orchards or from the twice weekly deliveries and there were plentiful groceries, hardware, pharmaceuticals and lots of toys. If anything else was needed, Ana Maria would place her order with her younger son, Mario, who would bring it back from Biri on the mainland, with the daily supplies that he fetched for their restaurant. The enterprising proprietors had even organized a once weekly dry-cleaning service for the island folk.

Two or three times a year the travelling gypsy salesmen would arrive, in old converted ferryboats laden to the gunwales with ceramic pots and urns, kitchen utensils, linen, plastic buckets, dustpans and brushes, cheap furniture, bicycles and even push chairs and prams for new babies. One of the larger boats boasted a 'garden centre' offering a variety of plants, small ornamental bushes and even olive and fruit trees, all bound together on the aft deck. They did a roaring trade in every description of farm implements and tools for the fields and vineyards, taking orders in advance for the next season. Any larger building items, or pieces of machinery, would be brought over in yet another rusty old tub, which had been adapted by a company on the mainland supplying all the islands down the coast and which looked as if it could sink at any minute.

The islanders looked forward to Biri's monthly market, which sold everything imaginable, taking the opportunity to catch up with news and to gossip with relatives and friends. On these days, the little café on the port supplemented its income tenfold! Boats would go back and forth all day between Biri and the island, packed with people, produce and even small livestock. Alicia wondered if the locals had ever worried about the officious new EU regulations for loading ferries! Gianni said that he thought the port police either turned a blind eye or bribed the inspectors to keep away on market days.

Nowadays, mature animals were shipped over in sturdier, specially equipped, boats. The locals had eventually accepted that horses, full grown cattle, goats and pigs, all without any proper holding pens, did not mix too well with the tourists on the journey, especially when the sea was choppy.

The meat for the village mostly came from the local farms. The farmers would bring it in, freshly butchered and collect their bread at the same time. Here again was an ancient practice under threat from the European Union with its new fangled rules and regulations on abattoirs. The islanders had been butchering their own meat for centuries, with no known ill effect on anyone. Indeed the extra meat brought in from the mainland was considered to be far inferior to their own.

An inspector, Giorgio, would come over twice a month to meet the farmers and to check all their meat for disease and standards of cleanliness. Mario reluctantly agreed to bring him across in his boat precariously squeezed in with his early morning supplies. Giorgio would sit uncomfortably surrounded by sacks and boxes. He didn't like the sea, or being on it. If he thought it was going to be rough he would visit the island by way of the small passenger ferry, which he considered to be the better option, even if he did have to pay the fare himself.

Giorgio was no relation for once, not even a friend. Worse, he was an employee of the State and considered to be thoroughly puffed up with his own importance. He was doing a job that the islanders thought a waste of time, paid for from the hard earned taxes they all had to bear. So he wasn't wanted, no one liked him and most ignored him, keeping out of his way. Ana Maria couldn't help feeling slightly sorry for him, when he arrived looking green and disorientated. She kept him plied with cups of coffee and sweet biscuits until he had recovered enough to start out to the old market place to begin his checks. Once he had finished, the men got rid of him as quickly as possible, after which the farmers would produce their better hung meat from somewhere around the corner! Any meat not immediately sold was frozen in freezers which were kept well stocked in wintertime, when the sea might be too unpredictable for travel or for fishing.

When Mario ferried the inspector back to the mainland at the end of the morning, Alicia wondered if Giorgio had any idea what all the laughter was about, as the noise must have carried across the water to the boat as it headed out of the harbour. She rather hoped he didn't, but Gianni laughed as loudly as any, saying that Giorgio was a miserable little man and came from a bad family in any case.

~

Alicia's favourite place on Delfino was the lovely shell beach that she had found on her first morning at the end of Gianni's own land. It was totally secluded and she enjoyed being alone there. But she also liked visiting the other end of the island, which was quite different: perhaps five or six hundred feet above sea level, it was more cultivated, the fields were verdant green and now that it was spring, the hills were clothed in a profusion of many, different coloured, wild-flowers. The scattered farms and small holdings were few and far between, surrounded by their own olive groves, orchards and vineyards. They were a picture to see in the clear, early, mornings or in the soft light of the evening. Alicia wished she'd brought her camera with her from England, but she'd forgotten it when she had left home in such wretched confusion.

Alicia would sometimes borrow an old bicycle and peddle away up into the hill country by herself. It was a hard climb on the outward journey, so she would determine to reach the highest point without having to dismount. Physical exertion seemed to help her mental state. This small goal achieved, she would allow herself a break and find somewhere quiet and out of the wind, to sit and think. She would eat the food she carried and stare out over the sea towards the mainland; if she could make her mind blank afterwards she would doze. When disturbing thoughts started to rattle around in her head she would move on once more. On these occasions she would return quieter than ever. Giuseppina noticed and made it her business to talk to the people who lived on the farms, asking those she knew and liked best to look out for the sad English girl. Alicia had no inkling of Giuseppina's kind interference and was rather surprised when the farm people began to stop her for a friendly chat.

She began to get to know and understand the people and their way of life and made a conscious effort to learn from them. They liked and accepted her with the generous capacity for warmth that Italian people so easily bestow, particularly responding to her interest in their homes and their traditional customs.

When the farm people were busy, or short handed, Alicia would help in whatever way she could. If she came across a herd of sheep or goats being moved from one pasture to another she would jump off her bike and lend a hand, blocking their escape routes in one direction or the other. Once she found two sheep caught up in some brambles and concerned for their plight, set about freeing the distressed pair with little thought for her bare legs and arms. The farmer appeared with his tractor and trailer just as the sheep delightedly regained their freedom. After checking the rest of the flock the young man insisted on his wife seeing to Alicia's scratches. He gave both Alicia and her bike a lift up to the house; but she was happy to have been of some use. She felt that these occasions brought at least some purpose to her life on their island. Her Italian improved with use and from memory, although she wondered if she was acquiring a 'Delfino' accent at which her aunt Caro in Venice would protest.

As time went by, Alicia found herself more and more frequently invited into the islanders' homes and being offered something to eat or drink, after the work was done. The island folk were aware of the unhappiness in the young woman. In accord with Giuseappina, they sensed that there was much more to Alicia's misery than one of life's accepted upsets. They were polite and sympathetic, yet chose, in this instance, to remain, at least outwardly, incurious. Alicia was no threat to them. They took her to their hearts, included her in their every day lives as much as possible and by so doing, hoped to make her life a little happier. The men couldn't understand how a woman like Alicia could still be unmarried and most wished that they could be held responsible for bringing a smile to her face.

The older Delfino inhabitants had heard much about and seen pictures of England, but although many of their summer visitors were English, most of the senior residents had never journeyed far afield. They had no wish or reason to travel. They were content; they had everything they needed on the island and were happy to leave the exploring to the young ones. The more advanced generation was not in the least bit interested in any 'change' to their lifestyle or their natural habitat.

Alicia read a lot, devouring the many books left behind on the guest house bookshelves by previous visitors. She found one that Guy had in his own collection at home, which startled her. She wondered who would have had this particular book on the island, of all places. It was an unusual book from a set on military strategy, with a subtitle about surveillance counter-measures, not at all what you would consider holiday reading. It was strange that someone else had stayed here, sharing a taste in such specialist books. She took it out and flicked through the pages. It had long lost its original cover, as had Guy's. It gave her an odd feeling. She shivered involuntarily and put it back in its place. What was the saying? 'A ghost walking over your grave?' Alicia turned quickly away, understanding the expression. 'How much Guy would love this island and how well he would get on with Gianni and his family', she muttered out loud, 'but where the hell is he?'

With the sea air and healthy way of living, Alicia finally began to sleep again. Life on the island was peaceful and calm and went at altogether another pace. She even swam once, as it was unseasonably warm for so early in the year. But only once, after being thoroughly ticked off by Giuseppina, who had spied Alicia returning in her wet swimming costume, marched her off into the warm kitchen and enveloped her in a huge towel, before sitting her down to a cup of hot, frothy, chocolate. It was almost as if her lovely refreshing swim had in fact been a dangerous ordeal! She had been told, in no mean way, that no self-respecting Italian would ever consider swimming off the island until at least July. Swimming at any other time of the year was for the 'fish, and the real dolphins', she was firmly informed.

"But I'm English," Alicia had protested, "and I enjoyed it!"

"Never mind! When I am in England," retorted Giuseppina, which was only once during the last twenty-seven years, Alicia had later discovered, "I am English. Here I am Italian," she concluded, as if that explained everything.

★★★

CHAPTER 5

Giuseppina and Gianni Vivarini's little guesthouse; an old farmhouse which had expanded into the surrounding buildings, was a haven of peace, encircled on three sides by the family vineyard. Alicia felt secure, cocooned in its midst. It had a cosy, family, atmosphere, was spotlessly clean, cheerfully decorated and smelled aired and fresh after Giuseppina had thrown open the windows each morning to let the mild spring breeze into the rooms.

The friendly dining room, with its red and white checked tablecloths, led out onto a tiled terrace shaded by a prolific vine which, later in the year, produced the sweetest of all the grapes on the island. Here the family cat would be installed in her usual place in the sun, with her kittens scrambling all over her. Giuseppina was proud of her vine, which she had planted when she and Gianni had first been married. Everybody had said that it wouldn't grow in the position she'd chosen, she told Alicia, but she'd proved them all wrong, which had been the best part: it had been her very first triumph after marrying into the family!

Giuseppina and Gianni used a big room behind the kitchen, opening out onto a separate patio surrounded by a trellis covered in seemingly perpetual flowering roses. The natural wooden staircase, made by Gianni's grandfather, led upstairs from a small hallway between the kitchen and dining room. At the top of the stairs, to the left, a door led to Giuseppina and Gianni's bedroom, with its huge bed covered by a beautiful white bedcover, handmade by Giuseppina's mother as a traditional wedding present. Gianni's grandfather had also made the carved headboard, now handed down to the third generation. All Gianni's family had been both conceived and born in that bed and they were all proud in that knowledge. Outside the bedroom was a small balcony, with wrought iron railings entwined by the sweet scented rose from the terrace beneath.

In deference to the English side of Giuseppina's nature and her insistence for the need to 'soak' in wintertime, the Vivarini's had their own very large bath tub; this provoked much light hearted teasing from the rest of the family, who considered it extravagant, although Patrizia, surreptitiously, had enjoyed it's benefits whilst heavily pregnant. Next door, was a little room, for visiting grandchildren, with scarcely enough space for the bed, amongst all the boxes of toys. Giuseppina loved to have the little ones sleeping near to her, but always said that it was to give the parents a rest at night, without them having to worry: not that anyone believed this! Behind a long red curtain, across the far corner, was Giuseppina's secret den where she kept all her sewing equipment. The many coloured bits and pieces were a constant source of delight amongst the younger children, who loved to help her when she was making something, but when they 'assisted', the work would, of course, take twice as long. Anything considered at all 'suspect', as far as the bambinos safety was concerned, she stored in bright boxes on tantalizingly high shelves, above their heads, to be stared at longingly by the little people before sleep finally overcame them.

A door on the other side of the stairs led to three further bedrooms, each with its own small terrace, but a different view of the sea. Alicia's room had windows both on the front and on the side, letting the light and sun flood in all through the day. The curtains were thin and faded, old friends, washed and dried in the sun countless times, she imagined. They were so feather, light, that the softest wind made them dance. She often stood on her balcony, breathing in the smell of the sea and gazing out over the vineyard or, if she turned, looking out to the little harbour on the other side with all the brightly coloured boats coming and going. Alicia loved the comfy, simple furnishings, with their gentle, bleached, colours. She wanted for nothing. She had a small, but immaculate, tiled bathroom with a shower, which proved surprisingly efficient. There were even two old fashioned radiators, one in each room, which clonked, clanked and hissed their way into action every morning and at night. They filled the rooms with heat so quickly that Alicia, unable to turn them off herself, would soon have to be throwing the windows wide open. She hadn't the heart to tell either Gianni or Giuseppina that, being English and well used to the damp and the cold, she really didn't need them.

Outside, the rambling outbuildings enclosed a well worn courtyard, with stables, cattle pens, storage barns full of wine vats, agricultural implements and even an ancient olive press. One of the barns had been made into an extra sitting room and play area for children, with a ping-pong table and television. Nowadays, however, unless there were family visiting or a party was being held, it was seldom used.

Patrizia, married to Gianni's younger brother Mario, ran the restaurant on the quay in Rosato. She also ran the 'fornaio' adjoining the restaurant. She and two other wives would start baking at dawn each day. The smell of fresh bread soon wafted over the whole village enticing the people out of their houses to collect their orders.

'Mario's' was the only real restaurant on the island, although in summer portable stalls of all kinds were set up selling local merchandise, produce, artifacts, snacks and delicacies. Over the years, the restaurant had become a general meeting place where the whole community could gather together to discuss Delfino concerns, sitting outside beside the water in the warmer months, or in front of the open log fire in the winter. Giuseppina often helped out, but how Patrizia managed to look after her four children and do all the cooking, especially in the busy summer months, Alicia couldn't imagine.

Giuseppina thought Patrizia was looking tired and voiced her suspicions! If Giuseppina was right, Alicia felt really sorry for Patrizia. How could she cope with yet another child? She was a remarkable woman with boundless energy. She worked so hard yet always appeared cheerful and happy. It was obvious to Alicia that Patrizia's family, the restaurant and the island were her life. Gianni told Alicia that Patrizia was earning herself the reputation of a very accomplished *'cucinare'* and it was time she put up her prices, at least to the tourists. 'She'd gained much of her expertise from Giuseppina and his mother Ana Maria, of course', said Gianni 'so they were at least partly responsible for Patrizia's success', he'd added with a satisfied grunt.

After returning from school on the mainland with the other children, Patrizia's two older boys sometimes helped their father in the fields or with his boat. They went by ferry across the water for their education, with their sister and the other older children. The only daughter, Anastasia, or Tarsia for short, who was twelve, loved to be left in charge of the shop when she was free and already made delicious sweet pastries for the restaurant, although this was not mentioned to the inquisitive food inspector.

Gi, the youngest member of the family, at four, was an angelic looking little boy with dark, tousled, hair and long curling eyelashes. Nobody could resist him. Whenever she was at home he would trail around after Tarsia, who spoilt him, especially when she was cooking. The other love of Gi's life was his uncle. As soon as Gianni was available, Gi would attach himself to his side. Nothing Gi did ever surprised Gianni in the least: he was a mirror image of himself as a boy. He adored his nephew and to his parent's frequent annoyance, always stuck up for the child whenever he was in trouble, which was often. Gianni laughed when little Gi was reprimanded and usually said that he would have done the same thing himself at that age, given the chance.

Mario's family lived behind and above the restaurant. The so-called 'garden', protected by an old dry stone wall, was more of an unkempt field, which served as a play area for the children, home to a few chickens and a place to dry the daily washing. With her English love of gardening Alicia longed to get her hands on it. Sheltered from the onshore wind and with so much sun throughout the year, she could picture it full of shrubs of every kind, with beds of exotic fragrant flowers around an orange grove in the centre.

'Mario's' restaurant opened onto a terrace, with terracotta urns and different sized pots around the walls, all planted with scented geraniums trailing down to the old weathered floor tiles that had been laid by their grandfather, obviously a man of many skills. The tables were shaded from the heat by an old vine, all tangled together with pink roses, climbing up and around each corner support and out over the overhead wires stretched between the walls. Alicia's loved to sit where she could look out over the garden on one side, or towards the harbour and the boats on the other. It was a lovely spot. No wonder people returned year after year.

The few, little, painted houses, clustered round the harbour, were inhabited by fishermen, again mostly Vivarini family relations. Dimitri, Gianni and Mario's elder brother lived there. He had been appointed harbour-master and was in charge of all of the fishing on the island. He told Alicia that the houses along the quay had originally been painted in bright colours for the same reason as those on Burano, off Venice; to help guide the fishermen safely home on a misty day. They had wanted to decorate them again now, but the busybodies on the mainland would not give permission. He and his brothers had agreed that they would do it anyway, in the summer.

Dimitri was a hugely strong man, taller and broader than his brothers. Once, so the story said, he had raised a car high on his shoulders saving the life of a man trapped underneath. He was a shy, gentle, giant who had made it quite clear that he had no wish to take his father's place as head of the family when Allessandro had retired. So Gianni, much better suited, took the important decisions on their behalf, although he always discussed the various ideas with his brothers after respectfully asking his father's advice first.

Alicia had seen Dimitri returning from fishing, wet and exhausted, yet still smiling, finding the patience to lift up his doting little fans, one by one, to show them his catch of squirming silver fish in the bottom of his boat. He was the only one as yet unmarried. The woman in his life, to whom he had been engaged, had been killed in a terrible car accident near Bologna some years before and he'd taken a long time to get over the tragedy. Giuseppina said that he was now 'seeing' someone who was eminently suitable. They were all delighted! 'The woman was still young enough to have his children as she was not yet forty', Giuseppina had added with relish.

Alicia was glad. Dimitri was a wasted man on his own and he obviously longed to have a family. Perhaps he shouldn't wait too long to pop the question, she thought, as she watched him busy mending his nets in the sun, after morning school, surrounded by the children as usual. If Alicia was doing nothing else she liked to join them. She soon knew them all by name and little Gi, though shy to begin with in front of the others, would eventually come to sit on her knee. They would all listen, in spellbound silence, to Dimitri's stories of the sea embellished with lots of extra little people from fairyland. He had a natural way with children and a special gift for storytelling.

Dimitri's audiences included adults as well. Nobody was ever too old for the stories, which were based on the island and its history. The women would either knit or sew, while the older men would prop themselves up against the side of a boat, smoking or helping Dimitri untangle his nets. Ana Maria was forever urging her older son to write down his stories but Alicia suspected that he might find that difficult or perhaps considered it unmanly and that he wouldn't have had the time anyway.

At first light each day, with the stars not yet faded from the sky, Mario would chug over to the port of Biri on the mainland, to fetch the restaurant supplies and to bring back the two young girls who helped with the cleaning and chores. The cocks would crow almost in unison. This was Alicia's wake up call and she would arouse, comforted by the sounds of this daily routine. As she regained her energy she would often get up early too, dress warmly and go out into the cool morning. Sometimes she would go to the beach to watch the sunrise as she had on her very first day. At other times, she went to the harbour and stood listening to the distant, receding noise of Mario's boat out across the water. If the sea was flat calm and she really concentrated, she could just hear him cut the engine as he arrived at the port. Maybe one day she'd go with him, but perhaps he enjoyed having this short time to himself. This Alicia could well understand.

The bakery was the only building lit at this hour. As she passed by, Alicia could see Patrizia already beavering away in preparation for her early customers. The village was quiet and the fishermen not yet returned. Alicia would sit, as in a time warp, waiting for the day to begin. She loved the feel of the damp, dawn, air on her cheeks and the smell of the sea strengthened, perhaps, by the slight hint of fish wafting up from a fishing boat left behind on this run. Memories of childhood and happy summer holidays, spent trolling for mackerel in Ireland, would come flooding back: A safe memory. She would thrust her hands deep in the pockets of her coat and breath it all in. 'Medicine. This had to be the best medicine in the world', she reasoned, basking in the simple luxury of having the magical place all to herself.

At mid morning, with much accomplished and still in her apron, Patrizia would sit down and take a break, probably, thought Alicia, only on the insistence of her protective mother-in-law. On fine days, she and Ana Maria would wander across to join Dimitri's eager listeners, bringing chairs, pots of coffee, sweet biscuits and drinks for the children. Alicia loved these impromptu family gatherings, which had a habit of going on well past noon, when some of the working men would appear after their morning's work was done. Then they'd all have a plate of Patrizia's daily pasta. Miraculously, no matter how many people finally sat down, Patrizia always seemed to have enough food for everyone.

Over the years Gianni and his family had been frequently approached by business men and developers evaluating the potential of the island, but none of them had ever been tempted. It was their island and, as long as it remained under the supervision of their families, it was secure and there was no danger of any upheaval to their idyllic way of life. They needed for nothing. With the help and support they all gave to each other when problems arose, the islanders shared a good lifestyle enjoying peace of mind in abundance.

All through the, long, summer days the island buzzed with tourists, but it always came back to its own after the sun went down and the last boatload of visitors had left the little harbour. In reality, each month was just as busy as the next what with the harvest, followed by the September wine making, then the ploughing and replanting in winter and early spring, not to mention all the cleaning, decorating, mending and general preparation for the next summer season. In the autumn, at Christmas, in the New Year and at Easter, the islanders gave thanks in their tiny little chapel, which would be full to bursting. Alicia had often been told that no where else in the whole of Italy could celebrate a wedding as they did on Delfino! Their festivities could last for at least a week! Needless to say the priest, Father Antonio, was also a Vivarini relation, Gianni's uncle no less, a well respected and very important man.

Alicia decided that even the priest must have an exceptionally good life, here on the island!

★★★

CHAPTER 6

Time passed, the days rolled by, healing and restoring, each similar to the one before. The weather remained constant, with the soft spring rain infrequent and usually falling only at night. After several weeks on the island, Alicia realized that she felt very much better. In fact, she felt quite different, strong and healthy again, at least.

She'd had two calls each week from Guy's cousin, Nick. Until recently he had reported little progress in England. In their last conversation however there seemed to have been a breakthrough and he sounded cautiously excited. Trying not to raise her hopes falsely, Nick had told Alicia that he thought that his contact within intelligence had some relevant information which he seemed unwilling, or unable, to impart. He wasn't sure which. At their last meeting the man, called Jonathan, had visibly flinched at the mention of Guy's name and the look on his face had spelt barely disguised alarm.

Nick, instantly alerted, had put in many hours working on this connection, outside his own business day, pretending friendship and a liking for squash, which he had soon discovered featured considerably in the man's life. Nick hated squash and hadn't played since school so hoped he wouldn't have to now, particularly as he'd had to make out that he was keen on the game himself. So far he'd managed to avoid a contest being booked and it had been a good talking point. When the two had last met up, in a bar after work, Jonathan had begun to unwind after a couple of drinks, mixed particularly strong under Nick's supposedly generous, yet calculated, guidance. Nick had felt sure that he was about to be enlightened.

Unfortunately, they were interrupted by a telephone call insisting on the young man's immediate presence elsewhere. The situation was particularly curious as Nick, listening intently, thought he caught his own name being mentioned on the other end of the mobile. Although distant, the voice was well articulated and carried. Jonathan had unguardedly raised his eyes to look at Nick as he spoke, giving himself away and then nervously jumping up and walking off to where he could not be overheard.

Nick watched from a distance, pretending disinterest, as he drank his beer, whilst his ears strained to hear more. Jonathan had turned his back for privacy, the mobile pressed firmly to his ear and covered with both hands as he took his orders. There was a clipped, hurried, interchange, during which he glanced once over his shoulder in Nick's direction. Nick looked away just in time. It was obvious they were talking about him and that he wasn't meant to hear, so he feigned ignorance once more, smiling at a pretty blonde girl sitting by herself at the far end of the bar.

Jonathan had returned embarrassed, excusing himself, saying that although he was supposed to be off duty, his superior had called and he was afraid that he'd have to leave. 'Once you worked for these people your life is no longer your own', he'd muttered, his tongue the looser for drink, as he shook hands and said goodbye. Nick drew his attention to the girl at the bar, made a mild joke about his evening having only just begun and Jonathan, looking somewhat relieved, promptly left. There was no doubt that he had been warned off from talking.

Nick went on to tell Alicia that he was going to arrange another meeting and had no intention of giving up until he had some information about whatever was going on, or proof that Guy was alive. It wasn't going to be easy, as alarm bells were now ringing, but Nick was now more determined than ever to find out what was being hidden from him. One thing was already certain: there had to be some covert activity in motion, for those in seniority to have proved quite so deliberately unhelpful. Alicia must try not to worry too much, a tall order he knew, until he could continue with his investigations and find out more. Nick said he was also in touch with her mother Diana, who was of the same mind.

A tall order indeed: Alicia felt a wave of excited frustration pass through her stomach. Nick had obviously touched on something extremely delicate that could possibly involve Guy. His questions weren't being appreciated within the very secret world of Intelligence. He had done well finding out this much. She had to trust his judgment and wait to see what happened next. There was absolutely no point whatsoever in her rushing back to England to rock the boat. Nick wanted her out of the way: that much he had made very clear.

~

Meanwhile, at home, Julian also was still out of touch. It was now several weeks since Adriana had heard from him, which was unusual in itself. It was the longest time they had ever been apart. According to Nick, Julian's text messages to his girl-friend had also stopped, although this hadn't seemed to worry Adriana very much. Apparently, Julian seldom used this method of contact. A decent signal was hard to find in the type of terrain in which he so frequently travelled.

Alicia couldn't help but speculate on whether there could be any connection with Guy's disappearance. Why should there be? Except perhaps because of their shared past. Nick had done his homework well. He had said that he didn't think it likely that the two situations were in any way related, but that he would look into it further, surreptitiously, without worrying Adriana.

Alicia had posted various cards home implying that she was feeling much better, which she was, physically. Her mother would read between the lines, but at least she'd be pleased to have some news. She'd received a letter each week in return, telling her about matters at home and Diana's own research, being carried on discreetly, through her now rather outdated military circles. Her last letter had said that, at a London cocktail party, she had met the son of an old friend, a young man she knew to be rapidly rising in his cho-

sen field of military intelligence. A single remark, indicating her disappointment that her daughter had been forced to postpone her wedding to Guy
Hargreaves on account of his enormous workload abroad, had produced an
instant reaction. Diana told Alicia, with some amusement, that she now had
her first experience of being 'literally dropped like a hot brick'! Alicia sensed
that her mother was pleased to be doing something to help and that now
perhaps, she might even begin to enjoy a little intrigue, particularly if her
husband wasn't in any way involved.

So, merely letting slip Guy's name at the party had produced the same result as that within Nick's diplomatic world: an instant closing of ranks. Both
Nick and Diana had been left with the distinct and positive impression that
someone, somewhere, did indeed know something of great importance to
them all.

Diana had spoken to Guy's elderly parents several times, but had merely
commented that their mutual children seemed to need a little more time
before they married and that Guy had been sent overseas on an important
job. They knew this already, but Diana made a mental note of the approxi-
mate date when they said they had last heard from their son, which tied
up with Alicia's findings. They had seemed to accept the situation and had
not questioned her further, only adding that they were worried about any
wasted wedding costs. Diana had immediately put their minds at rest saying
that there had been no expenses at all, knowing full well that both would
have been horrified had they ever found out just how much she had forked
out on the various cancelled bookings. She had also suggested to Alicia that
she might like to send them a card or two, to reassure them a little further.
When next she wrote, Alicia pointed out, with some irritation, that she had
already done so - three times!

Alicia told her office that she was putting together an article entitled
'Unspoilt and Idyllic Islands off the East coast of Italy' and would carry
out some research on the mainland as well, particularly on the best ferry
connections, which were not easy to find, even on the internet. Hopefully
this would keep the people in her department quiet for the moment. She

didn't want them to think that she was taking advantage of their generous support.

~

Night time was the worst and Alicia dreamt. No matter what she'd done in the day or how much exercise she had taken, she dreamt vividly. An overly active mind endlessly searching for answers, she concluded, it never let up, even when deeply asleep. She would wake with a start when the radiator, completely unasked, would throw itself into action in the early hours of the morning stifling her room. Alicia would automatically stretch out her arm across the bed to Guy for comfort, only to find a cold, empty space. She would turn her hand palm down and smooth the soft worn sheet, profoundly troubled, as she remembered her predicament yet again.

At such times, Alicia would get out of her bed, pull on a warm fleece and go out onto the small balcony, where there was a chair protected from the dew by a plastic sheet. Treading softly, she would remove the covering and place the chair carefully, aware that any noise would disturb the chickens or the birds and then the tranquility of the moment would be shattered. She'd sit huddled up, her knees drawn up to her chin, her hands clasped around them, as she listened to the subdued night sounds and the distant, muted, voice of the sea. It was warmer now than when she had first arrived, the early morning air no longer chill, with spring fast giving way to summer. 'A lovely comfortable climate to be alone in.' Alicia would say to herself, 'if you had to be alone'. Then, lulled into a feeling of relative peace once more, as she heard Mario's boat setting off to collect his supplies, she would return to her room and sleep late, somewhat heartened.

Giuseppina and Gianni watched with gentle and concerned interest. They were fond of the quiet, anxious, girl in their midst, but they sensed that they could do nothing for the time being, except to cater for her practical needs. Alicia was an easy guest. Spending most of her time outside, as summer approached, both felt that she was in the best possible place to recover from whatever was causing her such distress. They watched as her skin turned a better colour, the dark circles under her eyes started to disappear and her fair hair began to lighten in the sun and to shine again. The sea air had also done wonders for her appetite, thought Giuseppina, pleased. Alicia looked less angular and gaunt and was starting to fill out. Thank goodness she had not caught pneumonia trying to swim in the sea so early in the year, in her weak state. She had done right to put a stop to that!

Gianni saw to it that there was always plenty of his best wine to accompany Giuseppina's varied but simple meals. At night, he would leave an open bottle of *Amaretto* and another of homemade *limoncello* on the side, hoping that Alicia would help herself and sleep the better for it.

~

"It's time our guest saw a little life again," said Giuseppina awaking one morning, as if continuing a conversation already started. "Maybe a trip to the mainland would be a good idea. She could stay with Amalia and Stefano, then go on to Vittorio and Francesca and visit the Opera in Verona. The *Teatro Filarmonico* has good productions most of the year round. It's lovely and quiet there now, before the season at the Arena starts and a girl like Alicia must love our opera, don't you think? She could also shop. Verona has smart shops and all women like to shop and … she could check on Francesca for me," added Giuseppina as an afterthought with a wink at her husband. "Perhaps then, on her return, she will feel like joining us for the family party for the old ones' golden wedding."

"*Si, si*, a good plan, *amore mia*," replied Gianni, chuckling and seeing straight through his wife. She was longing for more grandchildren as she watched the little ones around her growing up much too fast. "I will suggest it, you clever woman!"

Gianni shook his big curly head and, with a twinkle in his eye, set off to look for Alicia. It amazed him that, after all this time, Giuseppina still managed to make him speak in English, unless he was too tired, when she'd grudgingly relent as he started tripping over his words, but even that only made her laugh. When this happened he'd become annoyed and would not speak at all! They'd come to an understanding, at the beginning of their marriage, but only after an immense struggle. Giuseppina had won the battle and taught Gianni English with much patience and even more laughter. She had also taught their children, although this had been a lot easier. Now the two languages mixed quite naturally and with little effort. There was no doubt at all that it had served them well over the years, particularly in the restaurant and now in the hotel, as a great many of their summer visitors were English.

The younger members of the island families also spoke the language reasonably well, especially the small children, most of whom were still taught by Guiseppina in the little kindergarten that she'd started many years before, beside the chapel. When they went on to the schools across the water, English was now one of the most important subjects. Alicia would drop in to help if she thought Giuseppina was overly busy, so that she could leave a little earlier than usual to help Patrizia, or perhaps to pop over to the mainland for a visit with friends. Alicia's pupils soon lost their shyness. She would make them sit around her, whilst she told them simple stories. She genuinely enjoyed her time with the children and especially with little Gi, who would sidle up and insist on sitting in her lap, 'as she was his': Alicia being his latest conquest!

~

Alicia welcomed the idea of the visit to Verona, although she looked forward to it with some trepidation, so the arrangements were quickly made before she could change her mind. She felt safe and secure where she was and loved her little island retreat and the calm, caring, atmosphere into which the family had made her so welcome. But, in her heart, she knew she couldn't stay and hide indefinitely and thought it might be good to enter the real world again, if only for a few days, happy in the knowledge that her room was there for her return, whenever she wanted it.

Teresa, the Vivarini's youngest daughter, was due home from her university in Milan, so Alicia felt that it would be best for the family to have the house to themselves for a few days, particularly as Teresa was said to be involved with 'an unsuitable boy.' According to Giuseppina, Teresa needed to talk to her father about it. This had been said with much feeling. Alicia had thought that it rather sounded as if they were expecting fireworks but Gianni had merely laughed, saying that whoever took on their youngest would have to be a very brave man indeed and the sooner the better!

Mario was to take Alicia across the water to Biri. Another relation would meet them in the port and from there would take her to their village in Northern Tuscany, not far from Bologna, where she would spend the night. It would be an easy journey by train to Verona via Bologna the next morning.

The day of departure dawned bright and clear. Alicia experienced a moment of panic. She didn't really want to leave this peaceful haven now that the time had come. Giuseppina sat her down to a huge breakfast, as if Alicia was travelling half way across the world and then presented her with her idea of a 'small picnic', in case she needed food on the way. Alicia felt slightly sick again, an unexplained queasiness in her upper stomach, but concluded that it was, more than likely, just nerves. It was time to pull herself together and get on with life now that she was in a better state.

She packed few clothes. She hadn't much with her after leaving England in such sad confusion. Now she could shop for anything she needed in the city, something to which she really looked forward. She did love shopping. She would buy some new clothes. It would make her feel better, more in control of things again. Alicia dressed casually, wrapping a warm jersey around her shoulders before setting off with Gianni for the village quay.

Mario was an identical, if younger and slimmer version of Gianni, who always seemed to be smiling and laughing. Nicknamed 'Doctor Mario', if anybody felt ill they were referred to him, 'pronto'. 'Go see Mario' they'd say 'he'll make you feel better!' and he usually did. When the real doctor came over from the mainland on his weekly visits he would say that he never had to worry about his Delfino patients, with such an excellent assistant as Mario! This had been proved to be true. Mario had once even delivered a baby before the midwife had time to arrive and the celebrations had lasted for three days, with 'Dr Mario' being made a godfather.

Mario was waiting, accompanied by two of his sons, with a large grin for Alicia and an endearing bear hug for his brother. His eldest child politely took Alicia's bag and stowed it carefully in the bottom of his father's boat as Gianni lifted little Gi up onto his shoulders. Giuseppina had been correct in her assumption. The Vivarini clan had all just been told that Mario and Patrizia were expecting yet another child. This one would be their fifth and everybody awaited the forthcoming event with much excitement. They really were the closest of families which was what Alicia most loved about them. After her time spent in Gianni and Giuseppina's household she felt that she'd known them all forever and was part of it too.

~

Gianni stood with the little boy, holding his hand as he watched Mario's boat disappear around the headland. He felt another strange twinge of apprehension crawl down the back of his neck and decided to ring his two sons-in-law again. They must look out for her. He turned away with a wry smile. He was treating this woman like one of his own, but she worried him very much. Something was wrong, very wrong indeed. He'd like to get to the bottom of it and wished he could get rid of his anxiety and an uncomfortable feeling of foreboding.

Alicia had received regular calls on her mobile. It never left her side and each time it rang she would rush to answer the noisy little object, a look akin to despair on her set features. Gianni didn't think these intrusions were business orientated, at least not all of them. He'd noticed her pacing up and down as she talked, usually just out of earshot, around the side of the house, but the situation obviously wasn't in any way resolved, because afterwards her face would be pale and she'd be lost in thought, almost as if oblivious to her surroundings. Often she would head off down to her favorite place, the beach, where she would walk for hours. Then, if Alicia missed a meal altogether, Giuseppina would worry about her even more.

None of them had ever seen a proper smile, a warmth in Alicia's eyes and a lift to her sensitive mouth in appreciation or gratefulness, an obvious friendly gesture to the family and others, yes: but never a real smile, a smile from the heart. She loved the children; that was obvious, especially little Gi. The two were close and Alicia derived much needed comfort from the little boy. Gianni could see it in her dispirited face. It would soften and change when she was with the child, as if she could put aside whatever was disturbing her just for a little while, when they were together. Giuseppina and Gianni both felt that she needed to talk, to let out her misery. She wasn't just unhappy, it was more, much more than that and they hoped that one day soon she would find a way to confide in them.

★★★

CHAPTER 7

Alicia enjoyed the sea trip with the sun and wind in her face. It took her breath away, cleared the cobwebs and whipped the colour into her cheeks. Once out of the harbour Mario roared over the water, laughing with exhilaration, as he warned her to hold on tight to the seat and the side of the boat. The voyage didn't take long at this break-neck speed and soon they were approaching the port of Biri. Mario throttled back as they rolled their way over the swell outside the harbour's protecting walls. He had been watching Alicia for her reaction and noted the sudden change, a glimmer of excitement and was glad. It was as he had intended.

When Mario had first ferried Alicia across to the island, some weeks before, she had been distracted and looked vulnerable and unhappy, frightened almost. He had said as much to his brother, on their arrival at the guest house, when Giusappina had taken her upstairs. As he'd walked away that night, he knew that he had left the distraught young woman in the very best of hands. Now he was pleased to see her looking so much better. Mario was a sensitive man and, in one so young, her obvious plight had touched his heart.

~

Alicia was feeling well rested. It was spring now. Nothing seemed quite so bleak. She experienced her first faint stirring of optimism, perhaps even hope for the future. New beginnings: after all, she'd only been here on this earth for twenty-six summers and she really couldn't spend every waking hour for the rest of her life worrying about what could or should have been. Coming to Italy had been the best plan she'd been able to devise so far. She loved this country.

She mulled over what Diana had said at the airport. 'Remember. If life throws chaos and disorder in your path, leaving indecision infinitum, get on with everything else as best you can, keep fit, busy, go away, just as you are doing, ... whatever... until something happens. Eventually the road will become clear again but when you least, expect it, you can be sure of that...' she had added, smiling reassuringly, as they kissed goodbye. Good advice, however difficult, Alicia thought now, for the umpteenth time. So, I am 'getting on with my life'.

Yet, there were many unanswered questions still buzzing around in her head. Little tit-bits kept coming back to her, as if teasing her brain for a possible clue; bits of conversation vaguely heard from that telephone call to Guy's mobile in the middle of the night. She must think back. What had she heard? If only she hadn't been so deeply asleep. It made her dizzy just trying to fathom it all.

One way or another, the riddle had to be unravelled and resolved. Patience was wearing thin. She wasn't going to sit around waiting indefinitely. Alicia was used to making decisions and acting upon them. Someone or something had taken control of their lives and turned them upside down, only now she felt ready to find out and do something about it. But exactly what? The way forward was still decidedly blurred.

Alicia was absolutely sure, now, that Guy wasn't dead. She just had to keep faith with that conclusion. Meanwhile she certainly did appreciate both this land and these people who had the thankless task of looking after her. Enough morbid thoughts! She was already enjoying this little excursion and it was great to be on the water again.

~

As the boat drew near to the steps Alicia could see Gianni and Giuseppina's son in law, Stefano, standing, watching them approach. Mario had told Alicia that Amalia had married a distant cousin, which explained the strong family resemblance. Stefano's stocky figure, curly dark hair and open smiling face, reminded her, even from a distance, of a younger edition of Gianni. Mario negotiated round the craft already on their moorings, shouting out a greeting to a passing fisherman.

Stefano stood grinning, his welcome while he waited. His teeth were so white in his tanned face that Alicia felt certain he could make a small fortune advertising them. Mario threw him the rope and Stefano helped them tie up the boat. Alicia stood gingerly and climbed up the old wrought iron ladder when instructed. She was relieved to be suitably shod as the steps were slippery and wrapped in seaweed from the last high tide. Further up they were badly eroded and heavily encrusted with barnacles; decidedly suspect. Stefano held a hand out as she neared the top.

"Be careful *Signorina*, these steps, very bad," then he laughed loudly as if the idea of Alicia going for an unplanned swim was very funny indeed.

Mario politely introduced Alicia, then suggested coffee before they all went their separate ways. She nodded, noting how pleased the men were to see each other as they rattled away in light-hearted camaraderie, with much back patting and laughter. Mario slung Alicia's bag over his shoulder and they all walked across to the café opposite. Meanwhile, at Mario's instruction, a young boy began loading the restaurant supplies into the boat from the stack made ready nearby.

A large cheerful woman, with the unlikely name of Clementina, came bustling out, calling "*benvenuta, welcome*" at the top of her voice, her face, alight with pleasure.

"*Mario, Stefano, come ti va? Signora inglese, buongiorno.*" She kissed Mario full on the lips while appraising Alicia at the same time. "*La Signorina e' carina, si Mario?*" She then enfolded Stefano in the same embrace. He was almost lost from sight altogether. "*Si bella!*" she pronounced staring unashamedly at Alicia again, nodding and roaring with laughter as she wagged a fat finger at the men. The men, obviously well used to this performance, ambled over to a table, pulled out a chair for Alicia and then sat themselves down, chuckling. Smiling to herself, Alicia had the good grace to study her feet while they all recovered and Mario told the remarkable lady what they wanted to drink. 'Prego,' said Clementina with authority and scurried away, vanishing inside the café, where her voice could still be heard booming orders.

"Well!" said Alicia "your wives had better look out!" The men burst out laughing, shaking their heads with mirth.

Mario then told Alicia Clementina's unusual story, sad, but with it's happy ending. She was a permanent fixture and had been there ever since either of them could remember. It was said that she had been found as a young girl, alone, destitute and without memory. She was brought to the port by one of the travelling boat men. One of the childless villagers in Biri had taken her in, educated her and given her a home. Clementina had worked hard, married well and bought the café, where she had remained ever since. Nobody had ever come to find her and nobody knew her real age. She had no idea herself and the rest of the village could only guess at her years. Alicia understood what they meant, the woman could have been anywhere between forty and sixty-five with an ageless brown face, generously crinkled, with laugh lines at the corners of her eyes and mouth. She had been married three times, Mario told her. Two husbands had died and she had born eleven children! Alicia wondered the poor woman was still standing!

Clementina returned with a tray laden with cups of espresso coffee and delicious *amarelli,* almond flavoured biscuits, which she handed around, teasing the men and winking at Alicia as she did so. She then left them in peace and shambled off to collar some potential new customers, busy parking their car by the water.

Mario and Stefano sat talking in a relaxed, easy way, with the odd sentence in English for Alicia's benefit. She loved to hear their native Italian. It was such an attractive language. She understood a fair amount, unless it was spoken really fast or with the island people's distinct 'Delfino' accent, which was very different to the one she had learned whilst with her aunt in Venice.

The main interest in the lives of these people was family and everything revolved around it. They loved life, enjoyed it to the full and were seldom in a hurry. *'Domani, domani,'* as she so often heard, being called one to the other, as people went about their every day chores. *Domani.* There was always *domani* and it could mean anything from tomorrow to a week's time, or more. She was used to this shift in pace now and basked in the rare luxury of being without her own busy schedule. She sat contentedly, dreaming in the sun, waiting until the men were ready to move on.

~

Miles away, deep in her own thoughts, Alicia stared out across the sea, sipping her coffee and nibbling on the sweet biscuits. She watched another fishing boat come in, with a host of gulls in pursuit, noisily announcing a full hold. She wandered over to the water's edge, fascinated by the thought of the shining, silvery, slippery, mass of sea life, pulled from the depths. The unmistakable smell of fish came drifting across as she sat on a bollard to watch. The trawlerman held a large squirming *'pesce'* up in the air for Alicia's inspection, implying that she might like to buy it. She shook her head and thanked him and when he made it clear that he would give it to her anyway, she waved again turning to rejoin the men. Italians never lost their charm she thought, with amusement and had always been the same, so far as women were concerned.

The incident lifted her spirits even more as she wondered if the other two would make fun of her if they'd witnessed the small exchange. Alicia looked into their faces as she approached and suddenly felt herself jolted back into the present: Mario and Stefano hadn't even noticed. The tone of their discussion had altered radically. It was no longer carefree and easy. She could tell that even from a distance. They glanced in her direction, smiled quickly and continued, confident that their conversation had not been overheard, launching forth in ever faster, more urgent Italian, as if it were of paramount importance to conclude what they were saying before she reached the table.

There was much gesticulating and Alicia heard Gianni's name mentioned several times. She was referred to as the *'signorina bionda'*. This much, at least, she understood as there were few fair-haired people on the island. She feigned lack of understanding and hesitated before joining the two men, to give them time to finish. Their faces were serious and she wondered what they were talking about. This was a discussion that she was definitely not invited to enter. When she reached them, they were smiling again, as if she had imagined the whole scene, but the strange atmosphere lingered. She sat down again, a slight sense of discomfort hanging over her like an ill-fitting piece of clothing, darkening her mood. Even in the warm sun she felt slightly cold and wrapped her jersey more tightly around her shoulders. She never used to be so nervous.

More coffee was ordered and the conversation took on its easy going, usual, banter once more. Stefano began to tease Mario about becoming a father again. Perhaps she was inventing illusory shadows. Alicia was certain that they had not intended to embarrass her, or cause her alarm. This interchange must have been about private matters; so she tried to convince herself that it had nothing at all to do with her. Even if it had, Alicia knew that everyone in this family wished her well, so whatever was being discussed could only have been in her own best interests.

Mario checked his watch and rose from the table. The boy had finished loading and was waiting by the steps. They said goodbye to Clementina, who waddled after them laughing, shaking her fist at Mario for pinching her huge behind as he left. Mario went with them to where Stefano had parked his shambolic old car, telling him that it wasn't fit for his passenger.

The back seat was packed high with sealed boxes, so Stefano squashed Alicia's luggage into the boot, which was stuffed full as well. It wasn't going to close without the efforts of both men. Alicia was able to assure them that there was nothing breakable in her bag, so they grunted and heaved and pushed it down until finally, with a whoop of triumph, Stefano banged the lid shut. He climbed into the driver's seat, revved up the engine, which back fired noisily making Alicia jump, then leaned across to let in his passenger. Mario turned to Alicia with a heartening smile, gave her a kiss on both cheeks and held the door open, closing it firmly behind her.

"We don't want you falling out of this terrible old wreck, do we *Signorina?*" added Mario for Stefano's benefit, checking again that the door really was shut. Then he stood grinning as he watched them set off, with Stefano muttering about the blessings of his beloved motor. At the corner of the square Alicia turned to wave, but Mario was already striding off towards his boat with his hands thrust deep in his pockets. He appeared distracted, not his normal, carefree, exuberant self, Alicia noted with surprise and she wondered again what the two men had been talking about so earnestly, in the port.

~

The journey took some three hours. As they travelled inland, away from the sea, the country began to change, becoming surprisingly green and hilly, with colourful old villages appearing out of nowhere. Stefano chatted away happily in his charming, broken, English, telling Alicia with great pride about his wife Amalia, his family and their hotel business.

The old banger rattled along at its own speed, with Stefano throwing his hands around while he talked. They stopped once on the way, when the engine seemed a bit too hot, at a small *trattoria* , belonging to a friend. They sat outside, had a beer and ate Giuseppina's delicious picnic, which turned into a feast as the café owners kept bringing out their own home-made specialities to be tasted. By the time they arrived in the village it was early evening. It had been a beautiful journey, which Alicia wouldn't have missed for the world and which had made her forget her earlier, darker, imaginings.

The few people around recognized the car and waved as they passed by. Stefano stopped once to take a heavy, string, shopping bag from an old lady, telling her he would drop it off at her home later. Her wrinkled face lit up and a toothless grin showed her gratefulness. She stood blowing kisses after them as they continued on their way. Stefano told Alicia that the old woman was so terrified of the car that he had so far failed to persuade her to accept a lift with her groceries.

The late sun still bathed the church spire with its warm light. The village looked empty and peaceful. Life up here in the hills, as on Delfino, also went at a different pace and it made Alicia's frenetic existence at home seem decidedly unhealthy.

~

The hotel 'Amalia', named after Stefano's wife, was just off the main square, an old building with an outside terrace covered by a colourful creeper and with a mature fig tree standing to one side of the open front door. As the car stuttered to a stop, hissing alarmingly, Stefano's family came running out, they must have been listening for him; no doubt that they'd heard the car from half a mile away. He greeted his wife and children as if he'd been away for a week, then proudly introduced them; two girls and a boy, all spick and span and very polite. Amalia, was vivacious, attractive and decidedly voluptuous, the result of having so many children Alicia suspected and perhaps of a well stocked restaurant larder: she bore a strong resemblance to her mother, Giuseppina. She greeted Alicia like a long lost friend and swept her inside and up to a room overlooking the church and a square with the hills still softly visible in the distance. The meal would be ready any time after seven she announced, until then, 'please to make yourself at home.'

Alicia looked around. It was a simple room with a natural wooden floor covered with rugs, an old looking bed with a dip in it and a white handmade bedcover, similar to the one on Giuseppina's bed. On the walls hung an array of brightly coloured, rather naïve, pictures which just could have been one of the children's artistic efforts. Through what seemed, at first sight, to be a cupboard door, there was a small, tiled, shower room. Everything was spotlessly clean and nothing had been forgotten. There was even a bowl of fresh peaches and a bottle of water on the table in front of the window.

After unpacking her few belongings and changing her shoes, Alicia, taking a peach with her, went down and out of the side door. As she passed by the family room she could see the children gathered around the television. Stefano's wife was busy in the kitchen but he was nowhere to be seen and the car must have been revived, for it was nowhere in sight.

In the middle of the cobbled square Alicia found a small fountain, surrounded by dancing cherubs and circled by very old, worn, stone benches. Nearby, was an ancient water trough fed by a pump. On closer inspection it looked Roman but she couldn't read the date, as the inscription was partly obliterated. She must remember to ask Stefano how old it really was. The water sparkled in the late daylight, giving the whole square a luminescent glow. There was no one about. She imagined that the people were inside now, the women preparing and the men anticipating the all-important evening meal. She sat for a while, eating the peach, savouring each mouthful, aware that the juice was trickling down her chin. There was no one to see and she could do as she wished, all was still and the silence interrupted only by the gentle tinkling of the cascading water by her side.

When the sun moved off the fountain, Alicia roused herself and rinsed the sticky peach juice from her fingers and face in the cold, sparkling water. Invigorating: Shaking her hands, the water dripping from her fingers, she walked out of the shade and into the sun again. Memories of blackberry picking as a child and washing off the evidence, in a gurgling Cotswold brook, suddenly sprung into her thoughts. Far away, in time and place, but still there: a nostalgic flash-back triggered by such a small action. So much had raced past since that particular day. Little did she, or her mother, imagine, some twenty years before, what the future had in store: Little did anyone know from one day to the next: Exciting or depressing? She wasn't sure which. Still, life continued, at least for the moment and she intended to make the best of it.

Alicia set off along a narrow street which soon petered out and became a well-used track leading out of the village, towards the first of the foothills which she'd seen as they had approached in the car and later from the window of her room. She walked slowly, enjoying the pungent aroma of wild thyme. It had been warmed all day by the sun, giving off its significant scent, almost in competition with the smell of the sweet, yellow, jasmine growing in the bushes on either side of the path.

The view was spectacular. The fading light played with the clean cut shadows over the vines and on the small farms scattered over the distant hills, bathing the whole scene in a freshly laundered pink. All around her the small, walled, olive groves were covered in lush grass, swathed with patches of blue wildflowers and speckled with bright red poppies, contrasting starkly against the bright, verdant, pastures. Under the trees, the earth had been carefully cleared and scratched in readiness for the olive harvest later in the year. It was a like a painting. Monet? perhaps or, certainly one of the old masters.

Finally, the sun sank altogether in a brilliant display of red, gold and orange, spread far and wide across the sky. Then, the air quickly cooled and the land in between began to lose its sharp detail and merge into the background, as the light dimmed.

Alicia turned back towards the village. The peacefulness was suddenly broken by a rustling sound and snapping of twigs in the undergrowth beside her. Immediately alert she stopped and waited, peering into the fading light, holding her breath, her heart hammering. Then she heard the bleating; it was only a small herd of goats bounding down from some rocks onto the path, returning home, after a day in the hills. They knew their way and set off in front of her, nibbling at the bushes within reach as they passed. The goatherd, in their midst, raised a hand in polite greeting and then also continued on his way. They'd all appeared out of nowhere and Alicia followed quietly behind, not wishing to disturb or hurry them in their timeless routine. Such a gentle atmospheric scene: it would remain imprinted on her mind.

Alicia followed the animals towards the village, then, watched them disappear into a farmyard. They had turned off the main track and so she took a different route back, intending to head for the central square by another road, so that she'd have no trouble finding the hotel. This street was cobbled and very narrow with the sound of voices echoing up from the far end, so

Alicia continued, certain that she was going to finally arrive in the square again. An old lady, in black, stood at a window and stared at Alicia as she went past. There was no pretence, so Alicia waved and called 'Ciao'. The old woman merely nodded, acknowledging her presence, a disapproving look on her face, then resumed watering her window-box. Dogs barked. She could hear a television somewhere from within and there was an overall smell of cat. She could sense muffled movement, people going about their business inside the houses, but, still, there was a comforting feel of normality to this unknown place.

The little street opened into a small *piazza,* with a café on one corner, from which all the noise was coming, a store next door and a laundry opposite. As she walked by the crowded bar Alicia glanced in, wondering if this was where the men gathered in the evening while their meal was being prepared.

In the uncertain light she thought she recognized Stefano, concentrating on a seemingly urgent conversation on the public telephone which hung on the dirty wall near the entrance. There were several other men standing around, smoking and looking uneasy. She wondered what could possibly have spoiled the tranquillity of the evening. She passed by unnoticed, a shiver running down her spine once more and hurried on back towards the hotel. What was it with her that she could have this sense of veiled threat even in this little town, somewhere in the middle of Italy? It was quite ridiculous.

~

With great effort, the church clock rustily clanged its way through six chimes. Alicia returned to her room, had a shower, contemplated calling Nick, then decided against it. He would ring her if there was anything at all to report. He'd said that he thought he might be able to find out if Guy's credit cards had been stopped and she was curious to know. This might at least give her some clue as to whether or not Guy was still of this world.

Adriana hadn't been in touch recently either, but Alicia knew she would ring in if she had any news to pass on. She suspected that her friend was leaving her in peace on purpose. According to Nick, Julian's office said that a problem had come up which had delayed him in Florida and that he'd then had to move on to South America for some reason. Rather quickly, Nick had remarked, as there appeared to be sudden political instability in one of the countries that Julian had wanted to cover. It was all a bit 'hush hush', hence the lack of contact. Even Adriana hadn't been given this information. Once more the man from the Foreign and Commonwealth Office had done well. Adriana was well aware of Alicia's unexplained predicament but she knew, instinctively, that Alicia needed time on her own to try to work things out and resolve what to do next.

Alicia supposed that her friend was used to Julian being out of reach. 'It's all part of the job, his being a foreign correspondent', Adriana used to say. 'There's really no point in worrying, he always rings me when he can and quite honestly I'd rather not know what's going on sometimes, at least not until he's safely back again.' Alicia would, in fact, have described Julian as a war correspondent: he was always to be found where there was trouble, although she kept her opinion to herself. Even so, she still thought it rather strange that Julian should also be completely out of contact just at this particular moment.

'I must stop this continuing speculation, it simply doesn't help', Alicia muttered for the umpteenth time, picking up her mobile and checking once more for messages. She turned it off and put it away in the zip-up compartment of her bag, electing not to look at it again until the following morning, at the earliest. It was time to take a break from the wretched little object, although she wouldn't have been without it for the world. It represented a lifeline, literally. Guy had the number of course and so she lived in hope that one day − perhaps one day - her mobile might bring her a miracle: the person or the news that she hoped for most.

For now, Alicia was hungry. A good sign she decided. Things were improving. It had been a busy day and she was looking forward to dinner. She put on a clean pair of jeans with her favorite, heavy, silver-buckled belt, a pale blue, polar-neck jersey and her beige suede boots: she was genuinely fond of the boots, she liked the feel of the soft suede and she felt secure and confident in them. She brushed her hair till it shone, made up her eyes, fixed her silver earrings and looked in the mirror. 'Knock 'em dead!' she said to her reflection, thinking that she looked marginally less anaemic. Pity there was nobody to agree. Bit of a wasted effort really. 'Still, think positive; you never know! What if Guy should walk through the door?'

At this imagining there was an uneasy lurch somewhere in her upper stomach, which then made its way to her lower regions. 'She would kill him; without doubt there would be a terrible murder, such as the village had never seen before and which would keep them all going in gossip for years to come'. God! She must stop muttering to herself like this. She wouldn't even go to prison, as they would say it was a 'crime de passion', or that she was insane. She looked into the glass once more. There was a gleam in her eyes and a flush to her cheeks. Anger, she realized, studying her face with surprise. But it had to be healthier than misery.

~

With these brighter thoughts Alicia leapt up from the chair, took her jacket from the cupboard and went down the stairs two at a time, ready for anything. There were people outside, some sitting perfectly at ease, some standing smoking, propped up against the wall and others just talking comfortably together. The little group near to the entrance, turned as she walked through the side door, had a good, unabashed, stare and then resumed what they were doing, as if accepting that she had every right to be there. Alicia, murmuring 'buonasera' several times over went to sit at one of the tables in front of the hotel, where there was now bustling activity. There were more people sitting under the old fig tree. One party of four were playing cards and drinking beer. There were children running around, cats hoping for snacks and one poor frantic dog, tied to a chair leg, longing to give chase. It was a normal scene and just what she needed: the village meeting place outside the restaurant. An aura of contentment seemed to emanate from these people and Alicia resolved to let it become infectious.

Her hosts were clearly popular. Stefano periodically swept out from his kitchen, now in his chef's uniform, looking very important and managing to have a word or share a joke with everyone, always passing by Alicia's table to make sure she had everything she needed. Could she have been mistaken? Alicia wondered. Stefano seemed to have a permanent smile on his face. Maybe it hadn't been him in the bar after all, but someone who looked like him from a distance, for he certainly had plenty to do here.

Amalia was equally good with all their guests. She was efficient and funny and had trained her children to perfection. They didn't miss a thing. Alicia liked them all enormously. When she was ready to eat she was shown to a table inside and served with an excellent glass of Chianti by one of the daughters. Sophia, the youngest daughter, would gladly have stayed for a little, to practice her English had her mother not moved her on, thinking that the child was bothering their guest whilst she waited for her meal.

Dinner in the charming little dining room, with its smart yellow linen tablecloths, was exceptionally good. Alicia was able to study the scene in front of her from her discreet corner table. Still early in the year and cool at night she was glad of the cosy open fire at her end of the room. The restaurant was almost full. 'Amelia's' must be the eating place in the village and probably the only one, except for the bar, which most likely produced little to eat.

Her fellow diners were an interesting assortment. The local policeman, the 'carabinieri', recognizable by the red stripe on his trousers, seemed to be thoroughly enjoying a glass of wine with everybody, while he moved around the tables, even carrying a couple of plates out of the kitchen for Amalia. Alicia was later introduced to him as Stefano's brother, Marcello! She immediately saw the likeness: they were a good-looking pair. She couldn't believe there was any reason for crime in this little place. Perhaps he was responsible for law and order in several of the local villages.

A fat man with a moustache, wolfing down a large plate of pasta with his napkin tucked into his huge neck, could only be the doctor, judging by the old fashioned medical bag beside his chair. This turned out to be correct, as an elderly woman soon appeared to drag him off to deliver her daughter's baby. There were more drinks all around, in anticipation of the birth, when the poor, expectant, father arrived to be kept occupied while the doctor and the women were busy, but he was soon 'well away' and not in the least bit worried about anything. There were several men, seemingly travelling on business, who left quite early and a pair of lovers, oblivious to everybody and even the food, which they virtually ignored while they ate each other, annoying Amalia so thoroughly that she had to be calmed down by her brother-in-law! The rest were mostly locals.

Alicia carefully chose a carafe of rosé wine, after looking to see what everyone else was drinking. She knew that it would be good and that it was often best to copy the locals' choice. The pasta was perfect, with a Genoese style sauce and a *radicchio* salad, followed by wonderful little fish, which she suspected had journeyed with them in the boot of the car from the port. She'd noticed a slight smell rising off her luggage on their arrival! The homemade Italian ice cream was out of this world.

The atmosphere was informal and easy, with the food and wine meticulously served. Alicia thought that she'd never sat anywhere on her own and felt so comfortable. If the restaurant was already so full at this time of year, there wouldn't be a spare chair when the tourists began to find their way here, in a couple of month's time, at the end of the school term. Perhaps the villagers kept away during the season to leave room for the holiday makers. But for now Alicia knew that it was special. The village still belonged to its inhabitants and she was flattered to be included and hardly considered or treated as an outsider; thanks, she suspected, to Gianni and Giusappina. She stayed late, waiting with everybody else, wanting to hear that the baby had arrived safely.

Marcello the policeman, who had been smiling at her on and off during the evening and had brought her the ice cream, was, she had to admit, not just good looking. After a few glasses of wine he appeared devastating. He finally managed to sit down at her table bringing her yet another *amaretto*, with coffee on the house, as an excuse. Knowing who he was, Alicia was delighted with his company. He spoke excellent English and was very funny. It transpired that he was actually on duty and not in the least bit befuddled. He must have had almost the same glass in his hand for the entire evening. She'd had plenty! His dark eyes bored into hers as he wanted to know everything about her. He was genuinely interested without being intrusive and wonderfully easy to be with. Alicia enjoyed his company. After all, he was 'family'.

As Marcello talked she listened and studied him closely. He was tall, much taller than Stefano and muscular, probably very fit. No doubt that he had to be, especially if the police were militarily trained in Italy, as in France. He had that easily tanned, olive coloured, skin and a head of thick, dark, wavy hair. His mouth seemed to be made upturned, as if he were often amused and his eyes crinkled at the edges as if in agreement. They were kind eyes, too. A gentle giant, she suspected, but she had no doubt that he was also an excellent policeman. As the evening wore on she began to find Marcello more and more attractive. 'This is getting dangerous' Alicia said to herself, beginning to loose her head. 'I've drunk far too much and have forgotten about everything else outside this room. That tell-tale sensation is beginning to awaken from within and worse still I know that I must be in a thoroughly vulnerable state'.

~

The baby was eventually born. Word was brought to the restaurant by a young boy, also a member of the family. The father was thoroughly congratulated, before being unsteadily escorted out by Stefano and several others, very much the worse for wear. Alicia hoped that he'd be in a fit state to kiss his wife and acknowledge the baby. When she conveyed this worry to Marcello, he laughed and assured her that the man would be taken home via the water tank in the square, then dried off and smartened up, before being allowed into his house. He was terrified of both his wife and his mother-in-law. What a wonderfully archaic remedy for sobering someone up, thought Alicia, with much amusement, but feeling rather sorry for the new father.

The families all left and when Amalia had cleared the tables, with the help of Alicia and Marcello, she said 'buonasera' with a twinkle in her eye and followed her children to bed. Alicia needed some air. She said 'arrivederci' to the policeman as best she was able, went through the house and then tip-toed out through the side door. She headed, a little erratically, but as quietly as she could, for the fountain in the square. Luckily, it was a clear night and easy to see the way.

He was there in front of her, sitting smoking, on one of the stone benches.

"*Buonasera*, again!" he said laughing and then, in his perfect English with the delicious accent, "you don't think I'd give up that easily, do you?" Alicia giggled weakly and sat down, cursing the stupefying effects of alcohol as she did so.

"*Le da' fastidio se fumo?*" He indicated the cigarette. Alicia shook her head. He was so polite.

"Come now, Alichia *bella, perche,* why so sad?" The way he said Alichia pronounced with its 'ch' was seductive in itself. Marcello pulled her gently down beside him, put his arm around and turned her face towards him.

"Shouldn't you be doing something more important?" Alicia asked hesitantly. He looked deeply into her eyes and answered in his endearing English.

"I am off duty half an hour ago and I have two days now. So what else could there be more important?"

He put out his cigarette, drew her face towards him, then placing his lips on hers so gently, tentatively, began to kiss her, opening her mouth with his tongue, stroking the back of her head up into her silky hair. He tasted mildly of smoke and smelt vaguely of something citrus, yet, at the same time deliciously masculine. His other hand stroked her neck and shoulders. As the kiss continued, his hand went slowly lower and strayed to her breast. She shuddered and sighed - a long anguished sound. He drew back immediately to study her face.

"Alichia, *per favor*, why tell me not of your trouble? This heavy thing on your arm, is it so bad?"

"Shoulders!" corrected Alicia squeezing his hand, glad to have the mood lightened, "it's heavy on your shoulders, not arm!"

"Then why don't you let me help you … does Gianni know about this thing that worries you so much?"

"No," replied Alicia, getting up, "I can't tell him or you either; can't tell anybody," and in a muffled voice, "nobody can help me and I must go in now … before we both have something to regret, for tomorrow I move on and all this …," she said waving her hand wildly and getting up, "will become a wonderful memory." She took a gulp of air. "Thank you, Marcello for somehow understanding when I can tell you nothing of my horrible situation." She took his hand in hers and wistfully held it to her cheek for a moment, then turned and walked quickly back to the hotel, sensing his eyes following her until she finally disappeared from his view.

Marcello put his hand to his face. It was wet with her tears. "Regret?" he muttered, "*Non mai*, Never!"

After an eventful day and a thoroughly emotional evening, Alicia returned to her room, confused by how quickly she'd become physically moved to such strong feelings for the good looking, caring, policeman. She was restless for some time, her body thoroughly unsettled. Thirsty from the excess of alcohol, she drank copious amounts of water hoping it would settle her head and cool her down. She wished that her circumstances could have been different and wondered if Marcello was thinking the same, or had he gone on his way, having forgotten her already, back to his girlfriend perhaps.

When she eventually slipped between the sheets, Alicia slept surprisingly well in spite of everything that had or hadn't happened. No ogres invaded her dreams, but only a gentle nagging wish for the release she so badly needed and an unfulfilled promise of so very much more. She was disturbed, only once, by the first train coming down through the hills on its way south.

★★★

CHAPTER 8

Early April in Italy, perhaps comparable to June in England: it was warm enough to eat outside. Breakfast consisted of freshly squeezed orange juice and sweet Italian croissants, with homemade cake. The enticing smell of the coffee drifting up from beneath her window had brought Alicia quickly down from her bedroom. She had plenty of time to sit and enjoy the simple, yet, mouthwatering spread before catching her train.

Stefano, carrying her small piece of luggage, walked with her to the station: she felt in control of herself once more and only slightly ashamed of her behavior the night before. A mild headache, but thankfully, nothing had happened to spoil a lovely interlude, albeit with its unfulfilled conclusion which had seemed disconcerting at the time. If the evening had ended as she might have wished in the small hours, it would only have only complicated her life even more. It really would have been mad to have entered into an affair so soon, with a complete stranger, however attractive, just because she felt abandoned and in need of comfort. Still, at least she had spent the entire evening thinking about something and somebody else, for a change. Perhaps she should keep a diary and list all the plusses each day.

The station was situated, on the far side of the square, away from the hotel. It was tiny, with one building, which Alicia imagined housed the stationmaster. In front was a well worn path, slightly raised, running alongside the railway line which she realized must serve as a very rudimentary platform. There was nothing else. Stefano told her to be sure to get into the right carriage on her return and she quite understood why! It was a tiny halt. The train duly arrived and, sure enough, a very smart looking stationmaster appeared from the house, adjusted his hat, brushed some crumbs off his chest and madly waved a flag. He had been taking a break for a snack: he must enjoy many during the day, judging by the difficulty he was having in doing up his jacket. The train shuddered to a stop, resting only just beside the rough platform. The 'Fat Controller' shook hands with Stefano, winked at Alicia as he gave her a ticket and then opened the door for her with a flourish. Stefano helped her in with her luggage, the station master blew his whistle and they were away. As Alicia looked back she saw the two men grinning and gesticulating: she understood perfectly well that they were talking about her and was amused.

The journey was endless, with much stopping and comings and goings, particularly in Bologna, where they hitched on extra carriages. Alicia's filled up, mostly with men glued at the ear to their mobiles and bonded firmly to that other compulsory accessory, the brief case. Attaché case would seem more appropriate thought Alicia, as the men seemed to be joined at the hip to the wretched things. To her a 'brief' case implied something slim and neat, not a heavy bulging leather piece of luggage, transporting computers, software, clothes and perhaps an entire desk top, to another location. At least here in Italy they were made of decent leather.

When she travelled by train Alicia liked to play a game of, 'guessing what they all did!' The man opposite her had a case with an intricate locking device. She imagined that, with a pair of hand-cuffs to the wrist, the crown jewels could be aboard. Perhaps he was a jeweler. The men, on the whole, looked casual but still smart, an understated elegance, as only the Italians seem to carry off with such panache.

There were two trendy young girls in the corner window seats, who never stopped chattering and were quite aware of the rise in male testosterone within the carriage which they had intentionally aroused. They seemed to be going shopping for the day from what Alicia understood. No doubt a suitable bar would be waiting at the end of the retail therapy session. Their long legs were sheathed in thigh length black boots, with little left to the imagination above. How did they manage to walk all day in those heels?

Each time the disapproving ticket inspector came past, the legs were languidly removed from the seat opposite, only to be returned once more, as he left the carriage. Two darker skinned, swarthy, men had leapt on at the last moment. Possibly Sicilians she concluded. They appeared slightly nervous and rather out of place in their sombre, dark, city suits. Perhaps they were going to a funeral. They kept glancing furtively across at her and she didn't like the look of them.

Alicia knew Bologna to be one of the main junctions for Northern Italy. It was huge, stark and impersonal and she was pleased that she didn't have to get out and change trains. The journey was tediously slow, both before and after the city, although the distance couldn't have been far. The driver and guard had friends in all the smaller stations at which they stopped and got out, indulging in long conversations while goods were being either loaded or off-loaded. Then there would be a frantic blowing of whistles, crashing of doors and they would be off again.

Surprisingly, in spite of the many stops, they arrived in Verona only a few minutes late, soon after midday. Alicia let most people get out. The two dark-suited men seemed to be hesitating: she experienced an uncanny and momentary feeling of threat. The *Mafiosa* look-a-likes were creepy. She jumped out quickly, almost stumbling in her hurry, glad to leave them behind.

She leapt straight into the arms of a man standing waiting on the platform. She looked up starting to apologize then stopped in amazement.

"Marcello! What on earth are you doing here?" He stood back, held his arms wide and replied:

"You see, Alichia *bella*, here I am again just like a bad pound, to escort you to your hotel." He bowed low before her, smiling broadly.

"Penny, not pound, Marcello!" she cried, laughing, genuinely pleased to see his smiling face.

"*Via*, come with me then. We'll take a taxi to the hotel Raffaele. I know that's where you are going!"

He spoke quietly but with authority. Marcello hadn't missed the two rather furtive looking individuals stepping down from the train behind Alicia. He steered her quickly away, occasionally looking over his shoulder whilst continuing a light hearted conversation, not wishing to draw her attention to them. They could have been following, albeit at a discreet distance.

In the taxi Marcello took charge, amusing Alicia as he ordered the man to take a series of quick turns: to avoid the busiest and most crowded areas, she imagined. He assured Alicia, that because of his choice of route, the journey to the hotel would be half the cost. How the taxi driver finally managed to arrive at the right place was nothing short of a miracle. Only by way of some of the most incredible manoeuvres, negotiating the small streets and one way systems, not to speak of the extra hazards around every corner, Alicia thought. She had clung on for dear life, not wishing to be thrown across Marcello's lap too often and dissolving into helpless giggles when she failed. He, laughing, also enjoyed every moment of the journey, but considered it far too short. Alicia hadn't noticed him surreptitiously checking the rear window.

Marcello told her that he'd had to come up to Verona for a meeting, so he'd decided to come to meet her, after finding out from Stefano which train she was travelling on. She felt a momentary sense of relief when he inferred that, in a strange city, she might need an escort. Maybe it was a good idea. He already knew that she was going to the opera in the evening and now he was insisting that she would have lunch with him the next day. How could she refuse? He was so sweet, so funny and such very good company. What harm could it do? So she readily agreed.

~

The hotel Raffaele, in its small shaded piazza, was quite unique. Set back at the front and facing the side entrance to a little chapel, it had a very important, newly painted, glossy front door, beside which were all the various

71

Italian award signs. There were two huge ceramic urns with climbing roses, well in flower, on either side. Inside, the next branch of the Vivarini family were waiting to greet her with the usual exuberant hospitality to which she was now becoming accustomed.

Vittorio was much quieter than the rest of the family. He was a thin man and looked worried and overworked, but still managed to make Alicia feel the most welcome of guests. They both knew and liked Marcello well. That was very obvious. Vittorio's eyes lit up with genuine pleasure when he followed Alicia through the door, as did those of his wife Francesca. She greeted Marcello with much affection and Alicia sensed, straight away, that perhaps, at one time, these two might have known each other rather especially well.

Slim, dark and attractive Francesca could only have been Giuseppina's daughter. Alicia could see her mother's mirror image as a young woman, very much more so than in her sister Amalia. She suspected immediately that Francesca ran things here. There were no children, as yet, but Giuseppina had assured her, before she had left the island, that they were 'trying'!

In the large, open reception area, everything was immaculate The hotel had modern furnishings and was brightly decorated, in light colours, with half of the wood panelling picked out in a deeper shade. The windows were long and many, all swathed in red velvet curtains. Considering the sudden quiet, when they had left the noisy street, they must be double glazed. At one side of the room, away from the desk, was a sitting area with comfortable, brown leather chairs all facing the compulsory big screen. This huge modern 'box' contrasted sharply with a large bowl of fragrant lilies set on the table beside, pervading the whole room with their lovely scent, almost as if in apology for the television's loud, ugly, presence.

Vittorio was called away to help an old lady to her taxi and, as Francesca was also caught by the telephone at the reception desk, she gave Marcello the key so he could take Alicia's bag up to her room for her. When they were alone he explained where they could meet the following day, after his meeting, in the old city near to everything that she should see. Alicia had already read a lot about Verona so she was really looking forward to visiting it all - and as for lunch? She had to admit that she was really looking forward to that as well. Marcello kissed her on both cheeks, wished her a lovely evening and went bounding off down the stairs, singing at the top of his voice. He had someone to see about an important matter to do with the village, he had told her.

Alicia sat on her bed contemplating the situation. 'I should have told him not to expect anything more than lunch. I hate to hurt such a nice man. Oh well. I'm hardly able to take care of myself at the moment, so I really can't be worrying about everybody else, after all', she convinced herself, 'he is a policeman so must be made of strong stuff'. The added bonus was that when she was with Marcello she felt safe. Safe from what she wasn't quite sure, but nonetheless it was a good feeling.

Alicia had been given the hotel's best room, at the back, which was considered to be the biggest and the most private, with two beds, a large old fashioned, dark wood, cupboard, a cane seated rocking chair and a table with all the hotel literature spread out on its shiny surface, beside a vase of roses. The walls were half-panelled, the same as downstairs. The lower panels were of darkly varnished wood and the wall above papered with a light aqua colour which contrasted well with the rather dreary, darker, tone beneath. The bathroom was modern and beautifully fitted in grey and white marble, with large, fluffy, white towels and even a towelling robe on the back of the door Alicia noted with satisfaction, thinking that the huge deep bath looked most inviting.

The bedroom overlooked a tiny, narrow, cobbled street. The window boxes, perched on the ledges of the houses opposite, were already overflowing with, brilliant, trailing flowers reaching almost to the floor below. Sheltered from wind, yet in the sun all day long, no wonder they were so prolific, thought Alicia, her gardening interest rising to the fore. Perhaps the plants were cut back and left in the autumn, as there should be no fear of frost here and the winter months would be short in comparison to

England.

She leant further out to see more. The usual wire lines of washing were strung across the street. A woman was busy rearranging her cheerfully coloured array, with the use of a long pole and an ancient ratchet system, which seemed to wind the line in or out with a lot of noise. There was an ornate wrought-iron balcony facing her, below which two dogs sat sunning themselves. Further along she could see the *panetteria* and a little further still a *macelleria,* the butcher's shop. At the end of the street, the fruit and vegetable stall, surrounded with buckets full of bright flowers, caught her eye. Looking the other way, Alicia could see a couple of restaurants at each corner, with chairs set outside, almost in competition, all ready for warm days and the expected influx of tourists.

Downstairs, in the breakfast room, off the reception area, a light lunch had been laid out, with the opera ticket beside her place. Alicia looked at the ticket with interest. Astonishing! She hadn't enquired which opera she was to see, on purpose, preferring a surprise and now she had one. What an extraordinary coincidence! With so many operas being performed throughout the world, it had never occurred to her that it might be the rather elusive Flying Dutchman being staged, here, tonight, in Verona. Her stomach turned a cartwheel and memories threatened her equilibrium as Alicia recalled the last time she'd seen this tragedy and who had been close by her side on that particular night.

~

Lunch was a kind thought and much appreciated. Alicia knew that the young couple didn't have a proper dining room and didn't really cater for meals other than breakfast. Francesca explained that, in a city, there were so many restaurants nearby it wouldn't pay to run one in the hotel and that it also would mean more work and more staff to employ, not to mention all the new E.U rules and regulations that they would have to get their heads around. Besides, they were so busy in summer that they felt they really couldn't manage anything else. Then she went on to say, shyly, but with shining eyes, that she hoped, soon there might be other reasons why she couldn't take on any more work.

Aha! Alicia thought, smiling gently and nodding her understanding. Giuseppina will be pleased.

After she'd finished eating, a free afternoon awaited her. She refused to dwell too much on the past; tonight and the opera was still some hours away. Her emotions, for the moment, at least, could and must be held in check. No distracting memories were going to spoil this visit. She would see the sights and investigate the shops.

Marcello had been despondent about his obligatory appointments and with Alicia's plans, which could not include him. He seemed most impatient for their lunch the next day Alicia realized with some satisfaction. She felt rather the same. However she wanted some time to herself, to buy things she needed and she wished to visit this particular opera alone.

~

With Vittorio's directions and a small city map, Alicia set off from the Raffaele, in its lovely, little, tree-lined piazza, towards the shopping streets. As she walked along in the spring sunshine she knew that had she not been taken to the heart of this family, she would never have found these, hidden away, places in which to stay. They were hardly advertised; they didn't need to be, only happened on, found or passed on by word of mouth and then revisited time and again. In her plight, Alicia had been fortunate enough to come to rest with the all embracing Vivarini clan. As she moved around she had been carefully handed from one branch of the family to another. It was just like a tree that over the years had gradually spread its roots everywhere. She was lucky to be here and glad to be far away from the land of her birth and the depressing situation that she had left behind.

She wandered aimlessly down the ancient, cobbled, streets, absorbing everything around her and watching the Italians going about their business. It was an intriguing city, with most of the roads in the old quarter closed to cars and only open for deliveries and shoppers on foot. She stopped to look in a window beside a restaurant, with an especially interesting display of sophisticated and unusual nick-knacks. There, tucked behind a photograph frame, she spied a pair of gleaming silver dolphins, caught by the light above, as the creatures appeared to dive into the sea together. Alicia decided, at once, they would make a perfect present for Gianni's parents' golden wedding on her return to the island.

They were such an endearing old couple. The dolphins somehow seemed so appropriate and Alicia knew that they had a small cabinet for treasured items that they had collected over the years.

Alicia entered the quiet interior. The owner nodded a polite greeting to which she responded. There were two men in the shop before her, with their backs to the door, who left as soon as she walked in, so she went over to the window to find the dolphins. Glancing outside, she noticed the two previous customers, across the street now, half hidden by a group of young students as they ambled slowly on, deep in conversation, but she couldn't see their faces. Even from behind they looked slightly sinister. With a shock she realized that they reminded her of the two dark suited individuals on the train. The shop keeper watched, her beady eyes missing nothing. She spoke to Alicia in excellent English.

"Those men, *Signorina, spazzatura* … rubbish," the woman said, indicating the two men who had just left. "They had no intention of buying anything, you know, that's not their business". This she said in a considered manner, shaking her head, her lips pursed in disapproval. Perhaps not wishing her opinion of the men to put Alicia off making a purchase, the woman continued, in a more friendly tone, as she came to help Alicia take the dolphins out of the window.

"I wouldn't have left them alone in the shop and I didn't like the way they were looking at you, *Signorina*". Alicia stopped and stood upright, a bolt of fear charging through her like an electric current. She stepped aside to make more room for the shop keeper and looked out after the men again, but they had gone, disappeared from sight, even though the streets were quite empty. Alicia understood that she wasn't alone in her uncanny, uneasy feelings. What exactly did the woman mean, 'that's not their business'?

~

The dolphins were a perfect present, the shining pair, side by side, were poised to dive together into a golden sea, hand painted on the solid wooden stand. The silver marks were easy to define and the gift was not too expensive, so Alicia bought it. She had seen real dolphins off the island, playing with the wash from the fishing boats as they went past. They were so beautiful. She knew that, here, in Italy, they were considered lucky and particularly so on Delfino Island, where there were so many. Gianni had told her that sometimes, in summer, Mario or Dimitri would take visitors out in their boats to watch them from close quarters. Alicia hoped that they would take her, once the weather had settled. Dolphins frequently featured in Dimitri's stories. He used to tell the children that he had swum with them as a boy and they believed him, as she did.

Alicia wandered on glad to have people around her once more, safety in numbers? She supposed it was true. She looked at the map and took a short cut, towards the main area, hurrying a little. It was easy to loose your way in the narrow winding streets, but then she arrived, suddenly, almost by chance on Via Mazzini, the serious, designer, shopping street. It was full and busy, reassuring in its normality.

She had saved up a fortune for her wedding and now she had every intention of spending some of her hard earned money, to hell with the extravagance. She brought a dress, in palest blue silk chiffon, by Armani. Soft and slinky, the skirt, varied from a lighter to a darker blue, which both clung to and swirled around her long slim legs. She would wear it tonight. To finish the outfit she bought French navy sling-back shoes with small heels, a bag of the same colour and a blue grey pashmina. Just right, she wouldn't have to take her coat to the opera house; the cashmere shawl could rest on her knee.

Alicia walked on. She found herself obliged to enter another shop because of it's alluring window. Ultra modern and fashionable, everything in it mixed and matched, beautifully displayed to catch the eye of even the most discerning shopper. She found a charcoal grey trouser suit, of a light-weight wool, that would be useful all year round, with several different tops to match. The suit had a wide leather belt, with cream stitching, which she knew made her waist look tiny. 'I shall wear this, tomorrow, at lunch', she announced, as she studied her reflection in the long mirror. How could he then resist her? And how quite delicious to have something new! The last item that attracted her attention was in the window of a leather shop; or she wouldn't have gone in, she told herself: A beautiful, long, silk scarf, draped across some impossibly high-heeled shoes. Only the Italians could produce silk in so many glorious colours. It would go with everything she owned; both here and at home, so would not be extravagant at all, she reasoned, talking herself into buying it as well.

Feeling thoroughly pleased with her purchases Alicia then set off back to the hotel, before she could spend any more, with all her shopping bags swinging along beside her. The afternoon's indulgence had lifted her spirits. She had enjoyed the last couple of hours and had managed to relegate her anxieties to the further recesses of her mind.

Men coming towards her stared quite openly, as continental people always do, especially when the woman approaching was foreign and of such star-tlingly fair colouring. The smart Italian women, seemingly oblivious, held their heads high and walked on by, pretending disdain, while taking in every detail of both her, dress, jewellery and overall appearance. A few, pride aside and unable to resist, quite openly glanced back behind them to have a bet-ter look at the *elegante*, vivacious, young woman strolling along with such obvious enjoyment.

To the man, following not far behind her, she was the perfect girl from the film 'Pretty Woman'. Her silky blonde hair caught the light and swung rhythmically from side to side with each step, in time with all the smart carrier bags. He kept up with her, but at a discreet distance, purposeful and rude, pushing those in his way to one side as he did so. He was swarthy, of dark colouring and wearing a badly fitting, shiny, black suit.

★★★

CHAPTER 9

The opera was due to start at seven-thirty. Vittorio had organized a taxi for he considered the hotel too far from the *Teatro Filarmonico* for Alicia to walk. Alicia would have liked the exercise, but she gave in gracefully. Presumably Vittorio did know best: it was night time and perhaps she shouldn't be wandering around on her own. A plate of parma ham and melon, some bread and a dish of fresh olives awaited her downstairs. A chilled bottle of Frascati was already open: just what she would have ordered, had they asked her. They were so thoughtful, bothering to prepare these ideal, simple meals for her on top of all the other work. No doubt Giuseppina was behind this arrangement.

Alicia couldn't fail to notice the open admiration on Vittorio's face when he helped her into the taxi, nodding and clicking his tongue, as he explained to her exactly where she was to find the taxi after the opera had finished. The new dress was definitely a success! She had been told, rather firmly, thought Alicia, to go 'nowhere else and with no one else, as a young woman such as she would always be at risk out alone in the night and that she was to let them look after her.' She decided that she hadn't much choice. This directive sounded as if it had come from Gianni.

~

The entrance to the theatre was off the main square, the *'Piazza Bra'*, through a triumphal arch, which also led to the Museum. The walkway was lit by lanterns, with beautiful stone relief work on impressive statues to either side. They looked Greek and Roman from the inscriptions, which Alicia could just see, in the uncertain light, if she stepped off the path to look more closely.

Inside, there were already many enthusiastic opera buffs gathered, mostly locals she guessed and all talking at the tops of their voices. There was excitement and chaos, some people arguing, trying to buy or change tickets and others standing talking in groups, drinking champagne. Her *biglietto* was checked by the usher, torn in half and another man came forward, designated to politely show her the way. It must be obvious that she was a stranger.

Alicia looked around. The whole interior seemed to be made of light coloured, mottled, marble: the columns, statues, floors and even the walls. Alicia followed the young man to the bottom of a huge, ornate, staircase with iron banisters topped in glowing brass, where he left her, pointing the way up. She thanked him and started to ascend. The middle of the steps was covered with the same plush crimson carpet as elsewhere. Why was red thought to be the height of decorum and pomposity? 'Royal blue' she could understand. Bright, garish, red seemed somehow vulgar in this magnificent building. She found out later that it had been completely destroyed in the war and then rebuilt, albeit in the old style. It was early, so Alicia climbed, slowly, taking in the enormous paintings on each wall, thinking how badly they needed restoring. The chandeliers overhead sparkled brightly, as if matching the excited mood of the crowd beneath, outshining the older women decked out in their long dresses and jewels. All were waiting, in anticipation, for the entertainment to begin. The younger women were dressed more as she was: 'chic' she hoped, not remembering the equivalent in Italian. Some students, heading up to the Gods, wore their jeans while still managing to look, 'smartly casual', as her mother would say. The men, mostly in jackets with open necked shirts, came rushing in, after a last smoke outside, when the bells rang to announce the performance.

Alicia couldn't help but wonder what on earth Verona would be like when the summer season started. There would be twenty-five thousand people, congregating in the Arena at the old Roman amphitheatre on the other side of the square, for the bigger productions. What a ghastly thought. Where would they all stay, for goodness sake? Verona seemed much too small to house such an invasion. She made a mental note never to attempt a visit after the high season had started. But for now, this evening was as it should be, an evening for the Italian people, not for the tourists, thought Alicia as she arrived at her allotted row. She bent her shiny, blonde, head and, apologising profusely, squeezed past those already seated to her own place.

It was a magical evening. There is nothing to match an authentic, local, Italian production. The atmosphere in the little opera house was electric, the Flying Dutchman without fault and the performance superb. Alicia sat as if in a trance, captivated by the story and assailed by memories of another time and another place.

~

Alicia and Guy had seen the 'Dutchman' once before, on the night he had proposed to her. They had spent a surprise weekend together in Florence: his surprise. She had no idea where they were going until they had checked in at the airport. On their second day he'd taken her to Pisa and then that night to the little opera house. He had already brought her the CD, for her birthday, so he knew that she would recognize the music when she heard it live for the first time. It was then that Alicia realized just how extensively Guy had travelled throughout Europe. He was so well informed. He seemed to have been everywhere. He had often said he preferred the smaller opera houses as they were more spontaneous, less contrived, with the repertory company tailoring the evening's entertainments to suit the local community. On these occasions there was the added bonus of tickets being available at a reasonable price.

Alicia had adored their night in Pisa, not just because she was with Guy and he had asked her to marry him, but also because she agreed that the less well known productions were so much more intimate and real. They were meant for the normal working people. So very different from the performances given at the very elite, newly renovated Covent Garden, in the flamboyant La Scala, monopolized by the smart, rich set, or even at the more modern Bastille in Paris.

When the final curtain came down, there was a moment of total silence before the applause started, soon rising to become a standing ovation. Afterwards, when people around her began to collect their belongings and move, Alicia sat still for a while letting the atmosphere and the resonance from the last, lovely, aria linger with her as long as possible. She was filled with emotion. The story, beautifully depicted, was so sad. She remembered how even Guy had tears in his eyes at the end: he had loved the drama as much as she had.

~

It was as if something clutched at her heart. Why she turned her head at that exact moment she never knew, but something caught her eye. As the people hurried out to beat the rush she was certain that, for an instant, she recognized a familiar, dark, head amongst the crowd far below her. The face had already turned away but it was the slight lift to the left shoulder, caused by some youthful accident that she remembered so well: it was Guy - it had to be him.

Alicia stared after the man's retreating back but then, frustratingly, her view was blocked and she couldn't shout after him, there was too much noise in the theatre. She couldn't be mistaken, but why ever else would she have been drawn in that way and at that very moment? What was going on? She stood up and hurried through the crowd, as quickly as she could, towards the exit. She pushed as much as she dared, but there were so many people hampering her progress. The figure that Alicia had thought she recognized had soon disappeared and she searched in vain.

It must have been the music which had quite overwhelmed her, reflected Alicia, willing her heart to steady. Her hands were cold and clammy, and she really felt quite shaky. Not surprising, she supposed, given the circumstances. People were shoving and jostling as the crowd surged forward. Somebody close by, reeking of garlic, coughed near to her face. Everyone was talking loudly and some were getting out their cigarettes, ready to light up as soon as they were in the street once more. She was hemmed in: a slight sense of panic, a claustrophobic queasiness was beginning to overcome her. She needed some air but the exit was still a long way off. Alicia slowed down, edged away from the thronging mass of people and leant against the wall for a moment, her hands flat behind her for support. The wall-paper was red, as well as the carpet, a gaudy, burgundy, brocade cloth, flecked with gold. It made her feel dizzy, everything seemed hot and red in front of her eyes and her heart was pounding. Somebody, with concern in his eyes, asked if she needed assistance. She shook her head and mumbled her thanks, then, as if by magic, she spied the ladies room across the corridor. A woman had just come out and the burst of light from inside had caught her attention. With relief, Alicia forced her way through the crowd and pushed the door open again. There was no one inside, a welcome refuge. She went to the basin, cupped her hands and took a drink of water. She raised her head to the glass above and studied her face. Pale, wide, frightened eyes. This was pathetic: it was time to take a grip of herself. She washed her hands, took a few deep breaths, waited a few moments and then, feeling better, returned to converge with the exiting crowd.

Alicia walked quickly down the floodlit path and thankfully regained the street. As she stopped, looking around to get her bearings, she fleetingly caught the eye of a man, standing alone, watching her from underneath the arch. He seemed to be hesitating, agitated, as if waiting for someone. He bore a strong resemblance to one of the two forbidding *mafiosa* look-a-likes from the train and in the shop that afternoon. They seemed to be everywhere she went. He somehow appeared rather out of place amidst the chattering groups of people and she didn't like the way he was staring after her. Illusion again, she decided and her present unsettled existence; nonetheless, it was another small incident which sent a tremulous quiver down her spine. Alicia turned quickly away and hurried on to find her taxi.

She soon found Paulo, waving his hands around, fending off traffic police and other would-be passengers. He was exactly where he said he would be. He had turned his light off but the people still persisted, trying to get in. 'No! No! *La Senorina Inglese!*' she could hear as she approached.

In the secure warmth of the taxi, which seemed to have been heated up like a hothouse, Alicia heaved a sigh of relief and regained her composure. Her imagination was merely running away with her, making her 'wobbly', quite out of character and she must put a stop to it.

~

Back in her room at the Raffaele, Alicia found another selection of specialities awaiting her, on a tray, together with a half bottle of cooled white wine and a glass of almond liqueur. She picked at the food but drank the alcohol and felt the better for it. After what really had been a lovely day, although maybe not happy in the true sense of the word, for her burden of disquiet never left however hard she tried, but nevertheless sustained, nourished and with that last beautiful aria still in her head, she went to bed and slept soundly: at least at first. Later in the night she awoke startled, the cry of a cat and a dustbin lid falling, she thought, but something else too.

She'd dreamt of a comforting touch and his warm breath on her cheek and felt the familiar stirring deep inside as they would then have turned to each other, both of the same mind. Then his face altered and it was not Guy, but that of the nasty looking Sicilian glaring after her outside the opera house. She cried out in alarm, but was immediately soothed as the man's dark face lightened and became that of Marcello smiling gently down at her, but from afar. She awoke and remembered where she was. Both men had been there, in her unconscious mind, muddled up together with the lovely music and the horrible Sicilian. Loving, frightening, then protecting and all three of them had seemed so real in the quiet, lonely hours of the night. A single helpless tear slid down her face and onto the pillow, she squeezed her eyes tight shut, turned over and determined to sleep again.

★★★

CHAPTER 10

In the early hours of the morning, Guy Hargreaves stood looking down on the city of Verona from the hill above the old theatre, *Teatro Romano*, which was built into the Adige river bank. The city looked resplendent and somewhat mysterious in its strange, uncertain light, the silver water gleaming, flat and shadowy. The weather of the day seemed undecided. Despite the pervasive tranquility of the scene spread out in front of his eyes he had no illusions: destructive, inauspicious, wrongdoers were going about their ominous business under cover of darkness and Alicia was right there in the middle of it all. What a mess! Thoughtfully, he fingered the fire-arm fitting snuggly in his shoulder holster, almost part of his clothing. It's cold, hard smooth surface was reassuring under his hand. He hoped that he wouldn't have to use the lethal weapon, but, if it became necessary, he wouldn't think twice. He was trained to handle it, had no problem with shooting someone if he had to and had no doubt that he was still quicker than most.

Adrenalin was coursing through his alert, taught, body as he thought about Alicia, glimpsed earlier in the opera house and the affirmation of threat to her well being. It was the first time he'd seen his fiancée since he'd left for the Channel Islands and abandoned her: disappeared off the face of the earth to all intents and purposes. It was weeks ago now, another age, or so it seemed. So much had happened to change so many lives. He had gladly taken tonight's surveillance job himself. He needed to see her, for his own peace of mind.

In spite of what she must be going through, Alicia had looked fantastic, even from a distance and he'd fallen, lock, stock and barrel for her, all over again. He hadn't expected her to look so good. In fact had rather thought she'd reveal how she must feel: pretty miserable, he had supposed. He had been too far away to see her eyes, of course, but she hadn't appeared beaten down at all, resigned perhaps, but strong, resilient and delectable. Yes, that's just how she had looked. Absolutely and utterly irresistible: his feelings for her had been so strong that he couldn't believe that she hadn't been touched by the vibes emanating from his overcharged emotions, or would have at least, sensed his presence. He had longed to be closer, to be by her side and to experience the moving drama of the opera with her. He wanted to hold her and to smell the familiar fragrance of her skin. Most of all he wanted to make love to her and take away the pain that he had caused, but all he was able to do was watch from afar and make sure that his people were in place, to keep her safe. God! He'd wanted to make himself known to her so badly and explain why it had been necessary for him to vanish, turning her life upside down in such a horrifying manner.

Guy had seen the sinister looking thug creeping up on her as the crowd left the *Teatro Filarmonica*. Alicia's sudden dash to the wash room had been fortuitous. He'd managed to delay the man easily, with help from one of the others, without making himself conspicuous. The ominous looking individual had been left well behind when she'd stepped thankfully into the safe haven of Paulo's waiting taxi.

Guy was good at his job. He had to be, to stay on top. He was also tough, but when he saw Alicia go safely on her way, out of his life again, he thought that perhaps inside, where his heart lay, he would never be nearly tough enough.

He sat down on the uncomfortable, rough hewn, stone bench, pondering the situation, considering what had happened. The fates had dealt them a bad hand allowing Alicia to suddenly appear here in Verona, right bang in the middle of this particularly delicate job, but it was a heaven sent coincidence that Alicia had gone to Delfino. Gianni was one of his oldest and most trusted of friends. They had shared much over the years and had worked well together on many occasions.

If only Guy had been informed when she had first arrived on the island; he should have been told immediately: that had been an unforgivable and important slip by his department, made for all the wrong reasons. Granted, they hadn't wanted his private life muddled up with the present operation, but it hadn't occurred to them that Alicia might leave the island so soon, let alone travel to Verona. They must have thought her settled there and well out of the way. Bad mistake: Intelligence had been negligent; they should have known better and been ready, just in case, prepared for any possible change in her movements. He would have alerted Gianni immediately to the situation and this latest chain of events would never have occurred. Alicia would have stayed, safe on the island, well protected by Gianni and his people and far away from the current drama. He wouldn't have had to worry; to have this constant nagging fear for her life accompany his each and every move. Now, unbeknown to the poor girl, Alicia had, herself, created a very real, extra, problem, purely by her presence in their midst.

Guy had thought about enlisting Gianni's help, before Alicia had appeared on the scene, but then had considered it best to leave him out of it, now that he was older, with the ever expanding Vivarini clan to look after. He hadn't thought Gianni's expertise necessary for this particular job. It had seemed clear-cut and straight forward, at the beginning. His mistake; he should never have ignored the need for Gianni's assistance, he required his experience and more of his contacts. Over the years he'd proved his worth more times than Guy cared to remember. Gianni had to be put in the picture at once and brought up to date.

And Adriana, how the hell was she going to cope with the grim news that she had coming? The whole ghastly situation was beyond the pale, as far as Guy was concerned, now that his private life had become involved. A wrong turn or unexpected upset at this time could bring about complete mayhem. Careful coordination was of paramount importance to ensure that this didn't happen.

In spite of the changing situation and the extra groundwork it had caused, everything in Verona was once more under control. For the moment, at least, Alicia was in good hands and would be out of harm's way again, back on the island, the following day. He had made it his business to organize her protection. Guy was confident that he had an efficient, dependable bunch under him. He would continue to remain out of sight while continuing to co-ordinate the action, so he must put Alicia and personal matters right out of his head, as he had been taught. Once she had him thinking about her he knew that it effected his concentration and, as of now, he needed to have his wits one hundred per cent about him. The operation, he hoped, was otherwise progressing as planned, but there was no one watching out for him. He was the one doing the watching for the time being. He had to have absolute control, both physically and mentally. His life was not his own to consider.

Guy felt a chill wind getting up and pulled his jacket closer around him. The moon was still up, but rain clouds were collecting. He could have killed for a hot bath and a shave. No such luck, he must move on as there was plenty to do and time was no longer his own either. Forcing his thoughts and feelings for Alicia to one side, he got up, straightened his back and flexed his tired, tense limbs. The blood began to flow more quickly with the sudden activity and he went on his way again, confident and with purpose.

★★★

CHAPTER 11

The next morning there wasn't a cloud in the sky and the sun shone unhindered. A light rain had fallen, in the early hours, refreshing the window boxes outside Alicia's room: she had heard it pattering softly on the roof tiles when she'd been disturbed in the night. The pungent aroma of hot coffee and freshly baked bread had drifted up from below awaking her from a deep, but finally trouble-free, sleep.

After showering and dressing, Alicia dried the chair on the balcony with her damp towel and sat watching a new day beginning, as she listened to the church bells, striking loudly on the hour. The ringing vibrated from all around, in varying tones and all slightly out of sync, almost as if in competition, each church with the other. It was already as warm as an English summer's day and the disturbing memories of the night before seemed to evaporate in the comfortable climate. Breakfast arrived, as if ordered, brought upstairs by a young girl who laid it out on the small table outside. Alicia sat, contentedly, drinking the hot, stimulating coffee and absorbing the noise, smell and the feel of the city. The view over the roofs to the river could only have been Italy. She shut her eyes and listened, then sighed nostalgically, reminded that the Adige flowed on from here to Venice, where it rejoined the sea. Her mind began to wander and her thoughts strayed back in time to the man whom she had met there during the magical time spent living with her aunt, now some eight years before.

~

It had been a youthful and forbidden experience with Marco, a much older man. At least, at the time, she had believed it to have been forbidden, little realizing that her dynamic aunt had actually condoned the liaison. She wondered where Marco was now and if he'd ever married again. His young wife and their baby had both died in childbirth, some years before he and Alicia had met. Unusual complications he had told her. What a waste of life, she had thought, feeling sad for him. He had obviously adored her. It must have been dreadful for him to have been deprived of both a wife and child at the same time: poor man.

Conte Marco Raimondo Foscarini was a close friend of Alicia's aunt Caro. Alicia often wondered if they'd had an affair when he was recovering from his loss. They knew each other so well, were so easy with each other and he was so utterly charming. It seemed more than possible.

Marco had taken Alicia under his wing and shown her the very 'soul' of Venice. He was well educated, cultured and a fount of knowledge, besides which he was also great fun with a huge sense of humour. Behind closed doors, in the privacy of the night, he'd shown her a lot more, of equal importance.

Marco had worn his heart and his admiration for Alicia on his sleeve. He wanted her for his own and was both fiercely protective and possessive. Each night he would sit quietly across the dinner table and seduce her. At first he would amuse and tease, then with smouldering eyes he would tempt and tantalize. When he knew she was lost he would lean across the table and whisper to her of the hidden delights which he planned to explore with her later. He was very experienced and taught her the very essence of varied and uninhibited love making. He made her feel as if she were the only woman on earth, as he wined and dined her in the city and discreetly took her to stay at his country estates. As for presents! Even Caro had been quite shocked, commenting, diplomatically, that his generosity would turn any young girl's head.

But when Marco had asked for her hand in marriage, Alicia had known it was time to go home. She had grown up, but was still too young to settle into a life with him in Italy, bearing the children for whom he so longed and needed to take over his inheritance. Caro had packed her off, back to England and was left to pick up the pieces with the distraught Marco.

Alicia reflected on the experience. It had been very flattering at the time and so exciting. How her life had moved on and changed since those care-free days, when, so young, she had believed the world to be at her feet with nothing beyond her reach.

~

Sitting on her little balcony and sipping her coffee, Alicia turned her thoughts to her imminent meeting with Marcello. She was wary. 'I must be careful today', she said to herself, 'very careful indeed'. The situation could ricochet out of control very easily, given the chance. 'I'm as vulnerable as I was then, with the physical side so badly lacking: I'm not used to living as a spinster!' Still it was only lunch after all and that had to be quite safe!

Vittorio and Francesca were downstairs discussing the order of their day when she finally descended, feeling energetic and, if she was truthful, more than a little excited about her own plans. Life must go on, she continued to reason to herself. I'm human after all and certainly in need of a little fun. There was nothing wrong with a little lunch with a stranger. At home she frequently had meals with business acquaintances, both men and women and sometimes at night: everybody has to eat to live.

After a certain amount of light-hearted argument, Vittorio and Francesca decided, themselves, on the most important things for Alicia to see in Verona and in which order she was to see them. Alicia told Francesca that she thought that she'd like lunch in the *Piazza Del' Erbe*, which unbeknown to either of them, was where she had already arranged to meet Marcello, although she thought it better not to mention this. Both Vittorio and Francesca seemed to think it a very good stopping place which fitted in well with the tour that they were proposing. They insisted that it was most im-portant to see the ancient Roman remains and palaces from the right place and at the right time of day for the light to enhance their *'grandezza.'* This was so typically Italian; the people were so proud of their city and they had good reason to be.

Alicia was pleased that she had decided to stay another day. It would have been stupid to leave Verona after seeing so little. She felt sure that the whole idea had originally been concocted by Francesca and her mother and she was delighted to go along with it. It was good for her to have so much to do and see, to take her mind off all her own troubles. She also decided to write some notes for an article about Verona which she could later send off to the travel department in her office at home. It would be a fun project.

She wondered, had Gianni's family known, what they would make of her arranged meeting with the friendly policeman? Quite a lot, from what she knew of Giuseppina. As it was, she was looking forward to the day ahead and lunch with Marcello as well! There was no hurry for her to go back to the island and as for returning to England, that was, as yet, far from her intention unless there was constructive news. She'd had a couple more text messages, from both Nick and Adriana, with nothing much to report. There was still no point in rushing home.

The first thing that Alicia did was to buy a good camera: she liked taking photos. It cost her 'an arm and a leg', but she didn't care, revelling in the luxury. She was in the mood for extravagance anyway. She could take some pictures to send back to England with her article. The morning was spent wandering around, appreciating the ancient culture with all the various old buildings and remains of Roman monuments that had been so faithfully pointed out and marked on the map. Alicia took many pictures, some for her work, but partly for practice with the new camera and because she was often lucky enough to have the places almost entirely to herself.

The famous Arena was more impressive than she expected; spooky really. You could still feel the atmosphere of the centuries and it was easy to imagine the cruel and barbaric scenes played out in front of thousands of people, all revelling in the gory struggles between life and death. Men being killed in their dozens: by beasts or, by each other and all in the name of entertainment.

Alicia climbed right to the very top of the circular stone seatings, from where she could see out across the entire city, with its layers of pink-tiled roofs, brightly lit by the sun. She could clearly make out the River Adige with its shining, silver water, the Cathedral and the other churches which she wanted to visit later and, beyond, outside the city walls, she could see as far as the hills; a purple haze in the distance.

She looked down and held the camera to her eye to photograph the arena: there was one solitary person far below. She lowered the camera squinting against the glare. Oh! No! Not again - surely not? It just wasn't possible. Her heart beat faster as she stared down at the figure. The man was standing apparently looking up at her from the far side. She felt sure that he was looking directly up at her: there was nobody else anywhere near her. Why would that be? He wasn't looking around, he was watching her. No, he couldn't be, but he looked remarkably familiar and he was wearing a dark suit. Even at this distance she could see that. She shivered, took the picture anyway then, feeling slightly giddy, sat down quickly and dropped her head down to her knees. When she next looked up he was gone.

'God!' she muttered to herself, 'this place really does get to you, when a poor lone tourist becomes a rapist or worse'. But somehow he didn't look like a tourist and certainly wasn't dressed like one. Was it one of the sinister looking individuals she'd seen before? She got up after a minute or two and then went slowly down the steps, thoughtful, but with legs like jelly. She'd never liked heights. Yet there was something else as well, almost a sense of foreboding.

Alicia walked quickly out of the arena under the brick walled arches, built many metres thick and emerged, thankfully, into the bright light once more. Weird, really, how these ancient places could hold onto their atmosphere over hundreds of years: she was glad to leave.

Looking around nervously, to see if there was any sign of the dark suited man, Alicia saw only local people going about their business and a few early tourists studying their guides. With relief, she walked on through the old streets in the warm sunshine, forcing herself to forget her uneasy feelings in the arena. After all, there must be plenty of dark suited men in any city on any given day. Why should she imagine that it was the same man again? He was much too far away to be certain. Even if it was, there was no earthly reason why he shouldn't have been sight-seeing as she was.

~

Alicia could have spent hours studying everything in more detail, but it was just not possible to take in too much in one morning, it was tiring on the eyes and on the feet. After the arena, she spent most of her time in St. Zeno. The magnificent basilica overlooked the tree lined piazza, where on appointed days, according to Francesca, a colourful market sold local furniture and bric-a-brac. Not today, though, the square was empty. The church was spectacular from the outside. Two lions supported the columns of the protryon above the huge, wooden, main doors. The protryon, in turn, boasted a statue of the Saint flanked by his knights and foot soldiers. The famous inner door was embellished with solid, hand worked, bronze plates illustrating stories from the Old and New Testaments. The interior was equally impressive, a haven of peace with a particularly good feel about it. But best of all Alicia liked the twelfth century Romanesque cloister adjoined to St. Zeno on one side, with its beautiful frescos and view of the bell tower.

Sant' Anastasia, another of Verona's famous four churches, was the largest of all and well worth the visit. Alicia loved the Veronese marble, the vaulting and especially Pisanello's fresco of St. George and the Princess, at the foot of the right aisle. The rest she didn't like as much as St Zeno so she didn't tarry long, she'd had enough culture for one day, besides which the church was likely to close, as it was nearly lunch time.

Just outside Sant' Anastasia, Alicia fell upon the hotel '*Due Torri Baglioni*', this luxurious building was one of the oldest and perhaps most eccentric of Italian hotels. Inside, she found yet more beautiful painted ceilings and frescoed walls. Old dowagers were sitting around gossiping, staring hard at each and at every passer by, their crimped and dyed hair matching equally

immaculate small dogs on decorated leads. Business men were beginning to
arrive, talking loudly on their mobiles in the reception area, as they collected
together for their lunch meetings and she couldn't help thinking how boring other people's work sounded, in such a public place.

Wishing to escape this humdrum reminder of her own professional life
back home, Alicia went down the stairs just inside the entrance foyer, where
a sign clearly marked the way to the wash rooms. Someone was singing and
she hesitated at the bottom, to listen. There was a long corridor with more
of the popular plush, red, carpet. Rooms led off on each side, probably conference or private dining rooms. The singing was coming from one of these.
It was a woman, a strong confident contralto voice; obviously practicing for
the next opera performance that evening. She recognized the voice and the
scene from which the aria was taken. Even without an orchestra it was star-
tlingly dramatic. Of course: the lead singers would be staying here, at one
of the best hotels in Verona. What a strange and lovely coincidence to have
walked in at that particular moment.

Even *'la toilette per signore'* was impressive: more marble, crystal chandeliers, ornate pictures and an enormous bowl of lilies, scenting the whole
restful area.

Alicia stood at the mirror listening to the voice and brushing her hair. No
longer short now, it swung at shoulder level and shone with good health.
She wondered if she should have it cut while she was in the city. Maybe
she'd just let it grow for the moment and not bother. Her skin also had a
certain glow and she wondered if that was for another reason. 'What am I
doing seeing this man?' she asked herself yet again. 'I shouldn't be so excited. I am not free, in an impossible situation and nothing is going to happen!' However on this particular day her spirits were high and the burden
of worry, sitting so uncomfortably on her shoulders, was perhaps not quite
so heavy. She suddenly felt quite reckless and not the least tired in spite of
such a lot of trudging along cobbled streets. Her shoes, thank God, were
comfortable, but she kicked them off to give her feet a well earned break
and wriggled her toes, which delighted in their freedom and the plush, soft,

carpet on the floor.

Alicia studied her reflection in the long ornate glass on the back of the door; the suit certainly was an excellent buy. It was a good colour; dark grey was so much kinder than black. The light wool cloth was soft to the touch and hung well. It looked good and very Italian. She had chosen a light blue top with three-quarter length sleeves, which she knew was the best colour to match her eyes and wore a wide belt around her hips accentuating her figure: she must remember to take the jacket off.

Alicia put on some pale pink lipstick and looked critically at her face once more. It was definitely less pinched and had some colour again. 'Not too bad. Anyway, this all has to be good for the morale,' she muttered, experiencing a small flutter in her stomach, as she sprayed some scent on her neck and put her things away in her bag before leaving the room.

★★★

CHAPTER 12

At twelve-forty five precisely, she was a stickler for punctuality, Alicia arrived in the long, narrow, *Piazza Del' Erbe*, named after the city's old herb market. She wandered through the stalls searching for the restaurant belonging to Vittorio's friend, where he'd said 'she was to relax and take refreshment in the sun'.

Francesca, interrupting her husband's directions, had insisted that Alicia must remember to take the time to study the calm smile of the statue of the 'Verona Madonna' which stands over the fountain and to look up at the beautiful frescoes on the buildings above. In the nearby *Piazza dei Signori* she was to make sure that she saw the statue of Dante, the medieval poet.

'The food and wine will be excellent', Vittorio had added, ignoring Alicia's cultural tour, while he told her in detail what he had eaten last time he was there! And as for the company that she had failed to mention? 'Well that would be excellent too', murmured Alicia with another small quiver of excitement! The rest of the sightseeing would have to wait for now.

~

Marcello had arrived first. As soon as he saw Alicia, he rose to greet her, from a discreet table in a corner, outside of the reastaurant. He came forward with a wide grin of welcome and customary kiss on both cheeks. He was dressed casually in light cords and an open necked shirt, with a dark blue jersey thrown over his shoulders. He appeared quite different out of his formal uniform, clean and fresh and smelling of exotic limes as before: delicious! She felt her stomach lurch. 'Oh my God! I'm not in control at all. I really shouldn't be so attracted to this man. I've got enough turmoil in my life already'. Alicia smiled an unashamedly guiltless smile and stifled a sigh of resignation. She was going to enjoy this afternoon, so she removed her jacket as planned and sat down in the chair being held for her. Marcello took the coat and hung it carefully over another seat.

"Alichia, *sei bella bellissima* and so smart today, especially for me I hope!"

"But, of course for you," replied Alicia quickly, hiding her agitated state and matching his mood. "I told you that I was going shopping yesterday."

He laughed good-naturedly, took her hand and stared at her.

"Both you and your suit are really beautiful and as for that belt, you know what I am thinking. *Voglio fare l'amore*," he said with a wink, "but you know that already."

She removed her hand from his. Taking the hint, he sat down, leant back in his chair and, never taking his eyes from her face, asked her what she'd like to drink.

Marcello had already taken the trouble to find out all about the specialities of the day. The waiter came across as soon as he saw Alicia seated and produced a bottle of chilled *Pinot Grigio*, as if by magic.

"If you prefer something else you have only to say, for today everything is for you."

"No, the white wine would be lovely," she said, "and you choose for me Marcello. You will know what's best to eat today. I like everything." The wine was meticulously poured and Marcello raised his glass to her as they both took their first sip. Then he bent his head to concentrate on the menu.

Alicia studied him as he carefully ordered their lunch, glancing up at her twice to see if she was happy with his choice. *Fiori di zucchini*, courgette

flowers stuffed with fish mousse to start with followed by *risi e risi*, a light sea
food risotto dish and then they would see. Marcello obviously knew the restaurant well, calling the waiter by his first name. When he was finished, the
young man refilled their glasses, thanked them and moved discreetly away.

"You really are so kind and thoughtful to me, but, you know, I have nothing to give you in return," she added quickly, looking down, away from his
searching eyes.

"Alichia, Alichia, look at me! Look at me please!" She looked up, shy now
that this was said. "I am asking for nothing but your company. You have difficult situations, I know. I just want to see you a little happy, make your life
better for you, just for the time we have together. Please believe me."

"I do and thank you," she answered quietly.

~

The tension lifted and they had a magical lunch. He was as good company as before and as funny, especially when telling stories about various
parties that he had been to on Delfino, revolving round so many of the
people she knew. She felt sure that her hunch about Francesca was correct,
just by the way he talked about meeting her at his sister's wedding. It was
obvious to her that they had had an affair, at some time.

He asked her what she'd seen in the morning and what she'd liked best in
Verona so far. "The two great doors of St. Zeno and also the frescos in the
Romanesque cloister, definitely … I felt safe in there," she had added with
feeling. Alicia preferred, as he did, the simpler cultural assets of the city. Some
of it even he found much too 'gothic'.

Marcello was instantly alert. With a slight frown creasing his brow, he
asked her what she had meant when she said she felt 'safe' in there. Alicia
told him of her strange feelings in the arena and how the atmosphere in the
old amphitheatre had affected her. Then she hesitated, not sure if she should
go on. He sensed her uncertainty and that there was more to come, encour-

aging her to continue. So she told him everything that had happened.

She described how the man in the dark suit had seemed to be watching her from below in the arena and how she felt that it was just possible that he and another had travelled on the train with her and visited the opera house on the same night as she had. Everywhere in fact, one or the other seemed to have been following in her footsteps. She had thought it odd, as neither behaved or looked like tourists. She added that she had actually taken a photograph, though it would surely have been too far away to see the man's face. Marcello listened carefully to this, looking wary and slightly concerned. Then he reassured her by saying that he suspected that it was mere coincidence. However, if she'd let him take the camera he would get the film developed and have a look. He'd have it returned to the hotel later.

She nodded, glad that he hadn't thought her ridiculous or to be imagining things and then, thinking that it was only fair, went on to tell him a little of her strange predicament. She felt quite sure that her confidence was safe with this amiable policeman. His face, as she talked, showed both sensitivity and understanding, which in itself was disarming.

The sun was warm on her back and made her feel lackadaisical and relaxed or maybe it was the wine! Lunch went on forever, their mutual attraction developing further, as they sat, with the table safely separating them.

By the time they finally left, the restaurant was completely empty and the staff enjoying their own meal inside. Time had flown for them both. Neither could believe that they'd only known each other for two short days and nights. Slowly they walked back beside the river, quiet, taking as long as possible, both knew what was coming: the inevitable.

It was easy walking here, not many people, yet such a lot to take in. Much smaller than Venice but very different, which reminded her that she would soon have to telephone her Aunt. Before she finally returned to England, she must visit Caro again in the city on the water that she adored and which held such incomparable memories. Alicia told Marcello of her plans, about her aunt, her superb collection of pictures and about her palazzo, itself almost a museum.

They stopped for a while on the medieval *Ponte Scaligero* to admire a distant view of the Alps. Alicia wondered when to say goodbye. Better not too near the hotel, she decided. They wandered back across the bridge, slowly, reluctantly, neither speaking much, the tension was there again and both were delaying the moment. He draped his arm loosely around her shoulders, as they walked, lost in his own thoughts. She pretended to be busy studying the local architecture as they passed. Then Alicia made up her mind and suddenly stopped. She turned to him and said, raising her hand to touch his face.

"Marcello, it's best if we leave each other now and quickly perhaps. I know the way from here," she hesitated. "You will never know how much you have helped me. You have given me back my confidence and my hope for the future. Thank you, *grazie mille per la sua gentilezza* and also for a really lovely lunch, *mi mancherai*," she finished quickly and looked away.

"Alichia come here, *baciami*," he said taking her gently into his arms and kissing her for so long that her insides were melting and her legs becoming useless. When he stopped she was unable to speak.

"*Capisci*, Alichia. Never forget, it's I who have you to thank for this time you have allowed me," he said concentrating hard on his English. "I shall always regret what we could have shared, but here," he said touching his heart, "you will always remain and here also," touching his head, "now go!"

With that he let her out of his arms, gave her a gentle push and turning, walked quickly back the way they had come. She watched him getting further and further away, willing herself not to call him back. At the corner of the street he looked back once, blew her a kiss and disappeared from sight.

'I can't believe I'm feeling like this,' Alicia thought, shaking herself. 'What is the matter with me? It was just lunch for heaven's sake'.

~

Marcello was much troubled. As soon as he'd turned the corner and was out of sight he took out his mobile, checked the street name and made a short call. He didn't like what she'd told him over lunch, which had confirmed his worst suspicions. There was no question that she was being followed. He needed to find out who the people were, what was going on and why they were so interested in Alicia. He minded too much personally now. It was no longer just a job for a favour. She was beautiful and he was going to do his utmost to make sure that she came to no harm. He made another call and then walked purposefully on towards his intended destination, a determined look on his face.

Deep in thought also, Alicia ambled slowly back towards the hotel and the shopping street where she had been the night before. She had very much enjoyed being with Marcello. They had much in common in the way they thought and in what interested them both. He was both funny and fun. They also had a very strong physical attraction for each other. She was glad that it had only been lunch, dinner and night time would have been much more dangerous. But it was over now and before anything had even started, so she must get her emotions back in control and move on again. Soon she would have to decide what to do and where to go next.

~

Meanwhile she must find some small present for Giuseppina. After all, Giuseppina had been responsible for the idea of the trip to Verona in the first place, so she couldn't return to Delfino empty handed. Alicia set off, resolutely, to find the shop where she had bought the dolphins. She had walked a long way since and all the little side streets looked the same, but with some trouble and a bit of luck she found it again.

Alicia was looking intently at a little hand painted mirror in the window, when she sensed, rather than saw, an aggressive movement behind her. Too late. A man lurched into her, grabbed her arm and muttered in a heavy, accented, middle European sounding voice, 'Come with me, *Senorina*, if you please.' Then, almost immediately another voice, interrupted forcefully:

'Attenzione, attenzione, senorina! Barstardo, ma va' all' inferno'. She hardly had time to turn before there was a huge bump, much more swearing in Italian and she was hurled to the pavement, where dazed and confused, she sat trying to make sense of what had happened. There was the sound of running footsteps and excited shouts as other people gathered around to help or merely to stop and stare.

"Are you alright? Are you alright?" asked the second concerned voice beside her. A young man was helping her up and retrieving her bag. "I saw the pickpocket make his move. *Sente qualche dolore?*" Are you hurt?" He repeated in good and educated English.

"No, no! *Grazie molto*," Alicia answered. *"Sto bene*, I'm fine, just a little shocked, that's all. *Sono di L'Inghilterra. Cosa sta succedendo? No capisco, no capisco!"*

"Non preoccuparti. Let me help you to your hotel, *via*, come," he said, gently taking her arm. He had taken control of the situation. He was kind and genuinely worried, or so it seemed and she was not going to turn down his assistance.

"Per favore, what did he look like?" asked Alicia of the young man, when she had her breath back. "What did he look like?" she repeated urgently. "Did you see his face?"

"Si, he was dark and ugly and dressed in a suit for a funeral: black." came the grim and half expected reply.

Alicia stood, too stunned to speak. When they arrived at the Hotel Rafaeli, the young man, handing her over to Vittorio, explained what had happened, said goodbye and left almost as quickly as he had appeared. A horrified Francesca took Alicia upstairs and settled her on her bed.

"Do you need a doctor?" she asked.

"No thank you, I'm perfectly alright, really," replied Alicia. "I might just rest for a little."

"I will bring you some English tea then, *Senorina,*" she said and went out.

It wasn't until that moment, when she was left on her own, that Alicia remembered that she hadn't told the young man where she was staying. How on earth did he know how to bring her here and why did the so-called mugger in the dark suit want her to go with him? He hadn't even taken her bag! More importantly, why was she being followed by these people in the dark suits? What could they possibly want of her?

Could it possibly, just possibly, have anything to do with someone else? someone else altogether?

***

CHAPTER 13

Later that evening, as Alicia lay quietly on her bed, occasionally dozing off, but mostly reliving the alarming incident, there was an urgent knocking on her door.

"Come in," she cried, thinking that it was Franscesca coming to see if she was alright. She started and then stared in astonishment as Marcello walked through the door, bearing an anxious smile and a glass of red wine.

"Marcello! What on earth … how did you know?"

He put the glass down firmly on the table and gathered her into his arms, whereupon she burst into tears.

"*Mi dispiace!*"

"There is someone following me around, I know it, I can feel it, *non mi piace*, it's these dark suited people and I don't understand why. What do they want?" she whispered into his shoulder.

"I know, I know," he answered gently. "You are coming with me, it's decided now. Don't worry, *tutto fila*. It's alright, Marcello will look after you. He is a policeman after all. No more of these now," he added, wiping the tears from her face with his hand. "What is it I do, that you always cry? Now pack your things please, we are leaving right away and there's some speed," he said, losing his English again.

"Hurry, not speed, Marcello," she mumbled. He laughed softly.

"Alright, my little English *professoressa*, but please do hurry a little, and wear the jeans too. *Adesso devo andare.* I'll wait downstairs as I need to ring Gianni to tell him where we will be."

"But Gianni doesn't know …"

"Yes, he does. Later, I will tell you all later. *Coraggiosa* Alichia! and drink the wine," he finished, pointing to the glass. "It is good, I know the vineyard!" With that he kissed her hand and went out of the room. She could hear him bounding down the stairs two at a time. What was going on and how on earth did Gianni know about any of it? She'd told no one, absolutely no one. Well, at least somebody was in charge and she knew that she couldn't be in safer hands than those of Marcello. He was part of the family and she was no longer frightened now that he was around. She got off her bed and started to put her few things together, experiencing small but persistent flutterings inside her stomach as the adrenalin kicked in and excitement took over. She was on the move, she was safe with Marcello and something was happening at last. In fact anything could happen.

When Alicia arrived downstairs, everyone was waiting, talking happily together as if nothing had occurred. After heartfelt farewells and 'please to come again for a better visit next time', Alicia and Marcello left the hotel. He had made her wrap her pashmina round her head to cover her *'bella* blonde head, just in case,' he'd said quietly 'and please pretend you're my girlfriend', he said seriously, wrapping his arm around her protectively and talking Italian to her as they went out through the side door.

The sky was overcast and heavy as night began to draw in. There was rain around and she was glad of the warm jersey she had thought to put on over her shirt. As they walked quickly along the side of the hotel they could hear Franscesca's voice laughing with a crowd of people at the front.

"Just little distraction," whispered Marcello as he wheeled his motor bike

away around the corner. He fastened her bag firmly on the back, handed her
a helmet, then jumped on and started up.

"Now, behind me, *andiamo!* Hold on very, very close, *per favore!*" he said
into her ear, as she got on; perhaps making the most of the urgent situation,
thought Alicia, unfazed.

As they sped away into the night, she couldn't help but feel exhilaration.
'What will be, will be, *che sera, sera*', she thought. 'What choice do I have?
He's like my saviour!' She held on very, very tight, relishing the sensual,
comforting warmth of his body.

They went quickly through the traffic, with very little to hamper their
progress once they were out of the small streets. Marcello was adroit at
weaving safely in and out between the cars. He headed out of the city and
way up into the hills. The city looked another world away as they stopped
once, to look down on the lights, twinkling far below. After a few more kilo-
meters Marcello turned down a rough, bumpy track. Alicia held on for dear
life and laughing, made him slow down, thinking her bones might shatter.
Finally, they arrived at a small farm house. Tucked away at the end of the
valley, it was surrounded by olives beside a shimmering stream, caught in the
luminous silver light of a full moon, as it suddenly appeared from behind a
cloud. Alicia got off, removed her helmet and shook her hair free. With the
engine silenced, it was so quiet you couldn't hear a thing, only the bubbling
water. She let out a contented sigh. It was perfect.

"Now you can relax at last, *mia* Alichia. *Uno promessa, tutto fila*, all is well
here. You have nothing to worry about. There is no one here, just us." He secured the bike and, taking their two bags, led the way into the house. 'That's
exactly what's worrying me', thought Alicia, following … the 'just us'.

Inside, the little farmhouse was cosy and warm as if it had been filled
with the sun all day. It smelt mildly of lavender. There was one large room
with a small kitchen at one end, a bathroom leading off the other and two
bedrooms on one side. At the far side, a stable door opened out onto a small

terrace.

"From here," Marcello told her, "there is a beautiful view over a wide valley, we are quite high. *Domani.* You will see in the morning."

"But who lives here?" asked Alicia.

"It belongs to a friend of mine. He's an artist and is often away with his work. When I'm off duty I sometimes come here. There is a woman who comes in once a week only. She came in today," he said pointing to the table which was laid for a meal. Alicia shivered. He noticed.

"*Freddo,* are you cold?" Marcello asked concerned. "Shall we light the fire?"

"*Si, per favore,*" she answered quickly, "that would be lovely." But she wasn't cold, it was something else altogether.

"It would be, wouldn't it?" he agreed, catching her eyes. "It's still cool up in the hills at this time of year and there's been much excitement today, hasn't there, *mia* Alichia?"

'Oh dear', she thought 'the tension is here between us again'. They lit the fire, which cleared the atmosphere a little, giving them something to do. Then, with a flourish, Marcello pulled a bottle of white wine out of his bag.

"*Voil,* is that what they say in France, *mia bella; voil?* Look what Francesca gave us."

"No! It's *voilà*," giggled Alicia. What a relief she thought. The wine should make things easier, though I had better make sure that he drinks most of it this time. They sat warming themselves by the fire, talking about this and that, his family and where he grew up and what he liked to do when he wasn't working, while Alicia waited for him to tell her what was going on.

She could see that he was biding his time, unsure of what to say or perhaps how much and waiting for her to relax. She couldn't relax. She was too keyed up with the day's events and with Marcello's nearness.

After a while he jumped up, held out his hand, pulled Alicia to her feet, and suggested that they eat. What a feast! They had local olives and *focaccia* bread. *Carpaccio* to start, followed by a tomato and basil salad, together with a wonderful dish of spaghetti with wild mushrooms, which Marcello cooked with much pride and a lot of banging around in the kitchen, along with much whistling and not a few expletives.

He'd not allowed her do anything but sit by the fire, while he prepared their dinner, so she sat quietly listening to him with amusement as he moved around, periodically appearing to show her something, or to give her more wine. She knew he would tell her eventually, when the time was right. There was no hurry. They would be going nowhere else tonight!

A bottle of red wine miraculously appeared, to go with the main course. It was when they were half way through the bottle that he finally started to tell her. Marcello was honest and straight forward and told her that, after the incident in the street, he had been informed straight away, on his mobile. That was why he had arrived at the hotel so quickly. Alicia was startled and began to speak, but Marcello held up his hand. He had only just begun to tell her what he knew.

~

After their earlier lunch, he'd been really concerned about Alicia's description and the three sightings of the dark-suited men.

"I am, after all, a well-trained policeman and was in the military before becoming a member of the *carabineri*. I have much experience in surveillance and some other things", he had said with a reassuring smile. "It is my job again now". Marcello got up from his chair and crossing the room, retrieved her camera and the photographs, which he handed back to her.

He'd had the picture of the man in the arena enlarged many times over by the police photographic department, who had then scanned it and checked against their records. Marcello had already been told by his own superiors that there was a raised level of intelligence activity in the area. It was all very hush-hush and involved the British; but they had refused to tell him what it was all about. When he had handed over the picture he had only done so on the understanding that he was promised a meeting with the department's commanding officer, as he knew that the others could tell him nothing.

The *commandente* had been pleased with the picture. It was obvious that the dark suited man was already known to him. He then told Marcello that Alicia had become involved purely by chance, because she just happened to be here, in the wrong place at the wrong time. But he had added that she also had interesting connections. At this Alicia felt the cold fingers of fear and apprehension slide down the back of her neck and she shivered visibly. Marcello, quick to notice and thinking her cold again, got up to throw another log on the fire, before continuing. So, the Italian police were already aware of who she was and what had happened. He was then told that it was likely she was being watched and followed because of her connections, indicating that the so called mugging incident, although unfortunate, was less of a mystery to the intelligence services than it was to him. These people weren't after money. Marcello's contact couldn't or wouldn't say any more than that and, when he pressed for more information, the conversation had been abruptly terminated and Marcello had been shown out.

What Marcello didn't tell Alicia was that, when he left police headquarters, he was in no doubt whatsoever that he had only been told a very small part of a much larger story and that the status of the mysterious operation in progress was tense and delicate. As yet unaware of the menace dogging her footsteps Alicia was in obvious jeopardy and this made him extremely worried.

He had been ordered back to his own department to receive further instructions, he told her. There he had been told to make certain that 'La Signora Spence' was well looked after, wherever she went and for the moment she was to remain in his safekeeping. No chances were to be taken with the safety of a British citizen. At this, he couldn't resist a rather self satisfied grin as he went on. They wanted her out of the city *'pronto'* and, in a secure place until whatever was going on was settled.

"*Quindi!*" he added with another grin, trying to dispel her disquiet. He had gladly taken on this responsibility himself. Hence the quick departure. He had also told Gianni that he would personally deliver her safely back to Stefano, when they were ready.

"And so," he said, holding his hands out, "I have you to myself for a little longer, *mia cara!* You are safe with me and the world is ours up here high above the Veneto."

"Thank you; thank you again, Marcello, both for telling me and for coming to my rescue. I don't know what I'd have done without you."

"Then don't," he said taking her hand across the table. "Don't do any of these things without me."

"But," Alicia said quickly changing the subject, "I still don't understand what these people want from me. What could I possibly have of interest and who are they anyway?"

"*No lo so,*" he replied, standing up "and if my superiors do, they do not tell me at this time," spreading his hands again. "Come here now, *non più*. No more worry, *rilassarsi*. Sit with me here by the fire, it's been a long day for us both. I'll get us some more coffee," he said, striding off to reclaim the coffee pot from the table. Subject definitely closed, thought Alicia.

~

Alicia sat, curled up against Marcello's legs, in front of the fire, digesting what he had told her, while he sat behind her on the sofa. He stroked her silken hair and began to kiss the back of her neck, until she could think no more.

For a long time they didn't speak and when she turned to do so, he took her face in his hands and pulling her towards him once again began to kiss her, softly and gently all around her mouth, opening it with his lips, touching her tongue with his. She returned his kisses, unable to resist.

"Let me take you away from it all, let me make you happy just for a little while, Alichia *mia bella*," he murmured. A sudden thought leapt into her head. She pulled away and looked up at his surprised face.

"Marcello, tell me … tell me the truth. Did Gianni ask you to get to know me so that you could look after me, from the very beginning? That first night in the village, tell me please?" He looked trapped for a moment, let out a sigh and then she saw him decide.

"Yes, he did ask me to take care of you."

"From the beginning?" she asked again.

"From the beginning," he repeated, "but … to Gianni you are like family and he …" He was unable to finish his sentence.

"So this …," she waved her hands around wildly, jumping up, "our lunch in the city and all of this is just part of the job." She looked as if she was going to hit him, then he saw her subside with something akin to despair and the tears spring into her eyes again, this time from anger.

"I'm going to have a shower, if that's alright and then I'm going to get some sleep," she said, as she trounced off to the bedroom where he'd put her bag.

Marcello put his head in his hands. 'But you didn't let me finish', he said to himself, 'for no one told me to fall in love with you'.

Alicia stood under the shower for a long time and felt better. How could she have let herself fall so easily into this situation. He must think her a complete fool. Well, she would just go to bed on her own and insist on leaving first thing in the morning.

Marcello meticulously cleared up the kitchen, turned out some of the lights and threw another log on the fire. Then he lay stretched out on the sofa, with his hands behind his head thinking that it really didn't always pay to be so honest.

Half an hour later, Alicia wondered if she dared come out in her towel to get a drink of water. She opened the door a crack. The lights were mostly off and the other bedroom door shut, so she thought Marcello must have gone to bed too. She crept out as quietly as she could and tiptoed across to the kitchen, feeling somewhat guilty when she saw how tidy it all was. He'd done everything. She was half way back across the room with the glass of water, when his voice reached her from the shadows.

"*Ti amo*, I was going to tell you that no one told me to fall in love with you, but you didn't give me a chance!"

Alicia stood rooted to the spot, her glass wobbling in her hand with fright, then let out the same sigh of anguish that he'd heard once before.

"Oh! Marcello, *Mi dispiace!*"

He was off the sofa and across the room in a flash, taking the glass from her hand, putting it down and picking her up in his arms, then returning to lay her carefully down on the sofa in the firelight.

"*Mia caro*, let me love you, just for this one night. No one need ever know. It will be just for us and will have to last your policeman for a life time."

Alicia had made up her mind. It was all just too much and more than she could bear. Better judgement put aside, her spirit overcame her. She reached up, took his face between both her hands and let her towel drop to her waist.

"Yes, she said and we'll make it last a lifetime for us both!"

He kissed her as if it would last forever, then knelt by the sofa, pulled the towel apart and began to kiss her naked body, softly and slowly. She reached behind his head and wove her fingers through his thick hair. His hand glided over her soft skin, touching, hesitating, then moving on again, across her flat stomach, down the insides of her thighs, circling that most secret of places. She pulled his mouth back to hers and at the same time began to undo his shirt.

"Slowly, *piu' lentamente*", he whispered as she unbuckled his belt.

"Remember this night must last for ever!"

Naked in the flickering firelight, he made her stay still and stroked and kissed her body until she thought she'd die with longing. Just when she thought she couldn't wait any longer, he took her nipples in his mouth and began to suck on them gently; then she was begging him to satisfy her craving.

He moved his lean, strong body quickly, but gently, between her long legs. She was rising up to meet him, quivering as he entered her; warm and welcoming. He recaptured her mouth and held her tight, moving slowly and surely, as she had already reached beyond that point of no return, tumbling over the brink, tossing her body as she was carried away on rapturous waves.

When she opened her eyes in question, he shook his head.

"Oh no! *Mia Caro*. For me, not yet, for I told you we have a long night ahead of us," but the next time their rhythm matched and they rode the primal sea of incomparable sensation together.

He made love to her in a way that defied all description. She couldn't believe afterwards that she'd been capable of so much and for so long. Their appetite matching, it wasn't until the dawn began to work its way up above the hills, that they were finally satisfied. Their night must end. In order to continue with the day, they must sleep a little. When they awoke, the fire was still alight. Marcello raised himself up on one elbow, gazed at the glowing embers and then, looking down at her muttered.

"The fire you have lit inside, it always will remain; Alichia *mia*". She nodded her tousled head.

"For me too, Marcello. For me too!" she whispered.

"But we cannot be sad. We have too much too remember now. *Giusto,* that is right my little English teacher?"

"Yes," she answered, sitting up. "Yes it is right" then taking his hand, she pulled him up off the sofa. "How about breakfast, I'm hungry."

"So am I. *Ti desidero,*" he replied immediately and followed her into the shower.

"Oh no! *non piu!'* No more. Please Marcello. I won't be able to stand."

"Then I'll carry you, *no problemo,*" he said laughing.

He turned on the shower and let the warm water drench them. Again they climbed the giddy mountain together as he took her standing against the tiled wall, with the water skidding off their shoulders. After the night they had already enjoyed, she couldn't believe that once more they could ride the flames of passion so high, so quickly and with such force.

~

It had rained in the early hours of the night, clearing the way for a soft, gentle day. Marcello dried the chairs outside and they sat languidly eating the toast he'd made with so much aplomb. He sat looking at her, munching, a twinkle in his eyes.

"Because I know the English like toast," he explained, holding it up, grinning.

"Rubbish!" Alicia replied. "You know you only made it because the bread was stale!" He laughed and wagged his finger at her.

"And what is this 'rubbish'?" asked Marcello. "The English grammar is a mystery. I thought that rubbish was something that you threw in the box."

"Exactly," giggled Alicia looking at him and getting ready to run.

"And it's a bin, not a box that you put it in!"

Marcello made a grab for her but she was too fast. Holding her towel around her with one hand she jumped off the terrace and was running in her bare feet across the lush grass to hide in the olives, laughing helplessly. But he was there, close behind her within just a few strides. She stopped, gathering her towel around her naked body and turned to him, the laughter dying as she saw the stricken look in his face confirming his emotions. The familiar tears pricked the back of her eyes and they became serious again as he caught her to him.

"*Via!* Come with me, Alichia *mia*. Let us be together one last time, here in the olive grove." He laid his towel at the foot of an old olive and surrounded by the damp sweet smelling grass they reached again for that which left them both speechless and overwhelmed.

~

The time eventually came to leave their idyllic haven and both were silent as they packed and tidied up the house. When they stood together at the door, to look back one last time, Marcello said, 'the woman will be amazed that the sheets are still clean'. They laughed and it lightened their mood as they shut and locked the door, returning the key to its hiding place under the rafters. As they rode away up the track Alicia looked back again. Blowing a kiss with one hand, her voice carrying on the wind, she called, "Thank you, whoever you are, for lending us your heavenly home, I shall never forget this place". Marcello concentrating on the rough ground muttered in agreement. "Nor me, *non mai,* never." Alicia laid her head against his back and held on tighter than ever, with her arms around his waist.

~

They travelled along the top of the hills, the *'Piccole Dolomiti'*, leaving Verona and the Veneto far behind, before winding down into a little valley, where Marcello said they could catch a direct train to Stefano's village, avoiding Bologna.

After stopping at a *panetteria* and buying a sandwich for lunch they boarded the train together. Marcello insisted on checking the carriages and called Stefano on his mobile as they settled down for the last part of their journey. The little train seemed to halt everywhere. The journey took a long time and they were both glad.

Having eaten her share of the sandwiches, Alicia put her head on Marcello's shoulder and went fast asleep. The next thing she knew was that he was waking her gently.

"Alichia, *mia* Alichia, *adesso devo andare.* It is the best for us I think."

"But where are we?" she asked, waking instantly.

"We are coming to the last stop before Stefano's village. He will be waiting for you, but I think it no good if he sees us together and my sister-in-law, she misses nothing! So I get off here." He stared at her sadly. "Perhaps we will see each other again, who knows, *sono fatalista,* but I will carry you with me always, here," touching his head, "and here" touching his heart, "for ever. But please too, you must remember, never let these two days we have had spoil your life in any way. They were a most special gift and for no one else, *mia cara*. Just, for us."

"No one can ever take the memories away," she replied. "They will stay with us always."

"*Si*" he murmured, stroking her hair one last time, as the train shuddered to a stop.

"Now I go. Have courage Alichia. If ever you have more trouble you know how to find me and I am there for you in the moment." He kissed her deeply one last time and was gone, before she could say another word.

'A second, Marcello, not moment', Alicia said quietly to herself, correcting him, after he had gone. The train moved on and she looked for him through the window, but there was no sign. He had disappeared already. She sat back with a sigh of resignation. 'What will be, will most certainly be, I suppose', she whispered quietly to herself, brushing a tear from her face.

Marcello had walked quickly through the side entrance out of sight. He leaned against the wall on the far side of the station and with his hand shaking, took out a cigarette.

By the time the train lurched into the next station, Alicia had managed to tidy herself up a bit and hoped that she looked at least reasonably normal. Stefano met her with a beaming smile and marched off towards the hotel at the same speed as before, with Alicia almost running behind trying to keep up.

'If he had any idea of just what I've been doing with his brother, he wouldn't go so fast', she thought grimly, somehow making her tired legs work. It was late afternoon when Alicia and Stefano entered the hotel Amalia again. So much had happened since she was here last.

~

There were the usual enthusiastically warm greetings from all the family. Sensing that Alicia was tired and needed her space, Amelia packed the children off to watch the television and picking up Alicia's case, took her upstairs herself. It was almost as if she knew to ask no questions and Alicia was grateful. No doubt she already knew about the so-called 'mugging' incident and most likely thought that she was quiet and tired because of it. She was so kind and made Alicia feel so much at home that she didn't even find herself feeling awkward, but she couldn't help wondering if her intoxicating lovemaking with Amelia's brother-in-law somehow showed in her face. Marcello was quite right: they could never have come back here together, for what they had found would have been obvious to the family.

When Amalia went back to her kitchen, Alicia sat on her bed to collect herself for a few moments. Marcello had left her with an overload of the sweetest emotion, which had washed away the extreme anxiety she had suffered before. In spite of her physical weariness, she felt strong and confident again. She agreed with Marcello. The time they had been given together had been without doubt *'fatalista'*, God given and as far as the future was concerned, who knows? Maybe their paths would cross again. At this moment in time she very much hoped they would. He had filled an enormous gap in her life.

Picking up a warmer jersey, Alicia left the hotel to explore the village again. It was best to keep busy before a poignant sadness set in. She had really hated saying goodbye to Marcello. They'd had so little time together. She went into the little church. It was very old and simple with just one lovely stained glass window and a beautiful, partly obscured, fresco over the altar. She sat for a while and then lit a candle for them all. Strangely enough she felt no disloyalty to Guy. Her time with Marcello had nothing to do with him or her feelings for him and it changed nothing - nothing at all. The last two days and especially last night she would hold precious for the rest of her life. Marcello had given her back her sanity, her balance and her strength. He had loved and taken care of her and given her the courage to go on again, for which she would be eternally grateful. These gifts were all of immeasurable value. And what had she given in return? Her life and her unrestricted love, for a day and a night. Nothing could change that.

She walked further up into the hills, untroubled, yet saddened that something so wonderful must now be relegated to memory, albeit a treasured one and one never to be shared. She wondered what Marcello was thinking.

On this occasion, as she walked around the village so deep in thought, she noticed that there seemed to be several people around. All nodded to her or smiled as if they knew her as she went past and this made her feel secure. It felt good to be back in the country, away from the unknown threat which seemed to loom over her in the city. There were certainly strange things going on there. She wondered what she had somehow stumbled across. Thank heavens for the young man and for Marcello! She had been cared for and protected, otherwise goodness only knows what might have happened.

She sat for a long time by the little fountain, feeling that she was sticking out like a sore thumb. Everyone must have known who she was ever since she had first come here. News of a stranger in their midst must have spread quickly through a village so small. Italians were terrible gossips and loved someone new, especially if that person was surrounded in mystery too.

She spent a quiet evening with the family. It was Sunday, so the restaurant was closed, but she was glad of the company and for the opportunity of another simple family meal, finishing with Amalia's much prized, homemade, ice cream. She and her children had remembered how much Alicia had enjoyed it on her last visit and had specially added it to the menu!

Marcello's name came up once in a while, but only in general conversation. He was obviously a very popular member of the family. After they had all finished dinner, Alicia excused herself politely and went upstairs to bed. She was tired out, both physically and mentally. Sleep came to her easily. Lying between the sheets Alicia felt the uncontrolled peace of total exhaustion flood over her and she soon drifted into an undisturbed oblivion.

★★★

CHAPTER 14

Marcello stood for a while outside the station, smoking, waiting for a return train and reflecting on just how much his life had changed in such a short space of time. His hand became steady again as he regained control, now that Alicia had gone.

It had certainly been a night to last them for a lifetime. He would never forget one single moment of it. He would relive it all time and again. Most likely that was all that he would have: the memories. Alicia had been as insatiable as he, but much more than that she was of like mind, which in itself he found stimulating. More important still, she had touched his heart as no other had before and he expected no other would. He couldn't remember ever feeling this way about a woman. Yet he knew that Alicia wasn't for him. Their worlds were just too far apart.

When Marcello's tempestuous affair with Francesca had ended abruptly several years before, he'd been sad, but not bereft as he felt now. She had been too volatile and needed too much attention. Alicia was something different altogether but, as he'd told her, he'd be grateful for the rest of his life for the short time they'd had together. He'd never before given himself so completely.

Now he must get on with his job, put his tiredness on one side and his feelings away into a private compartment. He had to find out exactly what was going on in Verona and just how much it involved Alicia. For, above all else he must protect her, if only from afar and at whatever cost to himself.

He must also report back in detail to Gianni. He would wish to be up-dated with exactly what the *commandente* had to say, if he wasn't already in the picture. Gianni seemed to have an uncanny way of knowing most things before anybody else, with contacts and friends in every field including the police and Intelligenzia. Marcello was certain that, over the years, Gianni wasn't only kept busy running his island. He'd always had an idea that a lot more happened on Isola Delfino than the general public would ever know. Perhaps he noticed things because of his own training. He'd been staying on the island with Francesca on one occasion, towards the end of their affair. Gianni had been too busy to join them all for the midday meal, engaged in a meeting with a so called 'food inspector' he was told, but the man hadn't been a food inspector at all: Marcello caught a glimpse of the visitor as he left the island. The man was from an elite secret world. Marcello had sat in on a lecture which the intriguing individual had once given in Bologna and so knew him perfectly well by sight.

He heard a train approaching, stamped on his cigarette, rearranged his thoughts and with a sigh of resignation walked back onto the platform. He looked both ways from habit and jumped on quickly through the first avail-able door. As the carriages pulled out of the station, Marcello stood to make sure he was alone, then sat down by the window, decided on his course of action, took out his mobile and slotted himself back into work mode.

~

Stefano and Alicia set off together, early the next morning, after breakfast, taking the car to the port. By afternoon she was safely back on the island, being welcomed once more into Gianni's family. The grapevine had been working overtime. The news of her unfortunate adventure in Verona had spread like wildfire and Mario couldn't hide his concern when he met them in Biri. As they crossed to the island he wasn't his usual ebullient self and kept muttering about the city being no good for single women and that she shouldn't have gone there on her own. Alicia really would have preferred to have been allowed to forget the whole sorry incident as it was now remote in both time and distance. Besides which, she now had other things on her mind. Unbeknown to the Vivarini family much else had happened in Verona besides the mugging incident.

Gianni greeted Alicia affectionately and, noticing with surprise the new, soft, look about her, merely expressed with passion his opinion of those who took advantage of young women. He then changed the subject, making it quite clear to Giuseppina that she should do likewise. He understood Alicia's need to forget the frightening episode. She was unhurt, she was strong, looked remarkably well and had obviously enjoyed the rest of her visit, which had done her good. It could have been very much worse. Gianni thanked the Lord above for blessing him with foresight; the young man in the city had been put in place just in time and had been quick to the rescue that day. Marcello had also proved efficient and dependable, as expected.

Gianni took Alicia into the dining room and taking a brown package from the table, said:

"This arrived for you this morning," as he put it gently into her outstretched hands. 'What could it be, on this day of all days? queried Alicia! She sat at the table and carefully opened up the parcel. Her heart stopped, for inside was a flat box containing a perfect bunch of dried spring flowers. Gianni watched with interest. Alicia raised her head and he looked on in astonishment. Her eyes brimmed with tears and her whole face burst into the most radiant of smiles that he'd ever seen. She mumbled something, jumped up from the chair, almost knocking it over in her haste and was gone in a flash, upstairs to her room. Gianni stunned for a moment, heard her door close then recovered his voice.

"Giuseppina, Giuseppina, my Giuseppina where are you? Come quick! *Fai Presto!* Where have you gone?" Gianni called urgently as he rushed into the kitchen to look for his wife.

"Whatever is it? *Che'ce'.* What's happened?" cried Giuseppina, alarmed, as she arrived running in from outside. She'd been busy with her chickens and had a bowl in her hand, full of eggs bouncing dangerously up and down, as she hurried.

"I've seen it," said Gianni raising his eyes to the ceiling, "I've just seen it!"

"Seen what? What on earth have you seen? For goodness' sake man, what have you seen?" exclaimed Giuseppina, crossly wiping her hands on her apron, now that she realized that the look on her husband's face was one of twinkling delight, not real drama.

"Alicia! She smiled, really smiled; she has the most beautiful smile and her whole face lights up like a Christmas tree, like the sun," finished Gianni reverently, "and I was the first one to see it," he added smugly and walked off with a chuckle, leaving Giuseppina shaking her head and muttering in pleased exasperation.

Alicia changed her clothes and took herself and the box down through the vines to the path that led onto the beach. She walked slowly as if in a trance, frequently stopping to remove the lid and look again upon the flowers, almost as if to reassure herself that they hadn't somehow been spirited away, whilst out of sight. But they were still there, safe in their nest of crisp tissue paper. He was alive; Guy was alive and had sent her flowers on her birthday so that she would know. It was a message. There could be no other explanation: it had to be him. There was no card. She put one hand up to her face. Her cheeks were flaming with excitement and she couldn't stop smiling. It was going to be alright. She knew it: he hadn't abandoned her after all!

~

Arriving at the beach Alicia kicked off her shoes and wriggled her toes, revelling in the cool feel of the sand working its way up between them. She felt like jumping up and down and shouting something stupid for the whole world to hear. But there was no one, just the gulls. Instead she stared into space, as if mesmerised by something far off on the horizon, while this small miracle began to sink in. Guy really was alive. It was as if he was aware of what she'd just been doing and had made himself known again to put an end to it. She thought of Marcello and her sated body, but no sense of guilt intruded and she was at peace with the situation. He, too, was a wonderful man and she regretted nothing.

Alicia shook her head as if to clear it and, clutching the box of flowers to her chest, set off across the sand towards the water like one possessed, lost in thought. She had a lot to think about. When she finally regained the path home she found Gianni sitting quietly on the rocks, waiting for her. She wasn't surprised to see him there. Her behaviour must have given him a bit of a shock. She went over slowly and sat down beside him. She suddenly felt emotionally exhausted; by recent events in her life and now by this momentous revelation. He put his large hand on hers and said:

"Now, *Mia cara,* I really do think it's time for you to tell me your troubles. I only want to help, you know."

"Yes," replied Alicia, "I know and you're right. It is time, long past really. I should have explained my predicament ages ago. How silly of me." As she looked up into Gianni's, lined, brown, face, tears welled in her bright blue eyes and slid gently down her cheeks. He opened his arms and she buried her head on his shoulder. Then she began to speak so quietly that he could hardly hear.

"You see, I wasn't going to tell you, but it's my birthday today. I'm twenty-six: very old!" Alicia sat up, as he passed over his freshly ironed red spotted handkerchief. She blew her nose and sniffed, then awkwardly handed back the sodden piece of cloth. Smiling apologetically, she continued hesitantly, "*Mi scusi.* You see - it's because of the flowers that I know for certain - for the very first time - that my fiancé – Guy – isn't – well - that he isn't dead." She stopped abruptly with a huge intake of breath followed by a long sigh. Alicia was so overwrought that she didn't notice Gianni's startled reaction. Then the whole sorry story slowly poured forth, missing out only the magical interlude with Marcello.

~

After Alicia had finished speaking, they sat quietly together, each immersed in their own thoughts. Gianni handed her his handkerchief again and waited for her to dry her eyes. He nodded, as if having made up his mind about something, took her hand in his and kissed it while she still struggled to regain her composure.

"That's quite a story, *la tua couraggiosa*. Now tell me: what is he like, this man of yours, who has had good reason to turn your world upside down so rudely?" Gianni needed to be sure.

She glanced at him enquiringly and then, with an adoring look on her face, went on to describe the man that Gianni knew and liked so well. He sucked on his lower lip and dropped his head to hide this discovery from revealing itself in his face.

"I thought so, I thought so," he muttered almost to himself. Then, seeing a slightly puzzled look appear on Alicia's face, he sat up and putting his hand on her shoulder added quietly, "he sounds perfect for you, *mia cara, assolutamente perfetto.*"

Gianni left Alicia to walk alone beside the sea again, where he knew she did most of her thinking. He understood that she needed the time to come to terms with this sudden turn in events and to regain control of her emotions. Ever tactful, he said that he'd return to collect her after checking his vines, which she knew had to be done, meticulously, every day. Never mind that he'd already done this much earlier. She didn't have to know.

Gianni also needed time to do some thinking of his own.

★★★

CHAPTER 15

Gianni's anxieties proved well founded. After Alicia's recent experience in Verona, various conversations with his contacts and now with the name and knowledge that she had at last entrusted to him, he knew for sure that this dangerous business, in which she had inadvertently become caught up, had everything to do with Guy Hargreaves - he was right there at the centre of it all. Of that Gianni was left in no doubt.

Both Vittorio and Marcello had been constantly in touch with Gianni, as they had been asked, reassuring him that Alicia was in good hands after the mugging incident, which had taken everybody by surprise. Yet Gianni had known that there had to be more to the assault than first appeared, particularly after Marcello had recounted the other incidents of Alicia being followed around in Verona. She was being watched for some, dark, enigmatic, reason.

After making a few of his own enquiries of a senior officer from within the Intelligenzia and after much persuasion and side stepping a considerable amount of red tape, Gianni had eventually managed to get in touch on the telephone with a reliable source. The man, using Alicia as an excuse, patronizingly launched forth in English, hoping that his command of that language would silence Gianni and put a quick end to the questioning. Gianni wasn't to be put off and was more than able to hold his own with the obnoxious individual, who finally admitted that there was indeed a highly sensitive, shared, operation, currently taking place between the British and Italians. It was concentrated on the Veneto area and involved top level surveillance. *La Signorina Spence* had unfortunately become entangled, purely through force of circumstance and no fault of her own. He could most regrettably give Gianni no clue as to what the operation was about, or as to why Alicia featured.

Gianni was then told that he should follow standard security procedures, as he had done in the past. He was either to keep Alicia there with him, safe on the island or, without causing her alarm, get her safely out of the country altogether. She could be better looked after at home by the British. The second would be the best option. Then she would no longer be their responsibility, thought Gianni with disgust. She was indeed being watched and followed: as if Gianni didn't know. The reason behind this unhappy state of affairs he was unable divulge. If she did go elsewhere, he or his department were to be informed immediately, as they needed to know her exact movements at all times. It was 'imperative', the man repeated, 'imperative' that she be kept completely in the dark. She was to be told nothing at all. If Signorina Spence started asking awkward questions it would jeopardize the whole operation and put her own and other's lives in imminent danger. At this point, Gianni deduced that the man must be stupid if he considered Alicia totally unaware of the threat surrounding her. Could he be fully up to date with the facts? Perhaps not.

The man wound up the discussion by assuring Gianni that they were intending to tell him more about these matters shortly, once the obligatory security checks on him had been completed. He must understand that these were necessary as Gianni hadn't had recent dealings with the current employees of the Intelligenzia. They did things differently nowadays, this objectionable voice declared, but now, of course, since Gianni had come to them through his own channels - his voice petered out and he didn't mention that he had obviously been ordered to speak directly with Gianni.

Gianni, well aware that the conversation was being recorded, just managed to contain his annoyance and to get in the last word. He responded by saying that he had been told nothing that he didn't already know through his own people and that, given his own experience with the Intelligenzia in the past, it was a great pity that they hadn't warned him as soon as Alicia had first become mixed up in their web of covert activities. Not doing so meant that she, an unwitting civilian, had been placed in unnecessary danger, a risk that would never have been taken in his day. He ended by saying that it was lucky that he had the insight to have taken certain precautions himself, when the young woman had gone travelling, otherwise he didn't like to think about what might have happened.

He had then replaced the receiver quickly, before he said anything that he might later regret. Gianni could picture the faceless wretch on the other end about to reply, full of his own importance, with the telephone still held close to his ear. He would deflate like a balloon when he realized that he was talking to himself. Gianni felt certain that this taped dialogue would go straight back to those with greater influence. The man's unprofessional bungling and blunt lack of finesse would land him in trouble. Serve him right, thought Gianni. Those in command would now be aware of his own involvement, that he was quite probably one step ahead and certainly more efficient than those whom the government were presently paying to do the job. He hadn't lost his touch and, thanks to Giusappina's teaching all those years before, his English hadn't let him down either. Gianni allowed himself a smug grin and a large dose of self-satisfaction.

~

Once more Gianni thanked God for his gift of intuition. From the very beginning he'd followed his instincts. He'd sensed trouble and had been able to alert his 'friends' and family when Alicia had gone to Verona. His hunch had now been confirmed: the poor girl's present predicament and unhappiness was obviously linked to Guy and with whatever he might be muddled up. From Alicia's description, Gianni realized it had to be him. Apart from which, whilst telling her strange story, she'd also mentioned Julian, the other half of the original team. He hadn't enquired of their surnames. There was no need. It would have implied that he knew more than he could tell her. For the moment he wished to keep all the hard earned information he had acquired entirely to himself, because there was nobody he felt he could trust well enough in the present Intelligenzia.

Gianni felt disinclined to share any of his misgivings and preferred to continue to use his own people to ensure Alicia's safety. The fewer people who knew the facts, the less likely communication would go wrong, an essential rule, once learnt, never forgotten. He would keep his deductions to himself and find out in his own way how Guy was currently participating in his country's undercover world.

~

Gianni, Guy and Julian went back a long way together. They were both friends and associates. They had all worked closely together on numerous occasions in the past. The three men were trained as three parts of a unit, each so highly tuned mentally as to be almost aware of the other's thoughts. The two Englishmen had been on his island several times. Gianni wondered if Guy, wherever he was presently, had any idea that Alicia was here on Delfino and just how urgently Gianni needed to speak to him. He rather suspected that he did, but was restrained from making contact; Guy would wish his fiancé as far away from it all as was humanly possible.

It had been a long time since they'd had a visitor needing shelter and protection on Delfino. The time had come around once more. He hoped that he could persuade Alicia to stay. That was by far the best option. She would be safe and Guy would know where to find her when the time was right. The island was secure. The islanders were as loyal and as tough as the generation before them had been. From past events, the Delfino's knew how to protect those under their care. No stranger stepped ashore unnoticed. The island haven was guarded jealously at all times, for it was both idyllic and unique and they all wished to keep it that way, although nowadays it was visited mostly by family, holiday makers, or people who had business to conduct.

Trouble could arrive when it was least expected and in the most unlikely of ways, thought Gianni, his hand in his pocket, fingering the ball of twine as it unravelled, twirling it around his forefinger. He had much experience to draw on, thanks to his canny old father's teaching. Now, as Allessandro had instructed many years before, he must stay well ahead, be prepared for the unexpected at all times and hope for a message.

★★★

CHAPTER 16

Life was unsettled everywhere as the storm clouds gathered and the likelihood of World War II became an appalling reality. No one had any indication of the speed at which stability all over Europe was to deteriorate.

As a young man, Gianni's father, Allessandro, had shown an unusually far sighted understanding of the crisis unfurling elsewhere. He was intelligent, enthusiastic and full of energy. He had made it his business to educate and inform himself on matters affecting his country and Delfino. While the world held its breath, as the dramatic events began to unfold, Allessandro prepared himself for action. He was passionate in his wish to do anything he could to help safe guard peace and tranquillity for future generations.

A childhood accident and a damaged leg had left him unfit for active army life, much to his bitter disappointment and that of his elder relations. Allessandro was mortified when other members of the family and all able bodied men had left the island for duty. He had a wife and their first child Dimitri, when he took over all responsibility for running Delfino instead. But it wasn't enough. Fate then had irrefutably played her hand and brought an unexpected enigma to the island's coastal refuge.

A stricken English submarine, which had foundered in rough seas on its way out of the area, had managed to limp into calmer waters off Delfino. Allessandro instinctively realized the delicacy of the situation. At his instigation the islanders had hidden the submarine and sheltered the entire crew. They'd managed the operation in complete secrecy, off-loading most of the men at dead of night; bringing them safely ashore, where they were taken in and cared for by the locals.

The British naval engineers took several days to get the submarine under way again. There was much coming and going as Allessandro organized the extra help that was needed. Regular sea traffic was diverted away from the deep cove in which the submarine lay concealed and which the Delfino fishermen had ringed with nets. Word was put out that a sand bank had moved and with it an old wreck which had now become a severe hazard to shipping. Anyone from the mainland, asking further questions, was told of increased fishing activity in view of the oncoming winter and possible escalation of the war. As to the extra food supplies that were needed, the islanders were said to be merely 'stocking up'.

The British were deeply grateful and, once the submarine was made operational again, they succeeded in stealing quietly away at night, before relations with their host country soured disastrously. As a result, amongst the elite in their intelligence world, Delfino had earned her reputation as a safe and much sought after sanctary. Allessandro had been in his element. He had enjoyed every moment of the adventure. He found that he was good at helping coordinate covert operations. At last, he felt he was able to do something useful.

Through force of circumstance the British weren't to experience the island's hospitality again for several years. During the war the Italians took their place.

~

Mussolini brought Italy into the war on the side of Nazi Germany in the summer of 1940, encouraged by the liquidation of the Netherlands. During this time Delfino was overrun with the Italian military, their needs becoming ever more frequent. Allessandro put up with the unwelcome intrusion only out of a sense of duty to his country and its cause. Apart from this, their numbers alone were a huge drag on the island economy.

When, later, Germany occupied the whole of Italy, the international situation increased in sensitivity. Because of the island's hard earned repute, the authorities decided that Delfino should remain discreetly independent from the country as a whole and could continue to be run by the Vivarini clan. It would become a kind of no man's land. Island life was to continue as before, but the Delfino's were to supply the occupying army, on the mainland, with an agreed quota of their produce, including wine! The locals had to suffer constant inspections and no one was allowed to leave without permission and papers. While the islanders complied with most of the regulations, they had no trouble, when necessary, in eluding the attention of the few soldiers left in charge of the port of Biri, which was considered too small to be of any consequence.

On the surface, it seemed that Allessandro did everything he could to help Italy's so called 'war effort', but he became expert at allocating the German army with the very worst of their wine and the oldest grain. He made sure that the inspectors had unpleasant crossings to the island and that they were made as uncomfortable as possible on arrival. They were plied with corked wine, good for nothing except cooking and certainly not for their stomachs, which often had to endure rough, return, journeys. As time passed the German surveys and examinations of supplies became cursory and inadequate. The officials hated the task and couldn't wait for inspection days and the dreaded boat voyages to be over. It was easy to deceive these unwelcome visitors and for the Delfinos to hide the best of their fare.

After the war, Allessandro was invited to a meeting, held at government level on the mainland, to discuss his island haven's possible part in covert activities, during peacetime. Largely due to his deft handling of the negotiations, a satisfactory agreement was finally drawn up, theoretically for the benefit of all the allies, stating that, in the pursuit of world peace, providing and for so long as the islanders were willing, Delfino could be used for occasional military purposes. As the island was privately owned, services would be paid for as and when provided. This money earned was ploughed back into Delfino and so she prospered. People would be sent for highly secretive reasons, during times of instability, when they needed a place to lie low for a while or as a base to coordinate movement elsewhere. Security would be of paramount importance. Allessandro, together with his island people, proved their worth many times over ensuring confidence that Delfino was a safe refuge in the true sense of the word.

~

Gianni and his brothers, as they grew up after the war, came to understand that, strategically, their home held a very important position on the world map. The Nato listening communications centre for the whole Western Mediterranean was set up on the island of Tavolara just off Sardinia, on the West coast of Italy; with the American 6th fleet base nearby, on Isola Caprera.

The British were frequent visitors during the cold war, using Delfino as a stepping stone for undisclosed activities elsewhere. At these times, they showed the Vivarini family and their people the utmost courtesy and respect, seldom if ever taking advantage of the islanders' goodwill, but calmly and efficiently getting on with the jobs they'd come to do. They would leave as quietly as they had arrived, with no fuss whatsoever and leaving nothing behind them as evidence of their stay. They were by far the most popular of Delfino's guests.

Post-war life also produced the Americans. They were different again from all other nationalities in their needs and life became full of the most unlikely problems! Allessandro would chuckle, an amused expression on his leathered, old, face as he remembered those days. His eyes would crinkle at the corners and he never tired of telling the same stories time and again. Gianni and his brothers would soon be holding their stomachs with laughter! They were appreciative listeners and their father was a great 'raconteur'.

The incident the old man liked to recall most was the one involving his own beloved wife, Ana Maria. Smiling tenderly, Allessandro would tell his sons with pride that, 'as a young woman your mother had the face of the Madonna; everyone thought her beautiful'. Then he would continue, his smile becoming ever wider as he warmed to his subject and began to tell his favourite story.

'One night, after too good a dinner, a certain American soldier became much too friendly and Ana had hit him over the head with a saucepan' he remembered; 'for trying to put his hand where he shouldn't have put it'. This was said for respectability in front of the boys! Incensed by the man's behaviour, Ana, 'quite rightly', had knocked him out cold! Unfortunately, it had turned out that the man Ana Maria had struck was a colonel. The present doctor's uncle had to be brought over from the mainland to see to the injury and there were unwelcome repercussions.

Poor Ana was threatened with the military police. But the understandably indignant Allessandro had made it quite clear to the Americans that if the police were brought in, then the advances on his wife would be made public, blowing the cover of their secret lifestyle on Delfino and that, if any such 'insulting action' was taken against his wife, the U.S would never again be welcomed on the island. 'That had been that'. Allessandro had framed the commanding officer's apology, which hung to this day in Ana Maria's kitchen and still caused amusement to the older generation. At the time, the islanders had all longed to know exactly how the report sheet handed in to the senior US officer had read!'

~

It was twenty years later that Gianni, after taking over many of the responsibilities from his father, had his first run around with the Americans. Delfino had suffered a bad week of winter storms. A group of senior U.S officers had arrived from the naval base and were co-ordinating some training manoeuvres offshore. After three days of continuous rough weather, with no boat able to put to sea, the soldiers had become extremely upset that they couldn't get their usual quota of supplies over from the mainland, in particular their chosen brand of ice cream. They were military men, not sailors and seemed unable to understand why the facilities on the island should be any different from those in New York! Gianni had been indignant over the fuss. He had already gone out of his way to help these people and so told them exactly what they could do with their ridiculous demands. Their own Italian ice cream, made by his mother Ana Maria was far superior anyway, but after all the bother it was not offered!

Allessandro, who had left Gianni in charge whilst attending to some official matters in Biri found, on his return, that the small matter had escalated out of all proportion. He had laughed and told his son that it was common knowledge that during the last war the US Marines had set much stock by always acquiring the best food supplies. Everybody wanted to be invited to their mess for dinner: it would be like a banquet compared to the rations the other nationalities were able to produce. The Americans would almost cease to operate if deprived their usual catering. Gianni had stumped off muttering that for the next visit, if there was a next visit, he would ask Giuseppina to impregnate their ice cream with a pepper sauce to take their heads off and hopefully render them speechless.

Allessandro hoped that his son would have benefited from this lesson in the perverseness of human nature and that perhaps he would have learnt to better curb his temper in the future.

~

Ever since Gianni's educative experience as a younger man, the authorized visits had continued spasmodically. The most recent, a couple of years before had been from some rather dictatorial individuals from the Italian Defence Department. It had turned out to be a very long and difficult day.

The visitors spent most of their time examining the island in minute detail, making unnecessarily rude comments as they toured around, whilst at the same time enjoying the islanders' generous hospitality. They indulged themselves in an excellent meal cooked by Patrizia, with copious amounts of Gianni's best wine, slurped back with no moderation, even though they were supposed to be on official business.

Their stay ended with the self-important, ill-mannered, leader of the group stating that because Italy was now faced with escalating terrorist problems, he 'expected', to be able to continue to use the island facilities in the future. He assumed that regarding matters of defence his department would have the Delfino's cooperation and that personal from military Intelligenzia, in particular, would always be made welcome. Adding ungraciously, before Gianni could get a word in, 'just the same as in the past, when Allessandro had been in charge,' making it quite clear that he considered Gianni a very much inferior person.

The infuriated Gianni had replied that it would entirely depend on their attitude when making future requests and on how they conducted themselves on the island, the sensitivity of the situation and on how detrimental the effect might be on the Delfino people to have them billeted there. He had fixed the man with a steely stare, willing him to dare to throw his weight around further. He was not going to be pushed around and suspected that his father had given in far too much in past years. He was ever suspicious of these people and considered them neither genuine nor straight forward in the way they dealt with ordinary folk. They liked to be seen to enforce their will and use their considerable powers when it came to means of securing cooperation.

Gianni concluded by telling the visitors that they should consider themselves very lucky to be allowed there at all: Delfino was a privately owned island and that they had arrived without invitation on this occasion, when Italy was, for the moment anyway, thank God, at peace with the world. He made it quite clear that they should remember that he was under no obligation or duty to them whatsoever and that the original agreement no longer applied, the contract had only held good for five post - war years, after which it had been automatically terminated.

The party, headed by the imperious, fat, oaf in charge, had left disgruntled and slightly less sure of themselves than when they had arrived. Mario had made sure that they all got a fair amount of spray in their faces going back across to the mainland, arriving back in the port looking more like damp squibs than high ranking officials from the Defence Ministry. The people in the port, who had been led to believe that they were mere inspectors from the city, couldn't hide their amusement on seeing the wet, dishevelled boatload disembark, with Mario grinning from ear to ear.

Gianni's old father chuckled inwardly and secretly congratulated himself: he had taught his son well.

★★★

CHAPTER 17

Gianni stood looking proudly at his vines, every one properly secured and carefully tended. The grapes were already beginning to form. He picked up some pieces of cut twine from off the ground: he must have dropped them earlier. He tied them in a knot and placed them in his pocket with the unravelled twine already there. The spool needed rewinding. He must take it out later tonight, otherwise his job the next day would take twice as long: there would be plenty of 'tying' to do. The string was almost part of his clothing. He wouldn't feel dressed without it, or the old, worn, knife in the other pocket itching to be used at the slightest provocation, with its blade kept sharp as a razor ever since the day it had come into his possession, many years before.

The knife invoked memories, whenever he first touched it at the beginning of each day: memories he would rather forget, preferring not to think of some of the duties it had performed. Perhaps regrettably, 'execute' was a better word. Jobs long gone now; thankfully relegated to the past. There was no question but that his 'old friend' had saved his life on many occasions. And all in the name of peace - peace on earth, a rare thing, still much sought and strived for to this day, especially with the increase of that unquantifiable threat: terrorism. Nowadays, both he and his knife enjoyed retirement in the vineyard.

~

Gianni stared up into the blue heavens above, offering a silent prayer for clement weather; a soft and gentle breeze rather than a keen chill wind. It was time to return to Alicia on the beach and as he did so, his thoughts reverted to the present problem: Guy Hargreaves.

Gianni had thought that Guy's days in the British 'rapid deployment force' were also long over and was more than surprised to find him still operating. There must be some exceptional circumstances for him to be working again. The last time they had seen each other had been here, on Delfino, three and a half years before. Guy had dropped in when he'd been in the area on business for his legal firm. He had mentioned that, until recently, both he and Julian Birchall had continued to work on a reserve basis for their undercover unit, mostly instructing at the barracks, keeping themselves fit and helping out when manpower was short. They had both found it very difficult to keep up with the training, which was exhausting and extremely time consuming, making it almost impossible to hold down a normal job, let alone have a social life. Guy had gone on to tell Gianni that, when two very special women had entered their lives, they had both thought it time to pack it in altogether.

What an extraordinary coincidence that Alicia should be one of those special women and that she and Guy should not only have found each other, but that, after the miserable time she must have been through at Guy's expense, she should have found her way here, of her own accord, to Delfino island. The flowers were a clever, but risky, message thought Gianni, smiling and shaking his head, *'Che fortuna'*. That inexplicable force from above had miraculous ways of manoeuvring events.

It was becoming increasingly obvious to Gianni that, unbeknown to Alicia, something of enormous importance had happened. Guy had removed himself, apparently off the face of the earth: for very good reasons he felt sure. He had suspected that the two men were together when Alicia had mentioned that Julian also appeared to have gone missing. They were a particularly competent duo.

After this recent turn of events Gianni again wished fervently that he was fully in the picture. But he knew that, if he was needed, Guy would find some way of informing him and that the best thing that he could do for the moment was to take one big worry off his shoulders: Alicia. Guy would have no fear for her safety as long as she was with him on Delfino. The rest and his curiosity would have to wait.

But how to keep her here would be another matter. Gianni would do everything in his power to keep safe this young woman, of whom they had all grown so very fond. But Alicia would never sit quietly with them, here on the island, now that Guy had sent her the flowers. 'Hot headed fool, the Irish blood', Gianni muttered to himself, shaking his head. Typical: Yet he could well understand Guy wanting to let Alicia know, somehow, that he hadn't abandoned her and was alive: perhaps it was an indirect message to himself as well. Things were becoming clearer. He'd trusted his instincts which had proven correct so far and he was glad of some action. Guy must be in a desperate predicament to have this work so irrevocably muddled up with his private life. If Alicia was determined to move, then the situation would need careful handling, plenty of help and much organization, He was more than capable of managing all of this and without any condescending help from the present day Intelligenzia.

~

Gianni sat quietly on the rocks by the sea shore, waiting for Alicia to notice him. It wasn't long before she turned and waved. He went to join her. She was standing with her bare feet in the shallow water, holding her shoes in one hand and the box in the other. She was looking much happier and, he thought nervously, quite determined. They stood contemplating the sea together then she turned her face towards him, breaking his train of thought and he knew that she had already made up her mind. She stepped out of the water.

"Where do you think these flowers came from and how did they get here?" Her voice was strong again. She dropped her shoes onto the dry sand, opened the box and held it out for his inspection.

"A young boy from the village gave them to Mario early this morning as he was loading his supplies in the port," he answered and added, "he said that they'd been given him by a stranger and were for the beautiful young English woman on the island - and that the stranger was Italian," he finished quickly in case she'd thought that Guy himself was anywhere near. Little does she know what I know, thought Gianni grimly unhappy that he was unable to put her out of her misery and that he had to keep so much from her.

"They were sent by hand, but they are not locally grown. These blue ones here, you see," he picked one out, "they are not from Italy, they are grown in wide open spaces, fields, most likely in the South of France", he added thankfully with certain knowledge and a plan already formulating in his head.

"We have similar ones here, growing wild in our hills, but not as dark as these. These are cultured and used mostly in the making of perfume, probably in Provence, near Grasse perhaps, where they have the famous perfume factories, like Fragonard. They would know for sure," he finished looking at her wisely and thanking God that his other old friend and associate in the South of France had once explained all this to Giuseppina and himself whilst giving them a grand tour of the area. He hesitated for a moment.

"Alicia, you know that you can stay with us as long as you wish. You are absolutely safe here". She could see that he was concerned for her. "I would very much like you to stay," Gianni added hopefully, although in his heart he knew that she was already on her way and that there would be no stopping her without alerting her to the perilous situation. He wasn't in the least surprised that Guy had chosen someone not only beautiful and intelligent but with great courage and determination. She too should have been in the specialist forces. Alicia and Guy were perfect for each other.

Alicia looked up, Gianni was correct, she was leaving.

"No Gianni, I must go", she said. "I need to find out the truth behind Guy's disappearance: somehow I have to get to the bottom of it all, otherwise I shall never rest. I just know that he would never have left me like this, without a very sound reason. I can't begin to thank you enough for all that you and your family have done for me. I have felt safe here on Delfino. I love the island and the people. I have been so wonderfully looked after by you and Giuseppina, it's become like home. I feel strong and confident again now, a different person from when I arrived and ready to take on the world once more. I was so miserable." Alicia's startling blue eyes stared up at him. "But I expect you guessed that?" He nodded. "Anyway I am glad that I've told you," she continued "I must have been such a worry to you all. I'm so sorry. But I have to leave now and there really is nothing more that you can do to help; you have done so much already." She finished with a wry smile.

"Ah *mia cara,* you might be surprised how, sometimes, help arrives from the most mysterious of directions". He raised his eyes to the sky and she laughed. "Never be sorry for your sadness; it is a very human feeling, and you had much reason to be sad. When you are smiling again, it will be better than ever before and a beautiful girl like you, Alicia, should always be smiling!" He spread his hands wide. "But I wish also that you had told me before. As my Giuseppina says; 'the bigger the problem, the better to share it'. You must remember that in the future, for it is good advice. But, *'sono felice'*, I am happy to see you look so much better now, in spite of the unfortunate incident in Verona. I thank the one above and Marcello for protecting you. When you find Guy you must both return here together. You will be welcome here at any time, always."

"There is nothing on earth that I would rather do," replied Alicia, determined that he shouldn't notice the blush creeping up her neck to betray her guilty secret.

"But before you leave," continued Gianni, thankfully now staring out to sea, "you must promise me two things: first that you will not leave before the golden ones' party. Secondly and most important", he turned towards her serious again, "that if you are ever in any more trouble whatsoever, you will contact me immediately. I shall at all times know your movements for, you see, I do have friends in many places and some experience in matters of this kind. I too think that this Guy of yours has most likely moved out of your life for your own protection above all else. For any other reason he would be mad!" he added smiling at her and teasing to lighten the atmosphere. "*Non preoccuparti.* Don't worry Alicia. I feel in my heart that you will find your Guy eventually although perhaps we won't mention much of this to my wife, otherwise she will never let you out of her sight. That's for sure!"

Alicia put her arms around this kind caring man and hugged him, wondering as she did so how she'd ever leave them all. Gianni held her to him as if she were indeed another daughter of his own blood and said quietly

"There is no need to thank us, you know. You did that last night when you opened your package. That was more than enough - just watching your face," and seeing her confusion, smiling again he cleared his throat, stood up and holding his hand out said, "*andiamo, mia cara.* It's time to go back now. We have something to celebrate. Giuseppina will be pleased about your birthday, very pleased and so you had better be prepared!"

She looked at him for a moment, smiling warmly, with affection, then they walked slowly back to the house in easy and companionable silence. They stopped to pick up some more eggs from under a bush, which they both spied as they went past. Gianni watched, amused, as Alicia pulled out the bottom of her loose shirt and held it together as a means of carrying them safely back to the house without breaking.

"I used to do this as a little girl. I loved to roam free and was always collecting things," she explained. "My mother received many surprises this way, some good, some not so good," She laughed. "One particular time I remember she was so cross because I had filled up my white school shirt with loads and loads of blackberries. Needless to say the stain of the fruit never came out so the shirt had to go in the bin! After that I used to put leaves in the bottom first, to protect my clothes. Very thoughtful really, wasn't I?" Gianni laughed.

"I have no doubt that, despite the trouble, you also caused much amusement and much happiness, but I wouldn't have enjoyed the washing," he finished, laughing still and moving to one side to let her walk, ahead of him, up the narrow path.

Alicia thought how safe and comfortable she felt here. She secretly dreaded venturing out into the real and uncertain world again and wondered what on earth the next few weeks held in store. But at least she had reason to hope now and had people in her life on whom she could rely and she could turn to for help.

★★★

CHAPTER 18

Giuseppina was pleased, very pleased, to have Alicia's birthday to celebrate. Patrizia was summoned and all the family invited to dinner at the restaurant in Alicia's honour.

Alicia's mother rang on her mobile to say Happy Birthday. Alicia had already had her present: her open return ticket to Italy. She refrained from saying anything about her future plans or mentioning what had happened in Verona. There was no point in creating more worry. She just said that she'd had a wonderful time sightseeing. Diana, hearing the lift in her daughter's voice, waited for more, but Alicia, hating the intense feeling of disloyalty, changed the subject. Her mother would have had a fit, thought Alicia, if she knew what she'd been up to with Marcello.

Later that evening, as she walked into the restaurant with Gianni and Giuseppina, the whole family, already assembled, stood and clapped with a burst of enthusiasm and little Gi ran to her side, grabbing her skirt to lead her to her place. He planted himself firmly beside her, handed over a bunch of wildflowers that he'd obviously picked himself and refused to budge. Everybody laughed to see that he had bound the rather scruffy posy together with an old bootlace. Alicia felt very touched. He had become her shadow of late and she really loved the small child.

Patrizia had, somehow, found the time to make a huge cake, undoubtedly with Tarsia's help. The young girl had also made up a basket filled with orange blossoms and tied with pink trailing ribbons. Ana Maria and Giuseppina both gave Alicia lace: a beautiful tablecloth and matching napkins. Giuseppina told her that the old lady had said that they were to go into her 'wedding' drawer, whenever that might be mused Alicia, determined not to dwell on such thoughts.

When Alicia cut her cake, the Vivarini clan sung a very funny 'happy birthday' then they all got up and danced, making their own music. It was a happy evening, enlivened by the children's constant noise and entertainment. Alicia went to bed surrounded by her presents and three flower arrangements. The spontaneous party with the family had been unexpected: when she had woken that morning, except for a card and the telephone call from her mother, she had imagined her birthday would remain a lonely secret. Her last thoughts before drifting off to sleep were of Guy, somewhere out there, but she knew not where, closely followed by a recent, more solid and reassuring memory: of security, of laughter and a serene and sensual excitement. She missed them both, but perhaps for different reasons.

Gianni laid his plans for Alicia carefully. He decided that she should leave the island, at night, during the party for Gianni's parents. Nobody watching from the mainland would notice her depart, with all the comings and goings in the little harbour that evening.

Alicia was glad she hadn't told her mother that she was thinking of moving on. She thought it best that Diana still thought her to be on the island, with the Vivarini's for the moment. She rang her office to say that she would shortly be sending the travel department a piece on Verona. Then she rang Nick.

She waited to hear what he had to say first. He had depressingly little news. His contact, the man called Jonathan, had obviously been told not to make himself available any longer. None of his Foreign Office contacts were helpful any more either. In fact, nobody seemed prepared to stick their neck out and confirm anything, he said rather morosely. The bank cards, he had eventually found out, appeared to have been temporarily stopped. The word 'temporarily' said a lot, Alicia felt. Other than that, nobody would answer any questions at all. On two occasions they had merely cut him off and had rudely declined to answer any following calls, which he had thought more than strange. Quite obviously they didn't like his line of enquiry.

Alicia let him finish and then told him her news about the mysterious arrival of the flowers on her birthday. Nick was ecstatic with excitement. She could hear him almost jumping up and down at the end of the telephone. Alicia realized that he was beginning to become ever more fascinated by the 'secret' implications of Guy's disappearance. He had really done very well with his investigations, in spite of thinking he'd come to a dead end. Her news filled him with eagerness again.

Adriana on the other hand, was becoming increasingly worried as each day passed with no news of Julian. This, in itself, was odd. It had been the longest period he'd ever been out of touch, Adriana had told Alicia one evening. His office had heard nothing either. They were also becoming concerned and wondering just how long they were going to be able to keep the information of his 'unknown whereabouts' out of the press. So far they'd managed to stall.

Alicia thought it strange, to say the least, that both Julian and Guy seemed to have vanished at the same time. They were such very close friends and she now thought that perhaps they had shared a slightly suspect past. She decided she would have to continue the search on her own, with little to go on but a small glimmer of hope somewhere in the distance but, so far, a long way out of reach.

~

Once more Gianni came to Alicia's rescue, insisting that he just happened to have this wonderful contact for her in the South of France. He had arranged for Alicia to stay with his old friend, Jacques d'Aubert, who owned a prosperous vineyard in the wine country, up in the hills behind Nice. The d'Auberts had plenty of room and were used to having young people to stay and so, with a car, she'd be able to come and go as she pleased. Jacques and his wife would be delighted to have her: he knew this for certain as he had already talked to them both. Gianni was determined to continue to help and Alicia was amazed how easily and instantly all her travel arrangements seemed to have been organized. He really did seem to know a lot of people in a lot of places! Also, she was delighted not to have to stay by herself in a hotel, it would be too lonely.

Three days later, the evening of the party was set fair. The restaurant had been cleared, except for a huge table with food and wine down at the far end. Everybody had produced something.

Alicia had helped Tarsia make sweet pastries in Giuseppina's kitchen. Little Gi stood at her side longing for mis-shapen or broken pieces to come his way. With the child 'helping', the baking had taken twice as long and resulted in a lot of extra clearing up, but it had been fun. Meanwhile, unaware of the hilarity at the amount eaten by her small son before the party even started, Patrizia had been busy with everything else in the restaurant kitchen.

The family, even the children, were all dressed in their best and had decorated the room with flowers and golden balloons. There was plenty of noise and a great deal of laughter as everybody gathered together in the early evening. Alicia had a moment's panic when she saw Amalia and her children walk in, but she needn't have worried. Stefano was coming later and his brother, she soon gathered, was on duty and unable to attend. She suspected that Marcello had tactfully arranged his rota this way, but felt sad that she should be the cause of her policeman missing such a special family event. At the same time she was relieved, as perhaps her face might have given away how she felt.

Vittorio arrived with a radiant Francesca, who told her mother that she was expecting a baby in early August. She was already four months pregnant. How could she still look so neat? Alicia thought, wondering, rather sadly, if she would ever be in the same state. They were so pleased to see Alicia perfectly recovered, after the unexpected and unfortunate end to her visit with them in Verona. She couldn't but feel happy to see them all.

The celebrations really did start with a bang. The men had set up some fireworks on the quay which were lit as soon as the last guest had arrived and while the elderly couple were being escorted from their house by the three brothers. The party was no secret to them but, judging by their delighted faces, the fireworks certainly were.

After dinner, the singing and dancing began with Ana Maria and Allessandro leading the way onto the floor. Mario had a beautiful voice which brought tears to many an eye, particularly Alicia's, who was greatly moved thinking of her imminent departure. Mario sung his heart out and then got everybody to join in. They all got thoroughly carried away with the well known arias!

Alicia was thrilled that the elderly couple were quite so delighted with the dolphins she'd given them and she was touched when Allessandro insisted that she dance with him, while Gianni joined them with his mother.

The early evening flew by and when Mario told her it was time, she slipped back to her room, changed out of her dress and was downstairs and ready in a few minutes. Gianni and Giuseppina embraced her warmly and made her promise to keep in close touch, to call if she needed them and most of all to return to them all soon, 'preferably not alone', Gianni had added quietly, winking at her as they discreetly slipped away.

Giuseppina had been given a watered down version of the true story. Gianni was letting Alicia go only on the understanding that she'd leave after dark, just to be on the safe side and that she would be escorted all of the way out of Italy into France. On this he was determined and would brook no argument when she had questioned the need for a chaperone. He seemed to have an exceptional grasp of the sensitivity of the situation and although he played it down and was reassuring to Alicia, she knew that he was more than a little worried for her safety after the unnerving incident in Verona.

The moon was bright and the sea calm as Gianni pushed them out, wishing Alicia 'God speed' and '*spero che tu abbia successo*'. When Mario started the engine, Alicia turned and raised her hand for one last wave as they rounded the corner and left the harbour. Gianni wished that he could get some more information out of the Italian police. He'd kept trying, but they really were proving extremely unhelpful and continued to palm him off with the same line as before – 'it was considered better for everybody that as few people as possible knew exactly what was happening in the area and that he would only be told more if it was considered necessary'. Frustrating: to say the least.

Gianni stood listening until he could no longer hear the boat's engine. Then, with an anxious sigh and a heavy heart he retraced his steps back towards the sound of music and the party. It looked as though it was to be a long night and somehow he had to be seen to be enjoying himself for his parents' sake; but he knew he would be constantly worried for some time to come. How to hide it from Giuseppina was going to prove extremely difficult, of that he was sure. She knew him almost better than he knew himself. Now was the time to get in touch with some more of his so called 'old friends.'

In the South of France, Jacques D'Albert was already primed with the little information that Gianni had to pass on. The Frenchman had been so happy to hear from Gianni and even more pleased to have what he termed as a 'proper job' again. Alicia would be in safe hands with him, he assured Gianni, as he had an excellent man to watch over her. This was a huge relief, but Gianni was still perplexed. Guy was an absolute professional with a world-wide source of intelligence and so why had he still not managed to find a way to get word to him? He wished that he had some comprehension of the risks they were running and how the whole affair affected Alicia. What exactly was this unknown evil hanging over them all? How could he help when he knew so little?

Now that Alicia had left, he must recheck the immediate plans for her journey to the South of France, about which he had serious misgivings. It was a long way. He also assumed that he should inform the Italian police at some point that she was on the move again, though he trusted his own support team far better than theirs. Perhaps he'd wait until she was out of the country before telling them. Maybe he was being overly cautious, but he didn't want Alicia frightened unnecessarily and he wasn't taking any chances with the preparations he had made for her safe conduct being messed up by incompetent and over zealous, young, policemen with little experience. Even in his ignorance, Gianni preferred to rely on his own arrangements regarding Alicia's wellbeing.

★★★

CHAPTER 19

The moon lit an irregular path over the choppy water. Mario was adept at meeting the larger waves. The wash behind the boat threw up iridescent flashes of light, resembling a spray of diamonds, thought Alicia, her own eyes sparkling as she leant, trailing her fingers in the cool water. She was on the move again and she felt energized and positive. They made good time on the short crossing. Mario sensed the excitement in Alicia; it was as if she had come alive again and she looked beautiful under the stars. The ethereal glow from the heavens suited her, enshroud in mystery as he knew her to be. He was glad that his brother had organized her travel plans; she would be safe from whatever it was that threatened her. They were soon nearing the port of Biri on the mainland.

"Cover your head just in case, *Signorina,*" he said, as they made for a small landing to one side of the main harbour, where a lone figure was waiting. Mario stopped the engine and glided gently onto the steps, where Alicia immediately recognized Stefano's white teeth and beaming smile as he leant forward to help them. Now she knew why he hadn't come to the party. She greeted him delightedly. He was to be her chaperone.

"Shut your big mouth!" chided Mario good-naturedly, for this was surely a big joke between them. "Anyone can see you." Stefano chortled as he helped Alicia efficiently out of the boat, grinning wider than ever.

"It's good to see you again, *Signorina.*"

Mario followed her out of the boat, handed the hold-all to Stefano and taking Alicia's hands in his, wished her *'Buona fortuna, coraggiosa* Alicia, and may God go with you.'

Almost before Stefano and Alicia reached the car Mario was quietly making his way out of the port, heading back to the island. The moon was temporarily hidden as if to cover their movements. Alicia turned and watched the little boat grow smaller, its shape merging into obscurity. It's lights were two mere pinpricks, exposing a narrow pathway across the water. She could hear the distant, slightly, eerie, strains of music coming from the island, helping guide it safely home. They all seemed remarkably good at the cloak and dagger stuff, she thought, shivering unexpectedly. Stefano touched her shoulder gently.

"*Via Signorina,* come." They drove for an hour or so but Alicia didn't remember the way in the dark. When questioned, Stefano told her that they were travelling to Bologna from a larger station on the main line on this occasion. The smaller branch stations didn't function this late at night. Alicia nodded her understanding. It made sense. Nothing much operated in the middle of the night in England either. Soon she saw they were approaching a much larger town than on their last journey together. They arrived at the station where they parked the car and hurried over to a small siding. In a few moments Alicia could hear the train coming. It ground its way to a noisy halt.

"On time for once!" said Stefano chuckling, having gauged their arrival perfectly. He waited until the doors were being opened further along on the main platform then, opened the nearest door, swung her bag up and hoisted himself in. In less than a minute she was up beside him with the door closed behind them. When the train had started on its way again they walked through the luggage compartment and into the first carriage, which was empty. Stefano checked the two next carriages, both also empty except for a couple of railway staff returning home and then sat down opposite, smiling, once more advertising his teeth.

They talked about the family and Alicia told Stefano all about the party, which she was sorry that he had missed. There was always a party on the island for one reason or another, he reassured her. He would see all his relations when he returned to fetch his family the next day. He had actually enjoyed a bit of peace, catching up with the hotel accounts, while they were gone.

They had to change trains at Bologna. Stefano told Alicia that they would have to hurry as the connection time was short. He took Alicia's bag and walked fast with her away from the train and towards the main collection point of the station. The concourse was crowded, surprisingly, as it was late and as they slowed down to weave their way through the people, she heard a noise and rude exclamation of annoyance behind her. She turned around as she walked, to see what the scuffle was about and saw an elderly woman recapturing her belongings after being pushed aside and nearly knocked over by a man in too much of a hurry. The man was moving away and looking back over his shoulder. Alicia let out a gasp of horror as her eyes locked with his in recognition: he wore a dark suit. Stefano was right there beside her. He had heard her cry of fright. Alicia was pointing back.

"He's following me! Stefano, *quell uomo mi sta seguendo!*" Stefano was steering her away, cutting short her stuttering words.

"*Su, andiamo Signorina per favore, su.*" They hurried on down some steps, underneath the tunnel and up onto another platform, with Stefano talking to her, reassuringly, all the time as they walked.

"*D'accordo,* Alicia, now listen to me carefully, all is arranged. *Nessun problema.*" He slowed down and explained exactly what he wanted her to do. They were to walk further up the train and then, when he told her, taking her time, she was to say goodbye and climb on. As soon as she was aboard, Alicia was to walk quickly back down the inside and get out again at the very end, near the entrance to the platform, where he would meet her.

"Can you manage with your bag?" Stefano asked with concern. "And you will have no more than five minutes to get through three carriages before the train departs. If you are worried about the train leaving just open a door as you go past. They won't leave with one still open."

"*Certo,*" Alicia answered shortly. They walked on and stood talking on the edge of a group of people who were waiting as the night train took on the last of it's passengers. Alicia knew that Stefano was surreptitiously keeping an eye on both his watch and the people coming up the platform towards them.

"*Sono pronta,* I'm ready," she said, her stomach churning with nervous anxiety. She wanted to get on, worried about the timing.

"*Aspetta,* wait a little longer," he said quietly, then with a grunt of satisfaction, "*d'accordo* Alicia, he is coming now, I just want to make sure that he sees you and boards the far side of us. Don't look now: he is going past." Alicia dared not look anywhere; her heart was beating so fast she could hear its amplified thumping clearly. Then Stefano said louder:

"O.K, *andiamo, Ciao* Alicia, *arrivederci,*" he kissed her on both cheeks, whispered, *'a piu' tardi',* and helped her into the train, shoving her bag in after her, making quite a performance of it and shutting the door with a bang. Alicia started to move as quickly as possible down the train, bumping into people with her bag as they milled around finding their seats, hampering her progress. The first two carriages were very slow, but as she entered the third the people seemed to have settled themselves and were mostly sitting in their seats and so she was able to hurry through more easily.

Stefano waved once more, whilst watching out of the corner of his eye to make certain that her follower boarded a carriage further up. Once he had seen him do so, he turned and walked purposely back down beside the train, hands in his pockets. There were plenty of people waving and calling their goodbyes as Stefano disappeared amongst them. Time was running out, the guard was in position. Stefano couldn't see Alicia ahead of him so he opened a door himself, as he went past, hoping that she was nearly there and that he'd see her hopping out at any second. There was a shout behind him. It was the guard, hurrying to shut the door he'd just opened and swearing loudly. Stefano took no notice and continued down the train opening another door as he did so.

Alicia reached the end of the train almost at the same time as Stefano and just as she jumped down, the last door slammed shut, the guard blew his whistle, shaking his fist as he saw them and the train began to leave the station.

"Where was it going?" she asked as they set off again.

"Northern Germany," answered Stefano with a short laugh. "Now we have to hurry again to catch your real train." Even he sounded short of breath! They went quickly down the steps off the platform, passed back along the tunnel, leapt up the next flight of steps onto another platform and found the overnight sleeper to the South of France, also about to leave. They ran alongside to find her coach. Doors were slamming as he helped her up, she was breathing fast and the adrenalin was really working overtime by now.

Alicia suddenly realized that Stefano wasn't following her. He wasn't getting in, he'd tossed her bag and coat in behind her, shut the door and with more whistles the train was beginning to move already. She looked down from the open window, feeling totally bereft.

"Stefano, forza! Che c'e'?" But he was smiling and calling back to her.

"Non preoccuparti Alicia! Che Dio cia con te." He blew her a kiss, shouted something else that she couldn't hear, spreading his hands up towards the sky, something to do with God she supposed and then he was gone. Alicia let out a long sigh of distress; she was to be on her own again after all. Then a soft familiar voice spoke from behind her.

"Buona sera again, signorina, una problema?" She turned, her cheeks flaming, her heart lurching in excitement and her stomach turning a complete

cartwheel.

"Marcello! Marcello! No nothing's the matter, there's no problem, not now, *sono contenta*, but what are you doing here?" cried Alicia, relieved and laughing as she collapsed into his arms.

"*Alichia mia, Alichia mia, andiamo*," he spoke into her hair, his arm wrapped around her as he guided her along the narrow passage to her reserved sleeping compartment. He closed the door gently behind them, pressing the lock home, looking at her searchingly, his head on one side, the question in his eyes. She backed up against the door and nodded slightly, not taking her eyes from his and a half smile on her face, her arms stretched out to him. He took one step, enfolded her in his arms and seized her mouth, drowning it with his. Feeling her thumping heart underneath her jersey and pushing underneath her bra, he took her nipples between his fingers then bent his mouth to one of her breasts, pulling gently.

"*Ah cara mia* I have such power over you, no?" He undid the bra and removed her sweater.

"Yes," she whispered, already lost. Then he stood back and looked at her, murmuring endearments.

"*Sei bellissima Alichia, ti desidero.*" As her eyes, full to brimming, bored deep into his face, his hands moved to her waist and the buckle of her belt. They were undressed in lightening time, each helping the other. He made her stand where she was with her back to the door, as he stroked and kissed her ready body, her thighs and stomach, tasting and remembering her warm fragrant skin.

With the heightened adrenalin and emotion, Alicia could already feel the tidal rush beginning to envelope her. She moaned softly, helping him to a more comfortable position. He held her steady; they joined together easily and moving in unison she drew him ever further into those, familiar, hidden depths.

They rocked together matching their rhythm to that of the train. He covered her mouth with his as she cried out, begging him to travel with her once again on their indefinable journey together.

Afterwards they clung to each other, overawed by the speed and intensity of their desire, then, shaking and weak they sank down onto the lower bunk and were quiet whilst they recovered. Alicia looked into his face and saw that he still felt the same. She traced its outline with her fingers and placed her lips on his. He breathed life into her: there was simply no way could she resist.

"Marcello, you have no idea just how pleased I am to see you, *sono felice,*" then, with a naughty, seductive, twinkle, "are you my chaperone for the night then?" He nodded, smiling, watching her as she got up and moved over to the window to peer out into the rushing darkness. He stood also and moved up behind her his hands caressing the outline of her hips, then clasped her to him resting his chin on her shoulder as he too stared out into the night. One hand moved slowly round and across her flat stomach, while the other held her to him around her waist.

"I would gladly be your chaperone until the end of time, but that you already know, *Alichia mia.* Now stay where you are; I want you from here, *piu' lentamente,* just as you are stood."

"Standing, Marcello, not stood," she whispered with a giggle as she bent forward and offered herself to him once again. He laughed gently and replied,

"*Attenzione, mia caro,* for soon I will have you begging me to put you down on that bed. This night we will also remember for ever, *una promessa.*"

She placed her hands against the bottom of the window ledge and braced her body waiting for him as he, slowly, began again. She caught her breath and he held her for a moment without moving, waiting and savouring that which was to come.

"Continua, Marcello continua, fallo ancora," she sucked in her breath, but he didn't move.

"Ti amo Alichia, ti amo."

"Oh Marcello! I know and you know how I feel too, *per sempre*, forever, hurry please, *su per favore."*

He buried his face in her silky hair, inhaling the sweetness from the back of her neck, thankful that she couldn't see him and sighed softly. He still didn't resume, until her urgent movements made it impossible for him not to do so, then once again holding her tight against him, his energy and impetus returning, he began to push further still, into the very core of her being.

Alicia cried out. Swaying with the rhythm of the train as it rattled it's way on through the night towards the South of France, they took for themselves what once again seemed to be theirs by right, reaching deep within for those intoxicating summits of sensual satisfaction. Afterwards they stayed together again, unable to move. Finally, when they had regained their breath and their fast beating hearts had steadied a little, they fell onto the narrow berth and lay without speaking, both amazed, yet again, at how well they fitted each other's needs.

Alicia wondered if she could and should have stopped what had just happened, but, as she looked up into his gentle face, she knew that it just would not have been possible. Her fright and then the relief that followed, on finding him there waiting, force of circumstance or whatever, had made it inevitable. The electrical, sexual, attraction they had between them had simply overtaken them both, yet again.

They lay wrapped in each other's arms both thinking their own thoughts. Marcello considering the likelihood of this truly being their last time together: he would gladly never ask God for another thing in the whole of the rest of his life if he could just have this woman as his own. He loved her with all his heart now, this he knew for certain and thought that she must feel a little the same because of the way she gave herself to him so freely. But at the end of the day he still didn't think that she was for him, there was too much else to consider and there was Guy. God help him, but he shouldn't be hoping that the man had disappeared off the face of the earth, never to return again.

Alicia was contemplating an uncertain and a somewhat fearful future without Marcello. She knew that it just couldn't be, because whatever she felt, whatever happened, there was always Guy, somewhere out there and still right there between them, deeply entrenched in her heart. She had to finish that which she had set out to do: to find out the truth of what had happened to him. But how she would miss this man; so deliciously solid beside her, the safety, the security and the physical satisfaction. No matter what the future, he would always have a place in her heart and this she must tell him.

She wondered how they would ever say goodbye, once more, the next day: it was already the early hours of the morning. She turned to speak at last but Marcello, covering her mouth with his hand said,

"No, *Alichia mia*, there is no need for words. I am here again to look after you. Unexpectedly we have been given one more chance of being together and we must not waste it. What comes after '*sono fatalista.*'

"*Devo andarmene domani,*" she answered. "I always have to be leaving." He nodded.

"I know *mia cara, mi mancherai,* more than you will ever know."

"Me too, Marcello, me too."

"Now I will get us some coffee if I can find someone awake, so you stay there and be ready for me when I return," he said, kissing her, still hungry for more. He pulled on his trousers and a sweatshirt over his head and went to the door.

"I won't be long and don't open it to anybody but me, for they would have a big, wonderful, shock." He winked at her and went out laughing, shutting the door firmly behind him. Alicia sat back against the pillow pondering this remarkable man. She could sense that he was thinking along the same lines as she. If there was but a way - he made her feel so good, so extremely good. Was it possible to love two men at the same time? Yes, she concluded, it was. Never should her elusive fiancée forget that he was conspicuous in his continuing absence. She lay, waiting and anticipating what was to come next. *Domani* was still a long way off so it was best just not to think about it, at least not for a few more short hours.

There was a knock on the door. He'd been quick. She began to open it laughing, which instantly turned to horror as the door flew open with such force that she was knocked over backwards onto the lower bunk. She shouted.

"*Aiuto!* Help! Marcello!" As she fell, a strong arm was holding her down and a swarthy, dark, face with foul, garlic smelling, breath was staring into hers, growling in a thick accent.

"Your boyfriend, *Signorina,* your boyfriend: Where is he? Tell me or…" there was another crash.

"*Fermati!*" Marcello had arrived and, in one fluid movement dragged Alicia's assailant off and threw him with such force that the man hit his head hard, on the door, but he still fought on, grunting obscenities. As he reached inside his jacket, Marcello kicked him hard in the crotch, shouting,

"*Non essere un idiota,*" and hit him hard again in the stomach. The man crumpled forwards, swearing. Marcello removed the gun; he was furious.

"*Non me ne frega un cazzo.* I don't give a fuck, *sei proprio un bastardo,*" and hauled him out through the door, calling back to Alicia to keep it shut, no matter what. Alicia could hear the struggle continuing outside in the corridor. She sat, hunched on the edge of the bunk, her arms clasped around her bare breasts, willing herself not to scream. She wasn't hurt so there was no need, she kept repeating to herself. He'll be back, he'll be back, he must come back, she thought desperately.

The train was slowing for some reason. Alicia could smell the bitter smell of spilt coffee on the carpet and wondered, stupidly, where the cups were and if they had broken. She sat up looking down at herself. How much of her, nearly naked, body did the horrible *mafiosa* type see? Not much, she thought, in the dark and as if it mattered. She was unhurt, but Marcello - she stood up and drew the curtain back. There was no station and it was night out there. Most people must be sleeping, but somebody must have heard. Was anybody helping Marcello? Where was the emergency device? She looked around desperately but she couldn't see one. What about the guard? Where was he? Should she shout for help?

She was cold. She grabbed Marcello's discarded shirt and pulled it over her head. She paced backwards and forwards between the door and the window trying to keep calm, wondering what to do. She heard a door slam somewhere in the distance then the train began to pick up speed again. She made herself sit down, straining her ears and waited as she'd been told to do. Marcello had definitely won the battle, she was sure, but what was he doing now? Maybe there were two men in the dark suits, another one waiting outside for him, perhaps, with a gun or a knife. But that couldn't be possible she reasoned, as the other was on his way to Germany. But maybe there were three? What would she do if Marcello didn't come back?

A few minutes passed. It seemed like an eternity. With shaking fingers she carefully buttoned up his shirt. This small job took a ridiculously long time. Then there was a knock. She leapt up and pressed the side of her face hard against the door.

"Who is it?" she called.

"It's alright, *Alichia mia,* it's me, Marcello, you can open the door now." Thankfully she pulled the door open. He closed it quickly and wrapped his arms around her.

"*Tutto fila, liscio Alichia,* but are you hurt?" he asked worriedly, checking her quickly.

"*No, sto bene, mi dispiace.* I was so scared Marcello and it was my fault. I opened the door and you had told me not to." She was still shaking with fright. He gathered her into his arms and laid her gently on the bed.

"It's alright. Don't worry. He's gone!" She looked incredulous, and sat up.

"Gone? What do you mean gone? Gone where, with the guard? Did you get the police? Oh no! You are the police, how foolish! " He had an odd look on his face, almost mischievous and then she remembered hearing a door slam.

"Oh no! Marcello you didn't? "

"I did!" he answered her with a grin and flicking his hands towards the window. "I just helped him on his way, *il povero uomo,* the train slowed down most conveniently!" Alicia giggled weakly.

"I can't believe you did that!" She stared at him disbelievingly.

"What would you have me do then, *mia carissima,* with you like that? Would you have him join us in here for what I have in mind? " She laughed at last, getting up.

"Your right, I'm ridiculous, I'm going to have a shower and wash that disgusting man off me."

"Good idea," replied Marcello, "and I think I'll join with you, there's just room for us both."

"Oh no, *ancora*, not again!" said Alicia unbuttoning his shirt which she had put on.

"Oh yes, again, *cara mia,*" he answered, helping her.

Later Alicia slept a little under Marcello's watchful eye, with her head resting comfortably on his shoulder. They were disturbed only once and with many apologies by the ticket inspector. He'd obviously seen and heard nothing. They had no near neighbours. The train was quite empty and any other passengers would be in the privacy of their compartments. They travelled on through the night towards Genoa and the border, talking quietly together when they were both awake and not nourishing their rapacious appetites.

Alicia desperately needed to know what these people were looking for. She repeated the words she remembered being spat out, as the man accosted her, asking Marcello why he thought they wanted him. But Marcello explained gently that he was almost certain that 'the boyfriend' they sought was in fact Guy, not himself and that they were probably hoping that she could lead them to him or knew of his whereabouts. Why they wanted Guy, as yet he had no idea. But the whole episode shed a little light on the events which had taken place in Verona.

At Genoa they dressed and moved along to the restaurant car, where they sat side by side, neither feeling hungry in view of what was to come. However the coffee was good and Alicia managed to force down a fresh croissant, at Marcello's request, trying hard to put on a brave face. He was alert and watching at all times, once more the excellent policeman, meticulously doing his job.

The idea of soon being amongst strangers again was unnerving to say the least and the imminent parting with Marcello worse than awful. But Alicia knew that there was no way out: she had to continue her quest and she just wasn't free.

They sat quietly, Marcello smoking his first cigarette of the day, with his other hand on her knee, sensitive and understanding. Both were dreading the inevitable goodbye, yet again. After a while, Marcello arose abruptly from his chair and held his hand out.

"Come, *cara mia,* we have one more hour," and, indicating their fellow diners, "we are not needing all these people." She took his hand and they returned to their compartment. There they made love once more, slowly and surely, with the conviction that this would be for the final time and, without doubt, would have to last them for the rest of their lives. Alicia told Marcello that she would always hold precious the days and nights that they'd had together and that even with time, she would never allow the memories to dim.

"You have given me so much, so much …" as her voice broke. "I can't say goodbye again, I can't."

"Then don't," he answered, staring at her intensely.

"I have to Marcello, I'm not free." Then she said, placing his hand on her heart:

"Ho un dolore continuo. I have a pain here already, wherever I am, *mi mancherai, amore mia."*

She didn't know how to begin to thank him for the way he had cared. He'd possibly saved her from rape, kidnap or even worse. He stopped her mouth with his, then, told her that there was no need for words: she knew how he felt and that would never change. She also knew where to find him. The time that they had together had been 'given by God' and he refused to say goodbye. So he kissed her finally, until their time ran out, then merely said over and over again, 'non si sa mai,' one never knows, and 'sono fatalista.'

When the two alighted on the platform at Nice, they were met by Jean Pierre Beiron, the d'Aubert's all round helper, odd job man and much more. To him and any other stranger meeting them, Marcello was the 'chaperone' in charge and Alicia the woman being gratefully escorted – except, perhaps, for their eyes.

***

CHAPTER 20

Marcello handed Alicia over into the care of Jean Pierre Béiron, with a polite smile fixed determinedly on his face, as they exchanged pleasantries in English.

Jean Pierre was about nineteen or twenty, tall and dark, with mischievous brown eyes. He was athletically thin with that, typically French, olive coloured skin and a shock of very black, unruly, hair. No doubt he pulled the girls left right and centre, Alicia thought later, when she was in a better state to study him more closely. When they'd all introduced themselves he took her bag and placed it in the boot of the car that the d'Auberts had hired for her. He was obviously keen to get going.

Alicia and Marcello said their public goodbyes. Marcello took one of Alicia's hands in his and, as he held her eyes for a moment longer, she felt the folded piece of paper that he placed in the palm of her hand. He kissed her on both cheeks, as was customary, wished her good luck, good fortune and happiness always and helped her into the car.

Alicia had to exert every ounce of willpower to hold steady. It was one of the most emotional moments that she had ever had to handle, but they both played their parts perfectly. As her driver was settling himself in the front, Alicia looked out through the open window and, catching Marcello's eyes one last time, she saw him touch first his head, his heart and then his lips. And she, discreetly, did likewise.

Jean Pierre drove off swiftly. As she looked back one more time, Marcello was already striding away into the early morning mist, gone; gone forever she imagined. Alicia sat steeling herself in the back, wishing that she could disappear into a field somewhere and howl. She could almost drown in her unshed tears, or choke on swallowing them and as for the pleasant smile plastered on her face for John Pierre's benefit; it could well crack in two at the drop of a hat.

Jean Pierre was quite a chauffeur, with an interesting route of his own, and an equally unusual way of driving! He paid little regard to the one-way system around the station, or the struggling passengers, towing huge suitcases, crossing the road in front of them. He drove along the coast, turned off the *Corniche* and began negotiating the back streets, hardly altering speed. Alicia was looking around to see if there were seat belts in the car, when they rounded a corner and nearly crashed into a market stall of fruit and vegetables. The infuriated owner hurried over and shouted a string of abuse at Jean Pierre, banging on the roof of the car as he did so and periodically glaring into the back at Alicia, who immediately recovered from her need to burst into tears.

"*Je suis vraiement desolé,*" Jean Pierre kept saying, until the local farmer finally stepped back, then Jean put the car into gear and laughing loudly, shot off again leaving the poor man standing in the road shaking his fist and shouting, "*T'est fou! t'est fou!*" pointing at his temple. The amusing incident had saved Alicia from certain embarrassment and Jean Pierre obviously thought it very funny as well. He continued chuckling to himself, from time to time, throughout the rest of the journey.

They had turned away from the sea now and were heading up into the hills above Nice, to the village where the d'Auberts lived. The signs to the vineyard and Chateau d'Aubert were everywhere. It was well advertised. Soon they were driving down a long, straight, private road, flanked on both sides by pollarded plane trees, towards an elegant, small, chateau with a walled garden and a large collection of buildings and barns to one side. As they drew up in the courtyard, a rather large, sophisticated, man with two spaniels appeared from one of the buildings. This could only be the very successful Jacques d'Aubert, Alicia thought.

Jean Pierre jumped out to open the door for Alicia and as Jacques walked over to welcome her, he was asking, 'how long then J.P.?'

"Forty-three minutes, Monsieur d'Aubert, not good today," he laughed. Jacques d'Aubert took Alicia's hand, welcomed her, kissed her on both cheeks, then explained.

"Alicia, *pardonnez-moi,* Jean-P drives like a lunatic, I know, but he's always trying to break his record of thirty-four and a half minutes. I hope it wasn't too bad, but you should see him on his bike!" Alicia laughed with him. He spoke excellent and educated English.

"No, no not at all, but it was an interesting journey, wasn't it Jean Pierre?" she said turning towards him. He smiled in return.

"*Oui, mais très long* and please call me Jean-P or J.P. Mademoiselle, everybody does" and he gave a little bow.

"*Merci bien* then, Jean-P." They all laughed and Jacques walked her away towards his wife, Marie-Anne, who, hearing the dogs announcing Alicia's arrival had already appeared through an arched door from the garden.

"I think you're in there with J.P.," Jacques said, "though I dread to think how many of my countrymen he has nearly finished off on the way here. Come to meet my wife." Jacques was charming and just as Gianni had described him. A good looking man of about fifty or thereabouts, with light brown hair, a humorous face and a slightly freckled complexion. Only his rather portly figure showed his penchant for good food and wine! He wore an open necked shirt with a very English looking tweed coat.

Marie-Anne was petite, slim and very chic, somewhere between forty-five and fifty: hard to tell, Alicia thought as she was very well preserved. Her blonde hair, tied back in a neat pony-tail, looked completely natural. She had lovely, twinkling, cat-like, green eyes, with laughter lines etched at the edges.

Her face was beautifully made up; her creamy skin emphasized with a pale, pink lipstick. She held out her manicured hand, sporting a huge, flawless, diamond on her wedding ring finger.

Alicia could well imagine Marie Ann going out to a smart lunch party in what she had on; a light blue trouser suit, black silk shirt with matching leather belt and shoes, but hardly for doing things in the garden, even if only for giving orders.

The d'Auberts appeared to enjoy making Alicia welcome. Marie-Anne showed her to a lovely suite in one of the long barns, which had a sitting area at one end with a comfortable sofa, chairs and a coffee table piled high with all the latest magazines. It had been done up for one of the children, now grown up, married and expecting their first grandchild, she explained, "so soon I'll have to get some nursery furniture in here," Marie-Anne told her with a sparkling smile, "and that will be fun. I shall spoil the baby mercilessly and Jacques will be very cross. I thought that you would feel more independent out here, rather than in the main house, with all the constant interruptions and comings and goings." Alicia was delighted; she would have some space and not feel that she was in their way.

"The meals, in the house, are moveable feasts at present, except when we have our wine tastings, when we have to be very organized and on very best behaviour. No two days are ever the same here and there's never a dull moment either." She laughed. Marie-Anne evidently loved her life at the Chateau D'Aubert.

As she looked around Alicia commented on the beautifully restored and comfortable barn.

"There really isn't anything you haven't thought of. It's lovely and thank you so much for having me. I do hope that it's not too much trouble for you?"

"Good Heavens no, but of course not, we love having people to stay. We shall enjoy the company and my husband is much looking forward to hearing the latest of his beloved Gianni. The two were inseparable when they were together as young men. Please do absolutely as you wish here. Breakfast will arrive on a tray at whatever time you ask. Someone comes in from the village to help Madame Béiron in the mornings, so there are two of them in the kitchen gossiping away, with not enough to do between them. We have ours at nine, as Jacques likes to do his rounds first thing in the morning, before we eat," she paused and then went on, "just let Madame Béiron know when you need lunch, she's Jean-P's mother as you probably gathered. Today I thought you'd be too tired to want to rush off anywhere, so perhaps we could all have something light in the *orangerie* at one-thirty and then we can get to know each other." Marie-Anne walked towards the door and as she was leaving added,

"Jean-P will come to collect you. His mother makes up excellent picnics by the way, so when you would like one, just let her know the night before. Leave any laundry you have in the bath tub and the maid will take it, each morning, when she cleans your room. Otherwise we'll expect you each night for dinner at eight, to hear all the news! Now I'll let you settle in. I'll be in the garden if you need anything," and she swept out in a cloud of Chanel.

What perfect English Marie-Anne spoke and what an amazing hotel the Chateau d'Aubert was! Alicia flopped onto her bed and realized just how exhausted she felt. Now that she was left by herself, she started to think back over the last twelve hours. So much had happened in such a short time since she had left the island. She remembered how nervous she had been at the station when she was being followed. Maybe this was why, she excused herself, that she had so readily fallen into Marcello's arms as she boarded the train thinking that she was to be by herself.

Her pleasure in seeing him again had been genuine and not entirely physical. She liked being with him. They had plenty to say to each other. He was there for her when she needed him most, protecting her and looking after her as well, taking someone else's place and watching over her. So no wonder she had turned to him for comfort. She'd been very frightened when she'd been attacked. Maybe it was the rush of adrenalin that had so enhanced their love-making for the rest of the night. It had been even better than the first time.

But now she was beginning to feel thoroughly confused. She had known, this time, that Guy was alive and out there somewhere, probably in some danger, yet still she had been unable to resist Marcello. The electric pull had, again, been too strong. Where did this leave her feelings overall? In a terrible tangle, Alicia surmised. She then remembered Marcello's note and went to retrieve it from her bag.

'Amore mia,' it read, 'listen to Monsieur d'Aubert's advice. You will be safe there. God go with you everywhere you journey through life, I will never forget you and our time together, *mai* - you know how to find me, *ti amo, Alichia*, M.' Alicia held the note in her hand and finally gave way to her tears. She sobbed until she felt even more drained than before, then lay on the bed, pulled up a blanket and went fast asleep.

Alicia awoke, with a start, when a dog barked somewhere outside her window. From the hissing and spitting noise it sounded as though one of the spaniels had cornered a cat. She looked at her watch. God! It was nearly lunch time. She'd been asleep for an hour and a half. She washed and changed her clothes. Deciding that she was too tired to dwell further on her complicated love life for now and pushing it to one side she turned her thoughts to her present situation. 'I must think positively', she said to herself 'and get to the bottom of the whole scenario. Then hopefully everything else will become clear.'

It had been a great relief to unburden herself to Marcello during the quiet moments they'd had together. He'd been understanding and sensitive. It must have been difficult for him having to listen to her strange story, featuring Guy so dramatically all the time, especially when he'd made it so very clear that he was in love with her himself.

Gianni had been so kind and helpful too, before she'd left Isola Delfino. Keeping quiet about her secret love affair with his relation had made Alicia feel guilty. What on earth would he have thought of her if she had told him? It was also good to know that she still continued to have care and protection here in the South of France. Alicia had liked the d'Auberts as soon as she met them and sensed that Jean-P, also, was a man in whom she could have confidence and trust.

So: with positive thoughts uppermost in her mind, when Alicia saw J.P. approaching across the courtyard a short time later, she walked out to meet him her head high and an unwavering smile fixed firmly on her face.

Lunch, as Alicia had expected, was delicious, light hearted and fun. They were served perfectly cooked entrecôte steak, pommes frites and a salad together with an excellent Chateau d'Aubert red wine, followed by tarte tatin and lots of strong dark coffee; enough to keep an army awake, had it been evening. She soon discovered that Marie-Anne's perfect English came from her time at university and that she had met Jacques when he was doing a year's exchange, also at Durham. Jacques had met Gianni when the Italian had been sent to Jacques' French university for the same purpose. According to Marie-Anne, the two hit it off so well that they soon organized to share digs together and became famous for their parties, alternating between French and Latin cuisine.

"Those student's who were lucky enough to be included into their elite circle, loved them both", she laughed, "for obvious reasons and you can just imagine how big-headed the two became, can't you?" she said, teasing Jacques, who looked at Alicia spreading his hands.

"What can I say," he answered, "it was probably true! But we had a good time together and enjoyed 'running things'. It was the start of a long- lasting and meaningful friendship." He went on to explain that after finishing their education they had both gone into the Army, in their own countries, but still met up fairly frequently as they both, coincidentally, had trained with the 'special forces'.

How very interesting, Alicia thought. No wonder everything had been so faultlessly co-ordinated.

After lunch, Jacques took her on a guided tour of the Chateau and its extensive grounds. It was magnificent and in immaculate order. Alicia couldn't help being amused by the complete contrast from her island. She decided that, for the next couple of days, she would rest and recover from a period of high emotion. In this, new, safe haven she would enjoy the hospitality of her delightful host and hostess.

The vineyard was also impeccable and the various stages of the winemaking fascinating. The d'Auberts, were cultured, well travelled and interesting people but, thoughtfully, left Alicia to her own devices in the daytime, which suited her well. There was a well-stocked library from which she read several novels, sitting in the small enclosed garden outside the barn, when it was hot enough. Sometimes, if they seemed happy to accompany her, she took the dogs for walks.

Before Alicia ventured out for the first time, she remembered Marcello's advice and told the d'Auberts of her plans for the day and that she hoped to take out the hire car, if that was alright. Jacques had called her into his study after dinner the night before, ostensibly to show her some family portraits and pictures of which he was particularly proud. Actually he wanted a private word he had said, shutting the door behind them. Ah! Alicia thought: this conversation will no doubt have been instigated by Gianni.

Jacques talked to Alicia about life in the Chateau through the years, particularly during the last war when his home had regularly been used as a base for Maquis resistance. His father, Jean-Jacques d'Aubert, had been a courageous man and had masterminded a highly successful escape route out through the mountains to Switzerland. His mother also had played a large part in the saving of many lives. His parents had been much loved in this part of France. When they had died, within a year of each other, if he hadn't seen it with his own eyes he would never have believed the number of people who attended their funerals. 'They were still much talked of to this day,' said Jacques sadly proud, 'and still much missed.'

He went on to explain to Alicia that the Béirons had worked for his family for many years and that his father and Jean-P's grandfather had become close friends during the war. They had started up the resistance group together. Jean-P's father Henri, with Jacques himself, grew up at the Chateau d'Aubert where they learnt the wine business together. At home they were treated as equals. They had worked hard side by side to prove themselves in the vineyard, to earn respect from the rest of the workers, which had been more difficult for Jacques as son of the boss.

While Henri continued to perfect his practical knowledge amongst the vines at home, Jacques had been sent away to university and then to other vineyards to continue his training and learn the administrative side and office routine, until it was time for him to join the army.

After his successful military career Jacques had left the elite French Special Intervention Force. Henri and he had spent many happy years at Chateau d'Aubert, where, with his parent's constant energy and guidance, they managed to raise the vineyard into one of the most respected and consistently best-named in the South of France. They were all extremely proud of this achievement.

When Henri had died, completely out of the blue, from a rampant blood disease, they were all devastated. Their boy, Jean Pierre, was only fifteen at the time, a difficult age to loose a father. At Jacque's insistence, Jean-P had grown up alongside his own young family, all of whom had always thought of him as a brother in any case. Jacques, for his part, had tried to fill J.P.'s father's place a little, making Madame Béiron's life easier at the same time. The Beiron's were family: one hundred per cent loyal and trustworthy.

Alicia guessed now where all this was leading. Jacques then told Alicia that whenever she left the grounds, Jean-P would go with her, but on his bike. Alicia started to protest, but Jacques held up his hand.

"No Alicia, I promised Gianni that I would look after you and I'm only being overly cautious, maybe, but I also know what happened in Verona and on the train coming here." She felt her cheeks reddening. Jacques smiled, luckily interpreting her embarrassment for all the wrong reasons.

"Yes, you are a brave woman, Alicia. Your chaperone of course reported to Gianni on the fight and how he disposed of that nasty individual, but we must take none of these incidents lightly." She heaved an inward sigh of relief. Of course Jacques would have been told of the uninvited guest on the train. He continued. "Don't worry about Jean-P. He will be very discreet. He won't be intrusive, or get in your way, but please show him where you will be going on this map and he will always be somewhere close at hand." He handed over a large scale map. "Sometimes you will see him in the distance, at others he may just appear, so take no notice. Take your mobile with you at all times please and give him your number before you leave. He will give you his. *D'Accord?*" Alicia nodded feeling slightly foolish, although she knew this was a good plan and would remove unnecessary anxiety on all fronts.

"*Parfait!* And you will have a lovely day and worry about nothing at all. *Allez-vous en,*" he said taking her arm. "Now come and tell me what you think about these pictures," he finished. He was so disarming. How could she protest! She knew he was right to be so cautious, for it was obvious that there was some real threat out there. A slight nervousness had come over her ever since leaving the island, except, during those few precious hours she'd spent with Marcello, after the attack on the train. Then she had felt completely safe.

Alicia explored the countryside nearby, watching the men and women working on the grapes. It was fascinating and in the evening she appreciated drinking the wine all the more. Sometimes, when she was out and about, she caught sight of Jean-P in the distance. Once she saw him on a track above her doing wheelies, for her benefit she was sure and it made her laugh. But he was discreet as Jacques had said he would be and actually it was reassuring to know that he was around.

On the third day, well rested, Alicia decided to drive down into Cannes and visit some of her old haunts. It was the best time of the year, before the music and film festivals started, after which Cannes became a place to avoid at all costs. She went down to the old port and wandered around the boats, remembering the last time when she and Guy had been there together. Then she went back to the shops where she bought a bathing suit and a couple of shirts. She couldn't face Guy's favourite restaurant, so sat at one of the many places on the beach belonging to one of the hotels. There were few people around and it was sunny and warm.

Jean-P was never far away, he was vigilant and proficient in his supervision. As she sat down he was already ordering a cup of coffee nearby. Alicia wondered if she should ask him to join her, then decided against it as the whole point of his job might be lost, so she merely inclined her head and smiled as she would to any stranger. She ordered a seafood salad and a carafe of wine as she thought about tomorrow and planned a trip into the hills, to do what she had come to do. She felt a quickening of excitement and wondered what she would manage to find out.

Alicia went back to the car, buying an English newspaper from the kiosk on the way and was soon heading back to the Chateau. Just as she entered the old wrought iron gates, J.P. roared past, out of nowhere, showing off his wheelies again all the way down the drive in front of her. When she stopped the car he was standing there waiting for her to open the door, grinning from ear to ear. "Jean-P, how on earth do you do that?" she asked.

"I'll show you Mademoiselle, if you would like," holding his hands out to her. Alicia laughed with him.

"No thanks, J.P. I think I'll give that a miss, at least for the moment!"

It was early evening when Alicia put her feet up on the big, comfortable, old sofa and opened the newspaper, thinking how nice it would be to have a peaceful shower before going up to dinner at the main house, to which, as always, she was looking forward.

She was really was enjoying her time with the d'Auberts. Jacques endlessly regaled Alicia and Marie-Anne with uproarious stories of his adventures with Gianni, when they had been students together. 'Some of these stories I've heard so many times before.' Marie-Anne had confided to Alicia the previous night, when she and the dogs were walking Alicia back to the barn after dinner, 'but he tells them so well that they still make me laugh, even if they are all thoroughly exaggerated. He seems to conveniently forget that I too was at Durham University and that I and my room-mates also had many parties, to which he was invited … sometimes!' She giggled at the memory.

"But you must have all had such fun," answered Alicia. "Our celebrations at St Andrews were pretty wild on occasion too!"

"Oh we did. *Mon Dieu!* We did! It was the end of the swinging sixties. We were so bad and a lot we got up to they never even knew!" Marie-Anne linked her arm through Alicia's and laughed with her. "They had no idea about some of the awful things we were responsible for and wouldn't like to admit to even now!" She turned to Alicia, with a far away look in her eyes remembering something in particular, then shook her head and repeated. *"Mon Dieu!* But we were bad!"

Alicia could well understand Gianni and Jacques being compatible and spending many happy times together in France. As for women? Marie-Anne said that the two must have been worse than a nightmare.

"We can only imagine! I kept well clear of Jacques in those days".

"At Durham, I asked her out many times", Jacques had told Alicia, "but she always refused. She was tantalizing and exasperating both at once,"

Jacques continued. "She would only come to our parties when there were many people. 'Safety in numbers, Jacques', she would say and she was so beautiful!" He chuckled, looking at Marie-Anne whose eyes were shining. "So very beautiful," he said, stroking her chin and staring into her face, "and she still is."

It wasn't until some years later that they had finally got together, they confided. Jacques and Marie-Ann had met again at a family wedding and discovered that not only did their families already know each other, but that they had also been brought up, not far apart, in France.

Watching them together, Alicia had thought what a wonderful thing to be still so much in love after three children and so many years.

Alicia turned her thoughts and attention back to the newspaper, skimming through the headlines. There was nothing of much interest, the usual political slanging and terrorist alerts, continuing unrest and worry in the Middle East, a film star having twins by she knew not who. Idiotic: how unbelievably degrading. Her attention began to slip, she flipped through the pages thinking that maybe she'd go and have a good, long, shower and a snooze when suddenly her heart stopped as a small paragraph caught her eye at the bottom of one of the centre pages.

Her hand starting to shake; with increasing horror Alicia read the heading,

'Julian Birchall, the war correspondent, dies in boating accident off the South of France.'

Julian, no, it wasn't possible. It couldn't be true. No way, it just couldn't be him. It had to be a mistake. She made herself read on, clutching the paper, her breath coming in short gasps, not believing what she was reading. It said that he had died when swimming with a friend between the Iles de Lérins. They'd apparently dived off the boat to swim, on an unusually warm day for so early in the year, without noticing that the self-chartered boat had no steps for them to climb back on board. The few other boats passing, some distance away, hadn't realized that they were in trouble and the two men had finally drowned, exhausted, after many hours in the water.

Alicia couldn't take it in. It was an extraordinary story and just not conceivable. Julian had been brought up by the sea. He understood it, he understood boats. They all used to go sailing together, for goodness sake. He was a strong swimmer and he would have swum to one of the islands here off Cannes. She knew them, as he did and they weren't far off the mainland. At the same time Julian hated cold water, a frightful wimp about getting in. They all used to tease him, because he was so tough in other respects. He would never have gone into these waters so early in the year. She remembered that from when they'd spent a week together in Greece, the year before. It had been early in the year, when the sea was still quite cold and Guy had eventually had to push Julian into the water. No it just couldn't be him. This article was definitely wrong. It had to be nonsense. Oh! My God! She suddenly thought. Who was the other man? She read the article through twice more, there was no name given for the friend; then she picked up her mobile. Nick answered immediately.

"Nick, it's me I've just read the strangest …" he interrupted her.

"Alicia where are you? I've been trying to get hold of you, but your mobile's been off."

Oh Heavens! Yes! She'd forgotten to turn it on since dinner the night before.

"Yes, your right, how stupid, my fault, I was going to ring you tonight. I'm in the South of France and just picked up a newspaper. There's this odd story, some mistake, pure coincidence, just happens to be the same name I know because Julian would never …" he cut her off.

"Alicia, Alicia, I'm so sorry, so very sorry, but there's no mistake. I'm afraid what you've read is true."

"No, no, Nick it can't be the same man, it's wrong, he wouldn't have been so stupid … and … and the other man … who was it?"

"Alicia, you must listen to me. Brace yourself. I've checked it out, it is true, Julian is dead, drowned and the other man was a foreigner, as yet still not identified." There was silence. Alicia drew a huge shuddering breath.

"You're sure?"

"I'm sure. So sorry, but I didn't know how else to tell you. Shall I come?" Alicia was completely numb and dumb as it all began to sink in. Julian … dead. Julian of all people: tough, strong and fit. Dead.

"Are you still there? Alicia?"

"Yes, it's O.K. I'm alright, at least for the moment. How's Adriana?"

"Not good, as you can imagine. She's gone up to his parents to be with them for the funeral"

"When is it? The funeral, I mean."

"Next week: Monday. Will you come? Shall I come to get you?"

Yes, of course I'll come, to be with Adriana. "But no, thanks all the same, but there's no point in your coming all the way down here to get me. There's no other news I suppose? Nick, Guy is his best friend and I just can't believe …," she stuttered, that … that, he doesn't even know? "

"I'm afraid not. I'll send you all the details by email or fax, whichever they have there and let me know anything else I can do, because I'll meet you in Scotland. I'd like to come up."

"Would you? Would you really? But you hardly know Julian." She just wasn't prepared to say 'knew,' not yet, at least.

"I know, I only met him a couple of times, but I'd like to be there. We can go together and I'll book you in somewhere to stay nearby."

"Thanks Nick, I'll text you the numbers." They said goodbye. Alicia turned the mobile off and slumped down. She couldn't believe it. Julian was dead. Where, oh where the hell, was Guy? She couldn't accept or begin to absorb this latest, ghastly, turn of events. The four of them had been together having dinner in London only a short time ago. They'd had a wonderful evening and she and Guy had gone to bed that night sure that it wouldn't be long before his old friend lost his bachelor status too! Poor Adriana. How unbelievably horrendous; what must she be feeling? What on earth was Julian doing here, in France? He was supposedly in South America, according to the last reports. The whole thing just didn't add up.

Alicia sat in a tight ball on the sofa, shaking, her arms around her legs as she rocked gently to and fro, trying to take in the news, still disbelieving and as yet unemotional. She considered her plan of action. First and foremost: Adriana. What could she do to help her? She picked up the mobile, then put it down again. She hadn't got the house number in Scotland. She should have got it from Nick. No, better to text Adriana, then she could ring when it suited. This she did, not knowing what to say. What could you say? She sent: 'I'm here and send my love.'

Her thoughts turned again to Guy and to her immediate relief when she'd heard that the other man was a foreigner. Then she felt angry, very angry, that he could let her go through all this without him, if he knew. Maybe he didn't, but, wherever he was, he would be devastated when he found out.

The funeral was only three days away and Alicia would have a whole day's travelling to get there. She had but one day left in the South of France. She rang through to the house and explained to Jacques what had happened, telling him that, unfortunately, she'd have to leave them earlier than expected to attend the funeral of her fiancé's dearest friend in Scotland.

They had, of course, heard the news of the accident already and were both sad to hear it was a friend and sorry to learn she was leaving so soon. They understood, of course, were more than concerned and offered their help with travel plans.

She'd only just put the telephone down to Jacques when there was a knock at the door and Marie-Anne came bustling in with a large brandy and some bath salts, which were, she told Alicia as they embraced, her own particular remedy in times of serious trouble, or sadness. Realizing that Alicia was in a state of shock, Marie-Ann made her sit and drink the brandy then, wrapped a soft warm blanket around her, before going off to run a deep, hot and delicious-smelling bath.

Marie-Anne is so sweet, thought Alicia numbly. I am so lucky, in spite of these appalling times.

That night, Jacques lit the fire in the Chateau and Madam Béiron set up a cosy table in front of it for the three of them. Alicia didn't have to make any effort at conversation. Jacques made it quite clear that he was well aware of her situation, without going into any detail. He knew about Julian and had been going to break the news gently to her that night. The fact that she'd brought a newspaper in the town was so regrettable: he felt really stupid for not having considered that she might do so. If he'd thought about it he would have warned Jean-P. Not for anything would he have been responsible for Alicia having to deal with yet another hideous shock.

"*Je suis vraiment affolé,* Alicia. What more can I say, my dear, except that you are young and life must go on? Come, another digestive, before my wife takes you across to the barn."

He pressed her shoulder with his free hand and then, taking her empty glass, went across to the drinks tray to pour the comforting liquid. Both Marie-Ann and Jacques d'Aubert were extremely upset for her.

It was not until much later, when she was tucked up in bed that Alicia began to query, in her somewhat befuddled mind, how Jacques seemed to know that Julian was such a very close friend. Coincidence? Strange if it was, but she was too tired and distressed to wonder further for the moment. The following day she must gather herself together in order to do what she'd come to the South of France for, in the first place, as time here was now so unexpectedly short.

★★★

CHAPTER 21

Although deeply shocked, Alicia slept surprisingly well; helped no doubt by the copious glasses of Jacques' excellent red wine at dinner, followed by the brandy brought her by Marie-Anne later. The stupefying effects of the alcohol had rendered her incapable of doing much and so she had thankfully given herself into the capable hands of her hostess who had virtually put her to bed. In these dire circumstances she had felt like a child again and in need of the tender loving care, so gently administered. Was there no end to this string of grim events?

Alicia had woken only once in the night, after a disturbing dream, which was easy to understand given her muddled state of mind. She'd dreamt vividly, of Marcello pushing Guy out of the door of the train then sitting beside her bed, smiling down and stroking her hair as he always did. The scene had then changed; they'd all been swimming together somewhere and she had panicked on realizing that they couldn't get back on board the boat, crying out in alarm and waking herself, with a start, in the early hours of the morning. She was instantly aware that there was yet another dark cloud enveloping her. Her bewildered brain cleared, all the real horror flooded back, and she felt as sad and dispirited as ever.

On her last day with the d'Auberts, promising to return early to spend her final evening with them, Alicia set off after breakfast, for Grasse and the Fragonard perfume factory. In spite of the awful news, she knew that it was best to keep busy and to try not to dwell on the events of the moment. She had to keep strong for Adriana and the impending funeral. There would be plenty of time afterwards for her personal grief to set in. As yet, she still found the unlikely accident unbelievable. She would keep her mobile switched on, willing Nick to ring her, to say that there had been a ghastly mistake. Until then she would try to concentrate on the job in hand.

Alicia took the box of flowers with her. She found Fragonard easily: it was well signed. Soon after her arrival, she was showing the flowers to one of the guides who conducted tours of the perfume factory.

No, it's not one of ours," the woman answered curtly, surveying the box and its contents. Alicia's heart sank. Madame looked up and noticed her disappointed face. "Although the flowers are from this area," she added more kindly, inspecting them further, then closing the box and handing it back. "However I do know someone who might help. I'll see if I can find her. *"Un petit moment, s'il vous plaît."* She strode off purposefully.

Alicia wandered around while she waited and inspected the beautifully packaged soaps and perfumes, tastefully displayed for purchase. The woman soon returned with a plump and personable young girl who said, 'yes', she thought that the flowers were made up by a small family business in a village near to where she lived, the other side of Mougins. Alicia thanked her, took the directions and, after buying a selection of the Fragonard soaps for Marie-Anne, returned to the car and continued on her way to Mougins with a twinge of excitement and a familiar motor bike not far behind.

~

On the map, the village she sought looked no distance at all. Once further into the hills the narrow, winding, road made the journey twice as long. When she finally drew to a halt, Alicia wondered if there could possibly be a flourishing business in a village so small, for it seemed only to consist of a butcher, a *patisserie,* a café, a church and no more than half a dozen houses. The only thing to do was ask.

The *patisserie* was somewhat larger than it looked from the street and had a lot more in it than just bread! Inside Alicia found an unfriendly, stout, woman restocking some groceries; she hardly bothered to look up as Alicia walked in; shot her a glance bordering on disdain then, immediately bent to continue her work, though with some difficulty due to her ample size! But, on Alicia producing the box of flowers, Madame was completely transformed. Her huge bulk wobbled and her florid face lit up with delight; she couldn't have been more helpful.

"*Ah! Oui, oui, Mademoiselle*", she exclaimed, looking Alicia up and down with interest, "*montez a l'église. Demandez Monsieur Gerard, le Prêtre!*" and she pointed out across the road with genuine enthusiasm.

In the little church nobody appeared to be around, so Alicia began to explore for herself. The old building was simple and charming, with beautiful windows, at their best this particular morning with the sun streaming through, now that an early morning mist and mild drizzle had cleared. As she neared the altar, with a growing sense of excitement, Alicia noticed two, large, arrangements of dried flowers similar to her own. Then she heard a gentle shuffling noise behind.

An old lady was quietly sweeping the floor, completely lost in her own world. Not wishing to startle her, Alicia approached slowly, then realizing that the woman was obviously deaf, waited for her to look up. When she did raise her head, Alicia was rewarded with an immediate, toothless, grin. On seeing the box she was carrying the brush was put down firmly and Alicia was escorted courteously to a large, arched, doorway nearby. The solid oak door was then ceremoniously pushed open while the old lady indicated for her to enter.

Inside there was a positive hive of activity: masses of dried flowers and arrangements all over the place, boxes of all shapes and sizes, similar to the one Alicia held in her hand and bundles of different coloured ribbons for tying, with an enormous pile of discarded rubbish lying, almost overflowing, in an ancient, old, wheelbarrow ready to be trundled out. Three, middle aged, women were hard at work creating and the priest was deep in conversation with yet another who, Alicia noted had an interesting tone of what could only be described as 'aubergine' coloured hair. How could she notice the woman's hair, for goodness sake, at such a time? Alicia experienced a spiral of excitement and coughed politely.

They all stopped talking, turned towards her and stared. Obviously not used to foreigners bowling up, unannounced, in the work place, thought Alicia, paying little heed, her resolve unfaltering. When she held up the box, their facial expressions instantly changed from curiosity to approval. She was bid welcome and the priest hurried over to introduce himself as Monsieur Gerard. Alicia launched forth and he answered her questions helpfully. The women all listened, unashamedly; nodding their heads in agreement, each time the priest spoke. Madame 'Aubergine' looked as if she would prefer to do the talking herself.

'Most of their stock went to the local markets in the area. Their market here in the village was last week and took place monthly. Private orders were telephoned through, but it was impossible to keep track of every personal purchase. *Mais oui*, yes, her little posy could have been made up there in the church by one of their group, however it would have been bought off the stall in the street or from one of the shops they also supplied'. Monsieur was warming to his subject.

'It could even have been brought from the kiosk outside where, after a certain hour, when everyone had gone home, they left an honesty box, the proceeds being gifted to the church.' This was said smugly, as the priest rubbed his hands together, passing his tongue over his thin lips and looking at her meaningfully. Monsieur Gerard wasn't about to miss an opportunity, Alicia realized! 'This box is meant for those visiting the church'. Now he made no pretence! 'And, of course, for the local workers on their way home for their evening meals: to keep their wives happy'. Then the bombshell: 'but also - they had other bases supplying the various airports in France.' Seeing the look of despair on her face, the priest finished his speech with a kind, apologetic, smile.

Alicia felt shattered and so disheartened. So near for a minute and now so far again. She'd drawn a complete blank. There was no way of telling if

Guy had been here after all. He could have seen the flowers in Paris and pre-ordered them to be sent from there.

~

Alicia walked back to the car, her energy level plummeting she took out Madame Béiron's picnic and walked across to the café she'd seen earlier. A young girl was busy cleaning the tables in preparation for customers. Alicia looked around and wondered if there would be any other visitors in this tiny community, but perhaps the locals came in the evenings. She ordered a large glass of red wine hoping that it might cheer her up. Even if she polished off a whole bottle and got drunk she knew that Jean-P was around, somewhere nearby and would scoop her up and see her home. She felt disillusioned and at a loss as to what to do next. After coming all this way she'd set her heart on finding concrete evidence that someone could actually remember Guy buying the flowers for her. Then she thought of poor Adriana and was at once ashamed.

Her wine duly arrived. She took a sip. It was rough and unpalatable. She put it down, pushing it aside with disgust and bit into Madame Béiron's excellent salami sandwich instead. A moment later an old man appeared and hastened over, apologizing. He whisked away the glass and called to the girl over his shoulder.

"*Non, non*, not that one. *La bouteille de rosé: la même que l'anglais a eu la semaine dernière,*" he shouted to her crossly, in French, continuing to mutter his apologies. Alicia, sitting bolt upright asked quietly:

"Excuse me, Monsieur but did you say there was an English person here last week?"

"*Mais oui,*" he replied, "and he enjoyed my best wine too, just as you shall, Mademoiselle." He turned away to make sure his waitress was doing her job. Alicia raised her voice to regain his attention.

"Monsieur, would you mind describing this man that was here last week.

You see, I think it might have been someone I'm looking for?" Alicia suddenly felt dizzy with the urge to know. Her hands, clutching the edge of the table, were white at the knuckles. Now she had the Frenchman's undivided attention. He studied the beautiful English woman's intent, upturned face; her cheeks flamed in her agitated state. He was disarmed.

"*Bien sur, Mademoiselle,*" he answered, bending down to the table for a closer inspection and the better to judge her reaction. He remembered the Englishman well for he left a very good tip. He commenced to describe Guy in perfect detail.

"For not many people come here so early in the year, especially the English," he was continuing, only to stop, transfixed by the rapturous smile on the lovely face in front of him.

Guy had actually been right here. Alicia was sitting back now in radiant silence and staring past Monsieur into space.

The old man watched, transfixed, until her eyes refocused and she suddenly seemed to return to the present. She jumped up, picked up her things, left ten euros and some change on the table, kissed his unshaven cheek without speaking and scurried off back to her car.

The great grandfather was left staring after her in utter astonishment, wondering what he could possibly have done to put a smile, of such pure sunshine, on such a beautiful face. Maybe he'd forgive his next-door neighbour, for having let his unsuitable bull get in with his pure-bred *charollais* cows, after all. He was eighty-one years old and as he looked around, he thought what a pity it was that none of his friends or neighbours were around to witness the kiss. They'd never believe him! He sat down in the chair, saw the ten euros, and started on the wine himself.

Later that night, when his neighbour, reluctantly, returned to apologise for his bull's escape and unwanted attentions towards one of the café owner's cows, he was amazed to find that he had been forgiven and was invited in.

Over another bottle of wine and in a comparatively short time an excellent agreement had been reached. They would both share the costs of raising any progeny and would also share whatever market price they were able to get for the calf in eighteen months time! Together they might even have perfected the beginning of an excellent new cross-breed!

~

Alicia returned to the chateau feeling a great sense of achievement after a day well spent. Jean-P arrived back behind her, churning up the gravel as he skidded to a stop. She'd hardly seen him all day, but had often sensed that he had not been far away, which had just been confirmed. She hadn't even noticed him in the mirror on the last stretch of road. She waved to him as she walked to the barn. He waved back and set about raking the gravel, before Jacques ticked him off.

Alicia found that her hosts had booked her airline tickets for the next morning, early, as she'd wished, because she had to change planes in Paris to travel on to Glasgow. They had insisted on making the reservations for her, understanding her need to get on with her own plans for the day. The tickets had been put, neatly, beside the telephone in her sitting room with a thoughtful note. There was also a tray, with white wine in a cooler and a plate of Madame Béiron's tiny, savoury, quiches, all covered with a clean, white cloth.

After packing her things and enjoying a shower, Alicia, gulped down a large glass of wine for courage and then did the thing she'd been dreading all day: she rang Nick again, her heart in her mouth as she waited for him to answer - waited for him to tell her that it was all a big mistake, that they'd got it all wrong. He hadn't rung all day as he'd promised he would with any fresh news. Perhaps, just perhaps, no news was good news? Maybe he'd been busy investigating the strange story - but she knew straight away by the tone of his voice; no, he had nothing different to report. The circumstances remained, horribly, the same. He was very sorry, but she must accept the awful fact that Julian was certainly gone; he was - dead.

With half an hour to spare, before it was time for dinner up at the house, Alicia walked out into the vineyard. The evening was still warm although the sun was already low in the sky. The last of the workers were tending the grapes with no regard for the time or their own plans for the evening. Everything that could be done would be done to ensure the best possible harvest each year, for all their livelihoods depended on it. Spring and early Summer were crucial times in this business: a frost now could mean ruination for the year's crop. It was a peaceful scene and she thought how much she would like to bring Guy here. It would be wonderful to be able to return happily together and to find that all the horror had just been a bad dream. She sighed as she thought once again of Adriana, of her own uncertain future and of Marcello. How would he get on here, she wondered?

Alicia now knew, for sure, that the D'Auberts were only too well aware of her present predicament. Gianni had obviously briefed Jacques and she felt convinced that they were in constant touch. Yet how either could possibly have known of her friendship with Julian was extremely puzzling. But she hadn't the strength, or the heart, to question Jacques further, besides which, she trusted both his and Gianni's judgement absolutely. They worried both for and about her and would tell her all that she needed to know. She was deeply grateful for all the trouble they took, realizing that she must have created much extra work for a lot of people. However, she would soon be off their hands.

Only two short months ago Alicia simply could not have envisaged the misery ahead, Guy's extraordinary disappearance, the likelihood of his dearest friend being pronounced dead, or the precarious and possibly life-threatening situation in which she now found herself.

There was nothing to be done for the moment though, except to get through the next few days, with the ghastly funeral looming up. What an ordeal, Alicia thought. But more than anything she dreaded it for poor Adriana. She had received two text messages from her, the last just to say, 'nothing to be done, longing to see you and with love and thanks.'

Her mother was another matter. Alicia couldn't decide whether or not to telephone her. She would be so horrified for her daughter to have to deal with yet another devastating blow. Diana would be expecting her to fly back for the funeral. If she didn't tell her she was coming there was bound to be somebody who would report that they had seen her. Diana would know that she would want to be there, for Adriana, never mind her own problems, which were so small in comparison. She knew that if she talked to her mother she would break down, which would only make everything worse and then she would want to come rushing up to Scotland to be with her daughter. 'What should I do for the best?' she wondered. 'I know', she concluded to herself, 'I'll ask Nick to call her, to tell her I'm O.K, that he's going to be there with me, that I'm flying straight out again and that I'll call her from Scotland.' Nick agreed wholeheartedly to put Alicia's mother's mind at rest, thankful to be of some use after the previous, grizzly, task he'd been given.

The next morning, after yet more farewells, they seemed so frequent these days and promising to return soon, Alicia drove to the airport with Jean-P, who must have been asked not to terrify the life out of her on the way. He drove so slowly that she actually suggested that he went a bit faster to take her mind off things, at which his face lit up and he immediately put his foot down on the accelerator and roared off. Alicia laughed, thinking that this small amusement would most likely have to last her for a while.

She said goodbye to J.P. at the terminal building. She liked him a lot. He had given her so much light relief. She wanted to give him a decent present to thank him for looking after her so well, but he didn't want to take the euros in the envelope she held out to him and was obviously embarrassed. Alicia insisted that he must have used a lot of fuel on her behalf and besides, he must need something new for his bike. Then he grinned from ear to ear and pocketed the envelope, thanking her profusely.

At the airport, Alicia posted a letter to Gianni telling him that she had found out where the flowers had come from. She didn't mention that she was flying to Scotland, or the reason behind it, not wishing to worry him more, but indicated a move shortly to Venice. She was unaware, however, that he was already in the picture after speaking to Jacques D'Aubert that very morning.

Finally, Alicia called Aunt Caro and asked if she could come to visit. The Contessa was delighted and told her to arrive whenever she liked and to stay for as long as she wished, that she only needed a little notice to be ready for her and in which to plan some wonderful 'entertainment'. Alicia laughed as she finished the call, knowing exactly what this would mean: the Contessa's social life was a whirl. She knew too that Caro would contact her mother as soon as she put the telephone down and Diana would be pleased to think that Alicia would be with her sister in Italy before long.

She felt she must also let Gianni know of her plans, suspecting that, by then, whatever had been taking place in Verona would be well and truly concluded. She would have travelled in and out of two other countries before re-entering Italy, but she still wasn't sure about revisiting Delfino quite so soon, much as she would love to see them all again. The village of Erizzo on the mainland, where Marcello was based, was just not quite far enough away. Alicia still felt so very vulnerable and in the back of her mind she knew that Marcello's magnetism would be just too strong to resist, if the opportunity arose again.

So, with a heavy heart, Alicia flew from Nice, via Paris, to Glasgow. The journey was uneventful and dull. There turned out to be plenty of time in between planes at Charles de Gaulle, with only a short delay, so she had a last decent cup of French coffee and something sweet and comforting from the *patisserie* to boost her low morale and to help prepare her for the miserable ordeal ahead.

★★★

CHAPTER 22

In **Scotland** Alicia was greeted by Nick Hargreaves with a hire car. She found him, without any difficulty, as they'd met at various family parties in London and so they were able to recognize each other. He looked apprehensive and very young, with his curly red hair and pink cheeks: a very English complexion and colouring. Guy always said that Nick was the rising star in his department in the Foreign Office, so he must be very capable. But he's worried now about how I shall cope with all this on top of the rest, she thought.

"It's alright Nick," Alicia said patting his knee as they left the car park, "I'm O.K. Really. You don't have to worry. We'll talk about everything tomorrow and it's sweet of you to come. I do appreciate it." He looked relieved and started to chatter away about other things as he drove carefully out of the airport then turned south-east and headed for Berwick-Upon-Tweed. He told her that he'd booked her in at The Fisherman's Inn and hoped that would be all right, as there didn't seem much choice. He was staying with an old girlfriend nearby. Alicia turned down his invitation for dinner, saying that she was too tired and thought she'd have an early night, if he didn't mind. She secretly thought that dinner might have been rather an effort and also had the feeling that the girlfriend might not have been an 'ex' at all. As they said goodbye, Nick certainly didn't look too unhappy. He arranged to pick her up the next morning, if she didn't need the car that evening. Alicia was going nowhere, but wondered who was going to pay the car hire bill!

Berwick was both on the river Tweed and by the sea; it would be pretty if the sun was out and her mood different. Alicia went for a walk before it got dark then had a lonely dinner in the hotel's little restaurant, which seemed as cold and damp as it was outside. If she had kept the car she might have tried to find somewhere else; it was a depressing place. 'If I ran this hotel', she muttered, 'I would certainly have lit the fire'. It might have cheered up the other few rather solemn looking diners. One couple didn't seem to speak throughout the entire meal and both this and perhaps the sudden cooler and unattractive climate seemed to reflect the sad purpose behind her visit. Maybe they were there for the same reason as she was, but then, after sur-reptitiously studying them further, believed that wasn't the case at all. They were merely just fed up to the teeth with each other! God, how dismal and why didn't the awful, sour woman with the wart stop sniffing all the time. Alicia felt like handing her a handkerchief and telling her to go out and blow her nose.

After a lukewarm, boring meal Alicia decided that she really couldn't bear looking at all the miserable faces any longer and standing up quickly, tak-ing her very English coffee with her, she went upstairs, sat on her bed and promptly burst into tears! It was the first time she'd cried since she'd heard the news about Julian. The protective numbness must have begun to wear off a little, now that she had accepted the cold, hard, reality of his death. After ten minutes of uncontrolled sobs she felt better. She thought that she would like to ring Adriana to try to give her a little support for the next day but, on second thoughts, she didn't feel she should disturb the family at this particu-lar time. Anyhow, she was in such a horrible mood herself it might be best to send another text message. Then she would just go to bed and have an early night, as she'd told Nick she would do.

The room felt fusty and it smelt. The blankets were none too clean and Alicia wished she had her own pillows instead of the hard and lumpy hotel offering. She would rather not think about the number of heads that had lain on them. She decided to fling open the window while she prepared for bed, but it was too cold while she was getting undressed. She turned on the antiquated television to watch the news, which was a mistake. It couldn't have been more disheartening. Terrorists blowing up teenagers from many countries in a nightclub in the Far East: it might easily include someone's child she knew. What a pointless, cruel tragedy and what a sick, sick world we all live in she thought sadly, turning it off before getting into her cold, damp bed. Alicia decided that she'd never felt quite so depressed in her entire life.

~

The next morning was dark and drizzling, with a typical fine Scottish mist; almost to be expected given the purpose of the day ahead. After a surprisingly good breakfast and glad to be on the move again, somehow waiting for the awful things in life seemed worse than the doing, Alicia left with Nick, allowing plenty of time to buy a warm sweater and large scarf from the tweed mill in the High Street. She still felt cold and stiff after such a gloomy night. Nick waited outside in the car and read the paper but was rewarded for his patience. Alicia had bought him a dark blue, pure cashmere, scarf and a bottle of malt whisky from the gifts department next door.

"A small thank you," she said giving it to him with a kiss on the cheek, as she got in. He went pinker than ever, but was obviously delighted.

"And this we'll put over here," he said, taking the bottle and stowing it in the back. "We might well need a swig, after it's all over."

"Definitely," agreed Alicia, "possibly even before, the way I feel this morning. Now I need to find the flower shop. There's one half a mile down the road, apparently, on the left and around the next corner."

She chose a huge bunch of mixed tulips and daffodils and wrote a card saying: 'In sad disbelief and love always Alicia'. What else can I say? she thought. I can't even add Guy's name because I just don't know what's happening. Quite simply, I don't know anything at all for sure.

Alicia had put on her new sweater underneath her long suede coat, so at least she felt snug. They drove westward towards the village where the funeral was to be held and stopped at a pub on the way for a sandwich and a much needed, large, glass of red wine.

"Dutch courage," said Nick raising his glass to Alicia and downing it almost in one as they talked about things other than the funeral and her own predicament. Alicia found Nick to be interesting and much more mature than he looked and she began to understand why Guy thought such a lot of him. He told her that when they had finished what they had come here to do, he wanted to have a serious discussion with regard to her future plans. He had some ideas, so perhaps they could go to a hotel he knew for a drink after the service, before he flew south again. The hotel, near to where the funeral was to be held, was an extremely smart 'Country House Hotel', well described in all the guide books. In view of the night Alicia had just spent in Berwick, he rather thought he should have booked her in there instead, but he remembered that it was very expensive. Alicia also wished he had, she wouldn't have minded the extra expense on this occasion, but readily agreed to the plan. She had plenty of questions to ask him.

They continued on their way and, although early for the service, found Julian's home village full to overflowing with cars left in every conceivable space. They parked in a farm gateway just outside the village. They both wanted a little exercise and Nick couldn't take the added hassle of trying to find a place any nearer, or blocking somebody's driveway. They walked up and into the churchyard and along the path, which was lined on either side by bunch upon bunch of flowers of all sizes and description. Julian must have been very much liked and loved, thought Alicia sadly. She put her own offering under a tree set back a little from the rest then, taking Nick's arm firmly, they went in together.

There were people from far and wide. A couple, two rows in front looked vaguely familiar. Maybe she'd met them with her mother, Alicia thought. I must remember to ring her. When the service started there was standing room only in the church. It looked as if the whole village had turned out. It was a beautiful and moving service and many tears were shed, some discreetly and some not so privately.

Julian's parents, whom Alicia had only met once before, were quietly courageous. His attractive Swedish mother was, quite simply, amazing. Surrounded by the rest of their large family she remained dignified to the end. Alicia could see that much trouble was taken to keep Adriana close beside them. It was obvious that they were all very fond of her and she noticed Julian's mother's arm go around her, at one point, as his father handed over a handkerchief. The address was given by an uncle, who must have known Julian very well and who looked much like his father. He even managed to bring in a little humour as he told a couple of childhood stories. At the end he included Adriana and all the family as he voiced everyone's heartfelt sympathy towards them at this appallingly difficult time.

Where on earth was Guy and why wasn't he beside her? He should have been here, Alicia thought, annoyed and even more upset to be doing this without him.

As the congregation filed out of the church Adriana came straight over to Alicia's side. She was so pleased to see her and insisted on both Alicia and Nick coming back to the house for tea.

Both were glad, again, of a short walk to Julian's family home. It gave Alicia a little time to compose herself and think about what on earth she could say to them all that might be of some small comfort.

As they turned into the drive, she saw a most lovely garden carpeted with spring flowers, raising their bright heads bravely in the chill breeze, almost as if defying the reason for all the people being there. The house too was spilling over with daffodils so that, although the day was so grey outside, inside it felt surprisingly cheerful and warm. Fires were burning in the hall and the two main rooms and the old furniture sparkled with years of polish. Alicia noticed the family photographs, including a recent one with Adriana and all with Julian beaming out towards the camera. His joy in living shone from his eyes and Alicia's heart contracted with grief.

She managed to convey her sympathy to Julian's parents, without making a fool of herself and with Nick standing staunchly behind. Then, thinking it unnecessary to foist herself on Julian's brothers, whom she'd never met, she went in search of Adriana who took Alicia to one side and told her how very glad she was to have her there. There were so many people but so few that she knew and the whole thing was just so unbelievably ghastly. Her long fair hair framed her pale, white face, making the freckles stand out in stark detail, with the dark smudges beneath her huge hazel eyes telling of too little sleep and of so many spent tears. Alicia's sympathy reached out to her friend. It was hard to know what to say to her, so she told her all about the island. Suddenly, Adriana, unable to contain herself any longer blurted out.

"Oh! Ally! None of us can even begin to understand how this terrible accident came about. Julian was brought up by the sea and he would never, ever, have been so stupid as to dive off a boat without steps. Besides it's much too cold to go swimming in the Med at this time of year and you know how pathetic he was about getting into cold water," she paused: "I wonder what really happened?"

"What on earth do you mean?" asked Alicia, taken aback and following her into another room, away from all the people.

"Well, something was definitely going on before all this," answered Adriana. "I nearly called you, but I just didn't want to add to your worries, as I had nothing concrete to go on. Julian was very uneasy and constantly in touch with Guy and now he's disappeared as well. I just find the whole thing impossible to accept. And you Ally, have you really heard nothing yet yourself?"

"Nothing for certain, but it's all very strange … very strange indeed, I do agree." Alicia looked at her friend's distraught, sad, face and voiced the idea that had been formulating in her head for the last few days.

"Adriana come with me, tomorrow, back to the South of France and maybe the two of us can make some sense out of all this." Adriana's face came alive for a moment as she thought about the idea.

"I'd really love to come with you, but I'm not sure if I can leave the family here quite so soon. You see I was the last one to see Julian and ..." she hesitated a moment, then continued, "he never even said he was going to the South of France, you know. It really is very mystifying and we were so happy together. We had planned to take a holiday and I thought then, that maybe ..." she stopped her face red. "S ... sorry," she stammered looking embarrassed. "I just, I just can't believe that I'll never see him again." The tears coursed slowly down her cheeks. Alicia pulled her friend into her arms.

"I know, Adriana. Believe you me, I understand how you feel, I really do. Look," Alicia said holding her shoulders firmly and smiling, "see what you can do. I'd love the company and I think it would do you good to get away. We'll do whatever you want and you can have a good rest at the same time. You need it." Then she added with meaning, "but don't say anything to Julian's parents though, other than that I'd like to take you away for a few days. I shouldn't even mention we're going to France. I'll check the airline for tickets. I'm sure it won't be a problem at this time of the year because it's early and there's no festival on at the moment, as far as I know. I'll be at the Fisherman's Inn, Berwick and wait to hear from you there and I'll have my fingers crossed!" With that she gave Adriana another hug, said her polite goodbyes to Julian's parents, as did Nick and then they left.

As they walked back to the car, Alicia blew her nose with a shaking hand, then turned to Nick and said,

"I don't know if you heard any of the conversation that I just had with Adriana, but it was certainly curious."

"Only the beginning," he answered, "before you went into the next door room. I didn't really mean to eaves-drop either, but I heard enough and you're right. I think it's more than strange, it's bizarre. Let's go to the hotel now, it's not far."

Melrose Hall was a lovely place, surrounded by a large park filled with magnificent, old, beech trees. The man at the smart reception remembered

Nick, and Alicia had to stifle a giggle when he asked after Nick's wife!

"Now I know what you get up to when you're away from home, wife my foot. Maybe they think I'm your mistress!" Alicia laughed as they went and sat in the cosy bar by the fire and waited for their drinks. "You should have seen your face," she continued with mirth, "it was so funny. Don't worry, Nick," she pushed his shoulder playfully, noticing his discomfort, "we need something to cheer us up, don't you think?" Then he laughed too, looking slightly shamefaced.

"O.K, O.K, point taken Alicia, but don't say anything to Jenny or I won't have a girlfriend either." Their drinks arrived. Nick took a large swallow of his and began. "Now, I think that there's probably quite a lot that you have to tell me, but first what I have to say is this ..." Nick had done his home-work in London. He went back over the facts of Guy's disappearance to date, then went on to tell her that he had discovered a new source of infor-mation through the Foreign Office, which had just come up with some very interesting results. The two most important things were that not only did the British Intelligence service know about the incident in Verona, but they also knew about her attack on the train, which meant that they were keeping tabs on Alicia's movements all the time and were most likely in cahoots with their Italian counterparts. 'Oh God', thought Alicia, 'do these people know everything?' Nick took another mouthful of whisky.

"But," he continued, pausing to make sure of her full attention, "I think that both Guy and Julian are agents for M.I.6." He stopped a moment for this information to sink in. Alicia was stunned as he had expected she would be. She was silent for a moment staring at him, her mouth slightly open. Then she looked down at the table and picked up her drink.

"That can't be true. They couldn't be Nick," replied Alicia, taking a reviv-ing swallow. Her heart was pounding with excitement. "I would have had some tiny little suspicion, surely? I'm not stupid, or naïve and we've been together for ages. Are you serious? Do you really think so and if so why?"

"You don't understand," said Nick, "if what I think is true then they are both professionals, through and through. Their normal jobs and life are a perfect cover. You would never have known, nor would I: if we did, then they wouldn't be any good at their work, would they?"

"God!" exclaimed Alicia, "maybe you are right. I had always assumed they were part of some crack military unit some years ago, but never for a minute more than that, or that they were still at it. No wonder nobody will tell you anything!"

"Anyway!" Nick continued, "the key piece of news is that Guy and Julian were certainly up to something together and highly secretive too. My boss gave me a couple of names in M.I.6 and permission to try to get them to see me. It took me some time to set up a meeting, the service doesn't encourage relations with 'outsiders' unless at their own instigation. I encountered extreme reluctance. When I finally met with them, both men were unhelpful, off putting and in a hurry to get rid of me. But I only had to drop a name or two and there was an immediate reaction. I had their full attention. They believed that I really was on to something. These people are usually dead cool, but I had them rattled. Their behaviour alone just about told me that we are on the right route." Alicia took a sharp intake of breath.

"So Adriana was right, but we still don't have a clue what it was all about and where I fit in." Nick shook his head.

"No, sorry, but we don't. My M.I.6 contacts clammed up altogether and because of the obvious sensitivity of the situation, they sidetracked all my questions and wouldn't tell me a thing. I reckon they'd been blasted by their superiors for having seen me at all. Then I got well and truly kicked out and told not to come back again. Charming lot they were, I can tell you!"

Nick looked as if he'd been thoroughly enjoying the intrigue, thought Alicia, as she sat silent considering what he'd just said. He must have given up hours of his time trying to help her. At least she felt they were getting somewhere at last. Nick, flushed in the face with excitement, went on.

"There's no question in my mind that Guy is alive and kicking, otherwise these dark suited people, whoever they are, wouldn't be after you. Whatever they want him for, he must have or know something extremely important to them and they think that you might know where he is. As far as Julian's death is concerned, I'm afraid I'm beginning to think it wasn't an accident at all. I think he was murdered. I'm sure that his death is in some way tied up in all this." And then he added with complete conviction, "there was no choice Alicia. Guy had to disappear and for your sake above all else." She nodded, thinking hard,

"God, Nick, I hope your not going to get into trouble over all this."

"No, don't worry; I've got plenty up my sleeve. What I want to know is what are you going to do now? I somehow can't see you sitting still, but you are going to have to be careful, very careful and sensible about where you go and …" seeing the expression on her face, "… I really do mean that Alicia. Now, tell me please what are you planning to do next?"

"Well, said Alicia I have this idea formulating in my head." Oh no! thought Nick. Here we go again.

~

Alicia woke next morning to the ringing of the telephone. The intrusive noise, somehow suggested there was life outside her dismal room.

"I can come!" Adriana said breathlessly. "It's alright, they are all so kind up here and think that it's a very good thing for me to go away with you and I really want to go to the South of France too. I want to see where it happened. I shan't settle until I do."

"Are you sure?" asked Alicia. "I don't want you to be even more upset."

"I won't be, honestly," replied Adriana. "You see, I need to know for my own peace of mind."

"Alright then," answered Alicia, "I'll make the arrangements and wait for you here. There's plenty of room on the flight this afternoon and we don't have to leave until two. Nick stayed another night and says he'll take us to the airport. If you could get here about eleven we could all have lunch together at the hotel where we had dinner last night, as it's almost on the way. This place is awful. I can't wait to leave."

"I can't wait either. One of Julian's brothers will drop me off, so I'll be there before you know it." With that the telephone was almost slammed down. She was gone in her hurry, but had a definite lift in her voice.

Alicia smiled to herself. She felt glad to know that she'd have somebody with her to whom she could talk but, she also thought that the plan would be good for Adriana. Otherwise, she would only sit up there in Scotland feeling utterly bereft and miserable. After Julian's two brother's went South to return to work, there would be no one of her own age around, but his two poor grieving parents, who might prefer to be on their own for a bit.

Nick had been brilliant the night before, his shyness disappearing as he had warmed to the subject. He'd been both encouraging and reassuring, and although five years her junior amazingly adult in his thinking, which belied his youthful appearance. They had sat so long discussing the whole situation that they had stayed there for dinner, which had been excellent. They'd both had so much to talk about that he'd missed the last flight south, so he had booked a room there for himself and rather guiltily sent Alicia back alone in a cab to the grim Fisherman's Arms. She'd had such a surprisingly good evening and so much to drink that she didn't even notice the uncomfortable bed! Besides which, Nick had got through so much wine he really wasn't in a fit state to travel any further that night.

Nick, for his part, had been riveted by Alicia's adventures in Italy and the South of France and loved hearing about the island of Delfino and about Gianni and all his family. She had to improvise a little over the parts involving Marcello and was thrown slightly off balance when Nick suddenly said early in the evening.

"Alicia, I can't understand it! You seem almost to have enjoyed all these frightening incidents. You seem to positively thrive on adventure, and you look absolutely marvelous." He was getting thoroughly carried away and much more daring, as his cheeks became pinker by the minute.

"No, no, it was all really frightening," she answered, "but I was safe with so many people looking after me and anyway I was just over the moon to have some action and no more time to just sit and think. The inactivity was driving me crazy."

Nick wasn't entirely happy about her imminent return to France with Adriana, particularly as they were intending to be independent now that there were two of them. But they were both intelligent and streetwise and Alicia promised that if there was any hint of trouble she would immediately get in touch with Jacques d'Aubert.

"I'm sure Guy would have a fit if he knew that I was letting you do this." Nick said rather worriedly.

"Well, it's not your responsibility," retorted Alicia. "I'm my own person, and God alone knows what he's doing or where he is and however you look at it he left me one hundred per cent in the lurch. I'm determined to find out what the hell has been going on. Adriana, I know, is of the same mind and she'll never rest until she knows the real circumstances of Julian's death. So we'll do it together."

"Alright, alright!" replied Nick holding up his hand "I'm not trying to stop you, just as long as you stay in close touch and promise me ..."

"Yes, yes, I promise you all those things ... Daddy!" Nick's face flamed!

~

Alicia and Adriana took off for Nice on the afternoon plane. The girls' mood lightened as they left yesterday's harrowing events behind them, in the depressing Scottish mist. The two women were glad to be doing something positive and to be together. Alicia had decided not to tell Adriana everything that had happened to her, for the moment, as she saw no point in unsettling her further and realized that Adriana must be utterly exhausted. However, they did discuss the, seemingly strange, atmosphere surrounding Julian before the accident.

"He was so distracted and ill at ease. Ever since Christmas really," said Adriana. "In fact, he was in a very weird mood each time he called me during that trip to Florida. I even wondered if it was something to do with me and yet in a funny way we were even closer; but I'm certain that he was terribly worried about something and I just can't understand all this happening in the South of France. He kept saying that he thought he'd be heading towards Central or South America. Never even a mention of France."

By the time they landed at Nice they had come to the conclusion that it was simply no good continuing to speculate for what hideous reason Guy had found it necessary to literally drop off the face of the earth. It was a mystery. As for Julian's 'accident', neither could say 'death', that was another inexplicable and horrendous event. But both young women were determined to get to the bottom of it all, for their own peace of mind if nothing else.

★★★

CHAPTER 23

They stayed at a hotel near Fayence, very small and quiet, except at weekends, when it was full to bursting because of its renowned restaurant, which was how Guy and Alicia had originally come across it. When the two girls drove up in their little hired Renault, 'le patron' and his wife, Monsieur and Madame Pinard, welcomed them warmly, remembering Alicia. They were given the two best rooms and told that the chef was already at work preparing their dinner! Before settling in for the evening they walked down the little road as far as the nearest farm, which Alicia could not have forgotten!

'Guy had run over a chicken', she told Adriana 'and he'd been made to pay for it, much to his disgust. He'd taken the dead chicken back to the hotel and insisted that Madame Pinard cook him coq au vin for dinner, which she had been delighted to do. Monsieur Pinard was furious with his neighbour and had set out, purposefully, to tell off the farmer for being so unfriendly towards their hotel guests! According to Monsieur, the farmer should have handed over two chickens and wished them *bon appetit*, instead of making unnecessary bother! For what's one chicken in the run of things? Pierre Pinard had finished with a very French grunt of disapproval'.

'No doubt', said Alicia, 'the whole incident had been the main talking point in the area for the next six months! Hardly surprising that she had been instantly recognized when they bowled up earlier!

The country was emerald green, with wild flowers prolific in the hedgerows, the trees far more advanced than in Scotland and it was warm in comparison too. Adriana was quiet. Alicia turned to this woman who, through tragic circumstances, had so quickly become an even closer friend joined, as it were, by their mutual agony.

"What were you thinking?" she asked. Adriana looked at Alicia and smiled.

"I was thinking how lovely it is here after those last, ghastly, days in Scotland and the funeral. It all seems another world away somehow, though I still can't believe," she hesitated, "that he's really gone, you know, dead and buried and all that. It's all happened so fast, but I'm so glad I've come here with you as there is nobody else I can talk to, who understands."

"I feel absolutely the same," answered Alicia. "You need time to come to terms with everything; so much has happened. I agree, there's nothing worse than not knowing what really took place, so I promise you that, when you are ready, we'll go to the *Iles de Lérins* together and find out for ourselves." They linked arms and in silence turned back towards the hotel, feeling a genuine warmth and reassurance in each other's company.

The next day was the First of May: a holiday in France. After a good night's sleep, the two decided to ask Madame if she would pack them a picnic so that they could go up into the hills to explore. Madame Pinard suggested a visit to the old walled city of Trigance for the May-Day celebrations, which seemed an excellent idea to both Alicia and Adriana. It was a lovely morning and, armed with their lunch and the bottle of wine which Monsieur had insisted on adding, they set off, determined to enjoy their time together and to try to leave all the sadness and worries behind them, at least for a few hours.

They drove slowly, each admiring the scenery, particularly beautiful at this time of the year. The hills were alight with so many different colours, the grass and trees everywhere as bright as they can ever be and so unspoilt in their freshness. As they approached Trigance, they could hear that the May-Day parades were already well under way. A band was playing in the distance and there were many cars and bikes already parked outside the walls. Alicia watched a young man arrive in style on a very fast looking motor-bike. She couldn't see his face; it was too far away, but he reminded her of Jean-P and she smiled to herself.

"What? What's amusing you?" asked Adriana.

"Oh! Nothing, really," Alicia answered, "just that man there," she said pointing. "He just reminded me of someone; someone who has helped me a lot and who you shall meet one day too, when our life is more normal again!"

"Not someone who …"

"Oh no!" Alicia laughed, "it wasn't like that, not like that at all!" And she drove on to find somewhere to park. They left their car amongst the rest and walked up through the archway into the old part of the city. All the shops were open and selling their wares, both inside and on the street. The children were all dressed up; some had their faces painted and were in fancy dress; some were selling little bunches of lillies of the valley, *muguets de bois,* their distinctive scent lingering in the air. There were tables of mouth-watering sweetmeats, pastries and chocolates. The local vineyards were well represented and free glasses of wine were being offered to entice prospective buyers. Several of the sellers already appeared well away! Everybody seemed to be having a good time, children and dogs included.

Alicia and Adriana wandered around enjoying the lively atmosphere. They laughed as they watched a large mongrel cock its leg on a huge bag of potatoes. Then a couple of minutes later a large, bossy, lady demanded to be served two kilos from the same bag. The cheerful looking man in charge gave the girls a conspiratorial wink as he suggested that the lady might wish to serve herself, as was the usual custom. They walked on, greatly amused. Alicia bought a little carved box, with a mirror in the lid, which she intended to keep safe until such time as she could give it to Giuseppina. Adriana bought a hand-painted scarf and some small sacks of Herbes de

Provence for Julian's mother.

"Don't worry, I needn't say I've been here. Could have bought them any-where," she added sensibly. They wandered until they became tired of the noise and bustle and then wound their way slowly back through the narrow streets to the car. They drove further up into the hills, where they found a quiet spot to spread the rug Madame had given them for their picnic. The two women chatted easily about everything they could think of, except the subject uppermost in both of their minds, which they left well alone. Eventually, probably because of the wine, both felt sleepy and dozed off.

Alicia awoke first, feeling cold. It was getting late and the sun was low in the sky. She looked across at Adriana, who, even asleep, looked strained and pale and Alicia couldn't but wonder how she would be feeling if she were in her place. How she wished things could be different. She gently woke her friend, then they packed up their things and set off, in the twilight, back to the hotel. Agreeing to meet again in a couple of hour's time for dinner, they each went to their own rooms.

Alicia opened her door and stopped dead in her tracks for there, on her pillow, was a bunch of muguets, tied with a ribbon. She heard a voice behind her. It was Adriana coming back along the passage from her room.

"Look what Madame has put on my bed," holding the same flowers up in her hand for Alicia to see. "Have you got some too? Good Heavens, what-ever is the matter? You look positively ashen!"

"Oh! It's nothing really, I just thought for a minute that maybe …" she hesitated, feeling wobbly and looked at her friend, her eyes full …".

" … That these might have been from Guy." finished Adriana for her. "He always used to manage to send you flowers from everywhere, didn't he?" Alicia nodded.

"Oh dear Ally, I'm so sorry! … and now I've burst the bubble, haven't I?"

"Never mind, it's not your fault", whispered Alicia, "only wishful thinking on my part and really stupid of me."

"Right!" said Adriana taking charge. "I vote a long shower, feet up for a bit then a good strong drink followed by an excellent dinner. How about that for a good idea?"

"Brilliant!" agreed Alicia and gave her a hug, cheering up immediately.

~

Alicia sat on her bed and smelt the flowers. It was just the sort of thing Guy would have done to surprise her. It was here, two years before to the day, that he'd given them to her, thankfully not in the same room, for that she couldn't have born. Then he'd explained to her the delightful French custom of presenting *muguets de bois* to a loved one. Given the present circumstances it was so unlikely to have been him and therefore so silly to be so disappointed.

How strong Adriana is, thought Alicia, in spite of everything that had happened to her. Her situation is so much worse, so final and yet here she is, cheering me up. What do I really feel after all this time of not knowing? Just so much has happened, but one thing is for sure: I miss Marcello more than I care to admit. I miss his company, his funny accent and sense of humour, but, if I'm honest; I miss an awful lot more besides. With these, pleasantly disturbing, thoughts she went to run a bath.

They sat for a long time over dinner, discussing and deciding their next plan. Alicia thought that Adriana was probably well able to cope with the truth of her own adventures, but she didn't want to overburden her grieving, friend too quickly and equally didn't want to push for a plan to visit the islands until Adriana suggested it herself. Nevertheless, by the end of dinner her staunch companion had done so and they got up from the table agreeing on a leisurely start for Cannes the next morning, with breakfast at nine.

As they passed the reception Madame Pinard was waiting to wish them goodnight. They thanked her for their excellent dinner and also for the beautiful flowers in their rooms.

"Mais non, Mademoiselles, les fleurs ne venaient pas de moi. They were delivered this morning after you left." The two girls both gaped at her.

"But who brought them?" asked Alicia when she found her voice."

"A stranger, on a motorbike, stopped the old man who brings the bread and asked him to bring them here to you. I kept them in water until I thought you would be soon returning. You obviously both have French admirers," she added proudly. Madame was positively glowing, sensing the intrigue.

"I think that perhaps we have," said Alicia, laughing as she looked at Adriana's astonished, face. They thanked Madame profusely, ordered their breakfast and went upstairs as fast as they were politely able.

"Well, what do you make of that?" asked Adriana after shutting the door to the room. "Do you think that Guy could possibly have … been here, or how could he know …?" Adriana hesitated, uncertain whether or not to finish.

"No, I don't believe we should think too much into it, however mysterious," said Alicia, "or we'll get ourselves tied in knots. But it's definitely time for more research and there's a bit more that I think I should tell you about too …" They curled up together on Alicia's bed and once again Alicia told her story, leaving out only Marcello. Adriana sat quietly listening. Then, later, she looked at her friend and said.

"The whole thing is like a movie: the odd links, unusual coincidences, the horrific accident; the frightening incidents. The only thing needed, is some good old-fashioned romance; a love affair, or have I missed something? You do look remarkably well considering all the ghastly circumstances …" Adriana stopped and was staring intently at the rising blush on Alicia's face.

"Sorry, Ally, oh dear I'm so sorry, I shouldn't have said that, should I?"

"No, no it's O.K, but I think, perhaps, you shouldn't." Alicia got up and gave her a hug, to cover her embarrassment, then went to put the lilies in water. The next morning, Adriana looked much better and Alicia knew that it was because she had enlightened her the night before. Adriana, too, now sensed intrigue. It gave her purpose and something to focus on. They drove to Cannes, which took longer than they expected. Alicia tried to remember the shortcut that Jean-P had taken down the hill, but they got lost and then muddled up in the street market. The road was closed and was supposed to be for pedestrians only that morning. They were told off; Alicia could have sworn that it was the same man that Jean-P had nearly run over

After going round and round in circles, they finally managed to extract themselves with everybody 'helping', including the police, children clapping and dogs barking and then left the market place which was, by now, in an uproar! By the time they had eventually found somewhere to park the car in a back street, they realized that they had both been drying their eyes, but this time it had been from mirth and not misery!

"How I wish Jean-P could have seen us," said Alicia getting out of the car.

As if by magic J.P. appeared, parking his bike a little way in front of them. Strangely enough, he didn't look surprised to see them.

"What were you doing, Mademoiselle?" he asked hardly able to speak, he was laughing so much. "I was a few cars behind and saw you take the wrong turn. You had so many helping already, I didn't come into the Square, and also I didn't wish to meet that 'orrible' store-keeper again. Two days ago he threatened to report me."

"Oh! Jean-P, I'm so pleased to see you, let me introduce you to my friend, Adriana. She's had such an 'orrible' time too. I just love the way you say that". Noticing the bemused expression on his face, as he shook hands, she quickly added. "Don't worry J.P. I'm only teasing. Heavens, it's just so good to laugh!"

Jean Pierre, delighted to see their cheerfulness, suggested a cup of coffee down in the old port, where they could tell him what they were doing. In the café, once they had recovered and caught up with the Chateau d'Aubert news, Alicia told J.P of their plans. He said he'd show them where they could enquire about boats to take them out to the island. He asked where they were staying as he was certain that the d'Aubert's, once they knew that Alicia had returned with a friend, would insist that they visit. Later, they said goodbye in the old port and Jean-.P went off to get the d'Auberts' shopping, adding that he was sure that he would see them both soon. Adriana was looking perplexed.

"What's the matter?" asked Alicia.

"Nothing really, I suppose," she replied. "It's just that, did you notice in the café when Jean-P asked us at which hotel we were staying that, he had already started writing it down before you told him: almost as if he already knew!"

"Yes I did," Alicia answered "and I think that the d'Aubert's know exactly where we are all the time. Don't worry," she continued seeing Adriana's still puzzled face, "we're being looked after, that's all. Come on, I'll explain later."

There were various fishing smacks moored against the harbour wall: the men were busy on their boats, talking or mending their nets. Alicia enquired if anybody knew about the accident a fortnight earlier, when two young Englishmen had drowned between the islands after renting a vessel. They all seemed to have heard about the deaths but didn't appear to remember the two Englishmen. It was really too early for tourists wanting boats, they said and the men who died weren't on a rented sailing craft from a flotilla but on a stolen yacht.

The two women exchanged looks. Odd, they thought, that the story here, as told by the fishermen, didn't tie up with the newspapers. After some time, they managed to persuade an elderly fisherman to take them out to the islands. He agreed gladly to Jean Pierre's suggested price, but first he had to sort out his boat, which was full of fish!'

The man tried hard to clean it out for them while they waited. He was at pains to explain that he had to use it for fishing in the winter months because he was unable to survive on his fares from the summer tourists alone. He arranged clean sacks for them to sit on, helped them in and they chugged slowly out of the old port. It was still cool on the water at this time of year but the sea was calm and breathtakingly blue. The sun was becoming warmer by the minute. They were lucky. The old man told them that, the month before, the South of France had been dogged by violent thunderstorms and most of the fishermen with smaller boats hadn't been able to venture out at all, so there had been a shortage of local fish.

When they rounded the first island, Cannes disappeared from view and the two girls were lost in their own thoughts as they pondered what had actually happened out here, on this particular stretch of water, a couple of weeks earlier. It was extraordinary that, between the two islands, at this time of year, the scenery was still remarkably unspoilt and quite remote, considering that the fleshpots of Cannes were such a short distance away, hidden behind them.

They moored on a little pontoon specially built to service the two restaurants: one of them famous and much visited by the rich and rare during the film and music festivals. The boatman said he'd meet them back there in one hour. They asked him how to find the local bar. He pointed along a path, and they set off towards it, in the opposite direction to the restaurants.

The bar was small and intimate and not much frequented by anybody other than the local people in the winter, judging by the silence and stares from the counter as they stepped inside the room. A girl came across to the

219

table where they had settled themselves and took their order. She was young and shy but tried, enthusiastically, to make up for the rudeness of the men at the bar who by now had resumed their noisy conversation. The girl came back with their drinks and half a *baguette* salami sandwich each and asked if there was anything else they required.

"Not for the moment, thank you.", replied Alicia. "We are here for a very sad reason. I'm afraid, you see, that it was the fiancé of my friend here who died in the drowning accident off the islands two weeks ago." The girl looked totally horrified, mumbled her sympathy and fled back to the safety of the bar.

"Oh dear!" said Adriana. "That didn't go down too well, did it?"

"No", said Alicia "but it's given the old men something to talk about. Just look at them!" The conversation at the bar was by now alight and the poor girl, who'd obviously been grilled, was looking both ill at ease and annoyed with the Frenchmen. After a while Alicia said,

"Let's call her back and see if we can find out what's going on". The girl duly arrived back at their table, red in the face and awkward.

"Please don't be embarrassed on our account", said Alicia slowly, in French. "I expect your customers are just curious about us being here, but would you mind very much telling us what they are saying? It's really rather important to us, I do assure you". The poor girl hopped from one foot to the other, debating what she was going to say. Then, looking down at the floor, she said very quietly,

"They are saying, Mademoiselle," then she hesitated and glanced at Adriana, "that your friend is much too young and pretty to have been going to marry... such a disreputable old man from foreign parts," she finished quickly. Alicia heard Adriana's gasp and quickly kicked her under the table, not daring to catch her friend's eye. Alicia calmly replied,

"I see. *Est-ce que vous pouvez m'aider?* Would you be so kind as to try and persuade one of them to come over here and talk to us. It really is terribly important ... and I'll buy him a drink," added Alicia as an afterthought.

"I'll try," answered the girl and returned once again to the bar.

"Try and remain calm for a little longer; I know how difficult it must be.", whispered Alicia looking worriedly at Adriana, by now almost green in the face. They sipped their wine, hardly able to contain themselves and pretending not to notice the gesticulation and argument at the bar. At last the eldest of the men got up and slowly shuffled over to their table. Alicia pulled out a chair for him and, in her reasonable French, chattered for a minute or two about trivial matters, before asking him if he'd be kind enough to tell them what he knew of the drowning accident between the islands. It transpired that this old man had been fishing close by on that particular morning, hidden from the police by the rocks and he'd actually watched the bodies being pulled from the water.

"I suppose you weren't close enough to be able to describe the bodies were you?" asked Alicia intently. She could feel the suspense radiating from across the table and couldn't risk even a quick glance in the direction of Adriana.

"*Mais oui,* Mademoiselle I was very near. I dared not even light up a *Gaulloise,* for fear of being seen." He leant forward, fiddling with the beret in his hands. "I could tell it was all very secret, but the men who died were foreigners, definitely: they were of dark colouring and as old as me, *très vieux*," he added, looking across at Adriana with a wink and a meaningful stare. *Ils ressemblaient des immigrants illegaux, Mademoiselle.*" He stopped as Adriana shot up, knocked over her chair and ran from the room. The old man gaped after her and started to apologize, seeing how upset she was.

"*Non, non! Il n'y a pas de quoi,*" Alicia reassured. "You have been a wonderful help to us, you have no idea. Please have another drink with your friends and pay our bill for us," and with that she thrust a twenty euro note into his hand and rushed out of the room after Adriana. She found her sitting on a nearby bench, white as a sheet, gasping for air, with tears pouring down her face, stuttering incoherently.

"Deep breaths now Ari, come on, deep breaths", Alicia commanded, trying to calm Adriana, rubbing her back, remembering a little of the first aid that they had been taught at school. Alicia also was shaken, although, obviously, not nearly as much as her bewildered friend; she put her arms around Adriana, gently helped her to her feet and led her slowly away from the buildings and down towards a quiet place on some rocks by the sea. There they sat, side by side, stunned into silence, trying to get a grip of themselves, whilst absorbing this momentous revelation; then when Adriana had dried her tears and was able to speak again, she uttered in a whisper,

"So my gut feeling was right all along: he's not dead, Julian's not dead Ally!" her voice was rising, slightly hysterically, "They're both alive and most likely together, but who … who on earth was that in Scotland … and … and … whatever do we do next? … Oh Lord Ally, sorry, but I think I'm going to be sick!"

~

They returned to the mainland, collected the car and drove back to the hotel, pooling their thoughts and ideas until they had an agreed plan of action: both were far too busy to notice the young man, on the fast-looking motorbike, following at a discreet distance.

First Alicia rang Nick who was shocked, for a moment, into complete and astonished silence. All he could say was, "God! Alicia, God! Alicia", and then "so our instincts were right, we were right all along, the whole thing was just too odd; too odd to be true. So … what's next?"

~

The decision was taken for Adriana to return to London. She felt that it was most likely that Julian, if he really was of this world, would contact her there, when he was ready. Nick was going to meet her at the airport, then return to his M.I.6 contacts to try to get this latest turn of events confirmed.

Alicia thought that she would go to stay with her Aunt Caro in Venice. She was already expected there: then she would return to the Island to await news and there she could also confide further in Gianni. The three of them would say nothing to anybody else for the moment, but keep in close touch with each other.

Alicia and Adriana decided on two more, quiet, days together, recovering and relaxing after this dramatic and unexpected turn of events. They had found a message from the d'Aubert's waiting for them on their return from Cannes, insisting that they have lunch or dinner with them the next day. Jean Pierre, would come to collect them, so they needn't drive and could enjoy the Chateau d'Aubert wine. They happily accepted, were collected by a delighted J.P. had lunch and then spent the whole afternoon at the Chateau.

After a really happy meal, while Marie-Anne showed Adriana around the Chateau, Jacques asked Alicia to his study once more, for another private chat. They had a long talk about the whole situation. When Alicia related the events of their trip to the island the day before and finished with asking Jacques why he thought that Julian's death might have been faked, she was left wondering yet again, just how much Jacques already knew of the whole story, for he was, as before, non-committal.

Alicia's intellect told her, that Jacques would tell her everything that he felt he could, but no more. As a close friend and associate of Gianni, she must trust the Frenchman and cooperate fully. She understood that there were some things he couldn't disclose, at this time, both for her own and Adriana's protection and because of Guy's own continuing, personal, predicament. She accepted this and told him so. Their discussion finished with Jacques only wishing to know what their next movements were to be. This time she knew perfectly well his reason for asking!

Adriana's strength and colour seemed to return with remarkable speed, which Alicia put down to that indefinable emotion called quite simply 'hope'. By the time the two said goodbye at the airport, two days later, they both knew that they had plenty of faith, much determination and that an especially strong and ever more enduring friendship had been firmly forged between them.

★★★

CHAPTER 24

Julian sat morosely, smoking, staring out at the Venetian skyline and kicking at some stones under his feet. He took off the padded outer garment which helped to change his shape. His head itched from the hot, dark, offensive wig. You really would have thought that by now the department's masters of disguise would have produced something better to keep it on. He had absolutely refused to stick it on with the glue stuff provided, which brought him out in a rash. A few pieces of plaster worked perfectly well and as for the ridiculous goatee beard he'd had to grow, it was disgusting. Guy had thought it very funny and never ceased telling him so. He'd had enough of being incognito all the time and was looking forward to being allowed to be himself again.

The whole situation had deteriorated beyond the realms of acceptability. Adriana had just lived through his funeral, for God's sake: he couldn't imagine a worse ordeal. And his parents and family: how would they ever recover? How could they ever forgive him? Never mind the fact that none of it was his fault and he had been given no choice. Or had he? If only he hadn't been so bloody inquisitive in the first place. If he'd left the wretched bag underneath the bush; if he'd ignored the raised voices which warned him instinctively of someone in serious trouble, needing assistance. Yet he could never have turned his back and walked away; he couldn't have lived with that either.

He stamped on his cigarette end and immediately lit another. He felt energized and impatient, fed up with playing this waiting game. It was simply no good to keep blaming himself for what had happened and no good continuing to speculate further either. What an ill fated piece of chance it was that sent Alicia here. He wondered how his old friend really felt inside. He seemed to be coping well, but then he would. When Guy was on a job you could never tell what he was thinking. Ever the professional no wonder the department didn't want to let him go. He also wondered if their relationships with the girls would survive when this thing was over, favorably, God willing. It was hard to believe that it was only a few weeks ago since the whole, bloody, nightmare had begun in America.

~

Julian had been minding his own business that afternoon in Florida. It seemed like an age ago now, because so much had happened since. Little Beach Island had proved to be exactly what he had been looking for. He'd had two days off after his last job, in Latin America. The assignment there had turned out to be pretty good hell, both uncomfortable and exhausting and he had been looking forward to a break. He'd allowed just enough time to look at the island before flying home from Miami. Little Beach was both private and romantic, or at least how he assessed something romantic to be and Adriana loved the sun and the sea. It was the most perfect place finally to pluck up the courage to ask her.

He'd had lunch in the excellent restaurant then wandered out and followed the path beside the sea that led around the island. The hotel rooms were in individual thatched cottages, all a good distance from each other and well away from the main hotel reception and restaurant. He could see the outside showers, enclosed in bamboo, on each balcony, straight out of 'South Pacific'. The gardens were beautifully laid out with exotic flowers through which the discreet, smart and friendly staff drove their little buggies down the winding paths attending to the needs of their guests. There was an elegant shop stocked with all the sort of goodies that Adriana would like. He'd intended to go past on the way back, to find her a present. When he brought her here, he would keep their final destination completely secret; make it all really special. Then she'd have to say 'yes'. He thought she would. Still, you couldn't be sure about these things. It was a pretty nerve wracking business because it mattered so much if she turned him down. Rather worse than being shot at, he assumed.

~

He fingered the bullet-proof waistcoat under his shirt. Made of light weight material these days, like a second skin, it even allowed him to sweat. So used to wearing it, he put it on each day out of habit now, when he was on the move. He really should take it off when he wasn't working, but he was worried about some nosy person finding it in a hotel bedroom and causing a commotion. If it was pinched he'd be in trouble. It was easier just to go on wearing it when he was travelling; at least he had constant protection from a bullet. Mending a broken heart on the other hand could cause him a bit more of a problem.

~

He'd walked on, leaving the inhabited part of the island behind and had finally sat down, under a palm tree, in a clearing surrounded by bushes looking out to sea. He had felt weary after a gruelling week with too many working nights and too little sleep. He thought about his work. He enjoyed being a war correspondent visiting all the so-called hot spots. The adrenalin fairly pumped when he rushed from one place to another never knowing quite what to expect. But Adriana had changed his life. He loved her, completely and utterly and he had to admit to himself that he no longer wished to live under constant physical threat, both for his sake and for hers. If she said yes, then he'd give in his notice. They wouldn't have to worry about money for a very long time to come he had been exceptionally well paid over the last few years.

Now that he had made these all-important decisions, Julian felt that he'd earned himself a short rest; he'd learnt to sleep whenever the opportunity arose. He shouldn't have had all that wine at lunch, but he'd been tired and relieved to have some time to himself, devoid of responsibility for a change. He had several hours before he needed to get back to the mainland, which was only a short crossing on the hotel launch. He then had no more commitments until he flew home.

As he made himself comfortable, his attention was caught by something pushed under a bush on one side of the clearing. It looked like a man's hold-all. Whatever it was, he'd have a look later, he thought sleepily, and if it appeared to have any value, he'd take it in to the hotel reception on his way back.

Julian was awoken abruptly from a deep sleep by raised voices; somewhere near, through the other side of the bushes. What the hell? He was instantly alert and looked at his watch, an old habit from former days. 'Record the time,' they used to be told over and over again. How could he ever forget? Then he strained his ears to listen, another habit. This was no ordinary argument between a holidaying couple. This was serious stuff, someone in trouble and being badly beaten up too, by the sound of it. He could hear the thuds and stifled screams.

He stripped off, devising a plan as he did so, thankful that he had on his swimming shorts underneath his clothes. He walked quickly and quietly into the sea. As he entered the water, the people he had heard were still hidden from view so he struck out to sea, then turned and swum along beside the beach, as if he'd been swimming down from the other end of the island, until the next cove began to open up. They still hadn't seen him. They were too busy with what they were doing; but now he could see them. Three men were brutally laying in to another.

Julian had a moment to decide what to do before he was spotted. He made up his mind, turned on his back and with his head low in the water continued to back-crawl nonchalantly alongside the beach, splashing, apparently as yet unaware of the men. They'd seen him at last, he could tell. They had stopped their assault on the limp looking man and were pointing and gesticulating in his direction. He swum on for two or three minutes to give them time to reorganize themselves, then turned in towards the beach, as if this was what he had been intending to do all the time. Out of the corner of his eye, Julian had spotted an extremely fast-looking speedboat, moored almost out of sight in the next bay down.

When he reached the sand, he stood for a moment and shook his head, put his fingers to his ears, wiped his eyes and walked slowly up the shingle. Only then did he pretend to notice the others and wave in a friendly manner. Two of the three men, who looked Italian, wore badly cut dark suits. The other, also swarthy looking, had his coat off and his sleeves rolled up. He was breathing hard, responsible for most of the violence directed towards the hapless young man, a well-dressed Arab, who appeared semi conscious.

"Good afternoon, what a glorious day," said Julian, raising his hand to the sun and sky; pretending he'd seen nothing untoward, as he took in the scene in front of him. The ugly wretch in shirt sleeves was rolling them down again, putting on his jacket and smoothing his hair. Strange place to wear a jacket on the beach, thought Julian. Their prisoner, aware of his presence, jerked awake, almost toppled off the tree root, on which he was sitting then, doubled up with pain moaning audibly. He looked all in and in an utterly forlorn state.

"Is your friend alright?" asked Julian politely as he approached, indicating the young Arab, as if he had just noticed him sitting there. "Is he sick? He doesn't look too good." The Arab seemed incapable of speech, so Julian looked around waiting for an answer. One of the other two replied just too quickly, in a heavy Italian accent,

"*Si, si,* yes, but of course. He has girl trouble; worrying too much and tripped over the tree root," waving his hand around indicating a rough pile of wood nearby, the other two nodded in agreement. The man continued in bad English, gaining in confidence. "He's not looking where is going, *'e ferito,* he's hurt just a little; stupid boy. He's sitting down for a while to recover, that's all." He laughed and gave his captive a false, brotherly, pat on the head. The Arab moved, as if brought back to life, ducking away from beneath the rough hand, at the same time moving to wrap his arms around his stomach again. He was obviously in agony. These people knew exactly how to beat someone up without it showing, since his face, although grey and perspiring, profusely, was, as yet, untouched. Julian thought it was likely that the thugs were armed and so knew that he couldn't take on the whole group at once, he had to get away and get help, fast.

"That's alright then," said Julian, ignoring the three in the ominous dark suits and going up close to the suffering, frightened, man, to make sure that he had his full attention, "but seriously, you do look in pain. Perhaps you ate some bad sea food? Is it your stomach? Why don't you come up to the hotel, at the other end of the island? I had lunch there, they are nice people and I'm certain that they would send a buggy and someone to help if you don't feel well. There will be an in-house doctor for sure." Julian's expert eye swept over their miserable victim assessing the damage as he spoke. The wretched man already had several broken ribs he thought.

"No! please," implored the young man, coming to and taking a deep painful breath with immense effort. "Leave us. I know these people well and they will look after me. You must go, really I mean it. Go back to your clothes and your bag and leave. You must go," he said again with stricken, bloodshot eyes. He was adamant as he stared back at Julian and it was obvious, even in his weakened state, that the words were spoken with a hidden meaning. "Thank you, but please get your bag and your things and go."

"Alright. If you are sure," said Julian, then turning and fixing one of the two heavies with a steely glare added "however I'll send someone down from the hotel to check your friend is O.K."

"That will not be necessary, *signore*, *nessun problema*, we take care of him." I'm sure you will, Julian thought worriedly.

"Well, I'll ask them to send someone anyway, just to be on the safe side," and turning to the young man he spoke quickly, trying to convey his understanding of the situation, "I think the trouble with your girlfriend must be very serious indeed. I'm sorry; I hope you feel better soon and please accept assistance from the hotel people, who will come soon, *Ciao.*'" He waved into the air to all of them as he walked away, trying not to seem in a hurry, heading back towards the bushes, where he'd left his clothes. There was silence as he did so. They were all watching him closely, but for different reasons. He could feel four pairs of eyes boring into his back. The thugs were wondering what to do now, whether they should have let him go perhaps.

Right, thought Julian, let's just hope that's sorted them out and stopped the violence until more help arrives. Presumably, the young man was also aware that his assailants were armed and that a three to one contest was out of the question; otherwise he wouldn't have been so keen for me to go. Extra help brought back quickly was his only hope. Julian's instinct and training told him the poor young man's time on this earth was running out and fast.

Julian returned for his clothes by way of the beach. He was uneasy and alarmed at what he'd just witnessed. 'Girl trouble': my foot. He must quickly send armed security from the hotel. Then he remembered the bag under the bush. He looked around as he dressed. The young man had almost begged him to go back to his clothes and his 'bag', stressing the word bag? He didn't know where Julian had come from or what gear he had with him. How could he? Odd that. The bag he'd seen before was still there in the same place under the same bush. He went over to look. It was a smart, leather, designer hold-all, heavy, with three different compartments. There was an expensive laptop computer in it. Who on earth would leave something like that behind? ... unless; he checked in the other side.

It contained a passport and a small flat package that felt like a CD. Otherwise there was nothing except a pen, a packet of chewing gum and a screwed up piece of paper. The passport didn't look right. He knew it wasn't right. He wished that he had a little more time and light to study the hologram. What's more, it was written in Arabic and sure enough, with the same tortured young man in the picture.

But it was the screwed up piece of paper that settled it. The name Elizabeth Mac, Key West, meant nothing, but the scribbled telephone number did. Julian recognized it instantly. It was a coded number he'd used on many occasions himself, a number in Maryland, a direct link to his own old department, through C.I.A headquarters. That particular number was never written down. It had to be learnt, literally engraved on the memory. Nobody, but nobody outside their own department should have it, so who on earth had given it to the young Arab and why?

Julian looked around but there was nobody in sight. He picked up the hold-all and set off speedily, back to the hotel. The receptionist was relatively unhelpful, at least to start with and he knew he hadn't much time. The main part of the hotel security system was set up on the mainland. That was where everybody left their cars and guests then took the launch across to the island. She could contact Sam, the guardian, who would be out and about with his mobile. He had a buggy and could soon get down to the other end of the island to help the young man if he really was in trouble. She looked as if she didn't believe him. Julian told her to reach Sam on his mobile fast, and then he took over.

Sam, thankfully, sounded reasonably intelligent and said he'd get down there as soon as possible, calling up support on the way. He told Julian that he had a portable medical kit and that they all carried a small hand gun.

Julian insisted that he was taking the bag and its contents back to the mainland. It wasn't going to be left with this reception girl who'd quite obviously hand it straight back to the three *mafiosa* types should they come there. Mind you, he thought, he wouldn't really blame her if she did; they were a nasty looking trio. He felt sure that the contents of the bag would be of great interest to GCHQ, the Government Communications Headquarters in England and also to the National Security Agency in America and ought to be examined as fast as possible.

As soon as Julian had given his credentials, Sam agreed to help without question and lost no time in setting off for the other end of the island to rescue the young Arab. He seemed thoroughly excited by the prospect of such unexpected activity enlivening his rather dull day. Julian made the receptionist call up the boatman and order the launch to be made ready for him immediately. The annoying woman had finally given up arguing and now listened to him, understanding the urgency. He told her that she must 'know nothing whatever about the bag'. If the three men came in, she must make sure that she wasn't on her own and say she had never seen him, at least not since lunch. He would deal with everything else when he got to the mainland. Julian also suggested that the receptionist should ring security there to warn them that he was coming, more for her own peace of mind than anything else. Mentally noting the number and thankful that she had, at least, declined from wishing him 'a nice day', he then hurried off to the hotel quay.

It was at this point, watched by three shadowy figures, standing under the palms, as he was being taken back to the mainland in the high speed hotel launch, that Julian knew that the urgency was real. He felt certain that the computer carried highly sensitive information. What happened next would depend on its contents and the Arab's identity. He also decided that, because of the highly confidential telephone number on the scruffy piece of paper, he'd hold onto the bag and its contents as if his very life depended on it.

The person he needed to help him coordinate a plan of action and who must be contacted without delay, middle of the night or not, was Guy!

~

It wasn't until Julian was halfway across the Atlantic later that night, that he'd remembered there should have been something else in his pocket: a card that he had written to Alicia sometime before and forgotten to post. He had intended to send it to reassure her that he would be back in time for the wedding to be Guy's best man; that he took his best man's duties very seriously and that Adriana would keep her up to date with his movements. It could only have fallen out when he'd dressed, in such a hurry, after the fateful swim.

He'd handed all their identities to the thugs on a plate. He'd named each one of them and even addressed the card, for Christ's sake. What an unmitigated disaster.

~

And this, thought Julian, lighting yet another cigarette as he demolished the pile of stones with his other foot, under the swiftly darkening Venetian sky, had only been the very beginning.

★★★

CHAPTER 25

Alicia, alone again, flew on to Venice, where she was met with open arms by her gregarious Aunt Caro, who'd brought her private launch to the airport island to meet her. After a call from Alicia's mother, Caro was both surprised and considering everything else she'd been told, pleased to find Alicia in remarkably good spirits.

She scooped up her niece and returned to the city at breakneck speed, at the helm herself, scattering all others out of the way in spite of the relatively narrow channel. Caro was obviously a well-known figure here. Alicia knew she had done much for the preservation and restoration of various ancient buildings in Venice, otherwise she simply couldn't see how the water authorities could possibly turn a blind eye to such high-spirited antics!

Alicia sat back, stirred once again by the breathtaking view. The afternoon sun bathed the distant buildings in a muted golden light. Reminiscent of a Turner painting, she thought, as ever mesmerised by the magic of Venice. It had been a really good idea to come here and she was thrilled to be returning to the city that she loved, with her Aunt whom she also adored. It held so many happy childhood and early adult memories and whatever the situation, who could remain depressed in Caro's company or not be affected by her infectious enthusiasm for life? Alicia studied her aunt as they roared across the water allowing no possibility of speech. Caro was exactly how she remembered, now probably in her mid-forties, a little plumper perhaps, but still elegant and as smart as ever. Her hair was cut short, fashionably tinted; enhancing her own dark blonde colouring, her face beautifully made up and her well manicured hands flashing a collection of rather ostentatious diamond rings; but that was her style. There was nothing inconspicuous about the Contessa.

~

Caro, very young and beautiful, had married a much older man: Count Carlo Cavaggio, good looking, sophisticated, tremendous fun and fabulously wealthy! Alicia's mother had told her that they'd met at a nightclub in the West End of London. Caro had been just eighteen and when she and Carlo had first set eyes on each other they had fallen instantly and completely in love. Carlo had charmed Caro's parents who were delighted that someone older and with plenty of experience was going to take their headstrong daughter off their hands. The wedding took place within six weeks, which had been just long enough to organize the most exquisically romantic marriage in Italy. Her parents had been much relieved when Carlo had insisted on paying the enormous bill himself. They had enjoyed a fairy-tale honeymoon in the best hotel on the island of Capri and then he had carried her off to his family villa in Brescia.

There they had lived an idyllically happy life together, in spite of failing to produce offspring, travelling the world incessantly and following the sun until Carlo's sudden and untimely death, from a heart attack, some years before. The story had it that he adored his wife, but was sometimes hard put to keep up with her physical appetite and ended his days with her in their bed!

"What a way to go!" was Caro's remark to a close friend when she had finally emerged from a reclusive and grief stricken six months, only to find herself one of the wealthiest widows in the country. Every penny however would have gladly been given up to have her beloved Carl restored to her again, for theirs was a special and enduring love affair that had continued to grow throughout their marriage.

After a year or so, Caro had found Brescia too lonely, with only a few elderly relatives with whom to lunch and visit the opera, as well as a huge villa with a large staff to run, just for her alone. There was little to do or to keep her amused, young as she was and alone. So she rode endlessly over her extensive lands, visiting her farms and spending her days and sometimes, at certain times of the year, part of the nights in the vineyards and buildings. There, Carlo's loyal workers, who were worried for their young Contessa's obvious unhappiness, took her to their hearts and taught her from the very beginning how their best wine finally found its way to her table.

Caro soon realized how much she'd taken for granted and began to understand, for the first time, just how much work really went into growing, then harvesting the grapes, filling and finally labelling the bottles ready for sale. As she tiredly sipped from her glass in the evenings, sitting alone with her dinner, the wine took on a whole new meaning and she'd feel that her day had been well spent.

She was an enthusiastic and hardworking student, who learnt quickly and after a while became extremely knowledgeable. At the same time Caro readily joined with her people when they were short staffed or at their busiest. She felt happier knowing that not one of them did anything that she didn't know how to do and hadn't done herself. Their standards became, if anything, even higher than before, out of respect for her.

She learnt the names of all her employees and those of their families and she enjoyed being with them, as they did with her, sharing in their joys and problems alike. But above all the work filled her days and she began to recover from her sadness.

The majority of her friends were international, like she and Carlo had been and were constantly on the move, going from place to place, dependent on the seasons. After a couple of years in her vineyard and after much soul-searching, Caro decided to move her base to her other villa in Venice, where there was much more life and a younger set of friends. There she quickly became immersed in a full and interesting life. Everyone loved her and she was invited everywhere! Her elegance and charm ensured that every party she graced was a huge success. With her boundless energy she soon became deeply committed to the upkeep and wellbeing of Venice. All those most worried for the future of their beloved city recognized her unusual capacity for being able to move heaven and earth, sometimes against enormous odds, to get things done. The very British committee for 'The Preservation of Venice' thanked their lucky stars for the day the Contessa had agreed to join them.

Many men had sought to end the beautiful Contessa's solitude, particularly after she moved to Venice. She may have had the odd discreet affair, but Caro was never even tempted to remarry. Her Carlo 'was more than enough for one person's lifetime' she would always say.

Even with her new life in Venice she never forgot her responsibilities in Brescia and returned there frequently. She kept in close touch with her wine manager, who was efficient and well in control of financial matters, not Caro's best subject! She liked to be there with her people for all important events; for the many births, marriages and, of course, their sad losses. The celebration that she loved most was for the end of the wine harvest, when all the months of hard work and worry were over. When the cork was finally put in the last bottle, after a good year, the atmosphere became like none other that she had ever experienced. It was at this time that she knew just how proud of them all Carlo would be and as ever, she would feel him close by her side, watching.

~

Alicia sat contemplating her Aunt, who was silent for once, as she concentrated on navigating her way around one of the island *motonave* ferries which seemed to be taking up more than it's fair share of the channel. The Contessa held her position and blasted the ferry with her hooter. Incredibly it moved over a little. Alicia laughed as Caro waved her thanks, which prompted a responding short 'toot', as she roared past. She had a way with people; they would do anything to please her. She could speak both French and Italian fluently, had powerful contacts everywhere and had more energy than a woman twenty years younger. Pointed in the right direction she really could do great things for England as well as Italy. Aunt Caro should be our Ambassador here thought Alicia. She'd be brilliant.

Soon they were across the open lagoon and had turned into the narrow waterways of Venice itself where, thankfully, Caro handed over the helm to her long suffering skipper. He at once dropped the speed to negotiate the canals and courteously avoid the endless stream of craft of all shapes and sizes. There were trade boats, water taxis, buses and private launches. The lagoon police were out, conspicuous in their fast, distinctly marked, *moto-scafi* vessels, all dressed in their smart uniforms. One of them actually saluted Caro as they went past: and there were inevitable gondolas all wending their way skilfully around each other. She wondered how on earth the lovely polished woodwork on Caro's launch had managed to remain unscathed so far, particularly as she was so often at the helm herself!

"Very tame and well behaved in here, isn't it?" announced Caro with a sparkle. "My present boatman only agreed to stay with the job if I handed over in here out of the lagoon. He said he'd heard of my driving reputation in advance. Isn't that right Alonzo?" she called. He looked at them and nodded grinning. "Lot of old women, actually, aren't they?" she added quietly, letting out a grunt of disapproval.

Alicia looked at Alonzo who winked at her before turning to concentrate on the difficult approach to the villa steps. The water was high. When the launch had been efficiently and quickly moored, Alonzo put out the duckboards so that both Alicia and her Aunt could reach the bottom steps of the villa with dry feet and then he followed them up with Alicia's suitcase and some of Caro's distinctive and expensive looking carrier bags.

The villa was a clever blend of ancient centuries and modern comfort, enhanced by a slightly chaotic appearance, which seemed in keeping with Caro's lively character. The elderly housekeeper and her husband the butler, both remembered Alicia well from her earlier visits and fussed over her as if she was still a small child and incapable of doing anything for herself. They were taken aback when confronted by the girl they last saw as a young adult, now grown into a beautiful woman. Alicia noticed straight away that a great deal of extra effort had been made on her behalf.

A young Albanian couple looked after the cleaning and shopping. Caro said that she didn't think they were married but what did it matter as they were very good and delighted to be out of an unstable Albania. There was also a wonderful new cook, 'Italian of course, but he has rows with the Albanians', she added with much relish.

Alicia was shown to the room that her mother had been given the last time they were there together, some years before. She looked at the lovely old four poster bed with its elaborate hangings and at the beautiful pictures and rugs wondering, once more, how future events would unfold for her. She sighed with nostalgia and walked across to the window. The room was high above her Aunt's suite and commanded a panoramic view over Venice and on, out towards the lagoon. She stood looking down on all the activity below her and watched the same sun go down yet again, this time over the *Laguna Veneta* and beyond, over another part of the Adriatic.

For dinner that night the Contessa had organized all Alicia's favourite Italian dishes. The *Brodo di Pesce,* a delicious fish soup, was every bit as good as she remembered. Pasta followed, then another favourite, *tiramisù.* She would have to watch her waistline, although her aunt assured her that it was only a light meal.

Caro amused Alicia with hilarious stories, spiced with all the gossip surrounding the elite Venetian aristocracy and various political dignitaries. She told Alicia that she expected her to attend the early summer masked ball, the *Fiesta La Sensa,* with her the next week. This Alicia knew, from past experience, was an order not an invitation, athough it could be a problem as she truly had nothing to wear this time. She decided to say nothing for the moment. Maybe she could borrow a dress from somebody. Until then, she would visit all her old haunts in the day time while Caro was busy with all her appointments. Then, Caro said, they would meet each evening for dinner, to catch up properly. The Contessa was still endearingly bossy. She hadn't changed and the routine was just as Alicia remembered.

~

May was the most perfect time to be visiting Venice: a surreal, dream-like, city of many contradictions, carrying its heavy burden of centuries. Beautiful and timeless, on the surface but, when the mist rolled in from the sea, the narrow streets and canals became shrouded in a ghostlike blanket, with an eerily sinister undercurrent threading its way through and around the ancient architecture; lending credence to the stories of cruelty and decadence during Venice's fall from grace.

It was as if another universe lay hidden beneath the façade of the one on public view. The aura of the city would enfold you, as would a cloak, thought Alicia, shivering; then it would move you on, back into the light and warmth of the familiar present world once more. She loved the feel of shifting centuries, the contrast of light and dark, warmth and cold, which, more than ever now, seemed to reflect her own changing moods and circumstances.

She visited all the places she loved most: the Basilica, palaces, churches, bridges, museums and art galleries. She knew them all so well. There were still a few familiar faces to welcome her in the various restaurants, some of which continued to be family-run. Also she shopped, for who could resist the shops in Venice?

Alicia visited the islands. She thought for one awful moment that she saw one of the *mafiosa* look alikes again, boarding the *motoscafi* with her to San Michele, which frightened her. Then he seemed to disappear into the crowd and she never saw the man again, so she decided that it was her imagination running riot once more. In any event, there were plenty of *Carabinieri* around, which was reassuring. Whenever she saw an Italian policeman she would be inwardly comforted and reminded of Marcello.

Caro insisted that Alicia tell her, each day, exactly what she had planned and where she was going. Strange, Alicia didn't remember her being overly protective last time she was here and then she'd been much younger and so much more vulnerable.

She went to Burano, her favourite island. She lunched in the sun outside

Da Romana, the fish restaurant, then wandered beside the canals and along the little, cobbled, streets lined by the prettily painted houses. The ground floors had almost all been turned into restaurants, or shops selling the endless variety of lace for which the island was famous. Alicia bought some handkerchiefs for her aunt and a few for herself. Finally she sat under the cypress trees and looked out at the view across the water and the skyline of Venice. The sun still shone, bathing the city in soft gold; it was so poignantly beautiful, but the gentle fingers of melancholia began to take hold. It seemed such a waste to be experiencing this all by herself. The familiar, unsettled queasiness began to weigh on her stomach and she didn't linger long. It was better to keep busy and on the move.

When the evening boat pulled away from the quay and began it's return journey, the light was fading fast. Alicia watched fascinated: the brightly coloured houses of Burano, although shrinking with the increasing distance, were still clearly visible. The fishermen would always find their way home, more easily than others on a foggy day, reaffirming the truth in the age old story. How sensible of Delfino to copy this ancient tradition.

Alicia visited Murano and the glass factory, where the same man as before tried to sell her sets of lovely, but heavily ornate, glass. She went to the island of Torcello and the cathedral of *Santa Maria Assunta* with its beautiful mosaics, for whose restoration her Aunt had been largely responsible.

She loved visiting the furthest islands, where the people, less frenetic, seemed in less of a hurry and where nothing was too much trouble. She liked the long boat rides and the feeling of space, which was such a contrast to Venice itself. The air, the wind and the sea gave her an appetite, so she stopped for many an *expresso* along with something to eat, whilst watching the world go by.

Caro insisted on a shopping spree to find Alicia a dress which had to be 'long and worthy of the ball', as she put it. She couldn't possibly borrow one. 'The celebration of Venice's marriage to the sea is one of the most important dates in a Venetian's diary', Caro told her, 'and one of the most romantic,' she had added with a chuckle! 'So watch out'.

It was a fun afternoon. The Contessa was treated like a queen wherever they went. The shop they were visiting would put up its shutters to other customers for the duration of their visit and they would be offered little *cichetti* snacks and refreshing *prosecco,* sparkling wine with coffee or water, all beautifully laid up on a gilded tray.

They finally settled on a lush silk dress of midnight blue with a low back, almost off the shoulder, with a sensuous sash of contrasting aquamarine that swirled around Alicia's hips, finished with a slit well up above the knee on one side. Matching silk sling-back shoes and a sparkling evening bag, completed the outfit. Caro then announced that Alicia was to wear her own family set of aquamarines as they 'would match the dress and her eyes'.

"With that blonde hair, fabulous figure and classical English good looks you'll knock them all for six!" said Caro. "You'll be the belle of the ball and I shall be the most popular woman in the whole of Venice for finding you!" and then happily insisted on paying the bill, without a qualm.

That night they went to the Cipriani for dinner. As they sped across the short piece of water, leaving St. Marks twinkling behind them, Alicia had some reservations. Her last visit there had been under very different circumstances, with Guy. The Cipriani was one of his favourite hotels. Occasionally he even went there on his own if he happened to be in the area. He would bask in the certain welcome and enjoy the sophisticated peace and quiet not always easy to find in such a very noisy country! The staff loved his Irish sense of humour and treated him like a king. Alicia remembered teasing him and laughing when he had been embarrassed by the attention lavished on him, in front of her.

As she was handed ashore after her Aunt, she couldn't help but glance up at the corner terrace window on the first floor where their room had been, when he had brought her here so soon after they had met. Guy had insisted on telling no one where they were, not even her Aunt; selfishly he had said that he wanted her all to himself. She had felt slightly guilty knowing how much Caro would have loved to see them, but she soon forgot. It had been a memorable weekend. Little could anyone have guessed just how far their affair progressed on those two particular nights, surpassing all that had gone before. Even after all this time her legs turned to jelly just thinking about it. How she missed him and all that they had in their life together.

Nevertheless, it was unnerving to think how quickly that physical gap had been filled by Marcello. And what about Marcello? When she was with him she was unable to exercise any control whatsoever. Yes, she missed him too and the tell-tale sensations of a sexual appetite so recently reawakened. Lord! What a muddle she was in.

"Alicia! ... Are you coming?"

"Yes, Aunt, sorry I was miles away ...," she replied and hurried up the path and into the hotel.

Once inside, the manager appeared and welcomed them politely, recognizing Alicia and asking after Guy. Luckily her aunt had marched ahead, so Alicia was able to answer gracefully and told him that Guy was well, but away on business and sad to miss this visit.

They sat down to dinner at a table overlooking the water. Caro, having ordered her usual champagne, watched critically as the bottle was meticulously opened and poured. Alicia, anticipating the first sip, delighted in the bubbles tickling her nose while she waited for her aunt to be handed her glass. Caro, satisfied that this most important service was performed as she would have wished and that the waiter had moved away out of earshot, looked across at her niece and with a strange expression on her face she said,

"It will all be alright, you know ... eventually, but you must have patience Alicia, for a little while longer." She paused, "Here's to you, my darling and hoping that everything sorts out. I'm sure it will. Now then, what shall we eat?" Alicia sat bolt upright, confused and was just wondering what to say in return when her Aunt continued:

"Come on now", looking down at the menu, "let's have something really delicious. We'll ask what the specialities are". She beckoned to the head-waiter. "All that shopping for the ball has made me thoroughly hungry, and you have no idea just how much I'm looking forward to showing you off! Wait till you hear who's on the guest list!" The strange moment had passed and Alicia shook her golden head, laughed and turned her attention to the menu. An amazing dinner: they chose the same; fresh asparagus to start with, served with a sauce produced by the chef from his own secret ingredients they were told. This was followed by pasta with tomato and basil, then a huge dish of mixed seafood. It was an enjoyable evening, with far too much wine and must have cost the earth, thought Alicia.

"Don't worry", Caro had said, lowering her voice, as the second bottle was being poured, "there's nobody important here tonight to tell tales. Not even my sister, your mother, to tell us off." They enjoyed each other's company. Caro had Alicia amused again by telling her of all the unlikely liaisons amongst some of the dinner guests for 'La Fiesta' the next weekend.

"Italian people think they are so discreet, but you can tell exactly who's off with who, just by looking at them. They wear it on their faces, except when they have the masks on, of course," she said with a twinkle.

"But not you Aunt, nobody would ever know what you got up to in that respect, would they?"

"Oh no! Alicia, I should be much too clever. Though no one could ever replace my darling Carl, you know, even in 'that respect' as you say!"

"Have you never even been tempted?" Alicia insisted, "I just can't imagine someone so full of life as you..."

"Oh yes, my goodness yes!" she answered. "Many, many times, but mostly in the mind," she said, tapping her head and producing a lovely low throaty chuckle. Aha! thought Alicia.

When they returned to the villa in the private launch, she wondered again at her Aunt's remarks at the beginning of dinner. Did she somehow know more than she was letting on? And if so, how was that possible? She'd only talked to her sister, Alicia's mother, Diana. As they motored, more slowly now, across the dark water the sky was alight with so many stars. Once again she felt that familiar tug at her heart, and a longing for that which seemed as yet so very far out of reach.

Maybe it was memories in this evening's surroundings. Where on earth could Guy be on a night like this when she needed him so much? Or, maybe it was the constant reminders of Marcello, her irresistible policeman. It was almost as if they were both near, watching and waiting for something to happen, an unnerving sensation. At this moment, she knew not what she wanted anymore, nor whom she missed most. But maybe it was just too much wine and the romantic and mystical atmosphere in the ancient city of Venice.

★★★

CHAPTER 26

The night of La Fiesta La Sensa duly arrived. Alicia had known, all along, that her aunt had something up her sleeve and had finally got it out of her. She had only invited Alicia's old boyfriend from long ago, with his rather difficult wife. Apparently he'd only managed to stay faithful to the poor woman for six months after they were married. Whether Caro had decided to invite the Count and his wife for her own amusement, or to take her niece's mind off other things, Alicia wasn't quite sure. At any rate the Contessa was incorrigible.

"Marco took a long time to recover after you left. What ever you did to him was without doubt terminal. I had one hell of a task cheering up the wretched man", she told Alicia pointedly, her expression suggesting that she had been perfectly well aware of their passionate affair whilst Alicia lived under her aunt's roof and guardianship. Alicia, in her extreme youth, had considered herself so sophisticated and discreet at that time.

"And now, he will see just how beautiful you have become and his wife will seem to be more boring and more ugly than ever," with that, Caro went off to change, her peels of her laughter echoing down the huge corridor.

"Aunt, you're the most terrible trouble maker!" Alicia called after her before going on up to her own room, catching Caro's infectious, uplifting mood.

Alicia walked through her bedroom door and stopped dead. A dazzling mask, of the same midnight blue as her dress, lay waiting for her on her dressing table. She had thought that she was to borrow one from her aunt. This one looked brand new and it was beautiful. She took a step back and gazed down at the sparkling gift. Odd, she thought. Her aunt would normally have packed it in an elaborate box with all the trimmings and given it to her very publicly, with much pizzazz. It really was most unlike her not to wish to present the gift in person.

Alicia wondered, again, at the curious remark Caro had made that night at the Cipriani as they had sat down to dinner. It was as if she were aware of the unfathomable goings on. Yet, she couldn't know anything. Or could she and if so from whom? Alicia had mentioned nothing of her present predicament and there was no one else who could have told her of the unreal sequence of events over the last few weeks. Perhaps it was simply her mother who had been in touch for the umpteenth time, asking Caro to try to reassure Alicia a little, so as to make her future seem less bleak. Still, it was her aunt's choice of words that had seemed strange at the time.

I actually thought I'd done quite a good job of pulling myself together, with Marcello's help of course; if it hadn't been for him I might have been the most God awful mess by now, thought Alicia disconsolately. Maybe for those that know me well, I haven't done such a good job after all. She studied her face in the mirror on her dressing table and decided that she was looking worried again. This just had to stop. She must get ready for the evening ahead. After all, both the dress and matching mask were sensational and she must do them justice.

This evening Alicia decided that she would enjoy herself, if only out of appreciation to her aunt for her endless generosity. She was also quite looking forward to seeing the Count again, if only for nostalgic reasons. He'd be forty years old by now, if not more. How would he react to her after all this time and in front of his wife? Knowing her aunt, Caro wouldn't have told him Alicia was in Venice. Her niece would be her surprise, her very own trump card. Caro loved any sort of intrigue, particularly if she was the cause.

Alicia lay in the, huge, old-fashioned bath, up to her neck in the warm, scented, water. She could only just touch the end with her toes. So big was the tub, a child could almost swim in it. Plenty else you could do in it also, Alicia thought, if the right person were here. She looked down at her body, now turning pink. She'd been in the water far too long. She'd shrivel up if she wasn't careful. Her face was quite probably rose coloured as well - like a lobster. She'd need time to cool down.

She did have plenty of time. Enveloped in the huge white towel, Alicia sat on the old stool by the bath and listened to the water gurgling horribly, as it raced its way down the ancient pipes. How long did it take to reach the dungeon level she wondered? Presumably it rushed unhindered into the canal far below with everything else that was discarded. If a leaf were to travel with the flood, where would it end up? Would it be nudged along into the Grand Canal and out into the *'Laguna Veneta'*? Then, would the tide take it further out into the *'Golfo di Venezia'* and from there to the Adriatic? An interesting thought: if the little leaf managed to avoid all the water traffic, there was no knowing where it might finally come to rest. Given this sort of project when at school, Alicia would have been in her element. The room was quiet again, the water had all disappeared and Alicia found, to her chagrin that, she was staring down the plug hole in fascination. Her mother would consider her mad.

She got up and went to dress, her thoughts turning to Adriana. She wished her friend was here; they would have such a good time together. She would ring her in the morning to tell her all about the evening and to find out if she had any news.

When she was finally ready, Alicia went downstairs, where her Aunt was waiting with the aquamarines glistening in their black, leather, box. Her own disguise and another were also on the table beside her. Caro watched her niece approach with pride. She did indeed look fabulous even before the sparkling stones were in place. Alicia stood, carefully positioning the earrings, while Caro, fixed the necklace clasp securely around her slender neck. Thanking her, Alicia then held out the blue mask to show how perfectly it matched. Caro, for a second, looked taken aback and started to speak.

"But where ...? she started, then stopped. Alicia, so excited, had moved away and was twirling around to show the staff; who were all lined up to see them depart.

"Look Aunt," she called as she held the mask up to her face, "how clever you were to find one the same colour as my dress and how mysterious I am! Nobody shall know what I get up to either!" Caro laughed with the staff and clapped her hands, but she said not a word.

As they left the room the second blue mask remained in it's place, on the table by the fire, discreetly hidden by Caro's best linen handkerchief. As the butler's wife went to pick it up and hurry after the departing women, thinking it forgotten. Fausto, catching her eye, merely shook his head.

~

The Contessa had decided to leave the launch and walk the short distance from the Canal Grande across the piazza to the palace where the dinner and ball was to be held. There would be too many people all arriving at the same time by the smaller canal. Besides, it was a lovely evening and Alonzo, the boatman, would escort the two women.

At the palace steps, they got caught up in a small group of revellers, who appeared to be carried well away, in their colourful costumes. The police were there watching, amused by their antics, or so it seemed, until one, dressed as a court jester, broke away from the rest. He came towards Alicia holding out a charity tin and beckoning most persuasively to her, almost as if he meant to speak. But, quick as a flash, one of the policemen had placed himself between the jester and Alicia, as if barring the man's way, leaving the way clear for herself and Caro to proceed unhindered. As Alicia followed her aunt to the bottom of the steps she turned to smile at the policeman.

"*Buona sera Signorina*," came that oh - so familiar voice. She hadn't recognized him in the evening light.

"Mar ..." but his fingers were to his lips and he shook his head, then inclined it slightly, indicating that she should go on, without knowing him. She stared, unable to move.

The court jester, behind, also stood as if mesmerized, as, almost imperceptibly, her policeman touched his head, his heart and his lips as he'd done before, then with his eyes told her to move on. The spell unbroken, Alicia did likewise. Then, as if in a trance, she turned and followed her Aunt up the stone steps, her heart pounding. Caro was standing halfway up with Alonzo, both were looking puzzled.

"Alicia, what were you doing?" The spell was broken.

"Nothing Aunt. I always make that gesture when I see the Duomo. It's so lovely from here against the night sky. I'm coming": and she walked on by, grateful to be able to hide behind her beautiful mask.

"Strange, but I've never seen you do that before," Caro answered somewhat uncertainly, but striding on with determination.

~

The Contessa was in a decidedly difficult dilemma. She had been speechless when Guy had walked through her door and had presented himself, the day after Alicia's arrival in Venice. Caro and Guy had never met. On this occasion Alicia had been out for the day, she had gone to Burano. How, had the man known that she wouldn't be there, Caro had wondered. When Fausto, her butler, had shown Guy in, she would later say that it was the first time in her life that she had ever been literally struck dumb.

She had stood up to welcome a strange man, but when he gave his name, she sat down again, very fast, absorbing the shock. Guy hurried to her side, but she had held her hand up to stop him while she took a moment to recover, to regain her composure. Then raising her head high, she looked him straight in the eye and said,

"Well, young man, I must tell you that I adore my niece and so your explanation for exactly why you have been putting her through such unmitigated hell had better be pretty bloody good. Now please sit down and tell me all. And I mean all!"

Guy had held nothing back. He had told Caro everything that had taken place, from the very beginning. He knew he must, in order to be in a position to ask for her help and so that she might understand the danger that Alicia had unwittingly brought upon herself, merely by her courage and determination, in never giving up her search to find out what had happened to him. The Contessa was brilliant, just as Guy had expected. The feeling was mutual; Caro had liked him enormously, admired his nerve and felt desperately sorry for them all being caught up in something so horrendous and not even of their own making. Of course, she would help them in every way she could.

Caro's worst problem was seeing Alicia sometimes so distant, confused and unhappy. Caro longed to be able to say something to ease her pain, but after Guy had explained the situation, knew she mustn't risk it. Meanwhile she made it her business to find out Alicia's plans in advance, as best she could and then pass on the information. The Contessa didn't enjoying spying on her niece but knew it to be only for her own good. She felt a certain relief in the knowledge that Alicia was to be spirited away to somewhere safer later in the evening. The strain of worrying about her would be no more, but she couldn't bear the thought of not being able even to say 'goodbye', just in case anything went wrong. And secretly, Caro admitted to herself, she would miss all the intrigue.

~

The palazzo, where the dinner and ball was held, looked as enormous from the outside, as it seemed inside, when they entered through the old, wooden, studded, doors. There were at least a hundred and fifty people attending the soirée. Again, Alicia recognized the different architectural styles blending so easily through so many lifetimes. These thick, ancient walls could tell many stories from past centuries and Alicia hoped that, if her Aunt and others following could keep up the good work, they would do so for many years to come. Pray to God that this beautiful city should never be allowed to sink into the sea, as the more pessimistic scientists were predicting.

The evening was typically Italian in its ostentatious decoration and flamboyance. This was in the old style of entertaining, a world apart from the time in which they now all lived. You could have been engulfed in a time warp, thought Alicia. It was lovely to witness. The older generation were all dressed up to the nines, the women wearing whole sets of sparkling jewellery, all continuing to keep up the highest standards, following the traditions as set down by their ancestors. Alicia was well aware of the envious glances directed towards her neck. The dinner tables were covered in cream linen and immaculately laid up; each with candelabra, fine china, Venetian glass and shining silver. The conversation was riveting, particularly as Alicia had been told all sorts of interesting information and gossip beforehand by her aunt. The other dinner guests were a complete mixture: friends, people from the government and even one of the Belgian princesses who just happened to be there with her husband, giving the Italians an excuse for even more pomp and ceremony.

The Count, Marco, her 'amante' from eight years earlier, had seen her as soon as she walked through the door. Caro was being welcomed by some important looking dignitary swathed in a crimson sash and Alicia had taken the opportunity to turn away and lower her mask for a minute while she collected herself after the incident with Marcello outside. She'd have liked to disappear to the ladies room, but after relinquishing her borrowed evening coat, her Aunt had marched Alicia straight ahead into the reception room. Alicia's hand was shaking. Marco spied her from the other side of the room and hurried over. He removed his mask to greet her and gathered her into his embrace, mistakenly believing her nervousness to be on his account - the very last thing Alicia would have wished.

"*Bella, bella, bellissima Alicia.*" He was older of course, but still fit and attractive looking and made no bones about being delighted to see her again.

Alicia was thankful for the diversion, drank a glass of champagne rather too quickly then found she was able to enter into the evening's celebrations much more easily. Caro soon came to drag her out of the clutches of the still ardent Marco and took her proudly around the room, introducing her only to those that she considered suitable.

Dinner consisted of many courses, all accompanied by different wines. Alicia thought it was the longest meal that she had ever sat through. The inevitable Italian expresso coffee was served with more pomp and ceremony in the same grand salon, in which the champagne reception had been held before dinner. She found herself much sought after by the younger generation, as well as Marco and even by some of the other older men, who were all thrilled to be able to show off to someone new. She was young and beautiful and, now that she had entered their social scene, the Italians had every intention of enjoying each moment of Alicia's company, except perhaps for some of the elderly and more staid dowagers, who made it quite clear that they thought their husbands were making complete fools of themselves, drooling over the young English girl with the fabulous aquamarines.

Marco was adamant that Alicia didn't need to meet his wife, which she found amusing, but faintly ridiculous. Nevertheless, Caro was delighted to point the woman out when she came into view, but was safely over on the far side of the room! Quite frankly, she looked like a right old dragon, even in disguise, but she'd given Marco the children for which he had longed to carry on his family name. Marco must obviously keep himself entertained and busy, away from the marital home, Alicia thought, judging by his behaviour towards her.

The dancing started promptly at ten-thirty. Alicia was swept up into the carnival atmosphere, as the masked dancers whirled her around and around, even though they were all virtual strangers. The men were so well disguised that unless they spoke she really had no idea with whom she was dancing. It was exhilarating and, together with the champagne was also dangerously intoxicating!

As the evening wore on, Alicia decided to escape to get some much needed air and to search out the bathroom. Funny, really, how the French and the Italians never seemed to have the need, in spite of all the wine they drank. She asked one of the staff near the entrance to the ballroom, who looked thoroughly disapproving. He showed her to a door off the huge hall, where she saw an arrow which she imagined was pointing in the right direction. She set off along a long corridor, with huge mirrors, interspersed with full length portraits of distinguished people looking both ominous and grim faced. I certainly shouldn't like to meet any of this lot on a dark night, thought Alicia hurrying past.

The arrows were few and far between, then completely petered out. After a series of turns she found a, worn, stone-flagged, staircase and imagined it must lead up to the old family guest rooms. Walking past still more pictures on the panelled walls, all too dark to see properly and most in need of restoration, Alicia climbed the many steps to the top. Eventually, after trying about six different doors – success! She found a tiny old-fashioned, picture on a heavy panelled door, of a lady making up her face. Inside was a solid marble bathroom with wonderful looking silver accessories and over-ornate gilded fittings. Alicia could hardly believe such a bathroom still existed. 'Lucky this isn't England,' she said to herself, 'these things would have walked, even at a private party.'

Alicia looked at herself in the mirror. Her cheeks were pink with all the excitement and her large eyes stared back at her, as blue as the aquamarines in her ears and at her neck. She fingered the sparkling stones, lost in thought for a moment as she continued to study her image. Her body felt vibrant and warm - alive again for the first time since - no she really mustn't think of where she had been such a very short time ago and with whom. But she couldn't help how she felt, he had such a physical hold over her and she just longed to be back with him somewhere, anywhere. Where was he now? Was he still on duty out there maybe and could he get away again, even for just an hour or so? God, what was wrong with her? She was behaving like the proverbial Scarlet Lady - only her dress was blue. She shouldn't be thinking of Marcello but of Guy. Both her aunt and her mother would have a fit if they could read her thoughts.

As for Guy? Well, he'd left her without a word. Surely whatever it was should be finished by now and he could have had someone bring her a message, whatever difficulty he was in. Alicia was even unsure about the flowers now. The whole thing was just too much and she'd just about had enough. How patient could any one person be? She wished that things could be different, especially tonight of all nights, with all those virile men down there, competing for her attention. The disguises were brilliantly colourful and undeniably alluring. She could tell the younger men only by their shape and the way they carried themselves. Even those with whom she didn't dance she found beguiling and couldn't help wondering what went on behind the clever masks. But she was aware of eyes following her around the room; she recognised the fragility of her situation and experienced a cold clutch of loneliness.

It must have been the champagne intensifying her feelings, after seeing Marcello again so unexpectedly, she couldn't help herself: she really wanted to be with him. He made her feel so good. She wished, at this moment, that they could just disappear together and be alone, away from prying eyes and back in the little farmhouse near Verona. He was so near and yet he seemed to have moved away, not just physically, but mentally, almost as if he'd made the decision for them both: that when they'd said goodbye, this time, he knew it to be the end and that their short, precious time together was over. He had been on duty outside the *palazzo* there just now and was doing his job. Yet, why was he here at all? It seemed odd that he should be in Venice at the same time as her and had even been given the job of policing the entrance to the palace and the steps, where she was to walk this particular evening.

She wondered, not for the first time, if Marcello also knew a lot more about what was going on than he had told her. How come whatever it was appeared to have followed her now to Venice? Was she really a large part of it? Was there still some lurking danger looming over her? If so; where on earth were the two men and why weren't they looking after and protecting their women from this unknown evil?

They are all very good at excluding me and Adriana from their plans, she concluded. Being kept in the dark, when something was going on that seriously affected you, had to be one of the worst experiences in life. She wandered how Adriana was feeling and wished fervently, that they could be together. At least they'd be able to talk about it all. She decided to ask Nick to step up his investigations. She felt frustrated and annoyed by her own inability to take any more action herself.

What was wrong with her? She had drunk a little too much, she thought, but then Marcello and Marco in one evening was really over the top. Marco really was becoming a bit of a nuisance. He was starting to add to her problems. She wondered if he'd continue his unwanted attentions after this evening. She rather thought he would. She must be careful downstairs or she'd be in some difficulty extricating herself gracefully and then Caro would be upset.

Alicia felt thoroughly hyped up. She held her wrists under the cold tap for a moment to steady her racing pulse then carefully dried them, not wanting to splash her dress. A touch of Guy's favourite scent: 'Joy' by Patou; as old as the hills and impossibly expensive. Perhaps now was the moment to get something new, symbolic perhaps that it might be time to move on. She needed some more, but Guy always gave it to her and she was afraid it might bring more bad luck, or something, if she bought it herself. 'How absurdly stupid' Alicia said to the mirror! 'I'll definitely get something else tomorrow, something new that spells excitement'.

She was fed up with the continual waiting: waiting for everything, waiting for anything to happen at all as far as Guy was concerned. God knows how long had it been now. Nearly three months she supposed. Well, she couldn't wait for ever and if Marcello did find his way to her side again, perhaps this very night, then 'what will be will be' and 'tough luck, Guy. This decision made, it was time to find her way back before she was missed and considered too English to be true for not being able to last the whole evening!

~

Alicia set off, with new resolve, back the way she thought she had come, then, soon realized that she must have taken a wrong turn as the music sounded even further away. She was just wondering which way to go when in the distance she saw a fellow guest, or so she presumed, who seemed almost to be waiting for her. A weird feeling shot through her stomach turning it upside down. How odd; it looked like that jester from outside. Had he been downstairs as well? Intrigued, she began to follow, if somewhat hesitantly, almost as if drawn. After all it was a private party, by invitation only, with a huge amount of security surrounding the glittering guest list and she could ask the mysterious harlequin to show her the way. As she reached the end of the long passage the figure she was following seemed to have disappeared. In which direction did he go? Alicia stood between two pillars deliberating and listening hard in the silence. Then she sensed a presence. But, before she had time to move, a shadow darted out from behind the pillar on her right and all in one heart stopping moment she was caught, pulled towards him, turned and once again enveloped by those, strong, so familiar arms.

"Mar ...," but before she could finish his name, or cry out with joy after her initial fright, her strangled exclamation of denial was swept aside, her mask pushed away and he found her mouth. Forcing his tongue between her teeth he began to explore and to kiss her with such intensity that her heart lurched in excitement, then, her brain cleared suddenly with shocked surprise, as she realized her mistake: it wasn't her gentle policeman.

The surge of adrenalin from her fear changed instantly to a rushing sense of such desperate need, as her insides began to melt and her legs to give way beneath her with overwhelming excitement. Miracle of all things, Guy was alive, here and making love to her, as if he'd read her very thoughts!

Somewhere in the outer recesses of her mind, she thanked God for the stupefying effects of champagne and sent a mental message, willing it to be received. 'Marcello, I'm so sorry but you have nothing to do with this. You and I and what we have had together is another story and never to be forgotten. You saved my sanity and my life. Forgive me! But this here and now is me, the rest of my life and my very reason for living.' She had never felt such energy surging through her body.

Guy held her ever tighter, safe within his arms, moulding his body to hers. The familiar sensations, so well practiced from before, began to overpower her. All worry and unhappiness seemed to fade into something inconsequential compared to this moment in time, when nothing else mattered but this compelling, intense, appetite they still had for each other. It had to be satisfied at all costs right here and now, without delay. No matter the danger or the urgency; if anything it merely strengthened their desire.

He picked her up and impatiently pushed a door open behind him with his shoulder. She heard the soft click as he kicked it shut with his foot and lowered her to the floor. His eyes never leaving hers he reached expertly up and underneath her silk skirt, moved the tiny silk covering to one side to touch and feel and stroke that part of her that he remembered so well and had thought of so much. Finding her soft and yielding he deftly pulled the delicate cloth down and away, she was shivering and her breathing became fast and furious. Still not a word was spoken as their passion continued to escalate.

She moaned as he pushed her back up against the heavy door for support. With his two hands behind and underneath he took possession of her writhing body as slowly as he was able, needing to savour the ultimate moment of his power over her. Then control abandoned, he thrust into the very core of her being and felt her close around him. With their mouths locked, their bodies as one, they climbed that mountain of sensation together, to the very summit where it hovered, held at the brink, soared, then, burst with joy into that other world of throbbing, pulsating, incomparable relief.

The urgent ferocity of unbridled passion left the reunited lovers dazed and shuddering. They held each other still, as if their very lives depended on never letting go again. They drowned in a wealth of sensation, tightly cleaved together as one half of the other, gently rocking in unison, catching their breath.

Time stood still, nothing else mattered now. He reached behind her with one hand to search for the door lock, finding it above her head, he rammed the bolt home. The shock of sound seemed loud against the silence beyond, yet, it merely heightened the already charged atmosphere within the room. Then, he was lifting her dress over her head and reclaiming her mouth once more. He could feel her quivering and tightening around him again. He felt her breasts, the nipples hard against his skin. He bent to suck and stroke and caress. Her smooth skin was like silk and the fragrance, which he remembered so well, made distinctive by her warmth. She made an incoherent noise from the bottom of her throat as with more force he continued to thrust deeper. Their appetite unquenched, merely paused and then, carried them further with renewed vigour, into deep primal expectancy. And still not a word had either of them spoken.

~

How long they stayed like this before moving to the floor and finally the bed, Alicia really couldn't remember. It seemed as if they were on a cloud somewhere else, high above the earth and out of this world, seeing it from another dimension. Finally, completely saturated with each other, both mentally and physically, they became themselves again and remembered where they were and what they were about.

When at last Alicia could speak, her face wet with tears of raw sensual gratification she began to question, but Guy stopped her and placing his hand gently over her mouth said,

"Alicia! No! My darling, listen, now listen to me carefully. I can't tell you anything at this time. One day I'll tell you the whole story but not now, there's no time, we have already used it."

He grinned and kissed her once more touching her face tenderly, then, urgently, as he could see her about to argue again he repeated.

"No, not now! You are in great danger and must leave here at once. Everything is arranged, you must go to the landing steps where your Aunt's launch is waiting." He paused. "It's alright. She knows." As this piece of information sunk in Alicia looked incredulous. "I have a note here for you from her. Read it on the boat. You will go to the airport where a small plane is waiting to take you somewhere safe and where you must wait for me. Now take this cloak. Your Aunt sent it. And wear your mask, it suits you, until you actually board the plane. Your things are already on it." She looked deeply into his eyes and realized that questions were useless. She understood the urgency but just one thing she had to know.

"Julian?"

"Yes, yes, Julian is fine and now Adriana knows as well. Get dressed before M.I.6 offers you a job too!" Her smile widened to encompass the whole room and she clasped her hands together with the loss of such a huge burden.

"I knew, in my heart, I always knew and so did Adriana, but ... but the funeral who ..." He cut her short.

"Not now, later. I know it's difficult but all will be revealed later." Smiling he helped her quickly, wrapping her in the cloak, then clasping her to him, said more earnestly than ever,

"Alicia look at me. Trust me for a little longer, my darling. You'll be quite safe where I'm sending you and I shan't have to worry." Then, very quietly, "I love you and until this is over ... you're always with me, here," as he took her hand and placed it on his heart.

"And I you and you too are here with me. You always have been, in spite of everything," she whispered with a sob, taking his hand to her heart, unable to look away, as her eyes spilled over with tears, willing this moment to last for ever.

But time was precious and Guy knew that they had no more to lose. He unbolted the door and opened it wide. They looked back together, then at each other, their love reaffirmed. With a catch in his throat he said,

"Now you must go, down those stairs," pointing to the stone steps hidden behind the pillar, "all the way to the bottom and there you'll find the boat with Alonzo ready and waiting, now go … and quickly".

He gave her a push in the right direction, hoping she'd understood and hurry. She started forward, heard the click of a door closing and, sensing the emptiness, looked around once, but he'd gone already, almost as if the whole interlude had indeed been a dream.

Alicia decided to try not to think for the moment but to concentrate entirely on what she'd been told. She went as fast as she dared down the old uneven steps, which wasn't easy as her legs were hardly able to carry her, reminding her that no dream could leave you feeling quite like this. As she neared the bottom she could both hear and smell the water and sure enough there was the boat, with Alonzo standing alert and listening, watching out for her.

She lifted her beautiful but crumpled dress as carefully as she could and stepped aboard, with as much dignity as she could muster. The engine was already running. Alonzo touched his hat to her in recognition and they were away, almost as if this was a perfectly normal journey across the water in the middle of the night to the airport, when in fact no normal aircraft would be flying over the city at this hour.

~

Guy sighed with relief as from a window above he watched the launch disappear into the distance. His darling girl would be safe soon. He'd taken immense trouble to make sure of that. Now it was time to meet Julian and together they must help settle this thing and bring it to its proper conclusion as quickly as possible. He couldn't stand being away from Alicia much longer. Tonight had been unplanned and incredible, but now he had to get back to work and fast, for he'd broken all the rules.

He was just about to turn away when a movement below caught his eye. Immediately on guard, he leant out a little further to see what had attracted his attention. How strange; someone was standing there, apparently watching, as he was. It looked like a policeman. He could see the uniform. It must have been one of the *folgore,* who was working with them. Well, he was certainly doing his job. Then, as he watched, he saw something quite extraordinary. The man touched first his head, then his heart and then his lips with his hand, then raised it out across the water as if in farewell and, as he did so, Guy could see his face under the street lamp.

It was the same man who had stepped into his path and stopped him approaching Alicia at the steps into the palace earlier! Now he had turned and was walking slowly away with his head down. My God! thought Guy. It's Alicia he's watching. He's saying goodbye to her, just as I am! He knows her and well, by the look of it. He grabbed his jester's hat and ran out of the room and down the stone steps two at a time. Then he hurried along beside the water to catch up with the policeman. Marcello heard him coming, turned around to face him and waited for him to approach.

"Buona sera, Signore."

"Good evening, *buona sera,*" answered Guy politely taking off his mask. They both stood, silently surveying each other and wondering what the other was thinking. Then Guy, having made his decision, held his hand out to Marcello and said,

"Thank you. Thank you for looking after her." first in English, then in Italian. What else could he say? Marcello took his hand, held it for some time then, answered equally politely.

"She's a very beautiful lady and needs looking after. You are a lucky man."

His eyes were dark and fathomless. "My good wishes go with you both. *Buona sera,* again *Signore,*" and with that he clicked his heels, saluted and walked quietly away.

"Wait!" called Guy. "Please wait a moment. May I know your name?" the policeman looked back once over his shoulder.

"Marcello," he said and continued on his way. Guy stood a few moments longer staring after him with his hat under his arm. Marcello. Was that the name of Gianni's man with Alicia on the train to the South of France? He wasn't sure, but thought perhaps it was. He cocked his head on one side to listen for her boat. A soft, distant, chugging could still be heard as it negotiated its way out into the open space of the lagoon. It was one of very few out on the water at this time of the night.

~

Guy decided then and there, he would never ask her, for he already knew the answer.

~

'He knows', thought Marcello, as he walked on without looking back again. 'He knows what Alicia and I have had together. She may be his now and in the future, but she had been lost to the Englishman for those precious nights. Both in the cottage and in the train she had belonged to Marcello. She had been totally and utterly his. There was no doubt about that.' Those two nights really would have to last him a lifetime. 'It was over.'

~

Alicia had looked back as the boat moved away from the side. She saw a man's head and shoulders framed in an upper window of the old palazzo, silhouetted against the dull light behind him and she knew it was Guy. She stared up, willing him to know she was reaching out to him.

Then out of the corner of her eye she, too, saw another movement, this time out of the shadows, beside the water's edge, near the steps she'd just descended. A man moved into the light under the street lamp, a policeman. It was Marcello. There was no mistaking him as she saw him move his hand and make the same gesture towards her disappearing boat as he had done earlier.

Alicia stood and stifling her emotion, took a huge gulp of air and raised both her hands, bringing them to her mouth and blowing them away again. She couldn't tell if either of them had seen her. She could only hope they had. As the boat turned away, into another canal, the two men were finally lost from sight altogether. She sank down exhausted. Alonzo, thankfully, was concentrating on the corner.

★★★

CHAPTER 27

G uy stuffed the farcical jester's hat into the bag with the rest of his discarded costume, slung it over his shoulder and, after taking a quick look to make sure that there was no one else around, set off at a slow jog back to his digs for a shower and then on to meet Julian. He was late, very late indeed, but it couldn't be helped.

He felt a lot better. Never mind his revealing meeting with Marcello; Alicia and he had found each other again. There was no question about it. God willing, it was going to be all right between them, in spite of their enforced estrangement and the damage done by the strange circumstances of his sudden and unannounced departure. Now it was back to work with a vengeance and extreme concentration on his part. His brain needed to stay alert and energized, even if his sated, body flagged a bit, after the unplanned, interlude with Alicia, it must restore itself quickly.

He hadn't reckoned on Alicia getting to grips with her detective work quite so well. If only she had just stayed quietly at home and waited. However he now accepted that this would have been entirely out of character. She wouldn't have believed that he had abandoned her without reason. She would never have just sat miserably at home after being left. He wondered how he would have felt had their roles been reversed. He would also have had to do something, anything, to find out what was going on and what had happened.

Little did Alicia know how difficult it had been for him to arrange surveillance for her safe-keeping. The team he'd organized had a hard task keeping track of her impulsive movements.

~

It had been Guy's telephone call from Julian from the US, in the middle of the night, that had been the beginning of the whole sorry saga. As soon as Julian had told him that the young Arab had their department's most recent emergency liaison number in Maryland and given him the details of the dodgy looking passport, he'd gone into action. He was inextricably involved from that point on.

His call to their old headquarters in Hereford and his subsequent conversation with the S.I.S, the Secret Intelligence Service, threw everybody into an instant frenzy. How had the Arab ever got hold of the number in the first place? Who on earth could have given it to him? And why was it written down? Nobody seemed to know, or rather if they did, no one was about to admit to this blatant misconduct. It was a breach of the department's most fundamental and basic rule which everybody had embedded in their brain, right from the beginning of their training. There had to be a bad leak which threatened yet another internal mole hunt.

The intelligence exchange between the two countries worked well and efficiently. Both services moved extremely fast. The young Arab's true identity, soon disclosed, made the bag and its contents of exceptional interest. He was a double agent with contacts in several key terrorist groups around the world, concentrated mainly in the Far East and North Africa, from whence he had come this time. The information he held was vital and it was essential that he was kept alive in order to be able to access his secrets quickly. The computer contained far reaching and momentous data, they were sure. It could be read, but this would take time, as the programmes were well encrypted and speed was of the essence.

Julian had been instructed to take the next flight home, bringing everything back with him. There had been a certain amount of dispute over whether the computer should be left with the National Security Agency in America, as it had been found on American soil, or brought home to

G.C.H.Q in U.K. England had won! Julian had been flown by helicopter to Miami from the hotel's base on the mainland, scrambled literally as he'd crossed the channel from the island, making his mobile calls as they flew across the water.

By the time he'd arrived at Miami airport, his travel, arrangements were already made. A flight, due to leave for Heathrow, had been held. He was met by two FBI agents, who had whisked him through their own private route and onto the plane. One had made the whole journey to England with him. Julian couldn't have been on the ground for more than ten minutes after leaving the helicopter. Once he and his companion had boarded, the big plane closed up its doors and took off. Airborne, the F.B.I agent had gone straight to sleep, a merciful relief for Julian. He wanted to be quiet while he assessed the situation and sorted his own thoughts into some semblance of order.

~

Guy had flown in from the Channel Islands, by private jet, to meet Julian at Heathrow. They had a friend living in Guernsey whose business was flying people to and from France. The man also did a lot of 'police' work, so was well used to undercover operations. Sworn to secrecy, he was happy to oblige with the unexpected trip to Heathrow. Guy had managed to finish his meetings before leaving Guernsey and even had the presence of mind to remember to send Alicia her usual bunch of flowers. The whole trip, up to then, had appeared normal and was right on schedule. She had thought him to be on his way to Paris as planned. That was the last time that she'd had news of him by text.

The timing had coincided perfectly with Julian's arrival from America. It would have been quite impossible for anybody to have kept up with Julian's sudden change of plans and his return flight from the U.S.

As Julian's flight came in to land, a conference was being set up on the ground at Heathrow. It was to be well away from the ordinary passenger terminals, attended by Guy, Julian, F.B.I, C.I.A and British Intelligence Agency representatives. On his arrival, the bag had been whisked away to G.C.H.Q in Cheltenham for its contents to be studied, while Julian recounted his story. Poor Julian: he had been mortified, when he'd realized, half way across the Atlantic that the post card to Alicia was missing. It really had been a terrible blow. Now they were all implicated. When he had written it, he had no inkling of any mission involving security and had no reason to give the card a second thought. The thugs would almost certainly have found it on the ground, whilst searching for the bag.

Whilst the clandestine group were discussing their future strategy, more news came in from America. The Arab had been found, unconscious and left for dead down the far end of Little Beach island. He was so badly hurt that it was unlikely that he'd ever recover consciousness. That was another heavy blow. The hotel confirmed that a business dinner had been booked in a private room that night at the Beach Hotel restaurant. So far they hadn't discovered with whom, as nobody had turned up. The booking appeared to have been made in the name of someone's assistant. The F.B.I thought that the information held on the computer was intended to be handed over that evening. Unluckily for the Arab, he had been trailed as he'd travelled from North Africa, via Europe and had been pounced on as he'd arrived on the island. M.I.6 verified that members of the Italian *mafiosa* were on the move and seemed to have been following pretty much in the young man's footsteps.

Once acquired, God alone only knew what the mafia intended to do with the knowledge from the computer. Its damage could be catastrophic: its value incalculable. It was of paramount importance to find out what data it held.

~

During the secret conference more dramatic news arrived from America via the F.B.I. An eminent politician running for Congress and his personnel had been assassinated on his luxury yacht off the Florida Keys.

Several, expertly linked, semtex bombs had been planted in the boat and detonated, with her owner and crew all on board. They had not a chance. The boat, with everybody and everything on it, was blown to bits. Even identification of those who lost their lives turned out to be a difficult and time-consuming problem.

It had been established, indisputably, that the politician had issued instructions, the previous day, for his boat to be made ready to sail to Little Beach Island that particular night. A mooring had been reserved, a private room arranged and a dinner reservation made under a false name. The boat, unsurprisingly, was called *'Elizabeth Mac'* after his wife and himself and its home berth was in the main Key West marina. The vital link had been revealed. With the politician gone and the Arab out of circulation, there was no way of knowing the content of their planned meeting at the hotel; except from the computer, which held the key to the enigma.

The connection had been made and the die cast, albeit too late for the prospective congressman and his unsuspecting crew. At least their deaths had been instantaneous. The horrific act was all over the U.S newspapers. The families must have been devastated. The mafia were already being accused, but the suspected reason behind the atrocity was being kept most thoroughly under wraps, at least for the time being.

After concentrating on getting Julian away and finding out about the young Arab, the Americans had bungled. They'd missed the link with the hotel and several lives had been lost, one, taking invaluable intelligence with him. Julian and Guy had both thought that the hotel guest list for the weekend should have been the first priority, particularly the dinner reservations. There had to be something else. It was obvious that the Arab hadn't planned his encounter with the mafia. He had been considered reliable, so it was more than likely that he'd had a rendezvous arranged on the island that evening. The F.B.I should have discovered who it had involved and that it was to be held at government level. Little Beach was in a perfect and secure location for a meeting of such importance.

As for Julian, he had been kicking himself for not having understood the second piece of information on the screwed up scrap of paper when he had found it. Every one of his summer holidays as a child had been spent mucking about by the sea, or on the water. He should have recognized that the name *'Elizabeth Mac*, Key West', must surely suggest a yacht.

The men who committed the murders had, for the moment, disappeared without trace. Their boat had been found abandoned. It had been hidden in a cove on another small uninhabited island near Little Beach, leaving no clue as to the whereabouts of the thugs. They could even have been lifted off by helicopter. The guardian, Sam, had thought he'd heard one as he'd rushed down the island on his buggy to rescue the Arab. By now they would be somewhere in or around Miami, lying low after the killings and collecting their people together, whilst formulating a plan to find Julian, who had vanished so completely. They would be wondering if he had any idea what he had, or just how revealing, explosive even, the contents of the computer might be.

The young Arab must have hoped that he had managed to convey the urgency for Julian to find and remove the bag from under the bush. Under extreme duress, he would have told the mafia where he'd left it, thinking perhaps, that this might be the last chance to save his own neck. The people into whose hands he'd inadvertently fallen were experienced and well able to inflict pain at its most excruciating level. The poor man must have endured terrible suffering.

When the killers had failed to find the bag, they would have picked up the postcard, which provided them with the vital clue. It was their easy way forward. Finding it would have saved them much trouble in learning Julian's identity and in tracing his closest friends and family.

~

The situation had escalated for the worse in a very short time. While the information on the computer was being deciphered, the two friends had simply been told that they must 'vanish' for a while. Guy could easily absent himself from Guernsey and Julian quite probably could 'cease to exist' altogether. This would be decided later; the department would 'work on a story'. As far as the world was concerned, for the moment, he was supposedly abroad with his job and incommunicado.

Guy and Julian knew the procedure from the past and had foreseen this dire turn of events. They had no choice but to agree. The waiting game commenced. Only time could tell what secrets the computer would reveal. The programmes had been expertly enciphered, making them exceptionally difficult to open and read. If only the young Arab had lived and remained coherent so much time would have been saved. Both men were told that Alicia and Adriana would have twenty-four hours protective surveillance, to be activated immediately. Their families also would be taken care of, if it was deemed necessary. But, no civilian was to have any inkling about the true situation. This was considered the safest course for all concerned. If things went badly wrong, what others didn't know, they couldn't tell.

As planned Guy and Julian dropped out of view to mark time, unhappily having to accept the agony that their families and the girls would have to endure. They were installed in a safe house in Switzerland, well known from the past. The men arrived there together and spent their time getting themselves back into peak fitness in the mountains. In the event of trouble they hoped they would be allowed to participate. If not, they joked, they were sure that the girls would appreciate them better anyway, never imagining for a minute what a long drawn out saga it was going to be. Surely Cheltenham experts would come up with the results from the computer quickly and the *mafiosa* murderers would soon be apprehended? Unfortunately, even with the speed and efficiency of the Intelligence Agencies on both sides of the Atlantic, it hadn't been that simple.

The computer codes had eventually been three parts broken and the programmes opened for thorough analysis. The first and most dramatic find was a comprehensive list of stored data giving the names and whereabouts of key terrorist organizations throughout the world, some known, some suspected but some completely new and of inestimable value. There was further information still to be decoded, thought possibly to be hidden files with lists of biological weaponry and even details of atrocities planned for the future. These now, hopefully, would come to nothing. Throughout the elite intelligence circles, worldwide, the computer with its priceless software was acknowledged to be a major coup for the British.

~

When Guy and Julian had been informed of Alicia's unexpected move to Italy, they could sit still on their mountain no longer.

Guy had been astonished to discover that Alicia had bowled up on Delfino Island, by way of her mother's friends. It had to have been the worst piece of luck, considering all the other places in the world she could have chosen. The possibility of harm coming to his adored fiancée while he was sitting on his backside, stuck up a mountain, was not an option, in Guy's opinion. Any man would go berserk, he argued as they drummed up support from their old bosses in Hereford to get back in action. After all, Julian had brought in the intelligence in the first place.

The Director Special Forces agreed to seek permission from the Chief of Defence Staff to allow them out of hiding and to become actively involved. It was complimentary and essential to the planned, secret operation, the Director had reasoned. With a well developed strategy, they could smoke out the murderers more easily for identification by Julian, while drawing attention away from the girls at the same time. The Foreign and Commonwealth Office's telephone line with the Chief S.I.S must have been red hot as they finalised the three way operation with their Italian counterparts, while keeping the Pentagon on side as well.

The nearer the two girls came to learning at least part of the truth, the more dangerous it had become for them. Unbeknown to the two friends they were drawing attention to themselves, making it easy to be found and followed. They could lead the mafia to their goal. Finding the postcard on Little Beach Island had been pure luck as far as the criminals were concerned because it was indicative of how closely the girls and both men were all linked.

With Julian in disguise, the two men then left their safe house and had flown directly to Italy in the small plane which had been put at their disposal. Whilst constantly on the move, they exerted all their influence and used all their associated contacts in Europe to coordinate a highly professional team to protect and look after the girls, wherever they went. Their early years of training in the S.A.S stood them in good stead. Both also had a long established and workable relationship with the Italian *Intelligenzia*. They integrated their own people with the undercover Italian *Folgore*.

Alicia put the cat among the pigeons when she left Delfino Island to visit Verona. She'd been absolutely safe there with Gianni and his family, although Gianni, at that time, was still unaware of the Intelligence movements in the Venetian area. There had seemed to be no point in worrying him. Their one big mistake had been not involving Gianni right at the very beginning. He would have made sure that Alicia stayed on the island. Guy was horrified when he learned that the Italians had turned up on her train. They must have been lying in wait for her to come back to the mainland; hoping that Alicia might be of use to them.

Guy had been allowed to take the surveillance job himself for the night of the opera. He had been determined to catch just a glimpse of Alicia to reassure himself that she was alright. He had been somewhat taken aback when he'd discovered that the opera to be performed that night was none other than The Flying Dutchman. It seemed particularly significant.

The 'mugging' incident was frightening and unfortunate, but at least there had been somebody in place, who went quickly to Alicia's aid. It also confirmed that the concern for her safety was very real indeed. From then on she was even better protected, in spite of the dramatic assault on the train, which ought to have been well covered.

~

With hindsight Guy knew he should never have sent the dried flowers to Alicia on her birthday, as this had prompted her move to the South of

France. He'd wanted to send her some small message of hope, of reassurance. But he hadn't realized that it would send her into an even more frenzied pursuit of the truth.

Guy was also greatly relieved to find Gianni had managed to persuade Alicia to stay with another of their trusted friends, the d'Auberts, when she had been determined to set off to the Riviera. Quite obviously, Gianni had worked out for himself the significance of the flowers. Between Gianni and Jacques, Alicia was as safe as she could be in the *Chateau d'Aubert* and better off out of Italy.

~

As they had been told would happen, Intelligence arranged Julian's 'final accident' in the South of France. That was the one thing that had turned out to be a lot easier than they had expected. Just before they arrived there, two Albanian refugees had stolen a boat from the old port in Cannes, taken it out between the islands and anchored; before setting out to get completely high on a large amount of alcohol and dope. It was thought that they'd eventually fallen over the side in a stupor. Both had drowned. Nobody had taken any notice of a boat moored out there. People often went to fish between the islands. With no passports or identification, French Intelligence was happy to help and to put out the story of Julian's unfortunate 'accident' instead of what had really occurred. Nobody saw the boat being taken; it had been moored away on its own. The local French police were also delighted to have the incident so quickly wrapped up and two more illegal immigrants dealt with so easily.

But the murderers of the American boat crew still had to be apprehended. British Intelligence and the Italian *Servizi Segreti* were searching for their lost quarry, who were obviously still lying low, after coming to a 'dead end', quite literally as far as Julian was concerned.

Believing the information still intact and theirs for the taking, the mafia bosses, were, by now, certainly demented with frustration. Their minions must have been in fear of their lives for having failed to find the computer, even with the help of their own underground network. They were employed by a powerful body of people who controlled their workforce's lives with terror and to whom failure was unacceptable and only answerable with a bullet.

Regrouped and collected, the *mafiosa* were eventually bound to come out of hiding into the open once more. The coordinated teams were counting on it. A deadly game of cat and mouse was being played out.

~

After the girls' adventures in the South of France, Adriana was easier to look after. When she returned to London she'd stayed quiet as she had been asked, whilst waiting for news of Julian.

Alicia was another matter. Guy had hoped that, after saying goodbye to Adriana in France, she would have returned to Gianni and Delfino Island. No such luck! When she arrived in Venice, she landed back in the middle of the hottest spot of all: wrong place, wrong time. Everybody was there! Just as Julian and Guy were hoping to wind up the whole operation quickly, Alicia's presence had created another huge problem, although her appearance must have seemed like a gift from providence to the villains.

At the first opportunity, Guy had organized his secret meeting with the Contessa. She was fiercely protective of Alicia, but once he'd said his piece, they'd got on like a house on fire, in spite of the sparky start.

The newly enlightened Gianni, together with the accommodating Italian *Intelligenzia,* had helped him coordinate a more extensive team, now spread over a wide area in the Veneto. The men enlisted were all well briefed and vigilant in their surveillance duties; keeping watch over Alicia and looking out for the Sicilian 'trash' as Gianni insisted on calling them. Guy could hear him spitting out the words down the telephone and no doubt gesticulating wildly as well, emphasizing his disgust. It amused Guy to hear him still use some of the slang he'd taught him in the past.

They had worked together on numerous occasions, dealing with many a sensitive issue. Guy and Julian used to laugh together at Gianni's efforts to conquer the more difficult English phrases. On Delfino, they both got into trouble from Giuseppina, who pretended to be furious with them, saying she couldn't imagine why she'd ever bothered to spend so much time and trouble teaching her husband English in the first place, if all he really wanted to learn was 'rubbish'.

Gianni was obviously very fond of Alicia and determined above all else to keep her safe. Guy felt a warm, reassuring feeling spread through him, as if he had just walked in from the cold and stood before a welcoming fire. Gianni had done well for them all. It was largely due to him and his extraordinary powers of intuition that his fiancée had, so far, remained unharmed. The two old friends had enjoyed their contact again in spite of their existing dilemma.

~

Now, they were all gathered in Venice together, being watched constantly, while the observers were themselves under close surveillance. Guy had made his plans to get Alicia out fast. Patience was wearing thin on all fronts: he sensed time was running out. But this last evening had been another matter altogether.

After all the meticulous planning to get Alicia away under cover and at night, Guy hadn't been prepared for his over-powering love for her as she'd unexpectedly stood so near to him, as he crouched in the shadows of his dark hiding place in the palace. Thanks to Alicia's chance search for the ladies room they were ahead of schedule: she had discreetly made her own exit from the party. With his own adrenalin running high, he'd made a split second decision and thrust his better judgment aside. He just had to set her mind at rest and make himself known. He quite simply couldn't let her walk right on by.

Their stolen half hour was something that was totally unplanned. He didn't regret one single second of their spontaneous lovemaking. On the contrary, now that she'd seen him he felt that she really would do as he asked. He wanted her far away and out of the firing line until this was finally over.

~

Guy knew that it was now up to Julian and himself to draw the assassins out into the open, so that they could be caught, identified by Julian and put away for good. Then, perhaps, all of them could revert to their normal lives again. About time too, thought Guy grimly. He certainly wouldn't want to go back into this work full time. Not for all the money in the world he wouldn't. Besides which, he'd broken rules. As a younger man this would never have happened. Yet, in his own defence, nobody dear to him had ever been involved with the shadowy side of his life.

When the presence of the three criminals was confirmed and the numbers of their aides assessed, the intention was that Julian, resurrected from the dead and undisguised, should blatantly go 'walk about'. This, their superiors considered, would flush out the murderers. It was hoped that total confusion would result leading to the *mafiosa* making a sudden and rash move. The *folgore* were in place, planted all around the city and awaiting their opportunity as soon as it arose.

Nonetheless, both Julian and he would have to be exceptionally careful how they handled this last and final part of the drama. Guy knew he was being followed. By now, he thought, his enemies must also be becoming slightly suspicious of the rather portly man constantly there, incessantly smoking, beside him.

He could sense that these violent men were getting reckless, as their methods of tailing were becoming sloppy and obvious. They had to finish their assignment and get away, back to their base, with the required information extracted by whatever means. When the *mafioso* had what they wanted he and Julian would be of no use to them alive: they knew too much. Unless these evil people were caught they would both be living under a death sentence.

278

When Julian reappeared, it would become apparent that he and Guy were no ordinary untrained citizens. How, otherwise, could they have managed to disappear so completely without trace, for so long? As for Julian's most efficiently faked drowning, what would they make of that? And the girls? Guy was sure that the mafia would begin to understand exactly why it had been so difficult to get near them and what they were really up against.

They would realize, no doubt to their certain horror, that the computer and its secrets was not just sitting forgotten in a cupboard in some dingy little flat, waiting to be taken, but that it was in exceptionally skilled and capable hands and undergoing detailed scrutiny.

~

Guy received more ominous news: already responsible for murdering the politician and the boat's crew, the vile trio were now also accountable for the young Arab's death. He'd died in hospital a few hours earlier, without ever regaining consciousness. The young man had been in an appalling state, beaten to a pulp, when he had been found on Little Beach. Sam the guardian, true to his word, with his basic training and medical kit had got there very quickly and had done his best. The mafia had gone, but the poor wretched young man hadn't had long to suffer without help.

God alone only knew what they had planned for Alicia if they'd got to her on the train believing that she could lead them to Julian. It had been at that point that it had been decided to kill off Julian. SIS thought that, with Julian out of the picture, the heat would be taken off Alicia and transferred to Guy instead. Even so, wherever Alicia had gone the killers were still never very far behind. After Julian had given them the slip they weren't about to lose sight of the others.

Guy heard the little Cessna fly away into the night sky and felt enormous relief that Alicia was out of it and well on her way. The future was, to say the least, uncertain. He thanked God for Julian's and his own crack training, for their expertise, their most efficient help and support and, for all their friends in important places!

★★★

CHAPTER 28

While Guy and Julian were carefully trying to manoeuvre events in Venice towards a satisfactory ending, Alicia was winging her way across Europe to yet another unknown destination. She was deeply affected by the sudden turn of events and if it hadn't been for her crumpled dress and gently bruised body, the euphoric but short time that she and Guy had just spent together could have been a dream. She wished beyond all else that they could have had the whole night to themselves and without fear; to have had the freedom to turn to each other in the early hours of the morning with renewed vigour and a quivering anticipation for more. She longed to sleep in his arms again and to awake with the knowledge that all was well. Alicia sighed, thinking that after another bout of love making she would never have made it down those unused, steep and slippery steps to the boat. As it was, Alonzo had to catch her as she stumbled aboard, as if drunk and thoroughly dishevelled. He must have realized that something had happened, but appeared to take it all in his stride, politely unaware of Alicia's embarrassment at her appearance.

Weak with relief and her trust in Guy restored, Alicia knew she must now do as she was told, for both their sakes. She was happy to follow instructions for a change, now that he had explained to her that the situation was so very dangerous for them all. She wondered about Adriana and what she must be feeling and wished they could have been together, both when it had been confirmed that Julian was very much alive and now, whilst the wretched waiting continued. Guy had told her that when she reached her journey's end, she could make a quick call to Adriana, on a mobile that would be made available to her, but that she was not to give any indication of where she was. He would have organized this by the time she arrived: she couldn't wait.

Wrapped in the warm afterglow of passion and its emotional release, Alicia laid her head back against her seat and watched the sky begin to lighten. As the little plane flew on through the awakening dawn, she finally began to relax and even slept a little, tired out, but fulfilled, with a new calm serenity softening her features, confirming the ending of a certain inner conflict.

~

Alicia awoke with the sun on her face, as the plane was beginning its descent. She thought she had indeed been dreaming, but her body soon reminded her otherwise and happiness filled her heart. As the co-pilot brought her a cup of coffee and some biscuits she turned to thank him with a radiant smile on her face, as she thought about what had happened the night before, at the same time thankful that he was unable to read her thoughts.

What an unusually beautiful start to the day, thought the co-pilot as he turned away; wishing the smile on Alicia's face was really for him. You just never knew what to expect with this job. That's why he loved it so much. Never two day's the same, but few started as good as this!

He had noted how exceptionally attractive she was, when she came aboard, in her sparkling jewels and lovely evening dress, in the middle of the night. She had appeared disheveled and exhausted; but, with an almost contradictory, excited, yet tranquil look about her that, no man could have misread.

As he walked back to the cockpit, he wondered what on earth had been happening to this woman to necessitate her moving out of Venice so fast. On this occasion he wished that he had been allowed more information. The young Miss Spence intrigued him, but he knew better than to ask questions.

Alicia raised a hand to her face to see if it was burning as the co-pilot

moved away. She had felt his direct stare and wondered what he was thinking. Oh! My God! The aquamarines! Of course she suddenly remembered,
touching the beautiful necklace. How could she have forgotten? Very easily!
And Caro would understand she felt sure! Then she recalled the note Guy
had given her from her Aunt. She searched in her bag until she found it.

'My darling child,' it said, 'forgive me for the secret I couldn't share. You
looked so absolutely stunning this evening and you are to keep the aquamarines as my wedding present. Have faith and be patient for a little while
longer. All will be well, as I said once before. Goodbye, *bon voyage* and with
all my love, Caro.'

How typical of Caro! Such an absurdly generous present, yet, Alicia knew
she'd have to accept the gems with a good grace. Once an idea or plan was
firmly planted in her Aunt's head there was no shifting it. What an amazing
woman she was: all this time she must have had a good grip on the overall situation while, Alicia herself, annoyingly, to put it mildly, was left quite
unaware. Except of course for that one, odd, remark at dinner: after their
shopping spree and, Caro's uncharacteristic insistence of needing to know
Alicia's precise movements each day. A couple of instances had made Alicia
just a little suspicious of her Aunt's ability to find out more than she would
have thought possible.

~

The plane landed smoothly on a small strip near Bern, where Alicia was
met by a private taxi, taken across to the station and given her ticket by a
smiling young Swiss woman of similar age, who then helped her to her place
on the panoramic mountain train going in the direction of Gstaad. She had
a first class seat in the restaurant car and tucked into an excellent meal. She
had suddenly felt very hungry indeed. After all the excitement, not to speak
of the exercise, she had been famished!

~

Alicia's carriage was virtually empty, with only a middle-aged couple their
small dachshund and a thick set young man sharing it. She suspected that the

single man was there for her protection, which was a comforting thought. He smiled at her, periodically, as if he might know who she was. She was getting used to having some reassuring presence near at hand. Someone up there has been looking after me, thought Alicia, as well as those on the ground. She turned to the little dog, which was determined to make friends, wagging its tail and staring at her for attention, desperate to come and say hello. Its owners smiled indulgently.

Looking back at that very first incident in Verona, she'd thought, then that it was strange that the man had been there helping her at the exact moment that he was needed. Somehow he hadn't seemed like a mere passer by. Besides, he had also known her hotel, when she hadn't told him where she was staying!

As for Gianni, he seemed to make rather difficult arrangements as easily as if they were an everyday occurrence, with contacts everywhere, particularly in all the places she seemed to be visiting. Alicia wondered about Gianni, not for the first time. What else did he do other than run his island? And as for Jacques d'Aubert: there were, as yet, just so many unanswered questions to ponder.

However, there was little point in trying to fathom out these muddling matters any further, as everything seemed to be well taken care of, for the moment and out of her control anyway. No doubt Guy would tell her the whole story one day and explain just how the whole jigsaw fitted together.

~

As the mountain train wound its way up into the Alps, the scenery was breathtaking. Snow still lay on the top of the furthest peaks, in stark contrast to the emerald green grass in the foreground. Complacent looking cows grazed, their heads almost hidden in the lush grass. The huge bells around their thick necks clonked in several different tones, as the beasts moved their heads with each mouthful. A full orchestra: those nearest the train didn't even bother to look up and continued eating. The window was open and as the train's progress was slow, she could not only hear, but smell the animals as well. A rich, sweet, smell: good and healthy looking cows, thought Alicia, no wonder the Swiss milk, butter and cheeses were so special. The cattle must lead a very different life from the huge dairy herds in England.

She had been told the time of arrival in the little skiing village of Saanenmoser and, true to the efficient Swiss rail system, the train was punctual as it glided smoothly to a halt in the station. A very smart, lady, station mistress appeared from her ticket office and was waiting to see the passengers alight safely. As Alicia stood, the stocky young man was already at her side and helping her with her bag, which she had found, neatly packed and ready waiting for her, when she had boarded the plane during the night. They walked across the tracks to where there was a pony and trap, of all things, waiting to take her up the mountain. The station mistress waved them off, then returned to see her departing travellers safely aboard. How lucky that Alicia had thought to change out of her dress on the plane and put the aquamarines away safely.

This last part of her journey in the sun and clear mountain air was exhilarating, something never to be forgotten! Alicia had only ever had winter holidays in this part of Europe, thinking that summer was only for the older people who liked to walk once their skiing days were over. How wrong she had been, for this was so very different from anything that she had ever imagined.

They set off up a small road beside the winter ski lifts and then wound up through the trees until it narrowed to a track, carpeted with dried pine needles and fir cones. The fresh, slightly medicinal fragrance, reminded her instantly of the green bottle of pine essence in her parents' bathroom. As a little girl, she had loved to be allowed to pour it into the great big tub, breathing in the strong scent and being fascinated when the water turned magically green, in front of her eyes. She inhaled now with pure pleasure and a sense of well being flooding through her body.

They met just one old man, bringing half a dozen goats down the mountain, so stopped and waited for them all to pass. Zak, her escort's name she had discovered, shouted a greeting, afterwards explaining unnecessarily that the old man, an uncle, was as deaf as a post. A stream bubbled down alongside, full to the brim with the end of the melt snow from above, cascading down over rocky, lichen covered, water falls. They climbed ever higher up the mountain. Cowbells could be heard in the distance as the herds moved about in their summer pastures and the birdsong sounded pure and full of promise. There were piles of fallen branches and some trees brought down in the winter storms, all waiting to be collected then chopped and stored until ready for burning next winter. Alicia imagined the warmth of the pinewood fires keeping everybody snug inside. Outside, on the frozen landscape; warm jerseys, boots, bright hats and scarves, pink cheeks and ice cold noses, would be the order of the day. At night, after plenty of exercise skiing or tobogganing on the slopes, there would be hot chocolate or intoxicating gluhwein, all combined with animated laughter.

Eventually they were on top of the world, or so it seemed! In the early afternoon light it was a most breath-taking view. The highest ski-lifts were now far below and there was no building in sight. They stopped several times for the horse to have a rest. It was cool sitting still at this altitude. Her breathing had become slightly more laboured and Alicia worried for the horse. What an effort it must be pulling the cart up the mountain. No wonder the animal looked both thin and fit. She hoped this form of travel was never attempted in the heat of mid-summer.

Zak had been brought up in these mountains. He explained that he was taking her to his parent's house. It was the highest habitation in the area and not a single person could get near without being seen. 'Mister Guy' was always trying, but had never yet succeeded! He added with relish. This was interesting information, thought Alicia immediately warming to her driver.

The track finally petered out altogether, but Zak seemed to know the way, as if it were clearly marked. Just when she thought the journey would never end and her bones never recover, they rounded some rocks and there was the house, nestling in its own little green valley below them, completely hidden from the rest of the world. The chalet wasn't habitable in the winter, she was told, because it was completely covered in snow. So much so, that you wouldn't know there was a building there at all. Off-piste skiers would ski right over the top, little guessing what was buried underneath. Alicia could well imagine this, for there were still small pockets of snow around on the very tops of the highest mountains.

As they approached the small farm they were met by two, extremely fierce looking, dogs. Alicia had no intention of getting down until they were safely tied up. Zak laughed and said that they were only ever loose at night. She noticed later with some relief, that, they were actually secured on long heavy chains.

Once inside, Zak introduced Alicia to his parents. His mother was red faced, solid, yet cheerful; but his father appeared the sort of man she couldn't imagine anybody taking on gladly. He was certainly a man of very few words. Neither could speak much English, but they spoke *Switzerdeütch*, so Alicia knew that she wouldn't be expected to make much of an effort. The introductions made, Zak took her to her room then, giving her the same instructions as Guy, punched in some numbers and handed her his mobile. Both Alicia and Adriana could hardly speak they were so overjoyed, so there need have been no worry about either saying too much! During the call Zak remained within earshot, although he discreetly, turned his back and moved over to the window; then, he reclaimed the mobile and left her, in private, to settle in.

The room was simple but comfortable, typically Swiss with its light carved pine wood and embroidered curtains. There was a tiny bathroom, in a cupboard. The bedroom had a second door which opened into a sitting area, which Alicia was told she could use if she wanted to be quiet and read or write. It was only ever needed as a bedroom if there was another guest, when the comfortable sofa turned into a bed. There were plenty of books on a long shelf, some in English.

It was heartening to know that Guy had been here before her. When exactly? Alicia wondered with a sense of intrigue and for what reason? This man of hers was certainly someone of many hidden talents. No question but that, both he and Julian were dark horses. Obviously he still had much influence around the world and a very secret world at that. Although neither Alicia or Adriana knew anything of Guy and Julian's earlier 'specialist army training' as it was described and imagined it had all ended some years before, Alicia now realized that they had both been quite wrong. It had never been in the past, she thought, with some trepidation, what on earth were the men caught up in now and why should it affect her so dramatically?

She felt free from harm, here in the care of Zak and his family. Alicia understood that they were all well experienced in looking after people with unusual requirements. The situation, cut off from the rest of the world as it was, had to make it the most perfect safe house. She shivered involuntarily, wishing she knew why she should have to take refuge?

Alicia contemplated questioning Zak about Guy. He spoke good enough English, but maybe it would be best to bide her time, at least until she knew him better. Once more she had to endure the frustrating agony of waiting for news. With too much practice now of 'biding her time', Alicia decided that she wasn't the most patient of people. She was so relieved for Adriana; that her burden of grief had been lifted. It had been brilliant to talk to her, even for such a short time, but she wished so much that they could have been together. For the moment she was looking forward to a good night's sleep, in this haven of tranquillity, on the top of the world, distanced from all the unfolding drama which enveloped those that she loved, in that far away, mysterious and beautiful, yet sometimes sinister, city of her dreams.

★★★

CHAPTER 29

Julian was getting really worried now. Guy was extremely late. Julian was alone, sitting outside Florian's café, and he felt conspicuous. He'd been followed there again, of that he was certain.

Even without their present problems, Julian was by far the most serious minded of the two friends. He was tall, with the blonde good looks and piercing blue eyes inherited from his Swedish mother. They missed nothing. Normally his fair hair flopped all over his face, out of control and when he was hyped up, as he was now, he ran his long fingers through it all the time, whilst he smoked incessantly.

Thanks to the disguise and the ridiculous toupee thing, which he longed to take off, he really felt thoroughly irritated and fed up. He missed Adriana, the home they shared and his family. He was a sensitive man and fretted over being, at least in part, responsible for causing everyone so much grief. He also yearned for his music, particularly at the moment, for it calmed him. None of the people with whom Guy and he were involved at the moment would ever believe that, in his time off at home, Julian liked nothing better than to play his grandfather's precious flute in a small local orchestra. Adriana would always come to listen. It was at such a concert that they had originally met.

His dress was casually modern, though sensibly discreet and his figure slight and naturally gangling, but not at the moment, thanks to the wretched padding. All in all, Julian was a deceptively gentle giant and the complete opposite from Guy.

Guy was more matter of fact and took things in his stride. What happened, had just happened as far as he was concerned. There was no point in worrying about anything, except getting the job in hand done. Unlike Julian, he enjoyed all the excitement, although it was tempered by the pain that had been inflicted on both Alicia and Adriana.

Guy was of a much darker colouring than Julian and tanned easily, with curling hair, brown smiling eyes and a great sense of humour. He was a brilliant mimic. This, Julian always teased was 'the Irish in him' and his quick witted clowning, attracted woman like flies. His clothes, although conservative, had leanings towards an understated flamboyance. For important business evenings Alicia insisted on choosing his tie. He used to laugh at her for minding, as, in general, he never thought about nor cared what he looked like: but he did love bright colours. Guy was the stockier of the two but, in spite of Julian's smoking and Guy was constantly telling him that he should stop; both men were strong and healthy.

Together, the two men were a well matched team. They complimented each other and were good at everything they did, especially now as they were, once again, as fit as fiddles. Not that Julian looked it at the moment in his particularly unflattering outfit, as Guy delighted in telling him. He never stopped making a joke of it. Julian, in contrast, rather minded what he looked like and was sensitive on the subject.

Guy was very late now. Julian guessed that maybe last night might not have gone quite as planned, or that it had all taken longer than expected. Perhaps he'd whipped back to his digs for a shower, maybe even a quick zizz. They were both badly lacking in sleep. Still, he'd like to have known if he wasn't coming and he just hoped to God that nothing had gone wrong with the plan to get Alicia away in the early hours of this morning. He'd listened for the little Cessna, then heard it leave, conspicuous in its solitariness. He had checked his watch and noticed, then, that it was a little late.

Julian knew that he'd been out in the open, sitting by himself here for long enough. His two companions from the next door table had moved on, little knowing just how important their cover had been to him. There weren't many people about at this hour. Now he felt even more obvious, in spite of the disguise. He remained seated and alert with nobody but the pigeons and a waiter or two around for company. The staff were busy getting the tables laid up for the morning coffee invasion. It must be hard work, constant all through the day, although just at the moment he rather felt that he would have liked to swap places with them.

Julian was well aware that the *folgore* were out in force, supplying back up and support but, he was used to having to look after himself, trusting and relying on nobody else. Maybe he'd move inside. Yes, that had to be the best idea: a quick visit to the gents and another cup of coffee. Then he settled himself in the corner facing the door and lit yet another cigarette. He really was going to have to cut down after this was all over. He'd seen nothing untoward so far today and, lets face it, he didn't even recognize himself when he looked in the mirror. Nevertheless, judging by the hairs standing up on the back of his neck, the enemy were certainly around. He could sense it.

The 'three W's', he and Guy called it: 'Watching, Waiting and Wondering'. This was what their quarry was presently about. They must be puzzled by all of their unpredictable movements. He guessed that the criminals were extremely impatient with the delay and must be getting a fair bit of flack from their superiors. They should have retrieved the bag with its contents long ago, or at least should have made progress in finding out where it was. They would be wondering just exactly who he was, this fat, ugly creature, so often in Guy's company. Where had he come from having dropped down as if from the sky? And where did he and Guy disappear to when they underwent their stint of enforced hiding before Julian's fatal mishap?

It was not surprising that the gang had latched onto the girls, especially Alicia, when she had unwittingly turned up. Thank God that so far they hadn't bothered anybody else in their search for him, particularly his parents.

Julian's mother would have been horrified, if they'd turned up on her doorstep. She would have sensed menace in the unsavoury looking characters and deduced it was something to do with the other, shady, part of his life. As for his brothers, they would have been more difficult prey. They lived and travelled to work together, were seldom alone and were also aware of Julian's secret lifestyle. Previously, they had both been given instruction on how to cope with unwarranted or suspicious questioning from strangers.

His father would have handled the situation well. If anybody had enquired, he would have shut the door firmly in their faces claiming ignorance as to his whereabouts, blaming his overseas job. At the first sign of trouble he would have then followed the emergency procedure learnt from the past, when Julian had been actively involved with the Special forces on a full time basis. The elder man would keep his cool and knew the drill by heart, just as long as he had the time to put it into practice.

Julian had argued about the truth of his faked death being kept from his family. It seemed such a drastic measure and so unfair to put them through such agony, but he had eventually understood the necessity. It was safer for them all to be left temporarily in the dark. Nonetheless his father wasn't stupid and might well have cottoned on that something fishy was going on, as he hadn't even been allowed to identify his son's body after Julian's so called 'accident' in the South of France. Supposedly his commanding officer had done that, given the 'unusual circumstances'. God almighty! What hell they must all have been through.

~

Intelligence surmised that, after their wholly unsuccessful period in London setting up a team of surveillance to watch the girls, the *mafioso* trio would have been ordered to cut their losses and return to Italy to regroup. They would have thought they'd hit the jackpot when Alicia arrived there as well, but it must have stopped them in their tracks when they'd heard about the drowning incident. Julian's 'death' had been well publicised both in the papers and on the television.

Even his friends considered him under the sod, thought Julian with disgust. He wondered how many went to his 'funeral'. Were they already over the tears and the shock, perhaps even now putting it behind them and getting on with their lives again? How long would he be sorely missed? What an appalling idea: contemplating one's own death. He really couldn't think of a worse scenario. As for his parents and Adriana? Well, he decided he really couldn't go down that route. At the present time these things were best not dwelt upon. It wasn't worth even trying to comprehend how they must be feeling.

~

Before Julian and Guy left the confines of the safe house, they had both been briefed in depth. Julian was given the disguise in a small squashy bag and told that he was obliged to wear it at all times, no matter what the aggravation. There was to be no risk of his detection; he was too valuable. Guy was not only his best friend, but now was to be his guardian. Julian was quite put out when he was shown his new identity, not helped by the fact that Guy couldn't remove the grin from his face whilst they were being given their orders by a solemn, ratty and mealy mouthed little man from the department. They were given hand written instructions, which once read had to be burnt in his presence. He was, irritatingly, thoroughly puffed up with the importance of his job.

Once the operation was activated, the two men moved often, never staying in one place for long. There was too much at stake. Julian was acutely aware that it was of paramount importance for him to stay alive. M.I.6 needed him to identify the guilty people, so nobody was to take any chances. A comforting thought, Julian decided, albeit begrudgingly.

Julian's description of the three men in Florida matched both Marcello and Guy's sightings in Italy. It was the same group, well known and long established. Unable to find Julian or Guy, the mafia had transferred their attention to Alicia, as feared, reporting on her movements on a daily basis.

Believing Julian to be dead, once Alicia arrived in the Venetian area, the thugs were hot on her trail. She was now their best lead to the whereabouts of the computer.

Julian was required to identify the three *mafioso* from Little Beach island before the security services could finish up their job. There must be one hell of a lot of dark suited, dark skinned, Sicilian looking Italians in Venice. He thought he'd seen the big, burly, individual, who'd taken such pleasure in beating the young Arab to death. He couldn't be sure: it had been too far away and the man had dived into a doorway. There was still no sign of the other two.

Maybe the thug on Alicia's train to the South of France was out of action. From the reports they'd had from Gianni's man, that brute should certainly have been left the worse for wear, hopefully with seriously damaged limbs. Julian was sure that the policeman looking after Alicia would have pushed him out of the train none too gently. The poor girl must have been terrified. Unfortunately, there was no report of anyone of the description given being found dead, or visiting a hospital that night or the following morning. The injured man must have been scooped up and spirited away by his associates, pretty darned quick.

These people were clearly clever, cunning, devils and completely ruthless. Julian knew well, from past experience, that life to them meant nothing at all. Never mind the cruelty; they simply enjoyed inflicting pain. Julian was quite sure that if they ever found him, they would be looking forward to treating him in the same way, to get the information they wanted and to wreak revenge. To date they had been made to look foolish. They were ignorant that they, too, were constantly being monitored by an equally ruthless, elite force of highly trained, ultra efficient and lethal professionals, Guy and himself included. Julian felt confident that he and Guy were still up to scratch.

The criminals must know that their time was running out and that in the right hands the computer would divulge its secrets before long. With Guy's exceptional powers of avoiding detection, Alicia slipping through their fingers and Adriana chaperoned in London, when Julian came back on the scene, their way would become clear again. He was the one person who knew, for sure, exactly where the computer was and so the villains needed him more than ever.

~

Julian lit another cigarette, feeling more at ease now that he was inside. There were more customers around, the earlier shops beginning to open. He checked his mobile again for a message. This time there was one: Guy was on his way. About bloody time too.

While he waited, he thought back over his conversation with Adriana, on the phone, a couple of days previously. She'd been extraordinarily brave and although she had been in an understandable state of high emotion when they had spoken, believing him dead, she'd managed to keep her head whilst they talked. He'd done his best to reassure her, both of his safety and his feelings for her, the former being thoroughly uncertain, as both knew perfectly well. He knew that as soon as the call was ended she would have burst into tears out of pure relief and joy at the contact. He'd heard the suspect, slight tremble in her voice. He hated the thought of her being on her own. How she'd managed to refrain from asking the questions that she must have been longing to ask, he really couldn't imagine and he'd admired her all the more, for it.

Guy, who had taken the lead throughout everything, had said merely: 'You have time enough only to reassure and tell her to trust the man named Drew and not a single word to anyone, 'not even the bloody cat,' he had added grimly. There should be no fear of a short call being traced.

"Thank God!" He could now see Guy, striding across St Mark's Square towards the open door, scattering the pigeons in every direction. He approached the table, taking off his coat and calling for some coffee as he walked.

"Where on earth have you been?" Julian started, then seeing the meaningful smirk on his friends face. "Jesus Christ! Need I ask?" he exclaimed. "I can't believe it!"

"No it's alright, really," said Guy, his head down and trying to suppress his grin as he sat down, "and now she's gone … and she'll be safe," he finished lamely, but not in the least ashamed. "It was just one of those things, couldn't help it, that's all.

Now," changing the subject rapidly and straightening the cuffs of his shirt, "back to business. I've talked to our people at the airport checking the early morning flights. They think, from your description, that all three of our quarry have now arrived here, and …," he hesitated, his eyes twinkling, thoroughly enjoying being able to impart this crucial piece of news … "the third member isn't likely to put up much of a fight, with one arm in a sling and a crocked leg as well, just as we hoped! He's been lying low, somewhere out in the country, probably trying to recover without using a hospital or qualified doctor. The man apparently looks very sorry for himself".

"Serves him right the bastard: pity he survived at all!" interrupted Julian with vehemence.

"I absolutely agree. Anyway," continued Guy, "they are all here now and with plenty of back up, as we know. So, as soon as you can give us positive identifications, the *folgore* will close in. Speed is all important, in case they get wind of our large presence and split up or disappear … and before they can get to you," he finished brightly, punching his friend affectionately on the shoulder.

"Thanks!" said Julian, forgetting once again that he couldn't run his hands through his hair in his usual manner. His head itched worse than ever. He felt hot and annoyed. Contrary to his friends last idyllic hour or so, all he'd had was a two minute conversation with Adriana, before which she'd thought him dead and been to his funeral. What a bloody fuck up! "Very encouraging indeed, so what next then?" he asked crossly, getting out yet another cigarette. Guy took no notice and went on.

"Our S.I.S controller wants a few days to finalise arrangements for the sweep up operation, then he wants us to go across to one of the islands, away from the main city, taking the bag with us. You're to be yourself again, you'll be glad to hear. They reckon that the Sicilians, once they are over the shock of seeing you, are bound to follow and then most likely make their move. We're really going to have to watch ourselves though; they are a nasty lot, with plenty of history. With new information coming in all the time this is becoming ever more apparent". Guy sipped his steaming cup of coffee while Julian digested the plan of action, then cleared his throat and continued.

"Their power base appears to have recently made contact with covert terrorist cells all over the place. The whole world and its mother have been after this particular group for ages, just waiting to get substantial evidence with no loopholes. Until now they have been too slippery, but thanks to your interference on Little Beach and your assistance now, we'll have everything we need to put this choice bunch away for a long time to come. On top of which our bosses are hoping that, once apprehended, these men will be persuaded to 'squeak a little' and maybe betray their superiors". He took another gulp of coffee, then grinned at Julian before finishing,

"Which, makes you my friend, not only the man of the moment, but, also, the most important person around."

"Just what I don't need," muttered Julian under his breath, unimpressed.

"It will however," continued Guy, still taking no notice of Julian's despondent mood, "make it much easier for the team if the trap is set outside the city, with not so many people around for them to worry about. We are going to need our firearms on this trip, so we need to get them authorised and have them checked."

"O.K. sounds exciting. Thank God I'll be able to get rid of this bloody awful thing on my head. Seriously though, I think time's running out. I have a feeling that this whole disguise thing is wearing a bit thin, so to speak," said Julian thoughtfully and cheering up at the possibility of impending action. "They don't know who the hell I am, but they're suspicious, because someone's definitely following me around now. The same man has been waiting by the paper stall near my digs the last twice I've been there and the *folgore* say he leaves only when I do. I brought my bag with me as I think that perhaps I should move. I have a feeling they're gathering their forces for a strike."

"Then you'd better come back to the Contessa's villa with me for the next few days." replied Guy. "Funnily enough, she already suggested that we'd be better off with her and it will be easier for us to finalise our plans from there." They left the money on the table, picked up their stuff and set off in the direction of Caro's villa. A bearded individual appeared from an alleyway as soon as they left the restaurant and fell into to step a few yards back. Julian stopped supposedly to light another cigarette but surreptitiously glancing behind him as he did so.

"This one appeared behind me on my way here." said Julian, "and while I was sitting waiting for you, I could sense that he was somewhere around. Lucky we are able to trust our instincts so well, isn't it? I can almost smell the nasty little shits when they're in the vicinity."

"Yes, well, we'd better lose him then, same drill as before, lets go," answered Guy shortly.

With that they walked slowly on down the cobbled street, leading away from St. Marks Square. A quick call on the mobile, then three minutes later they were ready. One word from Guy, 'now!' and they each darted into shops on either side, just as they'd done before. Once inside, nodding their thanks to the astonished storekeepers as they swept through, they went straight out the back, across another road, through a restaurant and a bar, then both doubled back into the bottom of the narrow street they'd first started along. There they turned the corner and met again at the steps leading to the water where the Contessa's boat was already waiting with the engine running and Alonzo at the helm, looking as if he was on a day's outing and enjoying every moment.

As they glanced back, there was no sign of anybody following and they laughed as they wondered where the bearded chap had ended up. One of the shops sold lingerie, with a very attractive Italian girl in charge and the other was a pet shop, full of squawking parrots and a huge amount of clutter! As they were whisked back to the villa Guy called across to Julian.

"I'd rather have the girls together now. Drew's going to bring Adriana out to Switzerland to join Alicia". He had to shout above the noise of the boat engine. Julian, still standing and holding on to the hatch door frame, looked back surprised, not bothering to check a relieved grin.

"Sorry, but I didn't want you to hint at anything on the mobile," added Guy, "just in case. Drew said Adriana's flat was definitely being watched before she moved and she will insist on going out at lunch time every day, leaving the office to get sandwiches, according to the chap he put outside there, apart from which ..." He added with a helpless gesture, "the poor girl's obviously thoroughly fed up with the enforced curfew and I can't blame her for that. She'll arrive at the house tomorrow evening". He looked across at Julian waiting for the pleased reaction.

"Good, I'm glad," smiled Julian, feeling much happier after a bit of good news for a change. "It's better for them and for us." He'd been worried about Adriana being in London on her own. Drew was still young to be coordinating the people looking after her and in his opinion hadn't enough experience.

~

The Contessa was sitting having tea. "Come on in then chaps. What's the latest?" she asked brightly and invited them to join her. Caro, immaculate as ever, was dressed in a sky blue light-weight trouser suit with a long matching scarf draped around her neck, fixed with an eye-catching diamond broach. Her hair must have just been done and her nails and make up were equally perfect. She looked, thought Julian nervously, ready for anything.

Guy told her their plans for the next few days. She'd been in their confidence for some time, ever since he'd first come to see her. It had become necessary as soon as Alicia had fetched up with her in Venice. The Contessa was stalwart, resilient and totally trustworthy. True to her character, she immediately insisted that she should join them for the final showdown and that she would take them to lunch at the Cipriani restaurant on the island of Torcello.

"It will look more natural. Less of a set up," she said with twinkling eyes. "It's isolated and quiet there too, not so many people around as in the city. Just the job, in fact," she added noticing their uncertain faces. "You won't have to worry about me and I'll keep out of the way when necessary."

Guy was thinking. He really didn't want her further involved, it was too dangerous, but she'd been marvellously helpful to date. He wouldn't have much trouble, he thought, getting the necessary permission and he had to admit it was a good plan. Also, he knew he'd have one hell of a job talking her out of it once her enthusiasm was fired and she'd made up her mind. She really was an indomitable creature. He knew that they were in for a long evening discussing their plans for the next week and even longer if he argued, trying to put the Contessa off from joining them.

★★★

CHAPTER 30

Adriana awoke to the sound of her mobile ringing. A sensation of excited energy flooded her brain as she remembered, '*He's alive, it's not a dream, he really is alive*' and she grabbed the phone.

"It's Drew", said the voice disappointingly. "Please be ready with a small bag and something warm. I'll collect you in one hour," and the telephone went dead.

'Thank Heavens for some action at last', murmured Adriana. She was fed up to the teeth with sitting around waiting, not knowing what was going on. She'd had a nasty feeling, for some time, that someone had been watching her when she'd left the office at lunch time each day, but she'd had to get out or she'd go mad! Anyway the whole situation was becoming thoroughly unnerving. She wondered where the two men were. She longed to see Alicia; they had only been allowed two minutes of uninformative conversation on the phone. Where was she? She knew that Alicia was somewhere safe, but wasn't allowed to communicate further. Adriana had been sent an odd looking new mobile but nobody rang in and she had been told that there was no facility for outgoing calls. Supposedly, so that they couldn't be traced, thought Adriana disconsolately. She felt trapped and very lonely.

The worst thing for Adriana was having nobody with whom to commiserate. It was also extremely difficult not knowing how to handle Julian's parents. Adriana was a literary agent assistant and his mother kept ringing her publishing house wondering why they couldn't get hold of her at home. Her boss was getting annoyed at her being constantly disturbed when she was supposed to be 'reading', so she wrote to them once a week just to put their minds at rest. She knew she couldn't help sounding so much happier herself and was simply longing to put them out of their misery; to be able to tell them that Julian was alive and well and that she had even talked to him. But, although she knew that to be impossible it was hard emotionally and very frustrating.

Adriana had been moved out of her flat for the time being. The office had been told it was being redecorated while she lived in a two roomed 'granny flat' adjoining a middle aged couple's family home in Richmond.

Robert Halter was tall, dark and very quiet. He had an air of mystery about him. Rob took Adriana to work each day and brought her home. He said it was on the way to his office, but she didn't believe it. She knew perfectly well that his was no ordinary job. She also knew that he had something to do with the new security man on the street at the entrance to her office. The man standing guard told her that he had been hired by all the different offices in the building, when she'd asked; but she'd never heard anything about it, so knew that wasn't true either. In spite of his suspect life style, the Halter's were both kind and decent people. Rob's wife, Vicky, was a good cook and often invited her to join them for dinner. Vicky was having their fourth child and Adriana was secretly terrified that, being near her time, Vicky might go into labour when she was the only one around. Adriana wasn't sure how well she'd cope with a baby being born.

Vicky was good fun and seemed completely unfazed and unflappable. She was always busy with one of the children, or taking the dogs out. She got in any shopping that Adriana needed and organized someone to come in twice a week to clean. Most importantly, Adriana had her cat and a television for company. The cat, very wisely, kept well away from the two boisterous, out of control, family dogs.

However trapped in a situation not of her own making; having lost her independence and unable to see anybody other than those at work, Adriana was thoroughly bored. Her friends must have thought that she had completely deserted them.

Now, with one telephone call, a growing sense of elation had flooded her brain and a new found energy was revitalizing her body. Everything had changed. Adriana leapt out of bed and into the shower. She dressed quickly, gobbling down an apple and drinking a mug of coffee, while she threw some gear together. Her passport, driving licence and some money were already stowed in the zip up compartment of her travelling case; they had been there for days, just in case. Next, she sent a text message to Rob, as she was allowed to do, although she was quite sure that he knew of her plans already. Vicky was off on the school run, so she wrote a quick thank you note, wished her the best of luck for the baby and stuck it up on the kitchen board with a pin. She left another note and some money to enable the cleaning lady to feed and look after the cat. By the time Drew rang the buzzer she was ready and waiting.

Drew was taken aback. He hadn't known what to expect when he rang the bell. Adriana Forbes was gorgeous and completely 'together' although he could sense an underlying nervous tension. Anyone would think that she was setting off for a perfectly ordinary weekend, not to heavens knows where!' She was about twenty-six or seven he thought, dressed in dark jeans, with flat heeled boots he noticed, thankfully. She wore a leather jacket over a high-necked black jersey, her long pale blonde hair still damp from the shower and curled around her neck. Her shining eyes were a deep, hazel, green and her skin clear except for a sprinkling of freckles on her up-tilted nose. Her mouth, my God! Her mouth, thought Drew, trying not to stare. She was without doubt one of the sexiest looking girls that he'd seen for a long time.

"Hello, are you ready?" he asked, clearing his throat and attempting to return to reality.

"Almost," she said, inviting him in as she went to retrieve her things and lock the windows. "Have I enough, do you think?" asked Adriana pointing to her small overnight bag, "and am I dressed alright? I didn't really know what I need?" She looked at the fair, curly headed, young man in question, not missing the admiration in his eyes.

"Perfect," answered Drew, meaning every word. "Come on then, we'll go." They left by the back door, through the garden to the little street, where he'd parked his motorbike under a tree and out of sight.

Flying along the M40 towards Northolt, sitting close up behind Drew, Adriana felt really alive again for the first time in ages. She wondered where on earth they were going.

"Somewhere safer," was all that Drew had offered when she'd asked, so she quickly understood that questions wouldn't be welcome, for the time being at least. If the truth were known, Drew was trying hard not to think too much about the near proximity of this overtly sexual young woman, close behind, with her arms wrapped around him and the warm heat of her body, penetrating through his jacket. Jesus! What did they expect of him?

On arrival at Northolt they went straight past security, with Drew producing a special pass and being waved directly onto the tarmac, where a small plane was waiting. Drew boarded the Cessna with Adriana and only when they were seated and with the engine started, did he speak again.

"I'm taking you to a special place in Switzerland where you'll have some company and can play Heidi for a bit!" he added with a grin. As the plane soared up into the sky Adriana's heart sang: she hoped and longed that she might be nearer to Julian and that the 'company' could possibly be Alicia. But Drew, with a twinkle in his eye, refused to be drawn any further. Instead, now that she was sitting opposite him, he could admire her properly.

Adriana enjoyed the flight to Switzerland. Except for a few bumps over the Alps, it was smooth and comfortable. Drew was a wonderful companion and very funny. By the end of the journey, however, she was well aware of a strong and very mutual physical attraction between them and was somewhat relieved that they wouldn't be going on much further together. This is what happens when these men leave us alone too long; it's just not natural to go 'without' all this time, thought Adriana crossly. Even some of the people in the office had starting looking quite reasonable lately and they were really a pretty average lot. These thoughts made her giggle with her hand in front of her mouth.

"What's so funny?" Drew had asked, as they began to descend. She'd laughed and answered looking him straight in the eye,

"Drew, you don't need to know what I am thinking at the moment. In fact it's a good thing you don't know, believe me." He looked straight back at her and replied,

"Ah! But maybe I can guess what you are thinking, and … maybe I was thinking similar thoughts!"

"Well, if you were thinking the same thoughts, then there's nothing to be done about it." She said firmly and turned away to look out of the window hiding a smile.

A pity, thought Drew with genuine disappointment. She was so sexy, brave and really good fun.

~

The plane landed safely at Bern. Following in Alicia's footsteps, Adriana and Drew continued their journey by the small mountain train to Saananmoser, with lunch on the way in the panoramic restaurant car. The meal turned out to be as much fun as the flight. Yet even more stimulating physically and without a single glass of alcohol either, thought Adriana with some shock at her own reactions. By the time Drew regretfully handed her over to Zak on the pony and trap, the day was closing in. The sun had already left the floor of the valley, for a final sweep over the higher slopes.

They took the same steep track up the mountain as had Alicia, some days previously. Zak was pleased to see that Adriana was just as animated as Alicia had been by the air and, the fantastic view of the further peaks, outlined, starkly, against, the warm, golden, light of the tired, dropping, sun. As they topped the highest point and looked down on the little house, safely nestling in its sheltered meadow below, Adriana could see a distant figure of a woman with fair hair caught by the last rays of the sun, bent picking flowers. She crossed her fingers and hoped. They came nearer. The woman turned and shading her eyes against the glare, looked towards them and waved. Adriana cupped her hands to her mouth and shouted as loudly as she could, her voice echoing across the valley.

Ally! Ally!" Then, asking Zak to stop, Adriana jumped down from the trap, crossed the track and started to run towards Alicia as fast as she could. When they met, they grabbed each other, nearly falling down and laughing so much neither could speak, so glad were they to be together again, with both their circumstances so unbelievably changed. Finally, they turned and with their arms linked started to walk slowly back towards the house, through the long grass covered with a bright carpet of many coloured wild flowers.

Zak, discreetly, took a more circuitous route giving the two friends some privacy and much needed space. Times had obviously been more than difficult for them both. He liked Alicia and he liked the look of Adriana too. Mister Guy had said to guard them both with his life and guard them he would. He took his time un-harnessing the horse, then turned her loose and watched as she rolled, shook, then galloped off to join the mare and foal, whickering, as they trotted across to meet her from the far side of the enclosure.

Adriana and Alicia sat quietly on the wooden steps to the chalet watching, in silence and with awe, as the sun disappeared behind the mountains, leaving a trail of brilliant colours in its wake, spread far and wide, clearly defining the horizon. High above their heads a pair of kites swooped and glided with the thermals, mewing to each other, seeing the earth from their own dimension. It was a beautiful sight.

Without the sun the landscape was darkening and the air cooling fast, but, the two young women were enveloped in a warm inner glow; so delighted were they in each others company. Obliged to withdraw for the time being, from normal life, they were both, calm, resolute and content, to wait out this period of seclusion together, but in one of the world's most remote yet spectacular of settings.

★★★

CHAPTER 31

At eleven o'clock precisely, on the final day of reckoning, the Contessa, Guy and Julian, greatly relieved to be dressed as himself, with the crucial Arab's bag slung over his shoulder, left the villa together. Alonzo was to pick them up in the boat in half an hour's time, at an allotted meeting place, giving them the chance to walk for a bit so as to advertise their presence to those who might be interested.

After a short night, the Contessa was going to take them for a cup of the 'best coffee in Venice, to get them all in tip top condition, before setting off', she'd said with a wry chuckle.

They had sat up late going over and coordinating the operation for the day in meticulous detail with all their back-up team, who agreed the detailed plan and would know their exact movements at all times. Caro had been a great asset with her local knowledge: she knew every inch of their proposed route and her cheerful and intelligent ideas, not to speak of her contacts at every level, were invaluable. She knew the Italian head of police, who had much admiration for her work on behalf of Venice and this had made it much easier for Guy to get the go ahead to include her. Although, at first, he'd been hesitant, Guy now realized how very much more difficult their arrangements would have been without the Contessa.

The day was clear and bright, with that extraordinary luminescent light so special to Venice. Later, as the Contessa threw her boat across the water at full throttle, all other shipping took avoiding action, except of course for the ferries and bigger craft on which Caro deigned to bestow a certain amount of respect, understanding their need for the middle of the narrow and shallow channels. Julian and Guy, in spite of what they were actually about, couldn't help but enjoy the journey.

By the time they arrived at Torcello they all felt positively invigorated and ready for anything. They had decided first to walk the quarter of a mile or so along the narrow tow path beside the canal, past the two restaurants to the monastery. Then, they were to take some time going over the lovely old building and absorbing its ancient atmosphere, like any tourist. This would give plenty of time for two more *motoscafi* ferry boats to arrive with both *bona fide* visitors and those of more unsavoury character and also to make their day out appear reasonably normal to those who they hoped would be watching.

Soon after they'd entered the monastery, Guy felt his mobile vibrate in his pocket, then stop, then repeat itself. At the exact time appointed this was the signal which meant that the plan that they had laid so carefully was working so far. The likely assailants were on the next ferry; after the one that was presently docking. The second vibration on his mobile meant that the Italian undercover police were ready and in their places. Now all they had to do was to continue as if they were on a perfectly ordinary day out with the Contessa, enjoying her company, until Julian could get a good look at their adversaries. Both men were alert and watching for anything unexpected to happen. They had not only themselves to look out for, but also their formidable companion.

Caro took the last piece of news as if it was the latest Test Match update and announced that she would shortly be extremely hungry and that perhaps it was time to venture along to the *Ostaria al Ponte*. Guy had decided against the well-known *Cipriani* restaurant, it was too smart and Caro was quite likely to meet people whom she knew. This could only complicate their situation still further and then, Caro would also insist on dressing up even more! As it was, she was wearing the most unsuitable shoes, dressed up to the nines, with diamonds flashing on her fingers and in her ears, as if she was off to a Buckingham Palace garden party.

As Caro and the two men walked, slowly, back towards the restaurant, they met a sprinkling of visitors off the first boat, mostly Japanese, regimented in a group. The men had expensive looking, identical, cameras hanging around their necks and the women had Prada or Gucci carriers swinging from their shoulders and almost to the ground because of their height. Both the men and the women were dressed in a similar fashion as if in uniform on a school outing. They were all talking nineteen to the dozen and were preceded by a little man with a cheer-leader's flag: as if they could get lost here on the tow path that only led to the monastery! The second ferry boat appeared in the distance and was approaching fast.

"We'll just amble along while it arrives and give everybody time to dis-embark. Then, when they are all on the path walking towards us and in full view, we'll go into the restaurant," announced Guy calmly.

A short time later the mobile in Guy's pocket shook again. This time he took it out to listen for a moment, then after a curt 'O.K', put it away again.

"They have been seen, getting off as expected," he told the other two.

"So far so good then," answered Julian.

"And I'm even hungrier. Reminds me of a war I was once caught up in Africa," added Caro with glee. "I'll tell you about it at lunch!"

It was easy to walk, talk and watch the people coming down the path towards them. There were more people off the second ferry than the first. The first batch was quite obviously tourists. They all began to march past, talking excitedly and consulting their guidebooks, as they went purposefully on towards the monastery.

Guy looked ahead and, with his trained eye, was able to pick out at least three figures from the last group of people who stood out from the rest.

Even from a long way off they were quite different, no matter how hard they tried to blend and they all wore unsuitable dark suits.

"Right!" said Guy, "the eagles have landed or whatever. Make sure you advertise that brief case a bit Julian, sling it over your shoulder and make it appear heavy. We'll continue walking for a couple more minutes, make sure they see us and then go into the restaurant."

"Gracious, you must have good eyesight," said the Contessa. "How on earth can you pick out the wretches from amongst all these tourists?"

"Practice," answered Guy, amused. "Now Caro, after this next lot of people have passed I want you to take a couple of photographs of Julian and myself outside the restaurant here. Try to include the last lot of people coming down the path towards us now, in particular those three in dark suits and make it look as if we're having fun, then we'll go in for lunch."

Amidst much laughter Caro took the pictures, making it all look as natural as possible. As she did so, she realised that this was certainly no ordinary camera. As she focused on the path, the people nearer faded and all those in the distance became magnified several times over. Even she could pick out the three men in the group that Guy had seen, in spite of their faintly ridiculous efforts to remain inconspicuous. They just didn't look like tourists.

The photography had drawn exactly the right amount of attention. People were looking at them as they passed by and the three men had also seen them, as intended. They had stopped, turned away slightly, having certainly recognized Julian and were now in deep discussion, pretending to look at a map.

"They're just waiting to see what we're going to do; whether we are going in or not," pronounced Guy. "Very satisfactory, lets go then" and he held out his hand for Caro to go ahead of him through the door.

"I'm off to the men's room," said Julian as Guy handed him the camera.

The restaurant was already quite busy so they were sensible to have booked. Caro and Guy were shown to their table and given the menus, which Caro immediately started to peruse after ordering her usual, large 'English' gin and tonic.

Guy ordered a bottle of *Prosecco* then, chuckling asked Caro "Why did you stress 'English' like that?"

"Because," replied Caro unhesitatingly, "it would otherwise be all tonic and no gin, like a *spritzer*, rather than the other way around," adding with a chuckle, "there are a few things that, even after many years, have never changed here."

Guy sitting, in the corner facing the exit, looked up as Julian came back across the room towards them, a grin lighting up his face.

"Well?" asked Guy.

"All of them, definitely and one appears more than slightly out of action you will be pleased to hear. Just as we'd hoped! His arm seems hooked up, as if it could be in a hidden sling. Well done Caro, you really have earned your lunch," Julian said. He bent to kiss the Contessa's perfectly made up cheek, then sat down.

"Here's to us and our venture then," said Guy raising his newly poured glass of wine and passing one to Julian.

The older woman positively glowed with her success. "I'm beginning to feel a little like Miss Moneypenny, but with a better dip in the action," she laughed. "Now please boys, can we order? Whatever happens I fully intend to enjoy some good food and wine. This is an excellent restaurant."

"We certainly can! It's up to the *folgore* now; we have done our bit and they have the info they want, thanks to you Julian," said Guy. "We can take as long as you like. We're quite safe in here with so many people around and might as well make the most of it." So, after tapping out a short message of confirmation on his mobile to their associates outside, the three of them settled down to the serious business of deciding what to eat, as if they were all on a perfectly ordinary day out instead of being involved in a dangerous game of cat and mouse.

The Contessa drank most of the wine and told her very funny story about the 'little war' in which she'd got muddled up, whilst staying with one of our ambassadors somewhere in Africa. Both Guy and Julian knew that it was of paramount importance to keep a clear head, just in case things didn't go quite according to plan and they were still needed. The three collaborators had an excellent lunch in spite of wondering how things were going outside. Yet with their engrained instinct never to relax until they were absolutely sure that the job was done and dusted, Guy and Julian unconsciously listened and watched all the time for signs, or sounds of anything untoward.

After they'd eaten, Guy looked at his watch and decided that it would soon be time to leave the restaurant, but first the Contessa must visit the ladies' washroom and reorganize her clothes as they'd planned. Julian handed over a carrier bag with the allotted vest, which they'd stuffed into the side section of the Arab's hold all. It had filled it out a bit, together with the useless old lap top they'd been given, to weigh the case down and, to cover any eventuality. Both men realized that it might have a certain bargaining power with the relatively dim witted *mafiosa* henchmen if they met with unexpected trouble.

As she left the table Guy, noticing Caro's frown of displeasure, took her arm and said firmly, "Caro you have to put it on you know. Please bring the carrier bag back empty. It's only a precaution, but essential!"

"Yes, yes, it's alright, I will," she answered slightly cross, yet resigned. "I told you I'd do as you asked. I only want to help, you know," she patted his arm as she walked away. Julian grinned and when the Contessa was out of earshot, leant across the table,

"She's only worried about it making her look less slim", he chuckled,

"Yes I realize that", answered Guy. "She really is an extraordinary person isn't she? Extremely good looking, as strong as an ox and totally unfazed by what we're doing here today, thank God. I tell you one thing though, I wouldn't mind betting that the Africans in her 'little war' were absolutely terrified of our admirable Contessa!"

Julian nodded in agreement and got out a cigarette, "Let's get some more coffee while we wait, do you think she'll mind if I …?"

He was interrupted by Guy raising his hand as his mobile reverberated in his pocket, against his leg, making him jump. He hoped this might be affirmation that it was all over. This time he took out the phone and raised it to his ear to listen intently for a moment. He turned to Julian.

"Everything's going as it should," he reported, "Some of the followers have already been rounded up in the city and the delay here is just that the *folgore* are waiting for a ferry load of passengers to depart before moving. It really shouldn't be much longer now. The three men are right outside, hanging around on the tow path, waiting for us to come out of the restaurant." Guy returned his mobile to his pocket. A small frown creased his forehead as he looked across the table at Julian, both silently agreeing that it was taking too long.

"Let's order that coffee then, shall we? Caro's taking her time, isn't she? Julian asked a little nervously, lighting his cigarette and looking around to catch the waiter's eye. Guy's pocket shook again, alerting him instantly.

"What now?" he exclaimed in annoyance retrieving the mobile and raising it again to his ear. Then looking up, as he absorbed the information he was being given, "Julian quick, get Caro! Christ Almighty! It's too bloody late!"

Caro had re-emerged and was arguing heatedly with someone by the washroom door. Guy could sense rather than see that it was one of the Sicilians, who must have come in suddenly through the back door and caught Caro unawares, just as she was leaving the washroom. Julian began to get to his feet. Guy immediately motioned to him to sit down and, feigning, ignorance, called:

"Are you coming Caro? It's time we were off."

"I'm trying to," she answered crossly, "but this unattractive individual here, behind me, seems to think I'm going with him". With that she was shoved forward into the room and Guy could clearly tell that there was a gun being held to her back. The few tourists left sitting in the restaurant turned to stare and the *capo cameriere*, with his waiters, were looking to Guy and Julian for guidance.

"Right!" said Guy loudly and with authority, standing up. "Might I ask just what exactly you think you are doing? Let go of my friend at once!"

"No!" growled the Italian. "You will come with me, all of you back to the boats, *subito!*" and he flashed a look of contempt and recognition at Julian, daring him to argue. "Again we meet," he said with a sneer and indicated with the gun for them all to move towards the door. Dead silence settled on the room as the rest of the astonished diners gaped.

"Right," agreed Guy thinking quickly, "but you don't need the lady."

"Yes, all: and bring the luggage," was the curt answer. The ugly individual, seemingly in charge, pointed to the Arab's bag indicating for Guy to pick it up, as he continued nervously waving the gun around. Guy reached for the brief case; whilst barely taking his eyes from the man's face he positioned the carrying strap carefully on his shoulder, suggesting the fragility of the heavy load. The Italian bully boy glared back at Guy and grunted with satisfaction. Good, thought Guy, he thinks he has 'the whole caboodle'.

"We have no choice for the moment," said Julian as they began to move, "and this of course is one of them. I won't bother to introduce you," he added, at the same time reclaiming and looking inside the discarded paper carrier, which was immediately grabbed from him and then flung to the other side of the room. Guy nodded.

"Nice," he murmured. "Empty?" he glanced in the direction of the carrier bag.

"Yes, thank God," Julian breathed.

As they reached the door, they could see waiters behind them quietly ushering the remaining people out of the back. The *Capo* was standing by the door.

"Thank you, *grazie molto*," said Guy. "I'm so sorry to have had such a marvellous lunch spoiled at the end."

"It's quite alright," the *Capo* replied politely, squeezing Guy's hand hard, "and I hope to see you again very soon, *Signore* Hargreaves." He dropped his voice "In a few minutes perhaps," then he smiled at Caro and kissed her hand, to lend reassurance.

Plenty of backup around, thought Guy with relief as they all stepped out of the restaurant into the bright summer sunshine. One of the other two crooks was waiting outside and immediately began to search Julian and Guy, who both tried to conceal their guns. Guy also hoped to hide his small mobile in the palm of his hand, unfortunately to no avail. They took everything, but Julian had surreptitiously managed to leave the camera behind on his chair.

They were wondering about the third man when they heard a commotion behind the restaurant. The people were being herded back and locked up somewhere, probably in the cellar, Julian and Guy guessed where they wouldn't be heard so easily. But it meant that they were unlikely to have any help from the *Capo*, which would be a problem. They'd also noticed that the telephone wires to the restaurant had been cut. When the third member of the trio appeared from the side of the building there was nothing they could do but to begin to walk back towards the boats, as they were instructed.

"This is the other one, I imagine?" asked Guy looking straight ahead.

"Absolutely it is," agreed Julian. "Out of action on one side as you can see and with a bad limp on the left as well. Attractive lot, aren't they?"

"Umm, yes, very." said Guy thinking hard. There were few people about now, as most were in the two restaurants or had left on the previous ferry to return to the city, but those that they passed paid them no special interest, too intent on enjoying their day trip to notice anything untoward.

Caro, recovering her equilibrium somewhat, began to prattle on about the rude ending to a lovely lunch and that they hadn't even managed to pay the bill. Guy and Julian were wracking their brains as to how they were to turn the tables now that their plans had gone so badly wrong. What had happened? There must have been too many people around and the *Folgore* had held on just too long.

They both wondered if Caro had managed to don the bullet proof vest before she was grabbed, or whether it was lying, discarded, on the floor of the wash room. Luckily she'd not been searched. With such a disturbance in and behind the restaurant, the thugs' attention had strayed. Perhaps it was because of the look on the Contessa's face, defying them to so much as touch her. Caro was wearing clothes which, although covering her voluptuous figure most decoratively, couldn't have disguised a gun, so maybe they just hadn't bothered.

Guy was well aware that modern day protective vests came in all shapes and sizes and had to be completely unseen on occasions such as this. He just hoped she'd had the chance to use it, because he certainly couldn't tell.

The sinister trio walked to either side of and behind them, looking both grim and tense, one with his hand into his side, barely disguising the gun. The one with the limp was sweating profusely and stank of garlic. He was nervous, Julian and Guy noticed and possibly still in a certain amount of pain from his arm, which had probably not been properly treated. It was becoming likely that they intended to requisition Caro's boat for their own needs. Guy wondered where exactly the Italian special police were placed along the way.

"It's really hot now, isn't it? Much more so than this morning," said Caro in her usual bright voice, shrugging her shoulders and with a knowing wink loaded with meaning. "Any idea what these unsavoury looking characters want? I'm not wearing the crown jewels, but do you think they'd like some money? Shall I offer?"

"Thank's, but no", answered Guy with relief, certain now that she had managed to put on the vest. "I'm afraid your boat is probably part of their plan," he answered.

"Thought so!" she agreed. "What a cheek!"

Throughout this short discourse the Italians had been having their own conversation and with some disagreement, it seemed. Although Julian's italian was quite passable, he found the thick Sicilian accent difficult to understand, but he had gleaned enough to know that they proposed to take Caro's boat across to the Russian tanker moored far out in the lagoon and that they were arguing as to the fate of their prisoners once this had been accomplished. Presumably their minders would have to await orders but, at this point he was glad that Caro couldn't hear what they were saying as he was pretty sure that he understood their intentions. They weren't very nice; she was considered to be a nuisance, but a very rich one and therefore had a substantial price on her head.

The Contessa's boat was tied up a little way away from the main ferry quay. As they came nearer they could see that her captain had been 'swapped' and that a member of the 'Folgore' was sitting now waiting for them on the stern of the boat. He was trying hard not to look a stranger. There were some people on board one of the moored lagoon water taxis nearby and Guy very much hoped that more help was amongst them. Maybe Alonzo was there too.

"Please board," ordered the assailant spokesman, who appeared to answer to the name of Luigi.

"Leave the lady," said Guy.

"No, all go, *subito*," he shouted and gave Caro a push, which she distastefully shrugged off and climbed in. Once again, they had no choice. When all were aboard the captain was told to start the engine and head out towards the tanker, in the distance. The engine started, stuttered into life and then stalled. He tried again with the same result.

"*Problema!*" said the new captain in his ill-fitting cap spreading his hands and making a face, indicating apology.

"Again!" barked Luigi, slapping him across the face and digging the captain in the ribs with the gun. The other two were beginning to fidget. The tall thin one was showing Guy and Julian that he also had a gun, pointing it at their heads. Rocco, the plump one with the limp, who disgusted Julian the most after he had seen him in action in Florida, was looking nervously towards the group of people getting off the water taxi and starting to show interest. Some were beginning to walk towards them.

"Can we help?" one of the men called from the quay.

"No, go away!" came back the rude answer, as Rocco waved them away dismissively, overbalancing slightly then wincing with the pain from his leg. The group continued towards them seemingly not to be put off. There was a sharp crack as Luigi panicked and aimed a shot in their direction, then turned and pointed the gun at the Contessa's head. The party on the side stopped at once. They obviously were the *folgore* or special police and were trying to assess the situation.

"Let me have a go!" interrupted Caro, pointing to the wheel," this is turning rather nasty. I do think we need to leave!"

"You're right." agreed Guy, then raising his voice. "The lady knows how to get the boat started."

Julian quickly repeated this in Italian, suggesting that Caro be allowed to take the helm. For an instant there was silence, then the gun was lowered and at Luigi's instruction Caro was roughly pushed forward by Rocco, with his good arm. She hit the start button once, then again twice and it burst into life.

"Do you think these boys are sailors?" she asked Guy quickly. "I could easily throw them around a bit, when you're ready."

"No, they're not," answered Guy. "I watched carefully as they came on board. No balance at all and, thinking themselves triumphant, their guard is lowered. Give me two or three minutes though to alert the other two." The noise of the engine easily drowned their voices as they edged slowly away from the side. Guy needed to get Julian's attention to warn him.

As they looked behind, a small crowd had gathered to watch. The civil Italian police, the *Carbiniere*, were busy herding the gawping people back towards another, newly arrived, ferry. It looked as though the *folgore* had re-boarded the water taxi and were intending to follow at a discreet distance, unsure of what to do next. Guy noticed a helicopter hovering out over the water. Their assistance from above was in contact, as somebody was talking on his mobile, standing and looking up at it.

Caro was heading slowly out in the direction of the tanker, as ordered, waiting her moment. Guy looked at Julian. He had to prepare him: he couldn't risk him, or the fake 'captain' for that matter, being knocked off their feet and rendered useless. All three of the thugs were armed. At last he caught Julian's attention.

"Do your belt up, old friend," as he inclined his head towards Caro and put one hand firmly on a stanchion beside him. Julian looked down at himself in puzzlement then at Guy again,

"What? Oh right," he murmured, understanding and fiddling with his belt. The captain nodded slightly.

"No speak!" ordered Luigi. They were beginning to relax a little as their goal, looming out on the horizon, came steadily nearer. The tall thin one was lighting a cigarette near the stern, watching the helicopter, his gun back in his pocket for the moment. Luigi was waving his gun around wildly, still trying to watch them all. Rocco, with the limp, was leaning against the hatch, pointing out the direction for them to take, his damaged arm hanging loosely at his side. None of them had any inkling of what their capable helmswoman had in store for them.

Caro had chosen her moment perfectly. She looked around once, then thrust the throttle violently, full ahead. With a throaty roar and in a cloud of smoke the boat half flew forward, throwing its bow up out of the water. The thin man at the stern, shot straight out and over, like a stone out of a catapult and disappeared into the wash. Rocco, still pointing out the way with his good arm, cannoned into the captain who grabbed him roughly by his bad arm; Rocco just had time to scream in agony before he was knocked to the ground senseless, all in one efficient movement. Luigi, with the other gun, also completely lost his footing, hit the hatch door hard and the gun went off.

To Guy's horror the Contessa slumped to the floor while the boat careered out of control in an endless and ever faster circle of rough wash. Julian threw himself on the now staggering Luigi, while Guy fought to control the boat before it turned over. Both the water taxi and the helicopter moved in to the rescue.

As the boat speed lessened and the hull began to settle Guy bent quickly to Caro, who was groaning, so at least she wasn't dead. He searched for signs to see where the bullet had entered and thankfully discovered it in the middle of her back where she was completely protected by the vest. He gently raised her to a sitting position, reassuring her as he did so.

"I suppose I'd be dead if it wasn't for the wretched vest?" she gasped.

"More than likely," agreed Guy.

"When it slammed into my back I must have fallen on the wheel and winded myself with the impact," she finished breathlessly.

"Yes, I think that's exactly what did happen. Now sit quietly and get your breath back; we have much to thank you for, you know," he replied kindly.

She patted his hand and smiled. *"Prego, prego"* she whispered. "All's well that ends well, that's all that matters."

As they turned back towards the quay the police were fishing the third member of the *mafiosa* out of the water none too gently and heaving him, choking and spluttering, into the water taxi. One of their launches was also approaching at speed from Burano. The people released from the restaurant were watching from a safe distance, where the tow path had been cordoned off with tape, the *Carbinieri* at either end. They looked both horrified and fascinated, all at the same time, thought Guy. Julian was standing staring out to sea, shading his eyes.

"Just look at that!" he said. They all watched as the Russian tanker pulled up its anchor and turned to steam stealthily away towards the open sea. The helicopter, joined by two others, was following at a discreet distance, escorting it out of the enclosed Venetian waters.

"There goes the life line of this motley crew," pronounced the Contessa with much feeling. Julian turned, thoughtful for a moment; as the captain and Guy covered the two villains with the captured guns, he picked up the dead Arab's brief case from the bottom of the boat undid the clasp and opened it wide. They all watched as slowly, Julian carefully, removed the phoney computer from it's compartment, then, holding it out for them all to see, with a meaningful glare at the thugs, he flung it far out over the side. There was a splash, then dead silence; the two startled italians looked dejectedly at each other, then at their feet. Caro gave a shout of delight and clapped her hands while the two Englishmen merely grinned at each other.

The police launch came alongside and offloaded the uninvited guests. The *Commissario,* Chief of Police and *Intelligenzia* exchanged a few words with Guy and Julian, who assured him that none of them were harmed, saluted the Contessa with the greatest respect, then left with a flourish in a fountain of wake.

"Well!" exclaimed that remarkable lady, "home for a cup of tea I think chaps and I'll let somebody else have the helm on this occasion. Just don't go too fast please, I've had enough excitement for one day," she added.

Julian and Guy looked at each other and burst into laughter.

★★★

CHAPTER 32

Alicia and Adriana were sitting contemplating the scenery below. They could see Zak digging in the vegetable plot. His parents had gone down the mountain in the pony and trap to replenish supplies. The two girls were now bored; bored stiff.

"Do you think that our men have forgotten us altogether?" asked Adriana of Alicia, a frown on her forehead.

"No!" answered Alicia, "but I don't know about you, I'm afraid I'm beginning to feel a bit tired of this particular mountain, the flowers, beautiful as they may be and the same, local, food every meal".

"And the terrific sense of humour with Zak's parents each night at dinner, kind as they all are," added Adriana.

Zak was really great and so conscientious in his job looking after them. At least he seemed to enjoy their company and their jokes: they laughed, remembering the night before when they'd been explaining one of them to him. His mother had at least appreciated that it was meant to be funny, even if she didn't understand much, but there hadn't been a glimmer of even mild amusement from his father who'd merely shaken his head and continued eating.

'Maybe the reason for taking life quite so seriously was all to do with protecting the secrecy of the safe house and worrying about the people in their care', Adriana had suggested when they'd gone up to their rooms.

"What, you mean like us? Alicia had asked grinning. "We must be one hell of a big problem then." They had dissolved into fits of mirth about nothing really, except the need to laugh and then had sat up late playing cards, with the pack they had found tucked away up on the book shelf.

They continued watching Zak below. He'd finished in the vegetable garden and was now driving out some protesting chickens. They sat silently for a while; each thinking along the same lines. Then Alicia turned to her friend with shining eyes and exclaimed,

"Ari: I know what we'll do and where we can go! To Gianni! Of course! Why didn't I think of it before? We'd be perfectly safe there. They're like my family and oh! It's so beautiful. I can't wait to show you and you won't believe Patrizia's pasta! You've never tasted anything like it in the whole of your life!" She jumped down from the rocks on which they'd been sitting and set off at a run down the hill with a determined look on her face, calling back to Adriana, who was breathing hard in the thin air, as she tried to catch up.

"Come on then, I'll get a message to them immediately!"

Zak wasn't happy at all. His job was to look after the girls and, although he didn't mind them using the mobile for a short call, when they announced they were leaving that was quite another matter. He knew he'd be in dreadful trouble if he went along with the idea, so his answer was very firmly 'no', they could not leave, without Mr. Guy's permission.

Later in their rooms Alicia wasn't to be put off. "Mr Guy's permission my foot! I vote we leave anyway! What do you think?" Adriana looked doubtful.

"Giuseppina and Gianni are thrilled with the plan", Alicia continued persuasively, I knew they would be and we can let Zak know where we'll be, in case of any news." That clinched it.

"Yes, Ally. O.K I agree," answered Adriana. "Let's leave at first light tomorrow, otherwise we'll never find our way down the mountain. What about Zak though, won't he get into trouble? And, what about the dogs?"

"They'll be alright," said Alicia, "I know them both well now and they are here to stop people getting in, not out! And as for Zak, don't worry, he's made of strong stuff."

~

Leaving a polite note for their sleeping hosts; the two set out at dawn, delighted to be on the move again, with their small bags slung over their shoulders. The dogs came with them a little of the way as if to see them safely off the property, then settled down to enjoy the pieces of bone and meat the girls had managed to hide from their last dinner, the previous evening.

It took them well over an hour and a half to get down. The beginning was the most difficult. There was a heavy dew, making it slippery on the rocks and loose shingle. It was hard to see in the early dawn and to remember the way, until they reached the end of the rough path and saw the first of the ski lifts below them. After that their route was clear and they had no trouble following the track down to the bottom.

They caught an early morning milk train to Bern, which luckily had a breakfast carriage, as they were feeling both well exercised and starvingly hungry and then the first businessman's flight on to Verona. There they left a message on the hotel Amalia's answering phone and then boarded the same train that Alicia had taken before, which went via Bologna and on to Stefano's village. After the telephone call, warning of their impending arrival, he was at the station waiting for them and with a beaming smile of delight, greeting Alicia and her friend with genuine pleasure. Taking their bags, he strode off towards the hotel with the two girls almost running behind him to keep up. At the hotel, Amalia and the children were lined up in welcome. A celebration meal had already been prepared.

"Does this sort of thing usually happen when you turn up?" asked

Adriana, amazed at their welcome.

"Ah just wait until you get to my island," answered Alicia with a smile. Although she was not quite sure exactly what they were celebrating, she decided that they should both bask in it.

The family didn't seem to be at all surprised to see them! Alicia was shown to the same room as the last time, with Adriana next door. They had time before dinner to walk to the square and for Alicia to show Adriana the lovely fountain, in the quiet of the evening.

Again, not a soul was in sight. It was still a strangely atmospheric place. Alicia knew that this little square would always be remembered with affection. It had given her such peace and calm before, when her mind had been so troubled. Now the whole situation had changed so incredibly and, although still uncertain, the future looked so very much brighter for them both.

The two girls spent a happy evening with Stefano and his family, who made them all laugh with endless stories of his childhood which, of course, included Gianni and Giuseppina and their children. They left the next day, after breakfast, in the dilapidated old family car. After an uneventful, but amusing, journey as Stefano was never short of words, they arrived in the port soon after midday.

Mario was in the café looking out for them. When he saw Alicia, he gave a shout of welcome, ran over and hugged her. She just couldn't wait to get back to the family. The day was golden warm. There weren't many tourists, as yet. It was still too early in July for most schools to have broken up. This part of Italy, away from the city, was still very much itself, thought Alicia, thankful and not many foreigners seemed to find the island, so far as it was from an airport. As the boat set out towards Delfino, with the open water to themselves, Alicia really felt that she was returning home.

They were all laughing together, at one of Mario's jokes, as they finally neared the quay. Alicia could see Gianni standing waiting and when she was near enough to see his face she knew his emotions matched hers. She wondered, again, just how much he knew of the continuing drama in Venice and what had befallen them all. She stepped out of the boat with tears in her eyes and Gianni immediately enfolded her in his arms. *"Mia cara! Mia cara!"* he whispered and Alicia knew that here was a home that would always be waiting. How reassuring!

Giuseppina had filled the whole house and their rooms with flowers and while she was busy making sure that Adriana had everything she needed, Alicia slipped out and went down through the vines to the beach. As she walked along the edge of the sea she remembered the terrible unhappiness and uncertainty from before as an almost tangible thing. But, although still unaware of the outcome of the unfurling drama in Venice, she also knew now that the feelings that she and Guy had found for each other were such as could never have been foreseen, for their love was, without doubt, something exceptional. She realized also that what she felt for Gianni, his family and for Adriana, was something equally special. Although a different kind of love, it was also to be treasured, found and strengthened by adversity.

And Marcello? Ah! Marcello! He would always have such a very large place in her heart. What they'd had together had been both inevitable and unforgettable. The physical force of feeling during traumatic times and in extremely unusual circumstances was a once-in-a-lifetime experience, not to mention the safety, security and comfort he had given her. He'd have her eternal gratitude, always. It was part of life's pattern, now slotted into its proper place and the odd thing was that he had reached there even before she had. It was meant to be, but simply not meant to be for ever.

Alicia stood by the edge of the water, in the peace and quiet once more, and stared out across the calm sea wondering what was going on over the other side. Was Guy in serious danger still, or had they managed to finish the thing successfully? She had to keep faith and believe that they had. Oh dear! This continual and interminable waiting was awful.

She took a huge breath, 'patience, bloody patience, Alicia,' she muttered to herself as she finally turned to retrace her steps, knowing, without looking up, that Gianni would be there waiting for her on their rock. There he sat, quietly watching the late sun catch the gold of her hair. What a beautiful picture she made as she came slowly nearer. If he could have chosen for Guy or Alicia, he would have chosen each for the other.

When Alicia finally stood in front of Gianni she raised her head, looked him full in the face and gave him the most blazing smile - a smile that as far as he was concerned, knocked the sun into insignificance and would stay with him for the rest of his life. For it was from the soul. With brave determination, this beautiful young woman had found what she was searching for: happiness emanated from her every pore. Gianni glanced heavenwards and was content; those under his direction had done a good job. His prayers had been answered. She was safe home. Alicia would always now be part of his family life, although not of his own blood, more importantly, she had touched and held his heart.

Gianni sat quietly, listening, while Alicia recounted the recent events which had so transformed her life, leaving out only her most private moments. After she'd finished, he merely nodded his head, as no more words were necessary. Little did Alicia know how much he knew of the story already and also just how much he'd guessed long before, for he was no fool.

As Gianni put his arm through hers, to walk slowly back together through the vines, Alicia knew that here she found the strength, wisdom and steady support that she'd missed so much after the death of her own father. Unlike her relationship with Tony, here was absolute unselfish and genuine affection, uncomplicated and constant. She loved Gianni, his family and she loved this enchanting island.

The atmosphere that evening was magical. Giuseppina and Patrizia, in spite of the impending baby, had laid on a feast in the restaurant, Mario was in full voice and even the elderly ones seemed to be celebrating her return, as the Italian family enjoyed yet another excuse for a party.

Once they had realized what was in the air, the two girls had dressed for the occasion, Adriana in a honey-coloured loose skirt, with a short sleeved matching top, which crossed over her breasts and tied at the side, showing off her figure to perfection. She wore a topaz bracelet and pendant that Julian had given her, reflecting the lights in her sparkling hazel eyes and her hair was loosely held back showing her skin, lightly tanned from the warm Swiss mountain air.

Alicia had put on a little weight, which suited her well and now, to Giuseppina's delight, she was a little more rounded. Her skin too, was a light golden brown and her eyes bluer than ever in the clear sea light. She wore her simple Armani dress. She felt the occasion merited it and she hadn't much else anyway. Judging by the pride and joy on the faces of Gianni and Guiseppina when they walked into the room that night they were more than glad they'd taken the trouble.

"*Bella, bella, bellissima,*" Guiseppina kept whispering as they approached. Gianni, safe in the knowledge that he kept to himself, just stood there, contentedly smiling.

★★★

CHAPTER 33

"Come on Caro, do come with us!" pleaded Guy. "Alicia will be so thrilled to see you and you'll love the island and everybody on it. And what's more …," he added with a wink to Julian, "even you really won't need an extensive wardrobe on Delfino, will she Julian?" Julian shook his head and laughed, but tactfully said nothing.

"Alright, alright! point taken. I'll get my maid to start packing," and out of the room she marched, mind made up and full of the usual vibrant enthusiasm with this next plan of action.

With the several months of tense drama and worry now over, the two men relaxed and discussed their hopes for the future, each with a well earned, large, glass of whisky. They'd had long conversations with their families, who needless to say were all in a high state of excitement. Both sets of parents had enjoyed visits from high-ranking intelligence officers, bringing them the startling yet thrilling news of Julian's 'resurrection', extraordinary explanations regarding their enforced 'vanishings' and admirable reports of their sons' work in bringing the whole affair to a satisfactory conclusion.

Julian's parents lives, having been so sorrowfully turned upside down, had now been set right again, although his father had said that he'd had a 'hunch' all along and had never quite believed in his son's death. His mother and the rest of the family were quite simply, overjoyed.

Julian and Guy now had the two girls uppermost in their minds and knew that they were most important to each of them, over and above all else. The way the two girls had behaved throughout, with unquestioning faith and courage, was really something to be admired. Their 'escape' from off the mountain, was typical and after the event, amused them both immensely.

Zak had rung through, in the early hours of the morning, in a slight panic, to tell them that Alicia and Adriana were on the move again. He sounded rather shamefaced that he'd been unable to stop them. Guy knew exactly where they were going, which was immediately confirmed by Gianni. So now there was no hurry. The two men and Caro proposed to arrive on Delfino before midnight, feeling sure that Gianni and Giuseppina's celebrations would continue well into the night. Guy knew from previous experience about Gianni's family parties! Add some romance and goodness only knows what he and Giuseppina had planned!

It was an astonishing chance of fate that had sent Alicia to Delfino, all those weeks ago and clearly she'd won all their hearts, which didn't surprise him one bit. Luckily, it hadn't taken Gianni long to put two and two together about Guy and Alicia and to realize that they were in serious trouble. His powers of intuition were as sharp as ever and he'd proved his worth again, a hundred times over.

The Italian authorities and *Intelligenzia* had been most professional and efficient in winding the whole affair up over the last few days, in cooperation with British Intelligence and the British Foreign and Commonwealth Office, though, if anything, they had all been slightly hindered when joined by the all-too-conspicuous CIA.

For diplomatic reasons and because the initial crime had taken place in USA, the European hierarchy had been instructed to keep the Americans involved. They'd had a difficult time dissuading them from sending their Delta Force to Europe to join the operation at the start. Horror of all horrors! What might have happened had they come into this sensitive situation with guns blazing. The successful outcome had been reached by a very different and calculated approach.

Julian had been summoned to formally identify the three men from Little Beach Island in Florida, which he had been readily able to do. The net had then closed satisfactorily around most of the other big and little fish implicated. Top intelligence and secret service agents from the various countries, with their minions in tow, had all arrived in strength, as had a multitude of lawyers, presumably to record the whole string of events and to begin to press charges for the many crimes already committed. With the information 'persuaded' from the captured group and from the successfully decoded data off the computer, world-wide atrocities planned for the future had been both discovered and foiled.

The Russian *mafiosa* appeared to have been deeply incriminated in the plot as well as their Italian counterparts. Unfortunately the Russians were untouchable. The security forces had nothing concrete that they could use without upsetting the comparatively new and warmer relations with the Soviet Union. Any dealings with the Russians were still politically sensitive. It was thought that the tanker had been waiting to take on board the Contessa and the two men. It had been lurking in the area for some time. The *mafiosa* from both countries had masterminded the final plan from the ship itself. Interrogations might provide further evidence, but the tanker would soon have reached safe waters. The Russian birds would have flown. At least they were certain to keep well clear of Venetian shores for sometime to come.

Most importantly the valuable information on the computer was intact, in safe hands and, thankfully, would only benefit the international struggle for world peace.

Much to her delight, the Contessa had been hailed a heroine and there was talk of a bravery award. Guy felt quite sure that, in the future, no water authority would ever dream of reprimanding her as she sped across the lagoon in her usual, gutsy, manner.

The press, who had cooperated and kept their silence during the operation, had been promised a conference the next morning with a panel of senior intelligence and police officers, where they were to be briefed on the full story.

Guy and Julian were both glad to be leaving the city. The Contessa was quite aware that her life would be extremely public for sometime to come, once the story hit the newspaper headlines. Secretly, she was quite looking forward to her new 'film star' status.

Julian's so-called death would be put down to a case of misidentification. Both men received hand written commendations from 'C', written in his unique green ink. Their credentials were updated and their identities protected just in case they could be persuaded back on a more permanent basis. Experience carried a huge value in all operations, but Guy had made it quite clear that they both intended to take a long sabbatical first, before considering any further involvement. They needed to sort out their private lives. They had other responsibilities and hopes for the future. Their offices at home had plenty of back up and their seasonal holidays were well overdue.

~

In the late afternoon the three friends sped across the lagoon for one last time, but this time to the airport. As usual Caro was at the helm. They flew in the same small Cessna to a former military airport near Ancona. Caro loved the journey and it was all they could do to put her off taking the controls of the plane. She argued that she would be 'perfectly 'capable', as it was similar to one she'd flown in Kenya, animal spotting, in her youth.

Vittorio was waiting for them. He had closed his hotel in Verona for the night and his family were already with Gianni on Isola Delfino. Francesca had filled the car with so many specialities from the city that there had hardly been room enough for the children. How the food had arrived in one piece was something of a miracle, he'd told them, grinning, his eyes raised to heaven.

The small party wound their way slowly down the coast road, arriving in the port in the soft light of dusk, during that strange hushed spell, that peculiar interval between the coming night and a tired, laboured, day, when the earth seems to pause on it's pivotal journey; as if holding it's breath for that which is predestined but, as yet, uncertain and unknown.

As they all sat in the little café, in the quiet mellow evening, Guy and Julian were thinking ahead with anticipation to their landing on the island. Both were slightly nervous, wondering just how it would be.

Caro was enchanted with the port. Vittorio, who had immediately fallen for her charm, was listening to her wonderfully musical, if cultured, Italian. She was telling him that she had friends who would love to come here to paint.

"Ah!" replied Vittorio, *"Pittore,* painting! But that's how it all began," and needing little encouragement he began to relate the story of his parents in law; of how Gianni first met and fell in love with Giuseppina on the *'magico'* island of Delfino.

'Gianni and Giuseppina had met nearly thirty years before. Giuseppina, so like his own wife Francesca, as she was now, was born and educated in England. She was of Italian extraction, but her dark features belied her perfect English accent. Her facial expressions brimmed with good humour. She'd been on holiday with her parents, all those years ago, when they'd come to the island for the day. "They would have taken a small ferry across to the island from the old steps", said Vittorio pointing. "The ones that weren't used any more, at the far side of the port. They would have planned to have lunch in the restaurant on Delfino. In those days Gianni's mother Ana Maria was in charge of the restaurant and she was *'famosa'* for her cooking". Vittorio smiled at them, he was thoroughly enjoying telling the story.

'A little time later, the unsuspecting and young Gianni was on the quay in the little island harbour, busily tying up his father's boat, when he noticed the little figure sitting painting quietly near the restaurant. It was early for tourists and few hung around long, after an exceptional plate of his mother's pasta: at that time of year they headed back for the shops and bright lights on the mainland. Most of them, he said seriously, didn't appreciate the raw beauty of Delfino, out of season.'

Gianni had picked up the large crate of silver fish and started back for the restaurant, pretending not to notice the unusual visitor concentrating hard on her work beside the water. The beautiful, dark, girl never even lifted her head as he passed. But he could tell that she was very beautiful indeed.'

Vittorio, Caro could see, was generously embellishing the story.

'Inside the restaurant it was dark, out of the bright morning light. Gianni's mother was deep in conversation with a couple drinking coffee in the corner. Maybe it was her parents Gianni had thought; they looked nice people. His father and brothers were nowhere to be seen, probably checking the lobster pots. He'd noticed Dimitri's boat was missing.'

Vittorio was now in full swing, gesticulating with his hands:

'Gianni had emptied the fish into the large, clean, enamel, bowl by the sink then set off back to the boat again, with the empty crate. As he passed by he'd stolen a glance at the picture. It was full of life, the water slapping against the boats where they bobbed up and down catching the light. So intent was he on looking at the picture that he jumped as she turned round and looked up at him. That had been it: he was lost forever. Humour had simply glowed in her deep, dark, eyes and the smile lit up her whole face. Gianni was in love ...'

Vittorio paused for effect. He had the full attention of his audience now and Guy and Julian were both trying to keep a straight face, Caro kicked them under the table. Vittorio didn't notice; he was in another world.

"Buongiorno", Gianni had sputtered, thoroughly embarrassed.

"Good Morning", had come back in the perfect English accent.

'All Gianni had wanted to do, as he stared into her face right then and there, was to pick her up and carry her off into the olive grove, never let her out of his sight again and forget all about the fact that he was due back at his army base the next day.

For Giuseppina it had been the same: instantaneous. She couldn't drag her eyes from his face; she knew immediately that this was forever and always: like minds and like souls. They were finally brought back to reality when her parents emerged from the restaurant with Gianni's mother, Ana Maria. The older ones had looked on incredulously when they saw the two young ones with their heads together on the quay. The falling in love,' Vittorio, hesitated, to establish his considerable knowledge on this subject then, repeated for affect, 'the falling in love, it had been in the twinkling of an eye, as you would say in English. The families soon knew that the future was a forgone conclusion and that their children's romance would lead to a marriage made in heaven!'

Vittorio, brushing a tear from his eye, looked at Caro to see if she was impressed. She was. Caro was entranced.

"Do go on, please! What a wonderfully romantic story," sighed the Contessa.

'They'd been married six months later, when Gianni had managed to arrange some extended leave on the mainland, where Giuseppina's father had most of his relations. They lived in the lovely, old, walled, town of Anghiari, East of Florence. It was situated in the peaceful valley of the river Tiber where for several generations they'd been in the traditional business of growing tobacco. The wedding celebrations had lasted for three days and three nights.'

"All of us Italians love a wedding," said Vittorio, "but a love match such as this was truly something to make the most of."

'Giuseppina's grandparents were delighted to have their 'English family' back in Italy again and for the next generation to be properly Italian. The Vivarini's had been equally euphoric.

Giuseppina had returned briefly to England before the wedding and Gianni thought his heart would break when she left the island. After that, they were separated only in the early days, when his army duties wouldn't allow for her to go with him.

When Gianni's time in the Italian special forces was finished; " *Very danger-ous work* ", said the storyteller, in a whisper for effect, 'Gianni and Giuseppina returned to the island and he began to take over responsibility from his father, enabling Allessandro senior to have a more restful life with Ana Maria, who at that time hadn't the best of health. Gianni kept himself fit and stong, returning to his nearest company base on the mainland at regular intervals, to make sure he was up to date with changes in equipment and training. Sometimes, he would join in the briefings, before an operation, or stay late into the night watching the outcome of some surveillance task on the ever-more sophisticated monitoring equipment.'

"For he was very 'big' and well respected in the army" added Vittorio with some relish, his English beginning to falter. He was quite obviously exceedingly proud of his father-in-law.

'When their children, the three girls, Amalia, my Francesca and Teresa were born, on the island, Gianni never left Giuseppina's side and no man had ever been so proud as he'd stood in the doorway of his house and on each occasion lifted each child high above his head to show the world. Never mind that they were all to be girls; as far as Gianni was concerned they were each a replica of his adored Giuseppina and his women meant the world to him.'

"As they still do," he said as he took a deep breath, straightened his back and concluding in a very serious almost reverent voice: "And I am very honoured to have Francesca as my wife." There was absolute silence for a minute.

"Well," said Caro, letting out a sigh, "what a marvellous storyteller you are, Vittorio. I thoroughly enjoyed it and just can't wait to meet them all. Thank you so very much indeed. I honestly think that you should write a novel, you told it so well!"

"Ah, no *Signora,*" replied the pleased Vittorio, modestly, "the real story-teller is Dimitri, Gianni's brother, who also you shall be meeting soon."

Later, much later, after several glasses of the local family wine, which also seemed to impress Caro, they heard the sound of music come floating across the water and with barely disguised excitement, the men began to stir. The party was well enough underway and it was time to take the little fishing smack, left for them tied up on the quay, out across the calm water to the island and there, hopefully, to pick up the thread of their private lives again.

★★★

CHAPTER 34

Alicia had found it difficult to eat. The hospitality, the genuine affection from all the family, the friendliness and courtesy shown to Adriana as they immediately included her in their welcome, was overwhelming. When she saw the emotion and love emanating from Gianni and Giuseppina she nearly burst into tears. It was all just too much! Later, as she and Gianni finished a dance, amidst much clapping and cheering, she said quietly to him. "Gianni I'm just going down to the beach for a while, will you please excuse me?"

"I quite understand, believe me," he answered immediately. "You go and stay as long as you wish, for it's the right place for you to be." She gave him a kiss and walked quickly away, once again thankful for his sensitivity.

Gianni watched her go, took little Gi by the hand to stop him following, then slipped outside himself. It was a bright, moonlit, night and easy to see. He strolled along towards the quay, listening. He knew it was nearly time, so he sat on an upturned, old, boat hulk and waited, until he could just hear the familiar soft put-put of Mario's fishing smack approaching.

"Ah: good! The timing is perfect," he sighed and went in search of Giuseppina, who was now busying around somewhere, quite certain that Patrizia was going to give birth at any minute, judging by the way she was dancing.

~

Adriana, too, was emotionally overwrought by being in such a place

340

and surrounded by such warmth. She wondered yet again where the two men had got to. Were they safe and what was happening? It had been ages now, with no word. Maybe something had gone terribly wrong and she and Alicia just weren't being told?

Adriana's imagination was working overtime. Alicia was nowhere in sight, so she left the party. She also wanted to be alone and quiet; she needed the fresh air and time to think. She went to sit by the harbour wall, half way down the little landing stage and reached her hand down into the water, where it slapped, gently, against the sea wall. It was cool and refreshing, snapping her out of her melancholic mood. Where the sea touched land the other side was not so very far and then on to Venice, such a short journey really. The worst, as always, was 'the not knowing', but this island was certainly a great place to wait for news and the people were lovely. She swung her legs and watched as the incoming swell covered the bottom rungs of the ladder beside her, then withdrew leaving a piece of bedraggled seaweed trailing, dripping, waiting to be released by the next surge of water. Visualizing its cold, slimy feel, she reached down to touch it, then, suddenly alert, she listened:

Adriana, too, heard the throaty little engine before she saw the boat and when it appeared through the entrance to the harbour, she decided that it was just another guest arriving late for the party. At least it's distracted my rather morose imaginings she thought, as she watched its approach.

As the vessel continued its way, steadily, towards the landing, the people in it were silhouetted against the dull glow of the entrance lights. Something made Adriana stand and, as she shaded her eyes to see better, under the harbour lights, one of the figures in the boat also stood and then she knew; she knew for sure; it was Julian. Why had she come out here? Sixth sense: and her heart reached out, drawing him back to her, across the calm effervescent water.

Gianni had returned and stood to one side, in the shadows, not wishing to intrude. Before the boat touched the harbour wall, they were together. He turned away and wiped the back of his hand across his eyes and then waited to give them time to walk away before clearing his throat and going quickly across the cobbles to take the rope from Guy to secure the boat. Guy took Gianni's hand as he leapt out, pulled him to him and kissing him on both cheeks, said gruffly,

"Gianni, my friend, thank you for this, for everything, what more can I say?"

"*Prego*, my friend, *prego*, you're more than welcome believe me!" then Guy looked at him, with a question in his eyes.

"She's on the beach," nodded Gianni understanding his hurry. "Take the path through the vines, then, down to the sea, you remember the way.

"Does she know?" he asked.

"No nothing. Now go, she's waiting and I'll look after the Contessa, don't worry," he added with a chuckle. Guy took Gianni's hand again, squeezed it hard then strode purposely off towards the vineyard.

~

Alicia stood looking at the sea, her shoes in her hand and her toes sinking into the sand. The soft breeze blew her skirt gently around her legs and moved her hair like a whisper. It was sensuous. The water began to lap around her feet. Tomorrow would soon be here, what would it bring?

She wished, Oh how she wished! But she just had to continue, just taking one day at a time and still keeping faith, somehow, that all might be well in the end. Gulls circled overhead crying and she looked up, then watched, as not far out the water began to ripple and they dropped to fish.

She started walking back; scuffing her feet and concentrating on dodging the shells, for some were sharp. Alicia looked up again suddenly as if disturbed. A movement in the distance had caught her attention. The rocks

- her rocks had moved! Somebody had been sitting there quietly watching and now they were standing and beginning to walk slowly towards her. Her heart told her before her head. His arms were now clearly spread wide under the moon.

Alicia began to run. Her feet were wet, the sand got in the way, clinging to her toes. She couldn't feel her legs, but somehow they propelled her across the beach with a mind of their own. Her heart unencumbered, free and certain of its direction; flew within her stumbling body across the space between them, as laughing and crying she finally arrived where she most longed to be.

Guy scooped her up in his arms in one easy, fluid movement, and against the pale light of a star spangled sky, their two halves merged as one.

~

Gianni was sitting by himself on the quay, smiling to himself. He was a contented man. He had, with God's help, achieved what he had set out to do all those long months ago when Alicia, so desperately unhappy, had first come to the island.

He'd seen her radiant, golden, smile; genuine and from the soul. He felt warm inside just thinking about it. Now he knew for certain that Alicia was to be secure and happy again with Guy. After what they had both been through, he thought that perhaps the two of them would never stop smiling. They would be living in permanent sunshine and the world would certainly be a better place for it.

Gianni was pleased in the knowledge that he'd played a large part in events. The biggest reward of all was that, by an extraordinary quirk of fate, this couple, whom he loved so dearly, should find each other again on his island. He could imagine them there now, the two of them beside the sea, silhouetted against the moonlit sky.

Gianni remembered his sense of disquiet, when he'd first noticed the lonely girl, newly arrived from England, by the waters edge, at dawn. Little did any of them know, then, what life had in store. He realized that, in spite of fate's twists and turns, they had come full circle. This strange, unsettled, period in time had reached its grand finale where it had begun: in his place, on the magical shell beach, his land and his proud home, Delfino Island. In his mind's eye, Gianni's view was enchantingly complete and he was so very glad for them all.

~

Aroused from his reverie, Gianni could hear a commotion at the entrance to the restaurant behind him. Something else was in the air. He turned to listen for a moment, to the excited calls and hurried conversation. From past experience, this time he knew, immediately, just what it was all about. Patrizia, with his next nephew and three weeks early!

The excitement was all too much for the mother-to-be. When he'd seen his sister-in-law at the beginning of the evening, he'd known she wouldn't last the night. She had what he called 'the look' and he'd told them all earlier that Patrizia had her timing wrong. His younger brother had laughed and walked away shaking his head, denying the very idea. Mario, wasn't quite ready, he was still struggling to finish re-decorating the family crib, but, Gianni's wife had caught his eye, imperceptibly nodding her head in agreement. It was going to be a long night ahead.

With his heart full, Gianni heaved himself up and set off towards the voices and the music. Still smiling, as if he too would never stop, he went to find his own, beloved, Giuseppina once more and, to help make preparations for the arrival of this next family member.

★★★

The End

Coming soon by the same Author

Synopsis

UNDER THE OLIVES

Under The Olives, is a present day story set on a fictional island in the Ionian Sea, off mainland Greece. Everything of importance happens in the strange, mesmeric, atmosphere amongst the olive trees.

Few people ever take the time to really look within these ancient plantations: the indigenous groves are not advertised. The local people, living alongside the olives are too busy, going about their daily routine, to see them as anything more than the provider of regular income.

Visitors flash by, without even a glance at the bewitching, almost eerie, light filtering through beneath the low spread branches of the knarled, old, trees. They remain unaware of the mysterious allure of the huge groves, in which there is another hidden world, waiting to divulge its secrets.

For the few curious enough to venture forth, on first entering there is a strange ambience; an overload of the three senses; a distinctive but pleasant, earthy, aroma; bright flickering light and a heavy, seductive silence.

At the beginning that is … for suddenly there is sound, the resumption of interrupted birdsong, the snap of a twig; then, as the eyes become accustomed, motion: movement in the distance, an animal perhaps?

But if you stay awhile, to linger, look and listen, if your mind is open and fertile, you might just come upon something quite unique ... and ... it could just change your life for ever.

~

Emma Brook, vulnerable and fragile, leaves a bad situation behind in England to explore the possibilities of a painting holiday in Greece for her travel agency business.

Underneath the olives, Emma does indeed discover a whole secret world, just as the stranger on the plane implied she would.

Who was the shy goatherd who never came out into the light? Why was he hiding?

Who was the beautiful, reclusive, woman? And who were the mysterious little gypsies playing amongst the trees?

At the Hotel Stavros Emma meets an intriguing mix of diverse, irrevocably linked, characters as she confronts her own destiny with visitors, both welcome and uninvited.

In the hypnotic atmosphere of the olive grove she encounters tenderness, tragedy and shocking drama. She unravels the answer to a gripping riddle from the past and discovers an unexpected magic for herself. .

~

VIRGINIA VERE NICOLL

Ginny was brought up in the Cotswolds and educated in England. She spent a year working in the U.S.A, before travelling extensively throughout America, Canada and Mexico.

A water-colourist, after leaving school, Ginny attended the Warwickshire College of art, and, more recently, studied both at West Dean College and in Italy. She exhibited, successfully, in the West End of London.

Ginny brought up a large, boisterous, family of four, based in London and in Sussex; in an old farmhouse, down a long, rough, track, in the middle of a large, derelict, plum orchard. Here, a few years ago, Ginny put aside her paints and started to write. She enrolled for an Arvon writing course in the West Country. It was winter and freezing cold, but taught by two well-published authors, she was filled with enthusiasm and given endless encouragement. In the beautiful, frosted, Devonshire countryside, she learnt how to polish and finish her manuscripts.

Passionate about travelling, particularly across Europe, either by car, train, or even by foot, she takes every opportunity, either alone or on business with her husband, to gather information and material, as she did when painting watercolours.

Ginny loves being surrounded by her family. But, whenever possible, re-treats to a refuge in the Alps, where she likes best to join the eagles, high up in the mountains, free from ordinary, mundane, matters and from where she can view the world from another dimension.

There, she finds her inspiration for the stories she has to tell.

~

Printed in the United Kingdom
by Lightning Source UK Ltd.
132433UK00001B/35/P

THE

PATMOS
ENIGMA

Quest of The Wandering Jew

KEN FRY

THE PATMOS ENIGMA
Quest of The Wandering Jew
Copyright © 2017 by KEN FRY

First Edition
v2.1

www.booksbykenfry.com

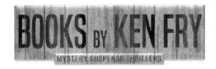

Edited by Eeva Lancaster
Cover Design and Book Interior by The Book Khaleesi
www.thebookkhaleesi.com

ISBN-13: 978-1975849030
ISBN-10: 1975849035

10 9 8 7 6 5 4 3 2 1

BOOKS by KEN FRY

The Chronicles of Aveline: Awakening

Disjointed Tales

The Patmos Enigma: Quest of the Wandering Jew

Red Ground: The Forgotten Conflict

The Lazarus Succession

The Brodsky Affair

Suicide Seeds

Check Mate

Is That You, Jim? (FREE)

AUDIOBOOK

The Lazarus Succession
(Narrated by Jack Wynters)

Join Ken Fry's Circle of Readers
and Get a Free Thriller

www.booksbykenfry.com

PROLOGUE

Beit-Guvrin
Judea, A.D.100

DEATH DESCENDED UPON him fast. Its blood lust grasped out to seize his lifeforce.

His heart hammered in his chest as he forced his exhausted body across an unforgiving terrain. He prayed for the courage to accept the kiss of his nemesis, and that its embrace would be short, sharp, and quick.

They were right behind him, gaining fast. He could hear their steel swords clashing.

Pushing himself forward, he gasped in pain. But … he must keep running. To stop would surely seal his fate. One swift blow and his head would be a gift to the sand beneath his feet. His sandals slipped and turned with every agonising stride across rocks and spiky shrubs. There was nowhere to go but upwards, and there could be no return.

His obedience to his mentors, the Guardians, had transformed him from law-abiding husband and father, into a man condemned. But he must obey his vows … must fulfill

1

his purpose.

Behind, an elite troop of armed Roman legionnaires were in pursuit. One mounted soldier astride a white Arab stallion urged his panting steed to a faster gallop, and began closing in on him like a cheetah pursuing a deer. From the way he pointed his javelin at Koury's sweat-stained back, his intent was clear. "Ya! Ya!" The soldier spurred his excited mount onwards.

Koury bit his lip and subjected his twenty-two-year-old body into extremes it had never experienced before. Zigzagging, staggering, and reeling across the stone strewn earth, he crashed through the thorny shrubs, ignoring the ripping of his flesh. He knew what they were after. He gripped the bag slung across his back closer to his body. Even he, Adil Koury, had scant knowledge of its contents.

He stumbled.

The stallion and the soldier brandishing his lance closed in on him.

Earlier that morning, before the sun's light consumed a stubborn moon, he had been at the Temple, preparing food for the community. The Guardians had recognised him as a loyal and devoted member, and had summoned him to their presence in secret.

He had sensed from the urgent and hushed tones of his Master that a cancerous fear had penetrated the sacred walls where God's altar stood. Like a reptile's unctuous tongue looking for food, foulness had seeped and wrapped itself into the holy place. It adhered to the walls like glue from gutted goats. It was in the air … a smell of dread had leached into the Temple.

In front of a small altar, lit by the oil of two small lamps, its aroma moving skyward to blend in with burning frankincense, stood his Master. The years had worn him down. A man who had seen too many of life's horrors. He wore a black linen robe, and around his neck hung the symbol of a fish. Watery eyes and a wrinkled skin enhanced his grave and perturbed expression. He handed Koury a small stone box. It had been sealed with great care, with a long hessian strap attached to it. The top was engraved with a winged crown.

He was to ask no questions, inform nobody, and bury the artefact in the underground caves, hidden from view in the distant hills. These were known only to a few, and Adil Koury was one of them. When accomplished, he was to report back.

His Master whispered in hushed and reverential tones, "In what you carry, hangs the future of mankind as prescribed by God Almighty, and the instrument from which Christ will return to deliver His promise to humanity. It is but a part, yet the most vital. We have concealed the others elsewhere. That is all you need to know. It is of the utmost sanctity and significance."

The importance and the honour he had been given was not lost on Koury. He swore in secret to himself that he would die in defence and execution of the Guardians' trust in him. As Christians, they had been persecuted by Rome, and for three years, he had followed and obeyed every doctrine and regulation the Guardians had given him.

He bent low in his acceptance of the task, and kissed the

feet of his Master. As he arose, he heard an enormous commotion from below, in the courtyard.

"Romans!" the Master shouted in a panic. "We have been betrayed and they're after our secret. There's a Judas in our midst!" He gave Koury a massive push. "Run, and do not stop! It must not fall into the hands of others. Take it to the place that only you know of and drop it into the eternal darkness. Do not fail! For the love of Christ … run like the wind!"

Even before he had finished speaking, Koury heard a heavy thump and a cracking noise. A Roman javelin had penetrated deep into his Master's back, protruding completely from the front of his chest, along with his bloody ribs, in a lung spluttering slurp.

The clatter of armour approaching from the bottom of the stairs grew closer. Koury needed no second bidding. He leapt from the window, down into the busy street, and began to run. Of what befell his Master, he had little doubt.

His own escape had not gone unnoticed, and a chase ensued.

For the first time in his life, Adil Koury experienced real fear. But he had become a courier of God, and the sanctity of his mission would give him the strength he needed to see it through.

The horse soldier closed in on him. He could hear and feel the rumble of the animal's hooves through the ground.

There it is… get up, get up! … only a few more yards. Please

God, let me make it for your sake!

The fissure, narrow and indistinct, beckoned him. He turned sideways and squeezed himself into the gap. The mighty sound of Roman steel smashed into the rock inches from his head, again and again. But, he had made it. Behind him, twenty Roman soldiers were struggling to fit themselves into the narrow opening. Koury knew that no fully armoured soldier would be able to follow him inside. He was safe for now.

Half crawling, half slithering, he pushed further into the damp shoulder-width passageway leading into the subterranean maze of twisting tunnels and dark entrances. The shouts of the soldiers lessened as he moved along.

It had not been long since the Temple of Jerusalem, as prophesied, had suffered its second destruction. He surmised that what he carried was in some way connected to that event. Many writings, parchments and manuscripts, had been saved from the Roman pagans. He was certain that what hung from his back was similar, but more important than the rest, for The Guardians to protect it with their lives. The Master had entrusted him with this task because of his knowledge of the cave system.

He paused and gathered his breath. From above, light streamed in from countless splits and crevices in the overhead rocks. He knew where he was headed, and he braced himself for the perilous path ahead.

For a moment, Koury thought of his wife and children. If captured, he would never see them again. If he wasn't careful, he might never come out of this cave. The corridors were riddled with endless labyrinths and rocky mazes. Skeletons testified to those who had perished in the subterranean darkness, unable to find a way out. It had been rumoured that riches were buried here, but Koury cared not. What he carried was priceless beyond the wealth of men.

He walked on, uttering a silent prayer for himself and his family.

The wall and rocks were chalky, slippery, and tight. So cramped, he had to flip upside down to continue.

When he reached his destination, Koury went down on his knees, giving his eyes a moment to adjust to the darkness. Then, raising his face to the stalactites pointing down at him, he gave thanks to God.

In a vast expanse stretching out to a great depth below him was a columbarium, now disused and forgotten even by the elders of his village, carved out when the Israelites had settled in the land as Moses had predicted. In the dim light filtering from above, he could not see the bottom. The light barely penetrated the blackness. He gazed down into the infinite expanse, and was suffused with the dark magnificence of it all. He, Adil Koury, had been entrusted with a mission from God. Unbelievable. He was unworthy, no better than a pile of pig excrement. *I am not fit for this task.*

Turning, his eyes increasingly adjusting to the sepulchral gloom, Koury paused, listening. There were no soldiers following. Only the odd drip of water disturbed the deafening silence.

Out of nowhere, a message filled his head. Persistent and urgent, he was being told what to do. Without thought, he retrieved a sharp flint from the ground, and began to scratch on the hard wall, writing what played repeatedly in his mind. When finished, he read it aloud and was pleased. He had done as he had been told.

Next, he took out the box from his bag and held it aloft. Where it was going, there would be no need for digging. Its mystery would be safe. *Great Christ be praised!*

He had underestimated the slipperiness of the rocks. As he lifted the box to drop it into the black abyss, his feet skidded on the damp moistness of the edge.

Without a sound, he fell … plunging into the deep and tarry darkness. Still, Koury held the box with a grip of steel.

No sound came from him.

He plummeted, the rush of air propelling him downwards into the depths, and out of sight.

Koury had accomplished his sacred mission, and for his courage and faith, he would be rewarded. To transcend death and guard the seal until the time comes for it to be opened.

His body would never touch the ground.

Chapter 1

Tel Aviv University
Institute of Archaeology
Israel
The Present Day

THE DEPUTY ARCHAEOLOGY Director barged into Professor Simon Rockwell's study and slapped a roll of papers across his desk. "I think we're on to something."

Rockwell raised an eyebrow. "What might that be, Julian?"

Dr. Julian Gallo had not been blessed with height. He was a chunky, well-rounded man with prominent, unkempt black eyebrows, brown eyes, and a fleshy mouth. His skin had an oily sheen.

Rockwell grabbed the roll and spread it across his desk. It appeared to be a map of their team's excavation sites. He stood and bent closer to look. Towering over Gallo by several inches, he was thin, with an athletic physique. A stark contrast to his deputy. Streaks of silver can be seen in his dark hair as he focused on the map, his dark blue eyes scanning the paper.

"It's a blueprint of our dig," Gallo said.

"I can see that. So, what's new about it?"

Gallo's stubby finger poked at the most northerly point on the chart. "Just eighty kilometres south from here are the hills and terrain of Beit-Guvrin. As you know, much of our excavation has been concentrated or near the amphitheatre, right here at this point." He stabbed at the location. "We know from our previous digs that a temple, albeit a small one, existed there until it was razed to the ground, like the Temple of Jerusalem and many others in the same period."

"Your point being?" Rockwell growled. As Professor of Ancient and Religious History and in charge of all things archaeological, he didn't need lessons.

"My point is, I had a phone call earlier this morning from Joshua. He has discovered a mass of bones, and an item he got excited about. He needs us to go there and examine them."

"You should have told me earlier. What are we waiting for? Let's go."

"I tried to, but you didn't answer your phone."

"Never mind that." He shouted into the next room, "Rachael, I'm off for a while. You can come along, if you want."

Dr. Rachael Carver, Rockwell's Assistant Director, had grown used to his sudden and unscheduled activities. "Hold on a moment please, Simon!" She stepped into his study. She was a pretty and petite, thirty something brunette, dressed in khaki shirt and army-style trousers. She bustled with energy. "How long are you going to be?" Even as she asked, she realised the question wouldn't be answered.

"How long, I've no idea. But we're going down to Beit-Guvrin now. C'mon, be quick." He gave her a grin, like a naughty boy being caught doing something he shouldn't and darted out of the room.

"I'm coming." She raised her eyes skyward and emitted an exasperated sigh. She liked him, and if pressed, would have admitted to more than that.

The Jeep, driven by Gallo, barrelled its way at speed down the main highway.

"Why's Josh getting excited over a pile of bones and a few religious bits? He must have seen enough in his time, Julian?"

"No idea, but boy, he sounded excited. All he said was this find was different from the usual."

"We've had plenty of false alarms before. I hope this isn't one of them."

The conversation came to a natural break and they sped on in silence. Rockwell was *the* acknowledged authority in his chosen field. At thirty-seven years old, his dazzling talents of observation and intuitive accuracy were legendary, and all at such a young age. His biggest discovery was a sealed urn found behind an ancient wall. Perfectly preserved, he had deciphered the manuscript inside, and it is now accepted by some as *The Gospel of Ephraim, Son of Mary Magdalene.* If speculation was correct, and Jesus did indeed marry Mary Magdalene, Ephraim would have been his son. That discovery, and its implications, had stirred scholars and the religious world into fervour. Of course, the Vatican and all other Christian denominations, barring a few fringe groups, rejected it. Not that Rockwell cared. He delivered what he found, and avoided subjective arguments.

An hour had passed before the Jeep finally rolled into the site's parking area. The three leapt out and were greeted by an excited looking Joshua Agar, the site and excavation supervisor. Joshua stood at around six feet, and had a Mediterranean appearance; with his tanned olive skin, dark wavy hair, and surprisingly green eyes. He shook hands with vigour, and began to explain the nature of the discovery.

"This way, please." He led them through rough paths and over low stone walls that were being excavated, revealing themselves after more than two thousand years of neglect.

Joshua stopped at a broad tented area, shielded from the blazing sun by an array of massive canopies. Inside, a dozen trestle tables were scattered, on which were displayed various packed, photographed, and labelled artefacts dug up from the site. On one table, conspicuous by its solitary position, sat a stone item that looked like an ossuary of some kind. Several photographs and bones of varying sizes surrounded it.

Rockwell's attention was captured. "Where did you find this?"

"In an area where there was an altar of some sort, wedged under a solid flat stone slab. My guess is that it has remained that way for two thousand years or so. It looked undisturbed and must have been there since the time it was placed."

Rockwell picked up the ossuary, and at once, he saw letters or figures etched into the stone. He produced a lens and peered at the markings long and hard. For a fraction of time, the hairs on his arms bristled. He gave a long low whistle.

Gallo remained expressionless. "What do you think it is?"

"It's a mixture of words and symbols; some Coptic, others Aramaic. I'll tell you quickly, offhand, and without real investigation, what it says and suggests, before we open it. This is it…

Blessed John, the leader of us Guardians, spoken to and delivered by Yeshua, tells you that the key is almost in your hands …

"The rest had been defaced or has worn away, and is unreadable. Who the hell the Guardians were, I've no idea. We all know the name Yeshua means Jesus, a common enough name at the time. Let's see if we can open this thing. Joshua, please …" He held his hand out for a scalpel. He gripped the instrument placed in his hand, hovering above the ossuary. "Someone start taking pictures, please … NOW!"

With a strange expression on his face, Gallo dug out his Lumix and focused in close on Rockwell's hands and scalpel, as the man probed around the ancient seal with utmost care.

Rockwell inched the blade along, and sensed the seal giving way. He couldn't help but marvel that someone had sealed it centuries ago, and here he was, opening it for the first time. He stood back and looked around.

"This really scares me, this sort of stuff."

By now, the word had spread, and a hoard of archaeology students had gathered round to witness the event. Gallo kept the camera poised and ready as Rockwell began to lift the lid, and minute pieces of debris said farewell to their ancient resting place.

The lid opened.

Inside were what looked like several metal plates held together by small clasps.

At that moment, the air changed, and for a minute, a blast of coldness blew with such force through the tent, it sent tables and chairs flying. Paper and anything on them were hurled across and out of the tents, threatening their stability. The observers looked astonished as they crouched and held on to anything they could grab on. In moments, it had gone as soon as it had arrived, and everything went still.

"What the hell was that?" Rockwell's brow was furrowed, his arm still around the ossuary to keep it from breaking. "Was I imagining it or what?" He looked around.

Joshua spoke, "No, it was real enough. I think we've upset someone, somewhere."

"Rubbish, Joshua. Anyway, it's gone, forget it. Let's see what this is. Don't anyone touch it, please!" He peered hard at the plates through his lens. "I would say, whatever this is, it's remained untouched from the day it was sealed. What it is and why it's been so carefully preserved, I can't say for now. If I'm not mistaken, that top plate looks as if it has a depiction of a crucifixion painted on it. What do you think?" He handed Gallo the lens.

Gallo was white-faced and grim, but his eyes held an excited gleam. "Astonishing! Good God, there're six clasps, and each with seven plates attached. They're not much bigger than a credit card. You're right. It's a crucifixion, without a doubt."

"Look," Rachael interrupted as she pointed at what looked like fabric of some sort, "there are strips of cloth here. They must be as old as the whole damn thing."

"This find could be of major importance, Julian." Rockwell quivered. This could be the dream find all archaeologists aspire for. He turned to Joshua. "Joshua, prepare this now. We are taking it back to the lab for testing and analysis.

Chapter 2

RACHAEL MARCHED DOWN the corridor to her counterpart's office. When she burst through his door, Gallo was speaking on the phone. At her unannounced entrance, he quickly rapped on the button and ended his conversation. He looked annoyed.

"Rachael, please don't barge in like that. I happened to be having a private conversation. In the future, will you please refrain from entering without knocking first?"

"Okay, Julian. Sorry." She had no interest in his complaint. "I just wanted to tell you that Joshua has delivered the reliquary, and Simon is already submitting it and its contents for C14 testing. He wants you and your colleagues to go over the findings.

"Well that's going to take a few days, so there's not much I can do until the results come in."

"There's something else you should know."

"What's that?"

"Those metal plates or tags are decorated with very fine paintings, a bit like the miniatures we associate with the eighteenth century. Each seems to depict a Biblical event. The reverse sides are inscribed, but we haven't translated them yet. They'll have to be checked. But here's the intriguing bit.

There's a set missing. The hinge clearly shows there was another set attached. We have forty-two, whereby there should be forty-nine."

The colour drained from Gallo's face, leaving it an ashen grey.

"Hey, you okay? You look as if you've seen a ghost."

Gallo pulled himself back to normal. "Don't worry, I'm fine. It's a regular thing with me … excitement maybe. What's missing, do you know?"

"Daft question. How would we know that? We don't even know what it is yet. It's interesting though, don't you think? The tags are two sided, so we may be able to work out what the missing plates could be."

Gallo gave an all-knowing smirk. "I'm sure you will."

"Well, when the test results are back, we're having a meeting to discuss what this discovery could be. I don't know what to do now, but I'm planning to check on some of those old prophecies these ancient Jews and Romans were always banging on about."

Gallo paused, his eyes held an odd glint. "Will they ever come true, or have they already done so?"

"Who knows?" Rachael replied. "But I bet for all the tea in China, that little find of Joshua's has something spooky to tell us."

"Rachael, I don't speculate. It's a futile response. I prefer facts. Now, if you will excuse me. I've work to do."

"God, Julian, you can be a right tetchy bastard at times. Don't worry, I'm off!" The door slammed hard as she left.

Gallo breathed a sigh of relief, stood, and then moved across the room and locked the door. He opened his desk drawer and reached to the back of it. Buried beneath a pile of papers, he detached a black velvet drawstring bag. Reaching in, he pulled out an ancient looking leather-bound booklet. The edge of the pages was crackled and discoloured to a yellow brown hue. He held the book to his lips and kissed it. Opening it with great care, he turned several pages before he found what he wanted. Producing a lens, he peered at the writing and copied it into his notebook. Then, he opened his computer, accessed a site that was not listed in English, and began to type in what he had written. When done, he knelt on one knee, and murmured a prayer.

Chapter 3

Patmos, Greece
1549 A.D.

THE SENESCHAL STEPPED onto the sacred soil of Patmos and knelt. Picking up a small rock, he kissed it with reverence. He had followed The Keeper's commands to the letter.

To this island, the blessed John had been banished by the Roman Emperor, Domitian, for preaching Christianity. On this very soil, the beloved disciple had received, in a sequence of seven angel-given dreams, the greatest of sacred revelations. He had been instructed by Christ to record and deliver them to the seven churches of the island.

He had said: *I will be hurt and I will bleed and I shall die. This I do for you all. You will scribe what I say, and when your writings are found, it will mark the final times.* This, the seneschal believed. He knew that John, fearful of the Church's collapse by the Romans, had the contents of his dreams depicted upon small metal tablets by two of his followers, Ephraim and Manasseh. There, they had revealed their understanding of the fate of humanity, measured not by events, days, weeks,

17

months, years, decades or centuries, but by millennia. The seven tablets or Seals, when broken, would herald the birth of a new world. Only the most favoured of men would be able to achieve this.

The two followers of John had returned to their homes near Jerusalem and took their secrets with them, but John's final words, he told them not. These he entrusted to a woman named Marathea, a descendant of Mary, to pass on to the accursed Guardians to ensure their safekeeping. When the times were in sequence with John's words and transcriptions, all would be revealed.

It had become perilous. Domitian was determined to wipe out the locusts of this Christian disease.

The seneschal knew of the seven churches, alleged to possess the sacred seals. Each of them had a characteristic synonymous with the prophecies. He searched, travelling to each location and making enquiries, but not a trace of the fabled relics could be found. They told him they never existed, and if they had, they had long ago been destroyed or lost.

But he didn't listen, and soon, his faith was rewarded.

While scouring the seventh church of Laodicea, the church that John described as 'lukewarm and insipid to God,' the seneschal found the only reference to the missing Seals. In a faded and almost colourless fresco, behind the altar and at floor level, was his first and only evidence. He became breathless. His hands trembled as he read in faded Hebrew:

אני השביעי שנמצא בבית גוברין

I am the Seventh and to be found in Beit-Guvrin

Supplanting it was an obvious depiction in faded blue and red, of some sort of scroll held by an uplifted hand.

Lukewarm and insipid to the Pope, but never God! He was overjoyed. His mission had not been fruitless. The Keeper would be pleased. Here was evidence that there existed a form of documented proof. What or where *Beit-Guvrin* was, he had no idea. It had taken centuries to find this one small clue, and it could take another century or more before another would come to light.

One Year Later
The Sistine Chapel, The Vatican
1550 A.D.

Standing under it, Cosimos Ricci felt the full significance of Michelangelo's *The Last Judgement* bearing down upon him from its divine throne. It didn't help the apprehension he felt for the meeting he had been summoned to today.

Behind the cause of his anxiety was the seneschal, not only of the Sistine Chapel, but of the clandestine society, *I Apocalittici Guerrieri di Cristo* (*The Apocalyptic Warriors of Christ*), of which he was a member. Their avowed intent is the destruction of the Roman Catholic Church, and existing world orders, no matter how long it would take. Their main interest is the implication of Christ's rule on earth, and to help bring about its devastation as foretold in the Book of

Revelation. They had been searching for the Seven Seals, for whosoever possessed them would wield power beyond the imagination of men.

To bolster their worth, the society claimed and tried to prove at every turn, albeit discreetly, that the Pope and his Church were instruments of Satan, preparing the way for the Antichrist. That if allowed, they would deviate people from the true doctrines, water them down, and allow heathens to open their mouths and preach from the Sacred Chapels of Christ in Saint Peter, seducing the masses with their blasphemous and vile words.

Cosimos worked as an artist with a burgeoning clientele. At twenty-five years, he had an enviable reputation, and had accumulated wealth at his young age. His forte was the depiction of notables set in scenes of rural idyllic. His recruitment to the Apocalyptic Warriors of Christ, or AWC, took place five years back. It happened the way all members experienced it; the casual encounter, the praise, an arranged meeting with someone of importance, the flattery, and then the subtle implantation of their ideas and philosophy.

Cosimos learned early on that any act that furthered the truth of the AWC was considered as approved by God. Second to that came complete obedience to their leader, The Grand Keeper. All unbelievers were considered poison. The Grand Keeper's identity remained unknown but to a small Inner Circle. His successor had always been appointed by his command alone. Nobody else possessed the authority to approve or disapprove any appointments to the society.

Cosimos had been flattered that a secret society, possessed of the highest knowledge and aspirations of men, should honour him with an invitation to become their disciple. He received a hidden thrill from knowing things, secrets and information that only the Apocalyptic Warriors of Christ knew of. They became integral to his life. He accepted and believed their tenets, without question. He had become close to the seneschal, but he feared him and his uncanny ability to see into a man's secret soul.

Waiting for his mentor in the half-light of the Chapel, Cosimos gazed around, feeling daunted by the overwhelming magnificence of the frescos. So different from his own work.

Soft footsteps from behind alerted him to the ghostlike presence of the seneschal. A stooped figure with a black cowl around his head, in the guise of a monk, beckoned him to a seat. His face, somewhat obscured, emitted an unmistakeable ageless intelligence. The seneschal stared down at the floor as he spoke, his voice curling around Cosimos like a wet tongue.

"Brother Cosimos, listen to what I say. As you are aware, the next part of your training is upon you. Few reach this point, and to do so is a high honour indeed. There have been but two others before you. The path is arduous and not without its dangers and heartaches. You may be required to do things part of you would rebel against, but are necessary to our cause. Yet, think again of what we will ask of you. If you decide to proceed, you will be taken from here to our novitiate, and you will begin the next level of your training. You will, of course, continue to paint. You will remain as Cosimos Ricci, the artist, to those who know of you. Perhaps, your hardest choice—" he stopped and seemed to stare at him from under his cowl. A few minutes passed before he continued, as if choosing his next words carefully. "You have a lover, Portia. You will be required to leave her. With what we have planned for you, you cannot be distracted by love and its ability to loosen willpower, dedication, and tongues."

Cosimos gasped. "How do you know about her?"

"We know everything about you from the day you were born. That is all I need say. You have three days in which to decide. To refuse will be considered as a request to leave us, and will activate the possible consequences that decision would incur. Is that understood?"

Cosimos understood the veiled threat. For him, there was but one consideration. Choosing between Portia and his Apocalyptic brothers.

He sensed that the seneschal wanted an immediate response. Hesitation, and the delay of three days would indicate uncertainty, indecision, ... not the qualities of a candidate destined for a high rank.

His heart lurched, like a log upon a block about to be split. Dizziness spun his head. Yet, there could be but one answer. Reaching out, he clasped the seneschal's tattooed, white bony hands in his own. With a low voice, he said, "I am yours to command, Master."

A thin smile crossed his mentor's face. "Congratulations, Cosimos. I knew you would not fail us. You have passed your first test. And now for the second ..."

Cosimos blanched at the seneschal's second demand. His hands shook. The seneschal's imperative made it clear to him that Portia was perceived as less than worthy, an embarrassment, and a hindrance to AWC's greater cause. In their battle with the evil descending upon the world, many unpalatable ordeals would have to be faced. Portia had become one such.

Before they parted, the seneschal had given the greatest promise he could possibly award the young Cosimos. Upon completion of his mission, he would get to meet the Grand Keeper.

Chapter 4

The Present Day

FIFTEEN MINUTES AGO, Rockwell had finished playing his piano. He played Chopin when he needed to relax, or to calm himself before a presentation. Today was one of those days. He left the house and drove down to the site to meet with his team.

The sun hesitantly arose over the camp as they made their way to the meeting area, under a large awning that overlooked the entire excavation site. On the table stood the subject of their meeting; a massive wooden crate, which housed the ossuary containing the metal tablets and the artefacts that had surrounded it.

Rockwell opened a computer printout and presented an analysis of the box, the tablets, and the bones and broken ceramics that had surrounded the find. He gazed around at his team.

"Friends, if the initial C14 tests are correct, we have hit the jackpot." He pulled the ossuary out from the crate and placed it in front.

"What do they show?" Gallo sounded cautious.

Rachael answered. "If we take the bones and pottery first, the tests confirm they are first century, and could be eighteen hundred to two thousand years old. As we speak, further DNA tests are being carried out on the bone fragments. What that will prove, I can't answer."

"This inscription on the surface of the casket could be a forgery." Rockwell stared at the writing once more through his lens. "But here's the shaker. The patina embedded into them is virtually impossible to fake. You can't get that degree or depth of ageing, as much as a faker might try. The tests confirmed that in age, it matches both the pottery and the bones, exactly."

Gallo's eyes widened. "Okay, we can go along with that, but what's important is what's inside. What does your report say about the tablets?"

Rockwell turned to Rachael. "Hold this, will you?' He handed her the thick file. "Let's have a further look then, shall we?" He opened the lid, and placed it with care on the table, before lifting out the metal plates and doing likewise. "Rachael, read the analysis for the tablets, please."

She read it aloud. "*Some of the metal pages are sealed and others are not. Each set contains seven metal tablets, and there are six in total, giving a total of forty-two pages. It is apparent, and is confirmed by metallurgical testing, that there used to be a seventh set containing seven more pages, which would have given a total of forty-nine pages. The corrosion, the oxidization present on the tablets, would be impossible to create artificially. The age of these artefacts is given confidently as first century A.D. The discovery is religious in content, and unless proved otherwise, very early*

Christian, and equal in age to any such previous discoveries."

"Wow." She looked startled. "Just what has Joshua found us?"

"It all seems to match up. What do you think, Julian?" Rockwell looked across to him.

Gallo didn't seem to hear. He had a faraway look in his eyes as he stared beyond the confines of the site.

The silence was broken by a loud shout from Joshua further down the slope. "Hey, you! Stop!"

They turned to see a small, dark, wiry man, dressed in black T-shirt and slacks, running at speed in their direction, and being pursued by Joshua and some other archaeologists. The man was zigzagging and brandishing a small pistol. There was the snap of a shot and one of the pursuers dropped to the ground as a bloody mess formed on his clothes. The man continued running and waving his gun. Both Rockwell and Rachael dived to the ground. Joshua and the others came to a halt with uncertainty on their faces. The man, with a glazed expression from bulging eyes, headed straight for the casket. He pointed the gun in every direction. Rockwell rolled over to cover Rachael and kept his head low. He didn't want anyone dying for an old relic.

Gallo hadn't moved. Standing between the artefact and the gunman, he stood motionless. His eyes fixed on the man as he stretched out his arm towards the reliquary. He spoke softly to the intruder, and the only indication that he spoke came from the movement of his lips.

The man froze as if in a trance.

Rockwell could only watch in astonishment with Rachael, who had lifted her head. The man raised the gun.

"Oh my God, no!" There was nothing Rockwell could do

but shout. There came the sharp sound of a gunshot.

But, it wasn't Gallo who dropped to the floor. The intruder fell to the ground in a messy heap. He'd blasted out his own brains.

"Don't look! Don't look!" Rockwell tried to push Rachael's head down, as he choked in disbelief at what he had just witnessed. "Julian's alive. But the man shot himself."

Rachael had to look. The sight of the dead man was not what surprised her. It was the expression she saw on Gallo's face. It was the same one she had seen when she barged in on his office the other day.

Gallo shouted down to Joshua. "Call the police and the ambulance. There's been an accident."

"Accident?" asked a shaken looking Rockwell. "The man just committed suicide. What were you saying to him for God's sake?"

Gallo turned. "Did you hear me say anything?" Without another glance at anybody, he sat down in a chair and answered the urgent tones of his mobile. The voice on the other line informed him his father had died.

The following evening, Rockwell, looking stony-faced, sat with Rachael in a nearby bar nursing a large Rusty Nail. She was having a Spritzer. There were no other customers.

Rachael looked around and spoke. "I think it's safe to talk here. There's no one around to hear us. I can't believe all that happened. Can you? Why did the man try to get hold of our find?" She shook her head. "It's made all the newspapers around here. Even the Washington Post called, requesting interviews and photographs. The damned thing's gone global. It's bound to set off a whole bunch of dealers, robbers, and Bible bashers heading in our direction."

"Right now, the artefact is locked up safely in our vaults. There's no way anyone can get their hands on it. But that's not what worries me. There's something very unusual here and I can feel it in my blood. Julian *was* speaking to the maniac, Rachael. I saw him, but he denied it."

"I agree. I saw his face and it was strange, to say the least. I'll tell you something else..."

"What?" He rattled the ice cubes in his tumbler and took a long gulp on his drink.

Rachael leant forward and whispered, "He told me some while back that his father had died years ago."

"What? But he's going to Rome to make the funeral arrangements."

"I know … Not much we can do about it now. He's on his way."

"We'll get to the bottom of it when he returns. I'm not letting him get away with whatever he's up to."

Hundreds of miles to the north, a private jet sped over the Mediterranean Sea heading for Rome's Ciampino Airport, the nearest to the Vatican City Heliport. Never a good traveller, Dr. Julian Gallo experienced a queasy sensation, informing him he could lose the contents of his stomach at any moment. He countered this by thinking of how he arrived at this situation in his life.

He had been drawn into the society many years ago, as if by chance. But later, he came to believe it had been ordained. He had been born of unknown parents and brought up as a Roman Catholic. The local Jesuits had been responsible for that. At one time, he had contemplated joining their elite ranks. But a conversation with a fellow brother had changed the course of his faith. He had been introduced to the study of the Book of Revelation, the Talmud, and other parallel routes.

Gallo had been searching for his life's purpose. For a short while as a young teenager, he had been a devotee of Opus Dei, and had happily worn the cilice. But their teachings had never been enough. It got close, but not quite.

He ventured into archaeology and had continued his exploration of The Book of Revelation and the Gnostic Gospels, and had published works on these topics, eventually gaining a reputation as an expert in Judaic and Early Christian Studies. His interests came to the attention of a mysterious brotherhood known as The Keepers, or *I Apocalittici Guerrieri di Cristo (AWC)*. His recruitment had been effortless.

His true and secret mission in life was to find and witness the opening of the Seven Seals. As a high-ranking member of the Keepers, he knew they were more than mere stories. A New World Order was just what this world needed. He believed that the Catholic Church was the enemy of Christ, and walked hand in hand with Satan. The sooner they were abolished, the better it would be for humanity.

The man who had introduced him to this knowledge had died long ago, but he always honoured his memory every 8th of May. That date had significance for the Keepers as well. It was the feast day of John the Divine, exiled to the island of

Patmos by Emperor Domitian around 90-95 A.D. It was there that he received and wrote the Book of Revelation.

There was an account of the miracle that occurred at St. John's grave. When over 100 years old, he took seven disciples outside of Ephesus, and had them dig a grave in the shape of a cross. St. John then went into the grave, and the disciples buried him there, alive. Later, when his grave was opened, his body had vanished. On May 8th of each year, dust rose from his grave, by which the sick are healed of various diseases. The Keepers saw this as their own, and a validity of their vision and movement.

An unexpected turbulence broke his thoughts and brought him back to the purpose of his visit.

His conversations on the phone was not what he had expected. There was an air of panic he couldn't quite understand. He fiddled with his briefcase which contained every photograph he had taken of the find. All that he lacked were the recent test results and analyses.

The suicidal runner should not have been at the site, and because of him, everything at Beit-Guvrin had gone wrong. Now, the whole world knew.

He bent his head in prayer, and on his finger, he twisted the gold ring shaped as a serpent eating its tail. He prayed that his master, The Grand Keeper, would know how to handle the situation.

The AWC was an ancient brotherhood, and they had encountered problems like this on many occasions. But like a phoenix, they had always prevailed and recovered. A small mishap would not be enough to divert them from their purpose.

All was not lost yet ... but Rockwell and Carver were

obstacles to overcome, before their great plan can move one
step forward.

Bishop Montefiore, solemn and unsmiling, was there to greet
him. The flight by helicopter had been short, and not a word
was spoken between the two men.

The rain lashed down hard. Montefiore took his arm and
steered him towards St. Peter's Basilica. Away from the
queues of pilgrims, and the ever faithful who would stand in
all weathers.

But would they be able to stand the truth? Gallo could only
wonder. He hugged his overcoat around him to keep out the
rain, and hoped the walk would not be much further.

A short and thickset man wearing a priest's collar and a
laminated Vatican ID lanyard around his neck, interrupted
their progress. His name showed him as Fr. Antonio Conti.

"Stop, please."

"What's the problem, Father?" inquired Montefiore. His
grip tightened on Gallo's arm.

"There's been a change in arrangements."

"I've heard nothing. What are you talking about?"

"You are not required, Bishop. Now, leave us." The butt
of a silver-plated Beretta M9 pistol revealed from a shoulder
holster was persuasive. "Go, please."

The Bishop seemed to understand. He nodded his head,
and scuttled away as if he had found a live fly in his pasta.

"What is this?" Gallo asked.

"You need know nothing yet, except that you are quite

safe. Walk in front of me and do as I tell you. *Si prega di comminare ora."* Father Conti waved his hand in a forward motion.

Gallo felt no fear. He knew too much, and his death would not help anybody. Whatever. He was an emissary of God, a member of *I Apocalittici Guerrieri di Cristo.*

They had not been walking long before a dark blue sedan drew alongside, and Gallo was bundled into the back seat. The driver swerved and manoeuvred his way through the crowded roads, tyres squealing, not stopping until he turned into the *Viale Bruno Buozzi,* where they finally stopped outside an unremarkable and unmarked building. Gallo recognized it at once. It had been twelve years since he was last there to complete his training.

"I know where I am, and I know why I am here. So, why the gun, Father?"

"You can never be too careful in Rome these days, Dr. Gallo. There were last minute changes to counteract possibilities of being compromised or spied upon. Does my answer satisfy you?"

"Perfectly. Now take me to him."

Father Conti gave a subservient nod of his head. "Follow me, please."

Chapter 5

Rome, 1550

AUTUMN ARRIVED LATE that year. Its drooping sadness gathered up and reflected the sorrow lurking in the heart of Cosimos. But, his course had been made clear.

Upon hearing his seneschal's second request, he knew he could not refuse it. At first, he thought he had misheard. He hadn't. It was repeated, so there could be no room for misunderstanding. As a faithful acolyte, he had accepted the first request. But the second stood as far away from his vision of potential beatification as he could have imagined.

It was a test, one he could not fail. He had replied, "Beloved seneschal, you once rescued me from despair and death…" he had paused, his heart heavy. Cosimos could not find his breath.

"Well, Cosimos?"

His reply was a strained whisper, "I cannot fail you. It will be done."

✝

The only sound he heard had been the flapping of a kit of pigeons taking off in the street below. From his window, Cosimos watched her walking up the steep cobbles to his studio door. Portia, without a doubt, was a beauty. The softness of her body rippled through the flowing material that clung around her without effort. At first, her parents had disapproved of her relationship with Cosimos. Artists were not to be trusted, they said. But his gathering success with distinguished figures and emissaries changed their perceptions. He became a welcome visitor in their home, and they began to consider their daughter's marriage to him.

Cosimos had set out his paints, brushes, and cleansers around the studio, as was his practice before commencing work. On this rare occasion, he had abandoned his working attire, and had donned the full regalia of the AWC instead. He wore a long shroud-like, monastic style robe and a full hood, which he left down on his shoulders. It was Tyrian purple in colour, with thin gold braiding on the leading edges. Before she arrived at the door, he knelt in a silent prayer for strength, courage, and to feel the warmth of his Saviour's hand upon his head.

Cosimos had struggled with the idea of how to perform his task. The seneschal had given him several suggestions. He opted for the least intrusive, least frightening, and that was as far as he could take it. It had to be done. He heard her gentle rap on the door.

Portia gasped when he opened it to let her in. "Cosimos, what on earth are you wearing?" Her jaw dropped and her eyes widened.

He gave a thin, tense smile, and leant forward to kiss her cheek. He imagined how Judas must have felt. She had to be one of a very select few who had seen the regalia. "It's to get me into the mood for painting today."

"You need *that* to paint me?" She tugged at the material of the robe and knew it was expensive.

He ushered her inside. "I need to start right now, my lovely. Everything is ready. First, take off the cloak, drape it across the arm of the chair, and sit on it."

She did. "Is that all?"

'No, it's not.' His voice quavered. "Next to you, you will find a table, bread, cheese, and a goblet of red wine with a bottle nearby. Behind, if you look, is a mural of Christ holding a cup of wine. You are to take the goblet in front of you, drink from it, and offer it up to Christ. Please look devout and awed to be in the presence of God's son.

"Cosimos, this is most strange."

"Far from it, my angel. For me, it is God's command."

A frown furrowed her brow.

"Portia, you're about to be placed in a masterpiece. You have been chosen, as have I." He made the sign of the cross. "Please. If you like, you can practice a little." He encouraged her with a smile. "But before you start, undo the fastenings around your neck and breasts. You are a rescued woman giving thanks to the Almighty. He will not be offended."

"Chosen? That's a strange thing to say."

He didn't answer.

Portia shrugged, unfastened her garment, and with a hesitant blush, allowed her white breasts to tumble into view.

He seemed not to notice. "That's perfect. Now drink and hold up the goblet." He poured her the wine. "I need to capture the emotion and drama of it all. Hold the pose as I make a rapid outline."

Portia's hand stretched out and picked up the goblet. She had posed for him on several occasions and knew the way he worked; quick sketches, words of command, and then a flurry of paints and brushes, then back to the poses. He would forever change her posture and body arches until he got it right. Tiring as it was, he was unlike the other artists she had worked for. She loved him.

"May I have a drink now? My arms are beginning to ache."

Cosimos took a while to reply. "Not yet." His heart lurched. He continued with his outlines, delaying its completion.

"Do hurry, Cosimos. You've never taken this long before."

"I know," came his strained reply. "I've never attempted a masterpiece before." He stood back from his draft, stared into her deep brown eyes, and took a long breath. "Take a drink now and offer it up to Christ."

Parched, she took a large mouthful of red wine, and allowed crimson trickles of it to drip down her chin and onto her exposed breast.

"Perfect." He watched the red stain trickle across her nipple.

She raised her eyes skyward towards the standing figure of Christ. As she did so, she experienced a warm, numbing sensation across her tongue and throat. It prompted her to drink another mouthful.

Cosimos closed his eyes. *"Madre di Dio!"* he whispered.

In minutes, Portia's skin had changed from a shade of mellow olive to a blotchy purple.

"Cosimos." She found it difficult to speak. "I can't move. What's happening?"

With a heavy clatter, the goblet dropped from her fingers to the floor. Her limbs stiffened, words refused to leave her throat, and her rigid body collapsed. Her unseeing eyes remained open, staring manically.

The belladonna had performed as expected.

Cosimos continued to paint in a whirlwind of drawing and colour. It was as if an unseen force possessed him. This way and that, paint cascaded around the canvas in a flurry of brush strokes. Only once did he look at the prostrate form of Portia. She remained still, a thin stem of saliva dripping from the corner of her parted lips.

Cosimos had been assured that she would feel nothing as her internal systems began to cease functioning. Death had arrived in minutes. He absorbed himself in his task, and did not feel the tears running down his cheeks. They were tears for the beauty of the work he created for God. Portia would be renowned, immortalised forever more.

When he had made the last mark upon the canvas, he stepped back and scanned what he had achieved. Undoubtedly, a masterpiece. He could produce no finer. As a gift to The Keeper, he could not give anything better.

The necessary precautions and arrangements had been made. Portia's body was never found, and there was no proof that she had ever seen Cosimos that day. The seneschal made the required arrangements, and Cosimos had moved to Florence.

The Keeper was impressed and in awe at what his artist had achieved. His task, one that most would refuse, had been performed with care and diligence. He had the material of a natural successor. Without a doubt, Cosimos had been chosen. With careful planning, all his descendants could form part of their quest to find the Seals … no matter how long it took.

Cosimos had acquiesced during their secret ceremony, witnessed by the Inner Circle of the AWC. He had never forgotten the seneschal's kindness to him in his early years, and the trust he bore. This was his destiny. There was no turning back.

The night following Portia's death, he had been wracked with shame, and yet, he clung to his belief that it was Christ's will. He had been released from mortal entanglements and their temptations.

Hardly a night would pass when what he had done would not embrace him. He had nothing to live for apart from The Keepers. At these times, he hated everything and everybody. His life was now plotted out. Daily, he would ask for Portia's forgiveness, but it never came … not even a whisper. He resigned himself in every way to the society. They became his entire life.

Chapter 6

The Present Day

SIX DAYS HAD passed since Julian Gallo left for Rome, and to date there had been no word from him. Rachael looked southwards from her Land Rover. Surmounting the valley stood a massive array of hills, topped with fortified ruins dating back to early Roman times. It took a moment to scan the horizon, but she had an inkling that there would be more here than met the eye.

The laboratory findings were complete, and Rockwell had spent most of his time going through them like a man on fire. At times like this, he became unapproachable, and she had learnt from experience to keep out of his way. Work obsessed him. He was due to call a meeting to discuss the laboratory findings, but stalled it until Gallo returned. He had also been working on the translations, trying to figure out what might have been written or not written. Some parts were unreadable, and he suspected, could be in code.

She shielded her eyes and looked out towards the hills. *If we are looking for something else, what are we looking for? It's out there somewhere.* The unremarkable hills of Beit-Guvrin, part of the bigger Beit Guvrin-Maresha National Park, were rumoured to contain hundreds of caves. Since the Roman invasion, they had been used to bury the Jewish dead. The whole atmosphere was unlike anything she had experienced before in any of her explorations. It had the mark of The Book of Revelation about it. The entire location reeked of buried kings and prophets from the Old Testament. Ancient villages lay beneath her feet, and that thought alone gave her a thrill, imagining what could be found.

She spotted Joshua's vehicle. He was kneeling on his hands and knees with several others, staking out a trench with bright yellow flags.

"Hi, Joshua. I didn't expect you out here."

Joshua looked up, and she thought she saw a look of awkwardness on his face. But he answered in his usual cheery way, as he brushed away soil from a piece of fractured pottery.

"Hello, Rachael. Until Gallo returns, what we're doing here is unscheduled activity, but Simon knows about it. All we can do is dig and hope to find more clues. There has to be something more here that can help us make sense of our find."

"What are we looking for, Joshua? Do you know something I don't?" This time, she knew she wasn't mistaken. He looked wrong-footed.

"Who knows? Something more to do with those plates we found. We've discovered a wall that runs through here. If you look back, you will see where the ossuary was found. The wall runs directly from it. As far as we can tell, it's as straight as a pikestaff, and heads up directly into those hills."

For a moment, she forgot his embarrassment. "Why

would anybody want to build a wall that goes nowhere?"

"That's not all. Every fifty yards or so, we come across the skeletal remains of a sheep, a goat, or an ox. They must have been ritually slaughtered, presumably as a sacrifice. But why, nobody knows yet."

"The locals say those hills are riddled with caves, catacombs and burial chambers from Roman times. Do you think this area could have something do with the find?" Rachael continued to survey the area they were excavating.

"Not sure. But I've not found a site yet that doesn't have a long line of attached coincidences around it."

"Well, the find is undoubtedly biblical in context. We'll have to wait for Simon's full report to know exactly what it's telling us."

"I know." He turned away from her and reached into his back pocket, pulled out a hipflask, and took a deep pull on the neck. Afterwards, he offered it to her.

She declined, and didn't ask what was in it.

Rockwell allowed the call to drop into voice mail as he studied the data that the find had delivered.

The second results came directly from the German laboratories he had designated for the task. He lifted his head and pushed the findings to one side, and with excitement brewing, stared out of his window at a landscape that now contained a million possibilities. One or two of which could be world shattering.

He had arranged for more C14 tests on the bones found

around, and the odd few from within the ossuary. The results had not surprised him. They had confirmed the first set of results. There could be no argument. Early first century AD.

What had ignited his expectations were the resultant DNA tests, plus the GenoScan analysis and the molecular microscopic interpretations. The strips of material proved to be coarse twill, impregnated with human hair. There was no indication of what they were doing there. Without doubt, the remains belonged to a man. The clincher was that the stains and hair were classified as predominant type Y-Chromosome. The findings had then submitted for genetic profiling, using computer algorithms designed to narrow down genetic lineage. The age came back as a male between thirty and forty years old and the man had been Jewish, of Ashkenazi and Sephardi descent. Those findings had startling implications. Whatever was to be deciphered from the metal plates, he didn't doubt, would add more speculation and controversy. Add to this the tantalising inscription on the side of the ossuary, and you had the makings of theological dynamite.

"C'mon Simon," he admonished himself. He was not a theologian. He only interpreted what he found. If the others wanted to squabble over it, so be it. The scientific evidence was indisputable, and that's all he was interested in. What followed was not his concern.

He leant back in his chair before reaching out for his copy of Bauckham's book, *The Theology of the Book of Revelation.*

Chapter 7

Viale Bruno Buozzi
Rome

THE GRAND KEEPER sat at the head of the semi-circular table watching every movement of Julian Gallo through his CCTV links, right from the moment he alighted from the vehicle. He twirled the gold ring on his finger, a serpent eating its own tail. Seated around him, three to each side, was The Inner Circle, never numbering more than seven. They were the elite members of *I Apocalittici Guerrieri Di Cristo* or AWC. Their identities, including that of the Grand Keeper, were unknown to most rank and file members. All of them enjoyed vast wealth and power. They had flown in the previous evening, answering the Grand Keeper's call for a meeting even with only two days' notice. None had dared disobey the summons. Their identities had been kept secret from each other until thirty minutes earlier.

Before they assembled, the Grand Keeper thought of what had brought the society to this point, and his pulse accelerated with anticipation of what the next hour would reveal.

When Cosimos Ricci was appointed as a successor to his existing Keeper, he had single-handedly transformed the Society into the clandestine but potent world force it had now become. He had officially proclaimed the doctrine of *Sacris Sancti Homicidium,* The Sacred Act of Holy Murder. However heinous, murder, if performed in the name of Christ's Second Coming, could only be considered a sacred act. Nothing could be allowed to stand in the way of their battle against false beliefs. Most Popes were wittingly or unwittingly servants of Satan. Their list also included John Paul I, John Paul II, Benedict XVI, and the present incumbent, Linus, who allowed blasphemous and alien religions to preached from the *Basilica Sancti Petri.*

For him and The Inner Circle, this confirmed the beginning of the end.

These events had been revealed to John of Patmos in visions and revelations as told by the Seven Seals in The Book of Revelation. The Seals had never been found, since no one knew for certain what they were looking for. But Cosimos' ancient seneschal knew of the metal plates, and had found a clue in one of the seven churches. He had directed Cosimos to where the Seals could have been hidden, beneath the town and hills of Beit-Guvrin. Even with that information, nothing had ever been discovered.

Whoever possessed the Seals, especially the Seventh, would have the knowledge and power to transform the world back to following Christ, and therefore, prevent its destruction. In their hands, the AWC would rule and ensure the right and proper course for all men. If lives needed to be sacrificed to achieve this end, then so be it.

The man they were waiting for, Dr. Julian Gallo,

seneschal for the Middle East and its surrounding territories, had important and transformational information. He made that piece of information known to the seated figures.

The Grand Keeper scrutinized the members of his Inner Circle, in turn, with a long steady gaze, as if he were preparing to paint their portrait. It was an unsettling technique handed down from Keeper to Keeper since the time of the illustrious Cosimos.

The first was Cardinal Francesco Riario, a wiry haired man in his mid-fifties, who had a solemn and inscrutable countenance. Attached to the Papal Household, he held the post of *Camerlengo* of the Holy Roman Church. In the event of the Pope's death, apart from overseeing all subsequent arrangements, he was tasked to remove the Fisherman's Ring from the Pope's finger. This ring was used to verify all Papal documents, and the Camerlengo was expected to destroy it in front of the assembled Cardinals. Thus, there could be no forgeries, and a new ring would be made. This would be a significant jewel in the armoury of the AWC, once procured. Until a new Pope was declared, during the *Sede Vacante*, Cardinal Riario would be the Vatican's acting head of state.

The second man, Xavier de Menendez, was a Spanish arms dealer who headed the giant corporation *Armas Españolas*. He was a man of small stature, had dark swept-back hair, and partial to wearing a red-lined half cape. His prodigious wealth ranked him in *Forbes* top ten wealthiest men on the planet. His financial resources and goods were irreplaceable to the AWC.

His eyes alighted on the third member next. Charles Salvador Woodford was an Americanos Meztizo from the Philippines. His companies owned sixty merchant banks scattered throughout South East Asia and Australia. A deeply devout and conservative Catholic, he ensured that all his employees were practicing Catholics, and not just on Sundays. He chaired numerous faith conventions, and fervently awaited the Second Coming. He also had prodigious wealth and influence.

Cardinal Ludovic Pacca, an energetic, lean, and hawk-nosed ruthless individual, sat to the right of the Grand Keeper. He was closer to him than any man alive. Part of the Papal Household and Prefecture for the Economic Affairs of the Holy See, he oversaw all the Vatican's finances, regardless of any autonomy claimed by those who spent the money. In that role, he had access to every balance sheet and budgetary formations. His contemporaries feared him.

Paolo Moro, suave in dress, deeply tanned, with atypical Mediterranean poise, and addicted to opium, had become a member of the Inner Circle ten years ago. As a politician, he had done well and rose to become a cabinet member of Italy's ruling party. His progress propelled him to the prestigious post of Italian Minister of Foreign Affairs.

His gaze then lingered on the daunting countenance of the sixth member, General Sir Gordon Anderson, whose lineage stretched back to King Henry the Eighth's reign and beyond. Devoutly Roman Catholic, his family had survived numerous persecutions, trials, and witch-hunts for five hundred years, yet remained true to the faith to this day. Anderson, deeply unhappy about the direction of the Church, had become a natural recruit to the inner sanctum. In his favour was his role as an attaché to the NATO Nuclear Planning Group (NPG) and Defence Planning Committee (DPC).

The Inner Circle were attired in traditional monastic style robes, all Tyrian purple, with the edges lined with gold braid. The only exception was his imposing robe, of purest white and, dazzled with black edging throughout. They all wore a gold ring of a snake devouring its own tail.

He allowed a thin smile to appear. Over the years, he had been judicious and meticulous in his selections and planning. The Inner Circle had between them awesome influence and power. In his choice of members, he had aimed for balance. Combined, they possessed a blend of religious, military, political, and financial influence and skills. He considered them the perfect mix. Above all, they had all sworn allegiance to AWC and its principal modus operandi: *Sacris Sancti Homicidium.*

Gallo was left standing in a corridor which had no doors. Before he could turn, the security man had vanished. In front and behind him stretched a panorama of white walling.

A voice sounded from nowhere. "Seneschal Gallo, if you turn around you will see what you require."

He turned, looking all around, and above him. The far wall at the end of the passage had somehow opened to reveal a small black metallic door. He walked towards it, but it had no visible means of entry. It had no lock or handle.

The voice spoke again. "Enter."

Before he could move, the door slid open and he walked in, not knowing what to expect.

Once inside, he stopped to see what confronted him. He stood in a large room, its walls lined with portraits in a variety of themes, ranging from biblical to modern. The largest of them was of a woman, her breast exposed, while offering up to Christ a goblet of wine. He had no idea who it represented. It stood raised above all the others and had a central position at the far end of the room, above a table where seven figures were seated.

"Seneschal Gallo, please approach and be seated."

Gallo had no idea who had spoken. The voice seemed to permeate from every corner of the room. He figured a parabolic microphone was being used to splatter the sound from every direction. He moved forward, discreetly scanning the men who sat behind the semi-circular table. He could not see a face. They were hidden behind hoods, and the only visible points came from the glint of seven pairs of eyes.

"Seneschal, you are most welcome. Your safety is paramount, please feel at ease." The Grand Keeper twisted his serpent ring around his finger.

Gallo focussed his eyes upon the white robed figure he knew to be the Grand Keeper. To be in the same room as him, was an unprecedented and rare honour.

"I believe you have news for us, seneschal. Tell us of your last message. Tell us all, and slowly." His sonorous tones filled the entire space.

There came a ripple of movement amongst the seated figures as they shifted position to lean forward, and await the information he had to relate.

"I am," he began with a hesitant tremor in his voice, and his eyes fixated on the ring around the Grand Keeper's finger, "the Deputy Archaeology Director at excavations in and around the ruins and hills of Beit–Guvrin, not far from Tel-Aviv University's Institute of Archaeology where I work, sponsored by the Israeli Department of Antiquities." Gallo went on to describe the circumstances surrounding the discovery. "I have here photographs of the find, and what it contained." He unlocked his briefcase, and produced sets of photographs of the exterior and interior contents. He handed them across for examination.

"The inscription reads, *Blessed John, the leader of us Guardians, spoken to and delivered by Yeshua, tells you that the key is almost in your hands.*"

Gallo sensed the level of excitement cranking up. He continued, "The remainder of the inscription is lost and obscured by erosion. Next, I have photographs of the metal plates. There were six sets of seven each, and we can tell there was a seventh set. That set is missing. Each set has an illustration, followed by inscriptions and writings that have yet to be deciphered. Some of the sets have been opened, although one or two remain sealed, probably more by oxidization than intent. My own opinion, which Professor Rockwell has yet to confirm, is that these plates are depictions of the Seven Seals of the Book of Revelation, revealed to John the Apostle in Patmos, Greece. They may even be the work of his own hand. Additionally, the find included strips of cloth. Initial C14 tests indicate the material and the bones are from the first century AD, and may predate the Dead Sea Scrolls." Gallo paused. The silence resembled a tomb in a buried city.

The Grand Keeper broke the tension. His voice crackled like sparks jumping wires. "Where is the Seventh? It holds the key to them all, and to the future of all mankind. Seneschal Gallo, we have known of the existence of these discoveries, but they have never been found, until now. We are in your debt. All praise to you. Our blood now flows thicker and stronger. *Sacris Sancti Homicidium.*" All the members repeated the oath and made the sign of the cross. "I can now tell you this, as all here have agreed. Our own research indicates that since the first century, there existed a clandestine group opposed to us who called themselves Guardians. As far as we know, they ceased to exist many years ago. The Seventh Seal was passed on to a member of theirs, and hidden in Beit-Guvrin. Romans had pursued him, but he evaded them in the hills, and both he and what we seek have forever been lost. This discovery brings us closer to the Seven Seals, closer than other Warriors has ever been. Today, you bring us joy. We honour you, Seneschal Gallo, and your rewards will be greater than you can imagine. Bring your chair closer and listen to what we must now do. What words are spoken here must never go beyond these walls ... ever!"

Chapter 8

Pontifical Biblical Institute
Jerusalem

BATHED IN A soft ray of sunlight, Rachael Carver sat at her reading desk, the light glinting off her small, rimless reading glasses. She was surrounded by numerous volumes and translations of the earliest scriptural findings, many of which predated the discovery of the Dead Sea Scrolls.

Pausing to rest her eyes, she looked around and felt a sense of the recent past. She had witnessed the death of her parents in a terrorist attack outside the gates of Jerusalem when only thirteen years of age. She would never forget it. They were both eminent archaeologists and researchers, and their deaths had shocked the academic world. She had made a vow to emulate and develop their work. It surprised nobody that she became renowned in her field, acquiring expertise in Latin, Greek, Aramaic, and Hebrew. Her reputation had begun to exceed those of her beloved parents.

Her line of research related to Old Testament prophecies, and how they linked up with the New Testament Jesus Christ, and The Book of Revelation and its pronouncements concerning the Seven Seals. Since her conversation with Simon back in Tel-Aviv, she had been aware that they were missing something about the significance of the find. Her determination to discover a link could be described as 'massive.' Rockwell had confided in her his suspicions of what the find represented, and had asked her to follow up on his line of thought, and all in strictest confidence. He had whispered the astounding possibility that the seals were actually the originals written of in the Book of Revelation. If proved correct, it would be the greatest discovery of all time.

The research had complexities. She opted to investigate the clear numerical patterning of the number seven.

Next to her, the porter had pushed a small trolley of varied volumes dating back from the Middle Ages to those of the earliest known writings.

"Dr. Carver, will you be requiring more?" He wiped the sweat from his brow.

She smiled at him. "I'm so sorry for making you work so hard, but I think that will be enough for now."

"Well, you know where I am if you want me." He scuttled off fast.

Working on her laptop, time lost its importance. Rachael was startled by a polite cough behind her. She jumped and looked up.

The porter was standing in front of her again with his trolley. "I am sorry, Doctor. We're about to close."

She gasped and looked at her watch. Five hours had passed. "Phew! Okay, that's fine. I'm done here now, I think. Thank you for your patience." She slipped him a twenty

Shekel bill.

Rockwell sat on the piano in his darkened office, playing several of Chopin's Nocturnes. He needed the maestro's calming music before he examined the initial translations for the forty-two tablets.

They were inscribed in a combination of mostly Aramaic, and a smattering of Greek. Due to the configuration of the markings, and the strokes, the three independent experts all agreed that one man had written them all. Each set had a painting on the topmost tablet, apart from the first set which had two.

He now had the complete results. Any further testing, he didn't doubt, would only confirm the initial trials. He had left nothing to chance. The transcripts of the plates were bound in a laminated folder, complete with enlarged photographs of the scripts and the paintings. Combined with the C14 and additional genetic laboratory tests, he had an impressive file as thick as a brick.

The door swung open and Rachael breezed in, her face creased with an earnest expression. They both began speaking at once.

"You won't believe what I found out!"

"You won't believe what the translations showed!"

Their sentences overlapped, causing them to stop and laugh.

"Rachael, you win. Go first."

She sat close to the lamp and produced her research,

slapping it with a sharp crack onto the desk. "I've been working on this through the night and it's an eye opener."

"C'mon, Rachael, get on with it."

"Everything we have here, and the result of my research, revolves around the number seven."

He raised an eyebrow. "What does that mean?"

She continued. "We have six metal plates, each with seven tablets, that equals forty-two. The missing set would make forty-nine. Every record I've looked at reaches a pattern based on and around the number seven, and culminating in forty-nine. The two names of Bethlehem are just a case in point, mentioned forty-nine times. The word 'parable' is mentioned forty-nine times, and seven times in the Book of Numbers." She stopped to gather her breath. "It goes on and on. *'Thou shalt number seven Sabbaths of years unto thee, seven times, seven years.'* That takes us to forty-nine again. There's also the Seven Churches of Asia. Believe me, when you read the rest of what I've found, there could be little doubt that what we have here is an artefact connected to the Book of Revelation and the prophecy concerning the End of Time."

He said nothing but his face had a curious expression. He pushed his file across to her. "Look at this. While you do, I'll make us coffee. Usual?"

"Usual, please." She muttered without glancing up.

For the next fifteen minutes, neither of them spoke, each examining the other's findings and sipping coffee.

He broke the silence. "What is not in dispute is the age and translations of the paintings and diagrams found on the plates. Without a doubt first century, and the fabric matches perfectly, as do the bones. The engraved side with the inscription bearing the name of Yeshua or Jesus is no fake.

Just look at it, will you?" He pushed a large photograph across to her.

"While the name was common enough in those days, you have to take into account the translation of what is written with it.

Blessed John, the leader of us Guardians, spoken to and delivered by Yeshua, tells you that the key is almost in your hands.

"I believe you, Simon. What's on the plates?"

"Apart from the first set, which has a depiction of a crucifixion on the front, with ancillary figures in the foreground, it has a picture of a white horse on the reverse side. A man is riding it, wearing a winged crown and carrying a bow. The other five each have a different picture. Let's deal with those first."

"Okay, I think I know what's coming."

"The second shows a red horse with a rider carrying a massive sword. Here's the blown-up image. You may as well look at these as I move through. The third, you can see, is ridden by a figure who carries what looks like a set of scales. Here's a scary one. A pale rider on the fourth horse, with a figure representing death or hell behind him. The fifth gets better. You can see figures in white robes, their arms and heads raised upwards, and emerging from what looks like an altar or grave, walking in a long line. That brings us to our last set. The sixth tablet is the strangest. It's just black, with red and orange streaks gashing across it." Rockwell sat back and looked at Rachael with questions in his eyes. "What do you make of these?"

"Well, we need Gallo here. He's the expert in ancient

Biblical icons and their deciphering. But it is eerily similar to the Seven Seals in the Book of Revelation, with the Four Horsemen of The Apocalypse and all. I bet the writing refers directly to Chapter Six of that book, doesn't it?"

"Possibly. So, do you think these are the works of John of Patmos?"

"I don't know, nor do you, although the scientific evidence is pointing in that direction." She grinned. "I've saved the best for last."

"Oh God, what are you going to show me now?"

"*The Pontifical Biblical Institute* was most interesting. I doubt if they truly know the importance of a lot of the material they're holding. It got mind-boggling." She paused, teasing him. "Deep breathing now, Simon ... I found an old text ..."

"Oh, here we go. You found an old text. Is this the beginning of some old wives' tale? You know I don't believe in superstition."

"Shut up and listen. I've photographed most of it, and without anybody noticing, I removed a page. Look, here it is. I can always go back and replace it."

"You what? You can go to jail for that. Oh my God, Rachael!" He clapped his hands around his head.

"Too late for all that ... it's done now. This is from the so-called Gospel of Thomas." She pushed the page towards him. "This was tucked in behind the title page. Better still, it states the time it was written: *It's been about seventy years since the Blessed Lord Yeshua was ...* It's the written testimony of a man named Ananias, the Olive Grower. I managed to translate bits of it, but there were pieces missing, and holes here and there in the original parchment. It says, ... *this was passed to me by a*

Guardian who witnessed the betrayal. Roman soldiers took our Master's body away. Before they killed him, he committed our dearest secret to the servant Adil Koury, who made good his escape into the caves. They captured him not, nor was he ever seen or heard from again.

"Then it gets difficult to read in places, but I'll continue with what I deciphered: *The Romans found nothing for they were seeking our Sacred Seal. They knew me not. I did hide them where no man would find them.*"

"Stop there," Rockwell interrupted. "Look at our box. Look at the inscription. Is this what this man Koury carried, do you think, or was it what the Olive Grower hid?"

"I think what we have here is what Ananias, the Olive Grower, hid. The man, Koury, must have carried the missing set. Without that final piece, our findings are meaningless. It's incomplete. Read that inscription again. It says, *almost in your hands.* If it's *almost,* then the message on the box, if it's to be believed, renders the contents as incomplete. Unless the translations of worldwide esteemed scholars are to cock? Everyone who has examined the plates said there's a set missing. If so, where the hell is it and why was it separated from this set?"

Rockwell leant back in his chair. "Let's slow down a bit on this for a moment. If it wasn't for the fact that we are scholars and researchers, I wouldn't give a damn about what all this means. It's an ancient mystery, I agree, but it adds no importance to the world we live in."

"There's a lot of people out there, and that includes some serious nutters, who would disagree with you. Has it occurred to you that if our discovery gets into the wrong hands it could be very dangerous? There's a saying, *He who holds the Keys to Heaven rules the World.* Isn't that what all this seems to be about?"

"Ruling the world? Bollocks! A set of seven metal plates won't give anyone the power to rule the world, will it?

"Who knows? But don't you agree that we are responsible for the knowledge we have gathered? If it falls into the wrong hands, who knows what might happen?"

"Nothing is fully confirmed yet. If this is, indeed, the Seals in the Book of Revelation, there will be theological storms unlike any we've seen in history. But that shouldn't concern us. We need Gallo here. When's he back?"

"There was a call from him earlier today. He reckoned, tomorrow, he should be ready to resume work again."

"What should we do about the anomalies in his history?" Gallo's recent behaviour still gnawed at Rockwell.

"I think we should just forget it, for now. Who of us hasn't had an anomaly or two in what we say and do?"

"Rachael, you're right. We have more important things to worry about. I won't say a word."

Chapter 9

JOSHUA AGAR SAT alone. Above him, the sky was dark, with only a crescent moon and a million stars shining as bright as the promise of life. Below him was the soft cooling sands as old as the earth itself. Much had happened around the site since he had discovered the ossuary. As the site supervisor, the academics leading the excavations relied on him for progress reports, and a synopsis on possible developments. The discovery had excited him much. For this, he gave thanks to the Almighty and prayed for a successful outcome. He had been instructed not to talk to anybody about the find, especially the media and any religious entity who might enquire.

He didn't have to be told that. He knew the implications.

Like the others in the team, he awaited Gallo's return. Joshua wanted to hear his interpretation of the materials. Much depended on it. In his heart and mind, he felt an overwhelming gratitude. He had been waiting for this moment for as long as he could remember … a major discovery. His grandfather would have been proud. Since he lost his parents when he had been four years old, his grandfather had cared for him.

He took in the nourishing cool night air, allowing a

satisfying shiver of happiness to pass through him. He thought about his grandfather, Nathaniel.

He had been a mysterious man and much given to academia, and his own personal interpretation of God. Nathaniel had passed most of his knowledge onto him, and that had a profound influence on his own beliefs. Nathaniel had died a year back after Joshua had completed his studies and was working in an important position for the University. He had bequeathed him a vast library of ancient books, texts, and cupboards full of scrolls and papyrus documents. Joshua had always been too busy to take the time to examine his inheritance. He was certain that if they had importance, the Ministry would have claimed them.

As he lay dying, Nathaniel had said to him, "One day, you will read them, and when that day arrives you will know who you are. We all live with and are surrounded by the ghosts of the past."

That statement had embedded itself into his mind. He did not know why, but it had a ring about it, and whenever it surfaced in his memory, ripples of curiosity ran through him causing the hairs on his neck to rise.

Members of the team had congratulated him on his discovery, and the professional manner in which he handled it. His grandfather, he knew, would have been delighted for him. What a shame he couldn't be here to see it. Maybe the time had come to look at his inheritance, but *manyana, manyana*.

He couldn't help but notice that Rockwell and Carver had become very tight lipped about their own research. That annoyed him. Importance and knowledge, in this field, should never be the prerogative of a chosen few. And what of

Gallo? What the hell did he say to that man who shot himself? He then denied that he had said anything. *But, I saw him speak!* Then he had departed for Rome, allegedly to attend his father's funeral.

Something very odd is going on around him.

They heard again from Gallo. He confirmed he'd be with them the following day, around lunchtime, and he gave them his flight number. There was to be no private jet on the return journey. All should appear normal.

Rachael turned to Simon. "I'd best be on my way. I need to collect some books I've ordered from the other side of town. I'll see you in the morning." She hesitated at the door, hoping he might suggest a drink or two … Nothing.

"Okay, Rachael. Sleep well. See you in the morning." He turned back to face his screen once more.

Feeling deflated, she marched at a brisk pace out into the grounds before heading across the campus towards the main gate. If only he knew how at times, when in bed, she yearned for the feel of his strong body pressed close to hers. *He had to be blind!*

Outside the complex, the streets were quiet as she walked beneath a colonnade that led to the main plaza. She never noticed the man watching her from a recessed niche, smoking a small cigarillo. He stepped out and followed her several paces behind. Halfway through the covered walkway, a delivery man with a sack truck piled high with boxes appeared to stumble, causing his cargo to drop across her direction. She came to a halt to avoid the obstacle.

As she did, a strong pair of hands gripped her shoulders from behind. "Dr. Carver. Please do not turn around," a sharp voice commanded.

The delivery man dropped his trolley and opened the double doors of his truck.

Rachael began screaming out loud, "Help! Help! Help!" At the same time attempting to resist the force pushing her towards the doors. But there was not a person in sight.

The deliveryman reached out towards her and clamped his hand across her mouth, while the man behind her pushed as hard as he could. Her left arm was twisted up hard behind her back. She had a brief glimpse of a small gold badge encircling a winged crown, and smelled the fleeting aroma of a cigarillo, before she passed out.

Chapter 10

RACHAEL'S HORRIFIED EXPRESSION registered with the man wearing a black fedora hat, a long brown coat, and smelling of hair oil and tobacco. She realised she was still inside the van and it wasn't moving. Where they were, she had no idea, nor how long she had been unconscious. Her back was pressed up hard against the metal side, and her wrists were taped together.

The man held his finger to his lips. "Sssh. Please do not make a sound."

She nodded her agreement.

"I have questions for you. They are not difficult and we want honesty."

She wondered who he referred to as *we*. The only other person involved was the deliveryman who had helped capture her.

"Dr. Carver, please be assured we have no intention of harming you. That is not our way. You may wonder how we know your name, but we know many things."

"Who are you and what do you want?' Any fear she had of sexual assault faded. Despite her predicament, her main emotion was curiosity, and not dread.

"Who we are is of no importance. What we want is."

"What is that?"

"You are Professor Rockwell's assistant, are you not?"

"Yes."

"A while back, an ancient artefact was uncovered on the site you were working on, yes?"

"Yes."

"The artefact and its contents had undergone extensive testing. Nod if you agree."

She nodded.

"That's fine. We think we know what the results are. There appears to be part of the jigsaw puzzle missing. Am I correct?"

"You are correct. How do you know all this?"

"We've known for centuries."

"What are you talking about?"

"Again, that's not your concern. You are planning to search for what is missing. Is that correct?"

"You seem to know you everything. You tell me."

"I admire your courage. Let me rephrase my question. It would be a careless archaeologist who did not follow up important leads, would you agree?"

Rachael nodded.

"An unknown man shot himself at your site. A colleague of yours spoke to him before he killed himself. The man who spoke, what do you know of him?"

Rachael, for a reason she couldn't understand, began answering the man as if he were an old friend. "His name is Dr. Julian Gallo. He's our Deputy Archaeology Director. He swears he never spoke to the man, but several of us saw him do so. He's flown to Rome to attend his father's funeral but he should be back tomorrow."

The man paused and a concerned expression crossed his face. "Rome, you say?"

"Yes, Rome. There's talk ..." She stopped herself from continuing.

"Why have you stopped? Please, carry on."

Rachael's voice stumbled and the next words came out in a rush. "Some of us thought his father had died years ago."

The man nodded in understanding. He asked no more questions. Twirling the small badge in his lapel, he stood, turned, and rapped sharply on the bulwark behind the driver's cab. The response came with the engine firing up, and the truck moving away from wherever it was parked.

Within ten minutes, it had come to a halt and the engine was switched off. The man reached out and untied her wrists. "Doctor, we apologise for our conduct, but there's a lot at stake here. Your replies have been informative and confirmed that what we suspected, I fear, is true. You may hear from us again, but we wish you no harm. I must warn you and your team to be on high alert. You could be in great danger. Now please, go."

He opened the doors and she stepped out onto the street where she had been taken.

Chapter 11

THE FLIGHT BACK from Rome went without incident. Gallo leant back in his seat, content in the knowledge that all arrangements were in place. More important was his unexpected elevation into a position of trust and responsibility. His star had risen. The Keepers had placed at his disposal the full extent of their capabilities. He'd been given a keyword, and upon its activation, Gallo only needed to ask and he would have the full support of the AWC. He had been treated as an honoured guest and that was the rarest of honours.

Now, the exciting task of locating the Seventh Seal lay before him. The history of the Six Seals had been explained to him, and he knew for certain that what had been discovered at Beit-Guvrin were the Six, written by the Blessed John of Patmos himself.

The find had been astounding, and in all his life he had never expected to witness such a discovery. It had earth-shattering consequences.

Stepping out through the arrivals lounge at Ben Gurion Airport, Gallo's sour gaze spotted Joshua who had arranged to meet him and take him back to the University, and then on to the dig.

"I'm sorry about your father, Julian. I hope the funeral went well?"

Gallo ignored the query. "Have we found anything new yet?"

Joshua raised an eyebrow, but guessed Gallo didn't want to rake through the ashes of bereavement. "No, we haven't. Simon wants us to meet and discuss our progress. He has the complete analysis from the scientific team. He wants your perspective on all of them." Joshua had grown accustomed to Gallo's caustic nature, and had never allowed it to bother him. But since the discovery, his attitude had got worse.

"Can't see the point of that. He'll do what he wants, as always."

Joshua wiped his aviator sunglasses and drew in a deep breath. "C'mon Julian, that's a bit unfair. Look, here's the Land Rover. Let's get in and drive back."

"Okay. Where's he keeping everything? I need to look at them again."

"It's all locked away in the records vault."

"There's a surprise. Any more ideas on the dig?' Gallo asked, although he seemed like he was detached from their conversation, his stony stare fixed somewhere beyond the horizon.

"That's what we'll be discussing. There's talk of bringing in ground scanners and penetrating radar."

"You can't get those into caves." Gallo couldn't keep the snap out of his voice.

Joshua raised his eyes skyward. *Bereavement can make you snappy, that's for sure.*

The journey continued in silence.

For a reason she couldn't explain, Rachael found herself unable to talk of her frightening experience earlier. That was just it. Her initial terror had evaporated like mist in a wind. Then, in an inexplicable way, she had felt … safe. *Safe from what?*

She thought back on all she could remember … the fedora hat, long brown overcoat so strange in this hot climate, hair oil, cigarillos, and that small, winged crown badge. Rachael also racked her brain about the delivery man. He had dark blue eyes, shaven head, wore overalls, and had thick grubby fingers. As hard as she tried, she could remember no more. Events had happened so fast. Her brain whirled. Abduction was a crime, but she had been treated with respect and then set free.

She couldn't bring herself to talk about it … yet. She forgot the books she was supposed to collect. Instead, she made her way home. Accompanying her was the oddest sense of peace. As if everything was as it should be. But she knew she was being irrational. The man had even intimated danger. *Why should there be danger?* She couldn't figure it out.

Once indoors, an enormous weariness assaulted her. Without warning, she began to sob. She cried like she had never done before, throwing herself on her bed without even removing her clothing. As soon as her head struck the pillows, she descended into a deep sleep. She dreamt much. Dreams are often forgotten upon waking, but this time, they stayed remembered.

She had been with the Virgin Mary, and she was not a

young virgin. On her hands and feet, she bore the bloody wounds of Christ. Around her shone an aura of blue light.

She had spoken to Rachael. "My child, my lovely child, you can help stop this. The time approaches and there is danger. Be wary, be vigilant, and act!" The vision, the dream, ended too abruptly. She grasped for it, but it had gone.

Rachael sat upright and glanced at the clock. She had slept for ten hours. *What the hell was that all about? Since when did Mary have the wounds of Christ?*

She went about her normal routine; coffee, breakfast, and then work. All the while, sensed Mary standing behind her.

Don't go ... Please!

A sense of comfort and reassurance filled her.

The morning of the meeting arrived, and Rockwell assembled his three-man team into the office. He had allocated extra places for a few promising students who could benefit from observing the proceedings.

Rockwell went to the safe lodged in the far corner and dialled in the combinations. Its solid metallic construction was at odds with the scrolls, dusty books, and assorted archaeological artefacts that littered the area. The door swung open. He reached into its yawning depths and pulled out the reason for the meeting. He placed the ossuary on the table in front of him, and several thick files containing the test results, all the bones inside and around the box, the strips of fabric, and samples of the surrounding soil.

He then proceeded to explain the test results in detail.

When he was done, he turned to Rachael.

"Tell the others here, what you discovered at the library."

Her tone was brisk. "There can be little doubt that the material we've found is first century in origin. What is not certain is whether what we found relates to the Seven Seals referred to in the Book of Revelation. The faded inscription on the ossuary could be interpreted that way. I found this at the library, and it's not a copy. I want no comments, please." She turned to her own file and produced the papyrus relating to the Gospel of Thomas. There was a collective gasp of astonishment.

"Please no, comments." She repeated her request with vigour and swung her gaze around all those present. "I found this tucked in behind the first page of the Gospel." She turned to the projector and brought up an image of the papyrus. "The document says Ananias the Olive Grower wrote it. This is what I was able to decipher:

> It's been about seventy years since the Blessed Lord, Yeshua was ...
> ... this was passed to me by a Guardian who witnessed the betrayal. Roman soldiers took our Master's body away. Before they killed him, he committed our dearest secret to the servant Adil Koury, who made good his escape into the caves. They captured him not, nor was he ever seen again.

"It continues ..."

> The Romans found nothing for they were seeking our Sacred Seal. They knew me not. I did hide them where no man would find them"

70

The room went quiet. Rachael continued. "I put it to you that what we have discovered is the ossuary of John of Patmos, hidden by this man, Ananias. The other man, Adil Koury, escaped to the hills of Beit-Guvrin with the missing Seventh." She faced Gallo. "Julian, you are the expert in Biblical icons and their interpretations. What's your take on this?"

Gallo's hands shook. He didn't look up but stared at the ossuary. Seconds later, he spoke. "I don't doubt it. It is true."

"But you haven't examined anything yet, Julian." Rockwell sounded perplexed.

"I don't have to. I know."

"How do you know?"

"The scientific findings are irrefutable. There is mention also of a brotherhood called 'Guardians.' That is rare. They were believed to be a secret society who reckoned they had claims over all relics concerning the Virgin Mary, Christ, and the Gospels. In truth, they were robbers and heretics who warped the true teachings ..." He stopped mid-sentence.

Rachael and Simon exchanged glances.

Gallo continued. "The Seven Seals are linked to the Seven Churches of Asia on the Greek Island of Patmos. Christ instructed John, his follower, through the intermediary of an angel, to write on a scroll what he saw, and send it to the seven churches. We know that Christ was referring to the Christian communities living there at the time. Each community supposedly had a particular characteristic, and its own guardian angel. Historians and theologians have frequently contested the true meaning of what is involved. In his visions, John saw Christ walking amongst seven lampstands with seven stars in his right hand. The stars are no less than the seven angels. Most of the symbolism revolves around the number seven. It is debated that each church, in some way, failed the angels. There exists a theory that the content of the scrolls was also recorded in tablets of steel or iron, should the scroll perish in some way. That may very well be what we have here." Gallo paused, swallowing hard.

Rockwell noticed the streaks of sweat running from his temples.

"On the opening of the scroll by the 'Lamb,' which we interpret as Christ, a series of apocalyptic disaster will occur. We..." He corrected himself. "I mean, some say they have already occurred; tsunamis, earthquakes, famine, etc. That the world is now waiting for the final Seal to be revealed or opened. But, some say that has already happened, and we're only waiting for the final trumpets to herald the end of times; blood moons, stars falling from the sky ... and so on. It was also said that whoever possesses the keys or seals holds the way to almighty power. Natural disasters are getting worse by the decade, which some say is because the Sixth seal has been broken. Hard to deny the truth in that."

Rockwell raised his hand and interrupted him. "Hold on a minute there, Julian. We're not here for a dissertation on religious beliefs. We're here to discuss scientific facts that are in the main, undeniable. What theories revolve around these items are fascinating, I'm sure, but have no part in our investigations. We're looking for a missing set of plates we believe is lost out there somewhere. I think we all understand what this fairy tale was meant to be. What interests us, and that should include you, is the historical importance of this find, and not the superstition that surrounds it, or what you think it might be. Belief is not scientific unless proved otherwise. In your opinion, Julian, should we or should we not continue our search for the missing set?"

For a moment, Rachael felt sympathy for Gallo. He had strayed into a separate agenda and it had no place in their activity ... or did it? She glanced at Simon and saw the firm set of his jaw and the light of certainty blazing from his eyes.

Gallo responded with the shaky voice of a man injured. "I wish we could all be as certain you, Simon. You, however, have a blind eye at times, I fear. That's not something to discuss right now. In answer to your question, yes, to locate something that had been missing for two thousand years is a great challenge. There exists a report that in the sixteenth century, a search found nothing on Patmos, apart from a carved inscription that cannot be verified. It suggested that the Seals, if that is what we are looking for, can be found in the Beit-Guvrin hills. It looks like we may have found them apart from the seventh. I heard that you're proposing the use of scanners, radargrams and echo sounders. That would help our cause for sure, but I will be amazed if you can get them into the caves." He looked around at all those seated, and wiped the perspiration from his forehead. "I will support you, whatever you decide." Picking up his notes and bag, he stood. "Call me when you need to." In a flourish, he swept out of the room and banged the door, a gesture that needed no interpretation.

"Simon," whispered Rachael, "you were a bit harsh on him."

"Not hard enough. I know I said I didn't want to go into his anomalies, but he annoyed me. Now more than ever, I believe something is amiss with him. That suicide, how can you forget that as though it never happened? Then he's got the bollocks to begin giving us some religious claptrap. Something is very wrong with him, and I don't know what."

"Forget it. Let's get going up into those hills. We'll have a better chance of finding what we want to find than sitting here with an agitated frame of mind." Rachael allowed the implications of Gallo's words to sink in, and she couldn't help but link them with her abduction the previous day. She looked across to Joshua and signalled for him to join them.

After thirty minutes, plans were in place for a systematic search across the hills and caves.

As the others left, Rachael spoke with an unexpected authority. "Stop, Joshua and Simon, both of you. Sit back down. There's something you should know, and I think it has a direct bearing on what we are doing."

"What's that?" Rockwell demanded.

"On the way to the bookshop yesterday, I was abducted by two men and bundled into a van."

"What!" they both exclaimed.

"They didn't harm me in any way, but asked lots of questions about the find. They were most interested in the shooting that day on the site, and Gallo."

She gave them the full details and descriptions of her abductors as best as she could. She included their clothing, jewellery … everything she remembered. To this was added her own feelings and sentiments.

Joshua looked thoughtful. "They sound like undercover police. That's the way they operate and it's quite common here."

"But there was one thing they said that was odd. The man knew every little detail about our work and the artefact. He even knew that a part was missing. He referred to it as *part of the jigsaw puzzle.* I asked him how he knew and he said they have known for centuries."

"Well, they didn't harm you. That's all that matters right now. There's little point in calling in the police, and who knows, they may have been policemen anyway."

"The man did warn us to be on our guard; that we could be in danger."

Rockwell looked rueful. "He may be right. We've had two deaths, an abduction, and Julian's father dies … or so we are led to believe. Not bad for a start, is it?"

"So, what do we do now?"

"We carry on as normal, but you, Rachael, are not to go out walking alone from now on. Understood?"

She gave a slight smile. "Yes, Daddy!" She laughed, but felt pleased at his concern for her.

Chapter 12

FOUR WEKS HAD passed since her abduction but Rachael had not forgotten it. What stayed in her mind the most was the dream she had of the Holy Mother, following the event. Her presence never went away. It wasn't intrusive, menacing or judgemental, in any manner. In fact, Rachael found in it a reassurance not available elsewhere. She was still perplexed at the clear stigmata on Mary's hands and feet.

As the team had suspected, news of the find proved impossible to keep secret. Such was the perceived importance of the discovery. Rockwell had received an invitation, direct from Cardinal Francesco Riario, the Papal *Camerlengo*, to discuss the details and relevance of the find. The Camerlengo had graciously given them full access to the Papal archives, including the Apostolic Library, if the team needed to extend their research.

It was agreed that Rachael should be their representative. Both Rockwell and Agar had deduced that the Vatican City would not be a conduit of violence. Gallo had also supported the move, and offered to help her in every way with his insider knowledge of both Rome and the Vatican. His enthusiasm seemed extraordinary.

Four days later, dazzled by the grandeur of ancient Rome, Rachael alighted close to Saint Peter's Basilica with its perpetual queue of pilgrims and the faithful. The sight of it all registered deeply with her, and she came to realise the importance of faith to those queuing, morning, noon, and night. It humbled her. Again, she had felt the presence of her vision, in the form of the Mother Mary.

A voice called to her. "Dr. Carver?"

She looked up and was greeted by a fresh-faced priest who walked with a limp and used a walking cane.

"Yes, Father? I'm Dr. Carver."

"*Mi dispiace spaventari. Sono* Padre James." With a broad grin, he broke into English with a heavy Irish accent. "I forgot your language was English, my apologies. I've been sent to accompany you to our office, where Cardinal Riario will meet you. He is very high in the rankings here and close to our Holy Father."

They shook hands. Father James was unable to walk quickly. He spoke faster than he walked.

"Your visit, and your recent discovery is the talk of the Holy City."

"Well, Father, I am here to tell you all we know, and we hope you can assist us also."

"We've had some mysteries here, too. Our Father had appointed an archaeologist, Dr. Luigi Bonelli, to examine and discuss your findings with us. Sadly, he died some days ago. He was found hanging beneath a nearby bridge … a crisis of faith, we fear. He had a history of depression. May Christ have mercy on him." He made the sign of the Cross. "A deep loss … a deep loss indeed."

"He committed suicide?"

"The police investigated, but there was no evidence of foul play. For his soul, it would have been better for him if he had been murdered."

By the time he had finished talking, they had arrived at the Cardinal's office.

"This way, Doctor." They stepped into an oak panelled lift and he smiled. "I hate these things. I got stuck in one once, and it was a very unpleasant experience." The lift stopped and the doors peeled open without a sound. With a sweeping gesture of his arm, he ushered her into a high-ceilinged office that looked startlingly modern, far from what she had been expecting. It had been divided into sections, each partitioned with glass panelling, bristling with computers and screens. From outside, she could see reflections off the River Tiber rolling past.

"The Cardinal's office is down the end here."

They reached the door and the Father tapped cautiously on the panelling.

"*Entrare,*" a soft voice spoke.

Father James pushed the door open and gestured for Rachael to enter. "Dr. Carver, may I present his Eminence, Francesco, Cardinal Riario of the Vatican City." With that, the priest genuflected before hurrying out, closing the door with a sharp snap behind him.

Riario's smile was cold and stiff, as if all warmth and tenderness had departed from him years ago. Wiry hair rested upon two large ears, and he was wearing a red cassock. Rachael leant forward, and kissed the ring that clung firmly to a bony finger as the Cardinal extended his arm.

"Be seated, Dr. Carver." He indicated a seat. "I trust your journey here has been comfortable. It is not often we have messengers bearing stimulating news. A most curious find, I believe?" A small twitch of his eyebrow crossed his mask of inscrutability.

She found something about the Cardinal's disposition she disliked, and her intuition about people was seldom wrong. It had never failed her. Riario was creepy.

With rapt attention, he listened as she detailed the operation and what they had unearthed. She omitted the suicide, and it struck her that there were now two connected to their discovery. She also left out the part where she had removed a page from an ancient book in the Jerusalem Library. The more she told him, the less she wanted to. *Mother Mary, where are you?*

She showed him the analytical and genetic profiling data, which he studied with the aid of a large lens. His eyesight had been failing for years.

"Remarkable, Doctor." He repeated the phrase several times, markedly impressed. "How may we help you further? As indeed, we must, for such a tantalising discovery."

"I need access to your earliest Jewish discoveries, materials on the Seven Churches of Asia, papyruses, scrolls, stone work, in fact, anything that will help clarify what we know you want to know. Without help, we could take far too long, and may never prove if we are right or wrong."

To her surprise, he agreed. "Of course. I will ask Father James to make the necessary arrangements. What you require are stored in the Vatican Secret Archives, as opposed to the Apostolic Library. They were separated in the seventeenth century. It's no longer so secret, but access is difficult for outsiders. However, you have been granted unlimited access."

"I'm honoured and most grateful. There's one last thing, Your Eminence."

"What is that?"

"You might like to see this." From her case, she produced a sealed package, heavily encased in bubble wrap, and beneath that, thick protective linen. She unfolded it in front of him, and extended both her palms in an open gesture. *"Solo per I tuoi occhi!"*

"This is …?" His words trailed away with a glazed expression. He knew what stared him in the face. *"Madre di Dio!"* He crossed himself and closed his eyes.

"This is the first set of plates. We were able to detach it without damage. We decided to bring this so you could see what we're dealing with. I guard it with my life. Here, a crucifixion is discernible on the first plate, and on the reverse, you will see a white horse ridden by a man with a winged crown, holding a bow."

As she said that, a shiver passed through her. She realised that the badge worn by the man who had abducted her had been identical.

"The First Horseman," he whispered loudly as his hands began to shake. "It is ridden by a Guardian."

This was not the first time she had come across that term. "Did you say Guardian?"

"A guardian angel, of course, of course."

Rachael thought he sounded unconvincing, and began to repack the artefact.

"When can we see this again, Doctor?" He had regained

his composure.

"Before I leave, and that depends on what I can find in your archives, Your Eminence."

"We're at your disposal, and Father James will be here to assist you. He knows his way around very well. I look forward to seeing you and your blessed treasure again very soon."

Once again, Rachael kissed the proffered ring, gave half a knee bend, and exited the office. It had been a difficult encounter for her.

Once the door was shut, His Eminence rushed to the phone, and processed a security call of utmost importance.

The following morning, Rachael paced around her room and continually checked her phone for messages. There were none. Father James was running fifteen minutes late. and the world seemed to be on hold. All she wanted to do was get into the vaults and archives, immerse herself in the vast treasures kept by the Vatican, and attempt to nail the enigma they had discovered.

Twenty minutes elapsed, before there came a soft knock on her door. She brushed down her clothes using her hands and opened it and saw a smiling Father James.

"All ready then?" He carried a pouch of small keys and plastic barcoded cards. No apology for lateness.

"No time to waste, Father. Let's just go, please."

The entrance lay opposite the Vatican Library, through the *Porta di Santa Anna* in the *Via di Porta di Angelica*.

After a series of small stairs and a lift descent, they arrived at their destination. The thought struck her. *I am under the Vatican and possibly St. Peter itself.* She held on to her case which contained the first set of plates. Rockwell's instruction was to never let it out of her sight. The lift door opened, and they were confronted by a set of extremely thick glass doors. Behind it, she could make out a panorama of dimly lit racks that appeared to stretch on forever. Her grip tightened on her case.

"Follow me, Doctor."

He walked up to a boxed panel and pressed his left eye onto a clear strip of glass. Without a sound, both doors swung open.

"Surprising, eh Doctor? It's the latest iris recognition system. We're not religious dinosaur's here. Only six of us in the Vatican have access to the archives. Without an approved scan, you cannot get in."

Rachael was impressed. "That's amazing! Can you get out without a scan, Father?"

"Yes, you can. It's designed that way. As so few ever enter this place, a power cut or failure could leave you here for weeks, and nobody would know. But we have a system in place to prevent that from happening. All six of us are aware that you are here, and after three hours, a check is always made. So, don't you worry. You won't starve to death down here." He chuckled. "Now, just a moment." He turned left, and within twenty seconds, he had activated a switch, and the entire area the size of several football fields lit up. "Where exactly to you wish to begin searching, Doctor? It's estimated that we have over eighty-five kilometres of shelving here, and over one hundred and fifty thousand deposits." He spread his arms open, and looked eager to please.

"I'm flabbergasted!" She put her hand up as if shielding her eyes from the sun. "Phew! I'd like to begin with first century scrolls and papyruses that have relevance to Judea and the Roman occupation at that time. Along with the Seven Churches of Asia."

"I think we have what you are looking for. You will find it in the long corridor marked with the letter 'J.' That's about fifty strides to your right.'"

"Thank you, Father."

"You are welcome. I will call for you in two or three hours?"

"Make it three, Father, there's enough here for a year or two."

With a grin, he bowed his head. "See you then. Don't starve now!" He disappeared the way they had come.

She stood still and took stock of her circumstance. A sweep of loneliness enshrouded itself around her. The environment was air conditioned, cool, too much so for bodily warmth. Endless gondolas of corridors oozed and stretched out in odd menace.

Silence … like a crypt.

A shiver, but not from cold, assaulted her. A whisk of fear brushed its dark colour through her entire being.

"Get a grip, girl. For God's sake, this is the Vatican, not Satan's dining room." Speaking to oneself was not unusual for archaeologist researchers.

Why the hell did I say that?

The area designated under the letter 'J' appeared endless. Rows upon rows spawned and seemed to go on forever. *Most of this should be in a museum.* She began from the sub-section beneath the letter 'A.' Locating the block referring to Asia, she followed through on the racks beneath *'Churches Of.'* Soon, she found *Patmos, The Seven Churches.*

This was exactly where she wanted to start. Numerous boxed containers confronted her, each containing scrolls, papyrus, and vellum parchments from the first century up, until the turn of the nineteenth century. Written in ancient Greek, Hebrew, and Aramaic, they stared up at her like Swiss Rolls and bolster pillows. *God Almighty! This material is priceless and beyond belief. Why are they being kept secret?*

As requested, she was wearing protective gloves. The first church was the one located in the Metropolis of Ephesus. She had done her research, and each one, she knew, had been given a reproach or a challenge as stated in The Book of Revelation. Following this was a promise.

All seven churches had the admonition:

He who has an ear, let him hear what the Spirit says to the churches.

Along each immense corridor, trestle tables had been placed at convenient locations. She lifted out the first scroll, and shivered. *Why am I trembling?* She held the scroll aloft, almost as an offering. The *Spirit,* she had interpreted as Christ, the Son of Man. With that in mind, she placed the scroll upon the table. As had been her custom from many years ago, when dealing with long past treasures, she offered her customary soft prayer. "Forgive this intrusion. I wish you no harm. I wish only to know your wisdom."

Soft hands then unrolled the centuries past.

Her camera went into overdrive. She could read parts, and it seemed to suggest the scriptures were full of liars and false prophets. The horseman was plain to see, carrying a bow, and identical to the one on the first tablet in her bag. Simon had suggested that it represented Christ, but that couldn't be correct. Wasn't He supposed to carry a large sword? She stepped back. confused.

She heard a crash and without warning, the lights went off, and she stood alone in pitch-blackness.

I don't believe it! The lights must have fused! Oh God, I hope I'm not going to be stuck in here for hours.

There was another loud crash, and she knew from a brief glimmer of light that the door had been opened.

"Father James, is that you? I'm in the first row in 'J.' What happened to the lights?"

There was no reply, and the sound of approaching footsteps was not encouraging.

"Father, please speak. I'm getting frightened."

Nothing.

She picked up her case, fumbled with the scroll, and rammed it back where it came from. There was a dim background of light, probably from an emergency source that activated itself when the lights went out.

Then, Rachael saw a dark figure heading in her direction … and it wasn't Father James. This figure didn't limp or have a stick. Instinct told her to get the hell out. She turned, and began to run. The figure matched her response. She reached the end of the giant bay, but he was gaining fast. Swinging around into the next bay, it stretched out forever, but at the far end she could see the glass doors. She ran faster.

The figure shouted, "You are not going to get away, so why don't you stop?"

Rachael carried on. She needed to reach the glass doors before he caught up with her. Gasping for breath, she came to a freestanding array of scrolls and ancient books. They were not stable. She turned and with one almighty heave, set one bay toppling, creating a domino effect straight down onto her pursuers head. He gave an almighty yell as steel racks and ancient writings crashed down on him, burying him out of sight. She panicked. Not a time to wait!

Grabbing her bag, she continued towards the doors. She was close and she could see that the doors were open. Upon closer inspection, Rachael realised why. A body lay between the doors, wedged half in the corridor and half in the storage area.

"Father James!" He looked dead. His walking cane lay broken beside him. She turned him over. "Oh, my God!" she shrieked.

His eyeball had been cut out to enter the area controlled by the iris recognition system. It lay in a squelchy staring heap on his chin. A bloody black socket stared up at her from the dead priest's face.

She couldn't prevent her next scream.

The security alarms had activated automatically since the doors had remained open too long. It didn't take long before in a whirlwind of movement, three armed, uniformed Vatican guards appeared. As they did so, there was a gunshot. Everybody ducked. They need not have bothered. The intruder had just blown his own brains out.

Chapter 13

BEING SHOCKED BY events figured high in the archaeological world he had spent most of his maturing years in. Joshua now experienced even more than he realised possible. The woman he had secretly admired and loved had, for the second time, been involved in a traumatic incident. Someone wanted the Seals, and had instigated some nasty events to obtain them. Rachael was fortunate this time. She had survived and had returned the first set of seven tablets for safekeeping. The sooner this search terminated, the better for the safety of all concerned.

The hip flask was empty. Picking up a bottle, he sat back and poured out a large scotch and added water. There was a nagging in his brain. It reminded him of a restless worm looking for home.

Joshua glanced at the shelves, and poking out were his grandfather's works, scrolls, and notes, all of which he had ignored. Amongst them was a black pouch, the size of a large tea tray.

"Why not?" He stood, and reached out for the bag that had become encrusted with long dead cobwebs and a flotilla of dust particles. He blew on them and wished he hadn't.

Two thick buckled straps secured the bag. He lifted the large flap and peered inside, exercising the care he had been trained to use. The first item he pulled out was a neatly folded purple sash of some kind. He held it aloft and it unravelled to a length of a couple of metres. Two gold emblems embellished its length. He squinted and examined the emblems, and the hairs of his neck bristled. Two winged crowns encompassed with circles of gold looked back at him. *Isn't this what Rachael described her abductor wore as a small badge in his lapel?* He took a photograph on his mobile phone.

What is all this stuff? His sense of exploration had been piqued. Delving further, he found small leather booklets, lots of notes, unopened envelopes, and a small silver crucifix. The last item he pulled out was a document that had been folded like a complex demonstration of origami. With great care. he teased the faded edges open, like a flower unfolding before revealing its entirety. He smoothed it out across the table and let his eyes travel its entire length.

Incredulity went to his heart like a dagger.

The Greek words headed the document, and Joshua, fluent in Greek, understood it with no trouble.

Οι Φύλακες

The lettering, written in a careful hand, spelt out 'The Guardians,' superimposed above a map of the Greek Island of Patmos, showing the location of the Seven Churches of Asia.

The closer he looked at it, the more he understood. It

represented a lineage. It seemed that several hands across the centuries had been responsible for producing it. A large fading red rose was positioned beneath the map.

With a shaky hand, he poured another large scotch and brought a spotlight to bear on the document.

Divided into three long columns, the first name stood paramount over all others. Boldly and centrally written, it proclaimed the name,

ΓΙΑΝΝΗΣ

Joshua almost dropped his scotch. *It can't be!*

The Greek word of the name John, and from it, running through every name thereafter, was a thin red line that twisted and turned from name to name, connecting all to each other in one undivided link. He guessed there were one hundred names or more.

This is unbelievable!

He had heard of the Guardians, and that they had disappeared in the distant past. This evidence revealed they had not. They were very much alive. Simon and Rachael had even mentioned them.

Joshua found the timing more than surreal. But, if he thought he had enough shocks for one day, he was wrong. With a muted reverence, he traced his finger through all the names towards the last few, until it brought him up to modern times.

"Oh, great Jehovah! Will you look at that?" His eyes went wide.

Staring up at him from the document was a name he knew well.

Nathaniel Agar.

"My grandfather … a Guardian!' His voice echoed around the empty confines of his room. "I don't believe it! He never said a word." He lifted his head back and hit the table with a clenched fist, unable to comprehend the significance of it all. "This means he headed up the organisation."

Joshua slumped on his seat, and tears trickled down his cheeks. He now understood his grandfather's final words …

"One day, you will read them, and when that day arrives you will know who you are. We all live with and are surrounded by the ghosts of the past."

He stood and paced for a few minutes, before he moved back to the document. He had missed one name … the last. Focussing the spotlight, on the end he saw what Nathaniel had written. His jaw dropped, and the world as he knew it ceased to exist.

Chapter 14

THE PRESIDENT OF the University, Professor Jacob Ahasver, had always been a scary individual … frosty, aloof, with a non-communicative persona. He stood tall, lean, hard faced; a grey-haired man in his mid-fifties. He carried a permanent pale, world-weary expression about him, as if he had been travelling too long and needed a hundred-year rest.

Academia recognised him as transforming the fortunes of the University, raising it to one of the top ten in the world. Forever traveling, he had an uncanny ability to conjure up funds from the most unlikely sources. It had even been rumoured that he had received direct funding from the Vatican. Ahasver never commented on such matters. Much feared, but respected, he forever rode roughshod over committees and projects he thought were a waste of time and resources.

The suicide at the site had not escaped his attention, and he had also heard of Dr. Rachael Carver's plight within the Vatican. Linking this together with the nature of the archaeological finds, he had issued a security injunction. It was simple.

Every location they worked on must be pinpointed and reported to security, and that included the twenty-four-hour movements of everybody working there. That meant where and what they were working on and any trips they intended to take. At no time were their mobile phones to be switched off.

He was determined to know the movements of everybody who worked on or around the project. Safety, he said, remained paramount.

The team considered themselves in a nanny nursery and resentment ran high. But they did as they were asked.

Rockwell steered the Land Rover up over the hills where the research team intended to dig next. He felt a tingle of excitement. He found a level section to park up where a lazy sun threw a seductive glow over the landscape of undulating hills and palm trees.

"That's so romantic," Rachael said, "and there's nobody else around."

"Should have brought some bread, wine, and cheese. But we are not here for that, are we?" came his gruff response.

"Now there's a surprise."

He ignored the sarcasm. He got out and went to the back, surveying the panorama that stretched in all directions. She moved beside him, holding a rucksack that he knew would be stacked with anything they could possibly need.

"Wow, that aroma." The air had the scents of pine, oranges and wind-blown olives. "It probably hasn't changed in two thousand years."

"Let's walk on further," Rockwell said.

"Where're we going?"

"I came up here the other day when Julian was away. Given what has happened of late, I've told nobody. You're the first." He led her up a rocky gulley that twisted and turned, the soft landscape surrendering to harder rocks and less accessibility.

"Now, stop." Rockwell held up his hand and she came to a halt. "Look at that." He bent his head lower and pointed at a faint etching cut into the rock face.

Rachael peered at the object of his interest and her blood started racing through her veins. She recognized it at once. It was an Ichthys.

The early Christians had used many symbols, and that of the fish ranked first in importance. This symbol's popularity among early Christians was due principally to the famous acrostic consisting of the initial letters of five Greek words forming the word for 'fish' (Ichthus). These words briefly but clearly described the character of Christ and the claim to worship of believers:

Ἰησοῦς Χριστός, Θεοῦ Υἱός, Σωτήρ
Iēsous Christos, Theou Yios, Sōtēr
Jesus Christ, Son of God, Saviour

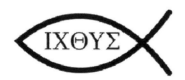

"Oh my!" she exclaimed as her hand covered her mouth. "It must be first-century."

"Without a doubt. Why would Greek lettering and symbology be cut into a hillside rock in Israel?"

"It looks as if it's pointing in an upward direction."

'It is. Let me show you more." He started walking.

"Much further?"

"Not much."

After ten minutes clambering, they reached a series of deep fissures that cut sideways into the rocky surface.

"Have you got the flashlight?"

Rachael already had it gripped in her hand, and she shone it through the gap. "Oh, wow! What do we have here?"

He squeezed in behind her and she felt the warmth of his body against hers. Not that he appeared to notice. She played the beam across the walls. They were decorated with murals, dozens of them, some looking as fresh as the day they were painted. Many looked indecipherable.

"They're all Christian. Look there." He pointed to fish symbols, crucifixions, Alpha and Omega letters, engraved Staurograms, and even the well-known Chi-Rho diagrams.

"My God!" Rachael exclaimed in an electrified whisper. "This is unexplored territory. I can't believe what we're looking at!"

"The passage goes on forever. It's full of murals. I think we have a major discovery here, Rachael. I've told no one yet. I wanted you to see it first."

Her heart rate speeded up. She was uncertain whether the discoveries or the closeness of him caused it.

"You're right. Let's get back and arrange a team to back us up before we go any further. What do you think?"

"Yes, let's go."

With breathless excitement, they started retracing their steps back to where they had parked.

Chapter 15

THE MILITARY STYLED Humvee pulled up close to the research facility. From it stepped three Dominican friars, who once assembled, began walking in single file. Their heads were bent, and prayers were intoned to the small clicking sound of their rosary beads. From beneath the black *cappas* worn across their backs could be seen the ripple of their white habits. Tucked in tightly to the cords that belted their habits, unseen at the back, each carried a suppressed Glock pistol.

A late Saturday afternoon, the Research area reception remained empty, apart from the presence of a burly security guard manning the desk. A nametag revealed his name as Henry. He looked surprised as the three figures made their way inside, and then alarmed as they ignored him and moved in the direction of the stairs.

"Hey there! Just a minute. Stop, will you?" He leapt to his feet and ran towards the friars.

The last monk in the file, turned, made the sign of the cross, and uttered, "*Sacris Sancti Homicidium,*" before he fired a single muffled shot.

The last thing Henry ever felt was the burning explosion in his chest.

He hit the floor, dead, the bullet splitting his heart.

The monk carried on walking with his brothers. They knew where they were heading. Up a few more flight of stairs and they reached a very long corridor. Their destination waited at the far end.

Rachael had always sensed that Joshua had a soft spot for her. She had found it endearing, but never in a romantic or physical way. He shared his concern for the project, and had invited her into his office to discuss the new finds that she and Rockwell had discovered.

When she arrived in his office, she immediately sensed his agitation. He was twisting the red scarf he forever wore.

"We have been in danger ever since we found those metal plates in that safe over there." He pointed at the steel structure in the corner. "Something is not right here. A worker was killed, a man committed suicide in front of us all, you are abducted, then somebody the Pope appoints to investigate our discovery was found hanging under a bridge, and then another attempt was made on your life, in the Vatican of all places. He failed and shot himself like the first man did, but not before a priest was brutally slain. Rachael, don't these events say something to you?" He tightened and untightened his scarf into small knots.

"Put like that, I can see what you mean."

"There's a force behind all this," he paused and looked up at her.

"What do you mean? You know there is, or you just think there is?"

"Have you heard of either the Keepers, or another society known as the Guardians?"

"Well yes, these names have cropped up ever since you dug up that ossuary."

"I meant before that. A society or secret groups?"

"Like the Freemasons, Illuminati, and Propaganda Due, for example?"

"No. Far deadlier."

"Are you trying to tell me something?"

A strained expression refused to leave his anxious face. "Forget it." He changed the subject. "When do we start looking at your cave carvings?"

"Why don't we go up tomorrow, all of us, and take a look?"

"Including Gallo?"

"Why not?"

"Okay, pick me up at about ten."

"See you tomorrow then." She smiled at him and left.

Joshua had not been able to bring himself to tell her what he found in his grandfather's documents. *How long can I keep this secret? Is it all melodramatic rubbish?*

He would have thought so, if the recent dramatic events around the Seals hadn't occurred. His grandfather, he knew now, had been the last in a long line of Guardians, whose lineage stretched back to the time of Christ's crucifixion. His documents revealed that they had been protectors of the Blessed John's Seven Seals. The revelation had shaken him and all his beliefs.

How could he have told Rachael what he now knew, but could only hint at? What would Rockwell and Gallo say if they knew? They would laugh me out of the research team.

The last name, on the lineage, and written in the unmistakable hand of his grandfather, hadn't been difficult to read … Joshua Agar … his own.

It couldn't be, but it stared him in the face.

He had found more. A gold ring, shaped as a crown with wings. It was identical to what Rachael had described her abductor had worn. If true, then the Guardians were very much alive.

In various envelopes were papers referring to an 'unholy' alliance known as the Keepers. The present incumbent's identity, the Grand Keeper, was a heavily guarded secret. Their aim was no less than world domination, and an overturning of the Pope and the Roman Catholic Church, all other faiths, and a return to the *One True Path to God*. A New World Order, no more, no less. This society believed that bringing together the Seven Seals would herald in the inevitable event. Christ will return, and whoever ushered in His Second Coming would rule beside Him as the chosen one.

The Keepers' lineage had many inexplicable gaps. It was incomplete, and stopped with the last four unknowns. The last known Grand Keeper was the deceased Nazi war criminal Heinrich Himmler.

To Joshua, it seemed preposterous. But in light of recent events, it couldn't be a coincidence. There was truth here. An inevitable destiny. His grandfather had been a highly respected man, and he would not leave a legacy of lies to his only grandson.

Another look at the Seals would be needed, and he had to do this alone.

Opening the desk drawer, he took the set of keys that would open the safe. He knew the combination sequence.

The safe incorporated thermal relockers in conjunction with those of tempered glass, which added protection against torches or thermal lances. Once he completed the correct sequence of procedures, the door swung open without a sound. What he saw inside startled him. The interior of the safe glowed. A soft blue light pulsated at regular intervals.

Joshua stumbled backwards. He slammed the door shut and began breathing at a rapid rate. *What was that? What on earth was that?* Maybe it was part of the internal mechanism of the safe once the door was opened. There could be no other explanation. *I must be going nuts.* For a moment, he thought it had something to do with the Seals.

Walking at a swift rate back down the corridor, Rachael found herself smiling at the thought of Joshua and Gallo's reaction when they saw their new find in the hills. She was on her way to the main reception car park where she had parked her vehicle. The three monks heading in her direction didn't surprise her. The University had a host of strange visitors and sights. Drawing level with each other, heads were nodded and small smiles exchanged.

She never looked behind. If she had, she would have seen them stop in front of the doorway she had not long stepped out of.

Joshua was contemplating if he should open the safe again. He couldn't help but think there was something very wrong about the whole proceedings. They were being led into an area few had visited. The more he thought of it, his conclusions dropped into the same direction as his grandfather's. The mystery had become very real. People were dying for it.

A sharp knock on the door broke his thoughts. He wasn't expecting a visitor, and assumed it was Rachael. Joshua smiled as he opened the door. The sight of three hooded monks was the last thing he would have expected, nor was the large ringed fist that smashed into his larynx.

A shrieking panorama of pain ripped through Joshua's neck and head, compounded further by a pistol butt smashing with force into his temple. He dropped to the floor, and heavy kicks from a black, steel capped footwear sent him into agonies of breathlessness. He tried to shout, but pain and lack of air jammed his vocal chords.

Two of the monks hoisted him up and threw him backwards into his swivel chair. A duct tape gag was wrapped around his mouth with speed, and his head was fastened to the back of the chair. Next, his hands were taped in hard to the chair arms, and in a similar fashion, his legs followed.

Completely immobile, Joshua's eyes swiveled back and forth, aware of burning pain rushing intermittently from head to toe.

After thirty terrifying seconds, the operation came to a

stop. Not one of them spoke. The first monk went straight to the desk drawer and removed the keys Joshua had used ten minutes before.

Restricted as he was, and overcome with pain, Joshua could still think. The men were unrecognizable, but they seemed to have knowledge of his office, the location of his keys, and the safe. They moved with purpose and familiarity. *How?* He attempted to struggle but the tape held him fast. One thing he knew, these men were not monks. They had physical strength and were etched with muscles no monk could achieve. He had glimpsed tattoos on two of them, a fish eating its own tail, and there was nothing pious or devout in their demeanours. They're here for one reason ... the Seals locked inside the safe.

Drenched in sweat and blood, he watched in terror as the second monk began to perform quick swivels on the large dial. *They didn't ask him for the combination. How can they know?*

At that moment, the General Emergency Alarm blasted out in ear-breaking decibels. Its raucous and rapid wail filling every floor of the University, and outside.

Rachael had clattered down the stone stairs of the building, until she reached the second landing where she had a clear view of the ground floor. *Where's everybody?* The place looked deserted, which was odd. She carried on down, and when she reached the ground floor, she knew something was wrong.

A pair of legs extended from behind the desk, accompanied by a widening red stain. She recognized a dead body when she saw one, but she had never seen one with a gaping hole in the chest.

"Henry!" she shrieked out loud. "Help! Henry's been shot!"

But there was nobody about.

All staff members knew the emergency procedures by heart. With a clenched fist, Rachael punched the fat red button sitting in the middle of the control console behind the desk canopy.

The result was instantaneous.

The sound blasted through the entire complex, signifying a potential terrorist alert.

Within a fraction of a minute, teams of armed guards, ambulances, and firemen, would descend on the Research Facility. She rushed to the exit as the wails of sirens got louder.

Then, she remembered. The monks! Those three must have been there when Henry got shot.

"Holy Mother!" Rachael's hand went to her mouth, and she rushed back to the reception console, crouching low in case they returned.

She knew where they were headed. Joshua's office. They're after the Seals. *Blessed Mother, please keep Joshua safe.* Rachael could only utter a prayer as she waited for help to arrive.

In less than a minute, there was a screech of brakes, and several vehicles packed with armed guards can be seen in front of the University entrance. The guards leapt out, and other vehicles can be seen cordoning the car park. The University was surrounded.

Captain Manovici, a squat and powerful man with no excess weight, crouched low, and entered the expansive foyer carrying a machine pistol. He saw Rachael next to Henry's bloody body.

"Don't move. Are you harmed?" he demanded.

"No. I'm okay. The guard has been murdered. There are three men dressed as monks up on the third floor. I think I know what they're after."

Manovici edged closer as she gave him an explanation. He nodded his understanding and gave hand signals, speaking softly into his mouthpiece for his men to cover the elevators, and for others to make their way up the stairway to the third floor. He warned them of the three men dressed as monks and armed.

The entire complex was now locked down and placed on high alert.

The monks had the safe door open. The blasting klaxon didn't deter them at all. Joshua watched one of them reach in and grasp the casket. This time, there was no blue light. The monk then dropped the item into a leather shoulder bag, and huddled. Joshua tried to listen in on their conversation, but they spoke in whispers.

Their meeting ended and all three reached for their pistols. One monk produced a knife and looked over at Joshua.

Joshua liked watching films, and in horror, he realized this scenario could only end badly for him. His heart rate accelerated, and vomit hit the back of his throat.

The monk went behind him and Joshua clenched his eyes tight, expecting pain. He prayed his death would be quick.

But there was no pain. Instead, he felt the knife cutting through the duct tape with ease, releasing his arms and legs. His mouth gag remained. Joshua almost wet himself in relief.

With great caution, they opened the door and pushed him into the corridor, using his body as a shield. He prayed to God the police wouldn't start firing.

They stepped alongside him and behind him, their Glock pistols pressed into him; two at his head and one into his back.

"Now, move along at a normal pace," one demanded. It was the first time they spoke to him. "Any stupid move or heroics and you're dead. If we are fired at, that will be your death warrant. Understood?"

Joshua could only nod his head, his eyes wide with fear.

Just then, the first guard appeared, holding a 9mm assault weapon. He dived to the ground, aiming straight at them.

"Hold it!" shouted the monk beside him. "There are three guns on this man. One shot from you or your men ... and he will die. You can't get all three of us at once, so if you want to save him, back off and go back down those stairs and we will follow you. All nice and slow now. One shot at us, and it will be over for your learned friend here."

The guard hesitated and spoke into his mouthpiece, lowered his gun, turned, and rapidly descended the stairs.

Joshua was propelled along by the monks, who circled him closely. At that moment, a memory flashed in his mind. He was five years old when he fell into a deep well. Terrified, he had shouted and shouted ... but nobody came. He'd been trapped for twelve hours, and thought death had him. Now, he relived that fear. From the corner of his eye, he could see uniformed gunmen everywhere; behind pillars, corners, even outside in the concourse. *Somebody's going to die today. I just know it.* All guns were pointed in their direction.

Captain Manovici had rigorously trained his men for moments like this. Now, a deadly reality stared at him. His breathing changed, sharpened as it always did when the threat is real. He'd learnt the hard way that terrorists and desperate bank robbers with hostages gave no room for compromise. It was a gamble that could easily be lost or won.

He glanced around the concourse and was glad to see his men positioned at every available spot. Amongst them were the force's best snipers and sharpshooters. He spoke into his mouthpiece and instructed three of his men to target one monk each. He assigned the monk they each should aim for, and reminded them to shoot only when he gave the command. All three shots were to come at once. One miss and Joshua Agar's life would be forfeit.

Captain Manovici could see the monks moving forward in an uncertain fashion, and he smiled when he realised they had made a serious miscalculation. *I wouldn't want to be in their shoes.* He focused his binoculars on them, and knew the three shots had to be fired before they turned left into the car park.

Determined not to fail, he clenched his teeth as he fixed his binoculars on the moving quartet.

"Number one, are you on your target?"

"Affirmative."

"Number two?"

"Affirmative.'

"Number three?"

"Affirmative."

"On my command, you will fire … One, two, three … FIRE!"

Nobody would have known that three separate shots had gone off. There was only one sharp audible crack, like a whip being flicked.

Joshua Agar was in shock, as he stood in a welter of blood and brains. Three monks lay dead in a manner they would not have believed possible. The bullets had struck before the sound registered with them. Each shot went cleanly through the head. The bag containing the six Seals lay undamaged at Joshua's feet, as if honouring him.

Over twenty armed men rushed forward.

Two hours passed before he could stop shaking.

Chapter 16

Rome

A WATERY SUN ascended above the Basilica, as the man pulled his topcoat tighter around him. He had no wish to get soaked from the threatening rain. He was disturbed. The recent events, suicides, murders, abductions, and the slaughter of three bogus monks had unnerved people. Questions were being asked about the shootings, and their possible connection to a rumoured discovery of huge religious importance.

He had slipped away from his base without notice. Business of the highest order required his attention. They didn't need controversy, and the situation had to be contained as fast as possible.

His affairs involved money, finance, and the redeployment of certain personnel. He rendezvoused regularly with Papal dignitaries, bankers, foreign ministers, and men of influence in international policy groups. He didn't doubt that his meetings would be successful, and funding for the proposed project would be substantial, given the rewards on offer.

At his chosen exit point, he found the midnight blue Mercedes waiting for him, complete with a uniformed driver. He slid into the back seat, and sat beside a lean, stern, middle aged man with wiry silver hair, wearing a scarlet cassock, sash, mozzetta, and biretta. The man stared fixedly to his front and clutched a tattered black briefcase.

"Master, I hope your journey was comfortable.

"Your Most Reverend Eminence, Cardinal Riario, a pleasure, as always."

"The answers to your questions," the Cardinal turned to him, "are in here." He handed him the briefcase. "The man who committed suicide in the Vatican museum had been unidentifiable, as expected. But the police are too inquisitive. What has been discovered is of major importance to Christians throughout the world."

"Camerlengo, I shall be the judge of that, not you." The car braked to avoid a bunch of nuns attempting to cross a busy Roman street. He continued, "There has been an amateur attempted robbery at Tel-Aviv University, I understand, and three legionnaires had been slaughtered. Unnecessarily, in my view. Where's Anderson? I need to speak with him. Please arrange it. At least he has a practical overview of events."

"We are close, Master."

"We would have been almost home and dry, with more careful planning. Heads will roll, and even worse, if this situation is not resolved soon. It's unbelievable that you failed to brief me on your operation, and that the seneschal was not informed. He doesn't know who I am, but I know he is a key component, and has excellent organizing skills. Instead, you chose to go off on some attempt at personal glory, and look what you achieved … zero, and three more soldiers down. Gallo must now be more actively involved. I trust him."

The Camerlengo bowed his head. "Agreed."

"Under no circumstances is he to know more than he needs to."

"That, of course, goes without saying. The meeting is ready for you. Do you wish to attend now?"

"Now." The Grand Keeper tried to reign in his boiling temper. The Camerlengo was not an ordinary member of the AWC.

The Mercedes slid into the Cardinal's parking slot, and both men alighted and headed to the Camerlengo's private quarters. His Swiss guard sprang smartly to attention, his back as straight as the decorative pikestaff he held upright in his right hand. The Camerlengo ignored him and swung the double doors open, and ushered in his Master.

The table had been prepared. It was heavy with flaming candles, and small vases of flowers stretched its length. Available were Havana cigars, decanters of the finest ports, and vast assortments of finger foods on gold and silver trays.

There were now seven of them in attendance, sitting in in a semi-circle. The Master, the Grand Keeper, sat at the head. The Inner Circle was complete.

He allowed his glass to be filled, then he raised it high in both hands, as they all did, and recited their oath three times.

"*Sacris Sancti Homicidium.*"

He remained standing as he gestured for the others to sit. Taking another sip of his port, he swallowed and allowed himself a moment to experience its warm glow before he spoke.

"I'm not here to praise you. We have been losing too

many legionnaires. The operation has become sloppy and the blame lies at your feet. To fix this, to possess what we seek plus the missing set, and for our plans to be put into operation, we will need financing. Believe me, unlimited power will be ours once we are in possession of the Seven Seals. But to achieve our aim, we need at least twenty million dollars, or the equivalent in Bearer Bonds.

"Twenty million!" Cardinal Pacca exclaimed. "We've had bankers hanging from under bridges for less. It's too much."

The Grand Keeper flung the crystal glass he was holding into the fireplace. "Too much? You sniveling penny-pinching cleric! And you run the economic affairs of the Holy See? How dare you tell me what is too much. I'll tell you what is too much. It's cowards like you who have consistently blocked our advancement. God's glory is in our grasp, and you dare question what we must do to bring it about? Do you really dare to do that?" He smashed his fist onto the table, turned his back on them, and folded his arms across his chest.

The room went silent.

"Of course not, Grand Keeper." The embarrassed Cardinal squirmed an apology. "I'm sorry, but it just seems such a lot of money."

"I call for a vote," the Grand Keeper said in a soft voice that unnerved the Inner Circle members. "Those opposed raise your hand."

Not one hand was raised.

"My request is carried. I want the money, one way or another, before I leave tomorrow. At no time are you to ever attempt another disaster like the one that just occurred. The Seven Seals are to be had in one swoop. Without them all, nothing is achievable. All you have managed to achieve is death and an increase in their security. I also wish to see each of you individually and alone, as from now. We have urgent plans to put into operation. You first." He pointed at their NATO representative, General Sir Gordon Anderson.

Chapter 17

I AM GOING to have to tell them.

Joshua Agar ran his hand through his dark hair. On the table in front of him, alongside the Seals, he had placed the relevant materials he had unearthed from his grandfather's effects. He laid everything out in a precise order, and so far, both Rachael and Rockwell looked intrigued. Gallo looked uneasy.

He lifted the Seals from their stone casket. Again, for a moment, they seemed to glow with a faint blue colour.

"They radiate a sort of power. If that doesn't make me sound crazy," Rockwell said with a gasp of drawn in breath.

"I've never seen anything so significant in all my work." Gallo bent his head as if in reverence.

Rachael could only comment, "The source of my recent misfortunes, here in front of me."

Joshua's pulse quickened as he leant forward and began to unravel his secret. "I have here the contents of my late grandfather's effects. I was astonished to discover they related directly to the find we see in front of us ... the Seals. You recognize this, Rachael?" He handed her the gold winged crown ring.

She jumped up and grabbed the ring from him. "My God,

it's identical." She referred to her abductor's badge.

He looked around at them all. Rockwell's jaw was set hard, and Gallo went white.

"Yes," Joshua continued, "my grandfather headed a long-forgotten society known as the Guardians, who were supposed to have been extinguished centuries ago. Not so, it appears. They had been tasked to preserve the secrets of the Seals that you see in front of you. Another highly secret brotherhood known as the Keepers have been attempting to locate all the Seals. They believe they contained untold power that will enable them to establish a New World Order, Christ's true kingdom on earth. They're prepared to destroy anything that stands in their way. They still exist. That's the reason Rachael was abducted, to warn her, and the reason for the bungled theft at the University. The Keepers need all seven to make it work. Think about it. Events here, of late, can only confirm that forces are after the Seals. Either to protect them, or acquire them. According to my grandfather, the Keepers have been in existence since the destruction of the Temple of Jerusalem. Their struggle has been continuous. They have an oath, *Sacris Sancti Homicidium* ... The Sacred Act of Holy Murder. That tells you much about them. My grandfather is now dead. With his death, the Guardians, who had been entrusted with the Seventh Seal, should have expired. Not so. It seems they number in the tens of thousands, as do the Keepers, now a very guarded and secret movement known as *I Guerrieri Apocalittici di Cristo*. Who leads it, is not known."

"This is a load of melodramatic Hollywood junk," Rockwell spluttered in an exasperated scientific outburst.

"I'm not so sure, Simon." Rachael looked heated. "Stop

being such an analytical prick. Everything points to something we know nothing of. The similarity of the winged crown, and everything else Joshua told us, could explain the suicide at the site, my abduction, the suicide in the Vatican, and the horror of Joshua's hostage incident. They were attempting to steal what we have here. Why? Simon, you can't just see everything in terms of $E=mc2$. It goes beyond what we know about. What do you think, Julian?"

Gallo's gaze was fixed on the ossuary and its contents. He didn't speak, although his lips appeared to move.

"Julian?"

He gave a start. "Yes, sorry. I don't like to speculate. Clearly, we have something here that somebody wants. If what you say, Joshua, is true, then we need to search for the missing Seal. Before I outline my ideas, can you tell us, Julian, did your grandfather's documents give any indication of who could be leading these Guardians, or the other group you mentioned?"

"None, whatsoever." Joshua lied.

Gallo nodded.

Rockwell interjected. "Rachael and I went way up into those hills, and found what looked like an entrance into a deeper cave system. This is what we found." On the large screen at the end of the room, appeared images of the Ichthys and the surrounding inscriptions. "I'm certain everyone here would want to explore further."

"Wait a minute." Gallo stood back from his chair. "I propose that I plan and execute this exploration, in conjunction with Joshua. We will set-up a team in this location." He waved a finger at Simon and Rachael. "You two are far too important to go climbing around in dark and deep caves. We have the workforce, the equipment, and the technology we need. Radar equipment here would be useless though. Only physical excavation has any point. What do you say?"

Rockwell stared at Rachael. She shrugged. He then looked at Joshua. He seemed unhappy.

"Julian is correct," Joshua replied, "but no more so than any of us here. We all have roles to play. What we are embarking on could possibly have worldwide significance. That is, however, my subjective viewpoint." Something had stopped Joshua from revealing the full extent of his grandfather's work. He had decided to keep some things to himself. His acceptance of his role as a Guardian moved one step closer.

"The Seals," Gallo said, "can be interpreted by different people in three ways. One, they have been opened, and we are in the final days of destruction. Each Seal can represent thousands of years. Two, they are yet to be opened. Some say that only Christ himself can do that. Finally, each can be construed as a metaphor, an acceptance of and demonstration of God's power. All will be revealed in the opening of the Seventh, and those who refuse to accept will perish."

Rockwell rolled his eyes skywards. "Well, we'd better get going then before the end of time arrives, hadn't we? Why don't we all go up to the hills and have a look around. We'll show you what we found, and then we can round up the team."

Rachael placed the Seals back in the ossuary. She had also noticed the faint blue colour, and it reminded her of the comfort she felt from her dreams of the 'stigmata' Virgin Mary, who had remained a close companion since then.

Joshua agreed to drive them, but for the second time that afternoon, he felt uneasy and he couldn't explain why.

Chapter 18

AFTER THE GRAND Keeper had finished with his interviews, there now existed a strategy that spanned every aspect of what he considered the imminent discovery of the final Seal. Economic, political, military, and social preparations were in place. The world would soon hear about the end of the Pope and the Roman Catholic Church. All other false religions would be required to surrender and return to Christ. The AWC, with the power of the Seals, would show them the way by fair means or foul.

Tomorrow I shall have twenty million dollars in Bearer Bonds. My monitoring of the University's excavations is going to plan. I know every move they make, even more than the seneschal. But he is vital to my plans. One day, he may access our Inner Circle.

He wondered if other members of the excavation team understood the true implications of what they were close to discovering. That didn't really matter at all.

At that moment, his encrypted mobile, a Silent Circle Blackphone 2, using three untraceable routers, gave out a text alert. It bore the number given to the seneschal. He had been commanded that it should only be used in exceptional circumstances. The Grand Keeper read the message, and it gave him cause to frown.

"Evidence of activity by the Guardians. Very much alive, I fear, and as close as we are. Awaiting instructions."

Deep in thought, he drank two full glasses of claret to calm his agitation. This had to be investigated and with care. He replied, asking for more information. Thirty minutes later, he had two names, Dr. Rachael Carver, but of most importance, Joshua Agar. Agar was as a prime suspect, having admitted that his grandfather had been the leading figure of the Guardians prior to his death. Carver was an academic, and like most, inconsequential. She could be a bargaining chip if matters deteriorated.

Chapter 19

IN SPITE OF Gallo's remarks that a radar equipment would be useless, a small unit was propelled into the back of one of the pickup trucks, together with pickaxes, portable trollies, trowels, brushes, spades, and powerful freestanding flashlights. Going with it were storage crates, polythene sheets, plus a compact generator.

"What we can get through the small gaps remains to be seen." Rockwell booted a tyre to satisfy himself it was solid. "What are you up to, Julian?"

He looked up from his mobile. "Just letting the President's office know where we are and what we are up to. Those were his orders, if you remember."

"I remember." Rockwell raised his eyes skywards. "C'mon, let's get these trucks rolling. I can't wait to see this again." He fired up his vehicle and Rachael got in next to him.

"You don't mind?" She smiled.

"Nope. Hope you packed a few beers."

"Would I forget?"

Gallo got in the other truck next to Joshua. "How long's the trip?" Gallo asked.

"Thirty minutes," Joshua replied in a flat tone. He had never felt comfortable with Gallo around. He started the engine and moved out, revving up more than needed to blot out Gallo's voice.

"Odd thing that, your grandpa being a member of some secret sect. What do you think about that?"

Joshua didn't want to talk about it, certainly not with him. "He was an old man. I wouldn't put too much weight on it." He lied. "Seems a lot of nonsense to me."

Joshua had more knowledge of the Seals than he had told anybody. He had found names, addresses, contact numbers, passwords and codes, and a story that went back to Christ himself. There were also procedures to be implemented if he accepted the role. If they heard nothing from him after a year, another leader would be chosen. The only person he trusted, Rachael, seemed agreeable to the whole idea. Her reaction to her abduction was a powerful indicator of that trust. Gallo didn't fit the pattern, far from it. He was hiding something, Joshua was certain of it. What startled him further was an evidence he found in the files linking the University's archaeology department and the Vatican. But that went back fifty years ago. The department would inform the Vatican of all finds considered of biblical importance, in exchange for helpful doses of funding. It seemed innocent enough, but the introduction of the Seven Seals, he suspected, would have caused a near panic in Rome. He would've enjoyed seeing their real reaction behind closed doors, after Rachael had showed them the first set.

The hand of God must have been at work for him to find the very thing his granddad had sought all his life, albeit incomplete. But Joshua now understood the danger. People were dying as a result of it.

The thought left him breathless. His grandfather had

referred to the violators as the Keepers, who had links back to the early first century, and were obsessed with the existence of the continuous presence of an Antichrist, now in the guise of Papal authority and the Roman Catholic Church. They had blossomed in the Italian Renaissance eras, under the leadership of the famed artist, Cosimos Ricci. Nathaniel's notes had indicated that there was evidence of the Keepers' presence in the university. But there were no specific names mentioned anywhere in the files.

Nathaniel Agar had written, as others have done before him, that real power, mystical and Godly, existed through the Seals only when they were complete and activated. If one believed the story, the implications were astonishing. It meant the Second Coming was at hand. Joshua wondered how it would come about. *Will Christ himself really return? In the flesh?* If all this was more than superstition and legend, power like that would enable anyone to change the world, one way or the other.

Gallo would be the last person he'd entrust with this information.

Rachael's brief abduction had seemed inexplicable, but not so when she had described the badge the man wore and the questions he had asked. She had a close encounter with a Guardian. They knew of the discovery, and after all this time, they were still protecting it.

If he accepted the role, he guessed there would be more to discover.

Joshua kept his eyes on the dusty track, ignoring Gallo's probing, tasteless questions. His dislike of him grew. Feelings that he didn't know he had, arose. He didn't enjoy the sensation, but he stopped short of telling him to quit nosing around. The more he thought of events, the more convinced he was that the Seventh Seal would be found ... and trouble will follow. There existed an air of inevitability about it.

Checking the rear mirror and watching the dust swirling around the Jeep, he noted the vehicle trailing them a hundred metres behind. It had followed them from the moment they had left.

Joshua dismounted from the vehicle when they arrived, and turned to get a better look at the Jeep parked way back, its two occupants taking photographs in their direction. It didn't surprise him. Gears in his brain, placed there by his grandfather, had begun to operate.

In one swooping moment of intuition, he saw it all. There existed a gigantic plot, and somehow the Seals had galvanized it. But by God ... it was real.

Standing there and looking across the pitiless landscape, Joshua reached a decision. By degrees, he would accept his grandfather's mantle. But he needed more time for the wet cement of the decision to dry. *Why did he choose me?* In that moment of his provisional acceptance, he bowed his head. *I am a Jew, as was my father, and his father before him. Christ, also a Jew, and controversy, had been a part of their lives. I wish to be part of theirs also. Honesty will find no disfavor with God!*

Rachael and Rockwell were waving for them to come up and join them. Gallo, not being too fit, was gasping for breath as they moved further upwards into the steeper parts of their climb.

Simon shouted out to the ascending duo as they got closer. "This fissure is where we found the first inscriptions and carvings. Look, there they are." He indicated a rock above their heads. Gallo began taking pictures.

They were bent double as they shuffled along in a wave of expectancy. The rock had whitened across the centuries, from rain that dribbled from the porous ceiling. Their flashlights had revealed a long-forgotten age. It became darker the more they navigated through. The entire proximity was awash with Greek, Latin, and Hebrew lettering.

When they realised the scope of their new discovery, Rockwell couldn't hide his astonishment.

"My God! This is phenomenal!" He shone his lamp around the deep shadows of walls and roofs, revealing more. The entire structure swarmed with icons and religious symbols of early Christian origin. "This looks unchanged since they were inscribed. It's a major breakthrough."

They stood in dumbfounded silence, as a fitful breeze murmured from beyond the rocks like a tortured soul.

Their feet trod through an abundance of broken clay pots, tiles, olive oil lamps, metal keys, and what looked like earrings. Together with these were scatterings of unknown bones.

Gallo raised his flashlight beam, searching the rocks as more inscriptions came into view.

"This place was once inhabited," Rachael whispered. "I agree, and it has remained secret for centuries and more. If you wanted to hide something during that time, something of value to the Christians, you'd hide it here, wouldn't you?" Gallo continued to swing the light beam to and fro.

"I've the strangest feeling that we are intruders." Joshua

looked dubious. "We must treat this place with respect."

"Of course, that goes without saying," Rockwell agreed. "We'll need a full team up here, but before that, we need to know what it is and how far this labyrinth expands. It could get dangerous."

"Just look at that, will you?" Gallo sounded excited and had directed his beam into the far corner where it was losing luminosity. In front, lay a chamber of circular design, with a natural high rounded ceiling that resembled a rocky opening. His beam shone through and what they saw caused a collective gasp. There could be seen the unmistakable form of a stone altar, surrounded with three crumbling crucifixes, around which stood unmistakable figures of the Virgin Mother and child. To each side of these stood carvings of angels holding trumpets. There were glints of gold, copper, and coloured glass. Against the walls, in neat rows, stood ossuaries and reliquary caskets. What they saw next was macabre. A skeleton was leaning onto the sidepiece of the altar, its skull broken in two places, yet it retained its hideous death grin. It stared straight at them as if the wait had been centuries too long. To the rear of him were numerous openings, passageways, and what looked like tunnels.

"We need more light." Rockwell slid the backpack from his shoulders. "Here, take this." He produced a battery-operated light bar that when switched on, flooded the space in a lemon and tangerine glow. All four of them spread out around the space.

"Where do we start?" Rachael had to ask.

"We don't," Rockwell answered. "This is far too important for us to go club footing around. We'll just make a preliminary assessment. Nothing is to be removed.

Understood?"

They all agreed.

"We'll take a few shots and have a look at those ossuaries, and then head back and make arrangements to divert all of our manpower up here until we decide otherwise."

"This is a site of national importance," Joshua whispered to Rachael. "Look, I need to speak to you alone very soon." In the strange light, he saw her eyebrow rise. *God, she looks so pretty!* Her reply surprised him.

"I thought you might."

"You did?"

"Sssh! Be quiet." She held her finger to her lips. "We'll arrange it when we return."

Gallo and Rockwell were on their knees with a large plastic sheeting underneath them, as they inched their way along the floor, marking areas of about three metres square with pegs and metallic tape.

"There's enough material here to fill a troop train," Rockwell quipped as he flicked a couple of Dinars into the air.

Gallo said nothing. His eyes, greedy with expectation, swiveled from object to object as if he was about to find what he had forever dreamt of.

Joshua watched him. As he did so, there arose within him a certainty that Gallo was part of the secret organization Nathaniel had documented. The Keepers. Something about the way he had behaved since they found the Six Seals, his loaded questions in the truck, and what were all those phone calls about? He had no family now, nor friends anybody knew of. He was a loner, but with a phone directory that would have filled four volumes.

Joshua *knew*.

He reached into his back pocket and pulled out his hip flask and gave it a mighty swig, before he stoppered it back with a snappy flourish. There, at last. One major suspect he had to watch. All that remained was his forthcoming talk with Rachael. From there, he'll see where events would lead.

Chapter 20

AFTER ROCKWELL HAD finished taking measurements, and Gallo had taken the required photographs, they all headed back to the concealed entrance, with their batteries fading fast. The wall art and murals they passed caused them to pause often. As they neared the entrance, the light became brighter, but because of the angle of their movement, they glimpsed yet another chamber to their right.

They headed straight into it. Again, it was circular and supported by natural columns of stone. On stone shelves that spanned the full circumference of the area, stood two rows of pottery jars; some with lids, some without. All appeared to contain scrolls.

Rockwell looked stunned. Scrolls, unburied, yet still intact? He daren't touch them lest they crumbled into dust.

Joshua felt awed by everything. *Whoever put these here would never have imagined they would be here for thousands of years.*

"Don't move. Don't touch!" Rockwell's command was muffled by the hand covering his mouth, as if his breath would cause irreparable damage to what they were looking at. "Julian ... photographs, now!"

The camera went into rapid action.

Bits of crumbly scroll littered the entire floor area like snowflakes.

"If we touch them, they'll fall apart. We're not yet equipped to interfere with them. This is a job for the laboratory guys," Rachael whispered, aware that her voice added to the violation of centuries of sanctuary.

"This is major. Let's get out of here now before we damage anything. But by God, we will be back!" Rockwell began pushing everybody out.

They made their tortuous way back into the sunlit entrance with its deceiving panorama of the plains.

Gallo had the expression of a man experiencing a bullet smashing through a nearby window. He turned his back on them and commenced talking at speed into his phone.

Below them, Joshua didn't fail to notice that at the same time, the two men clambered at speed back into their Jeep, and roared away in a swirl of yellow dust. With doubts growing in his head like a malignant worm, he looked back at Gallo who had closed his phone at the same time the Jeep scurried off.

Rockwell's mind raced with the myriad possibilities this place contained. The whole structure, unexplored, looked as if it had remained that way since the first century. They were the first eyes to see them since the last time anyone had used the place. There could be little doubt that it had once served as a secret Christian place of worship. What it contained, from what he had seen so far, placed it in the league of the Dead

129

Sea Scrolls ... or more. If the story behind the missing seal could be believed, then this had to be the most likely place such a thing would be buried. That servant, Koury, could be referring to these caves. On top of that came the added bonus of all the other items they had so far discovered. It would take months of excavating and cataloguing. God only knows what those scrolls would show, if indeed they could ever be opened without causing irreparable damage. The story about Guardians and Keepers seemed like fairyland. The only reference came from an unknown man, Ananias, the Olive Grower. The ossuary had to be a big plus in the story's favour, but only hard evidence would advance the theory. Having found what also looked like another ossuary, Rockwell guessed that the entire system could be part of a complex burial site, a catacomb. Many ossuaries had survived time, and numbered in the multiple hundreds. Of those, about twenty-five percent had inscriptions describing their contents. Illiteracy flourished in those days, so it was easy to establish a fake from the real article. As with the ossuary found by Joshua, the microscopic and laboratory analysis were clear. Scientific analysis was the only way to getting anywhere near the truth.

My God this is getting complex. Let's hope we have a breakthrough and this whole Seal business is sorted once and for all.

They traveled back at speed and in an excited silence. It would be a day or two before a fully-fledged team would retrace their steps.

That afternoon, the Grand Keeper received two encrypted messages. News came from his two legionnaires who had been detailed to follow Rockwell's team, and the other was from the seneschal. They were identical.

That pleased him. It displayed unity, and a common purpose. What their next steps would be required careful thought. He turned, went to the drinks cabinet, and poured out a large claret. As he sipped the wine, the thought crossed his mind that the wine drank at Mass was considered the actual blood of Christ. Transubstantiation, they called it, and the wafers and bread were supposed to be the Body of Christ! These antichrists ate and drank Him! It was ritualistic cannibalism. Satan had them duped.

Lighting up a robust looking cigar, he leant over his desk and jotted down the sparse information he had so far received. The best of that came from his seneschal. From the information available, there had been a major discovery in the hillside of Beit-Guvrin.

He lifted his eyes to the heavens and experienced the rush of sacred exaltation coursing through his blood cells, his brain neurons falling in rhythm with the universe. *The time is almost upon us.*

"And the Great Dragon was cast out, the old serpent, called the Devil and Satan, which deceiveth the whole world: was cast out into the earth, and his angels were cast out with him."

He could not be wrong, nor the long line of Keepers before him. He recalled the Renaissance under the grip of the blessed Cosimos, *whom he had mentored.*

He had placed himself in the very same line, not just of blood, but of ability and belief. It had taken many centuries. Now, as the Grand Keeper, he gasped at the enormity of what was almost within his grasp. The Keepers, with him as their beloved leader, were poised to demonstrate the full power of God's wrath upon humanity. *Me, a lowly servant, ordained by God, once cursed by Christ, will shape the future of mankind! How many centuries have I wandered this earth to await release? Twenty is the number, and I roam still!*

He fell to his knees and bowed his head, already brimming with plans to activate every sleeper cell across the globe.

He spoke directly to both Cardinals Riario and Pacca. "Your Eminences, I suspect closure is upon us. You are to begin gathering support and sounding out those within the Vatican who are favourable to our cause. I have spoken to important people across the planet, those who are prepared to join us. Those who do not will be denied a place in the new world we will create. One faith under Christ's hand will be inevitable once the Seventh Seal is found. The world will be changed for eternity. Are you now ready to commence your task?"

"I have always been ready," replied Cardinal Riario.

"May God bless us in our endeavours," Cardinal Pacca whispered in a voice trembling with emotion.

The seneschal's heart beat faster. With the instructions he had received, there would be trouble, of that he didn't doubt.

Preparations required him to be armed. He was equipped for that, as every seneschal and Warrior throughout the world would now be. He had kept a 9mm Baby Eagle handgun, often used by the Israeli army, locked away in his safe. He now strapped it to the small of his back, and covered it with an expansive kaftan style shirt.

The Grand Keeper had made known his command. Gallo, as seneschal of Israel and the Middle East countries, would set the process in motion once the Seventh Seal was found. From that point onward, they would begin establishing God's New Kingdom, with the Grand Keeper wielding the power that had lain dormant in the Seals since the time of Christ.

Chapter 21

LATER THAT DAY, Joshua returned to his living quarters and received another shock. The place had been ransacked. Furniture had been upended; books and papers were strewn everywhere. Pictures hung at crazy angles and his bed had been violated with the mattress standing upright against the wall, and the covers spread around the room like butter on toast.

The shock wasn't unpleasant. His reaction would have confused most.

Satisfaction.

It was a growing glow of confirmation, as what had been lurking in his mind began to expand. The important materials from his grandfather's legacy, and the scrolls and list of Guardians had not been touched. He had stored them away in his safe. Whoever broke in had done so for a reason, and it certainly wasn't for money.

Information.

Of that, they had found nothing.

Two hours later, he sat on a large rocky slab overlooking the town. Above him, as dusk began its descent, hung the stars like rows of broken pearls. Next to him, sat Rachael Carver.

"I know what you are thinking," she said.

"What's that?"

"It's about Julian, isn't it?"

"Yes, it is."

"I must admit that he's been acting strange since all this began."

"I'm going to tell you something that might surprise you."

"What?"

Joshua paused, distracted. Her sweet aroma had got to him, and she had the enigmatic scent only a woman could possess. *Attention, Joshua ... attention.* "My quarters were turned over today, but nothing was taken. Some people think I have something they want?"

There was a quiet moment as they looked at each other.

"You don't seem too bothered. Do you have something?"

"Yes, I do."

"Tell me." She placed her hand on his. He wasn't an unattractive man, far from it. *If Simon hadn't been around, well, who knows?* she thought. Josh had a gentleness about him. He wasn't the macho or tough type, and it made him seem vulnerable, bringing out in her a motherly regard for him. But nothing sexual or romantic stirred her feelings. She felt a connection with him. Ever since her continual experiences around the Holy Virgin, things had changed for her, unalterably.

"I don't know where to start."

"The beginning's a good place. I'm listening and I'll not

interrupt."

Joshua began to tell her of his early life, and his adoption by his grandfather. The wise things Nathaniel had said, his discovery of his grandfather's true identity; the last in a line of Guardians devoted to the search and preservation of the Seven Seals of the Blessed John. And how from that, he had found the existence of the Keepers.

"Your grandfather knew all this? So now that he's dead, what's happening to the Guardians? Who's leading them now. What about the seals?"

"Yes. He knew all this." "You haven't answered my last question." She gripped his arm.

"If all this can be believed, whoever reunites the Seven seals will obtain unbelievable power granted by God himself. Whatever it is, could shape humanity, one way or another. This world that we know of would cease to exist and a new age will be ushered in. Nathaniel wrote this."

"You're dodging my question. Answer me!"

Joshua couldn't look at her. He bent his head. "It's me. He wrote my name as his successor." "What?" Her grip tightened.

"Yes. I was amazed as you are. Your abduction, my ordeal with those killers, the ransacking of my apartment, think about it ..."

She interrupted him. "I don't have to think about it, Josh, I know. We both believe, don't we, that in some way, Julian is involved in all this. Am I correct?"

"Completely. What of Simon?"

"He thinks these sorts of things are rubbish. Put it the way you have told me, and I'm not certain he would be so dogmatic. What are we going to do now?"

The sky had become darker, the stars more brilliant, and the air had a chill that brought shivers to their skin. He moved closer to her.

"From Nathaniel's notes and writings, I have names to contact. I wouldn't be surprised if they included your abductors, since they wore the badge of a winged crown. That emblem is prominent in his legacy. It's also showed on the seals."

"You are in danger."

"We all are. I trust you totally, and I want you to persuade Simon as to what's going on. The Keepers are alive and active, as events have demonstrated. Gallo is not to be trusted, and can only be a cog in a bigger wheel. We must watch him closely. On my part, I must decide whether to accept my grandfather's mantle or not. He got me to this place, the loveable old fox, and I owe him much. He advised me to be armed and I now am. Do you have experience with weapons?"

Rachael didn't seem surprised. "Yes, my father insisted on it when I before I came to this country. I know how to use side arms and assault rifles."

"I find that reassuring for both of us. What of Simon?"

"I don't know. Nor do I know what we might be up against. But there is something very wrong here and we both know it. Simon half suspects it, but needs convincing. What do we do?"

"I need to look at the contacts locked in my safe. That, I think, was what they were after. I've been left passwords and codenames. James Bond, all is forgiven!"

Rachael laughed aloud and squeezed his hand. "You're a

lovely man. Josh. C'mon, let's head back. Danger has just begun." She kissed his cheek.

Chapter 22

FATHER LUKE TRAVELLED often between the Vatican and
Catholic Churches in Israel and Middle Eastern countries. As
an Emissary of the Vatican Council, he had an important role
in ensuring the smooth running of affairs surrounding the
Holy sites in and around Jerusalem. At forty-three years of
age, he was tall, with bright blue eyes mounted in a craggy
face and possessed of a commanding presence.

Rumours and stories often floated around, and he knew
most, and where appropriate, he got involved in them, if
nothing more than to bring them to a swift and decisive end.
He had been aware of the discovery at Beit-Guvrin. It was this
that had caused him sleepless nights. He knew a lot, more
than people realised, and what the significance of the find
could be.

Father Luke had a deep secret.

His closest friend died a year ago. His name, Nathaniel
Agar.

Since his death, and now, the discovery of the seals, the
very fabric of Christianity and all religions teetered in the
balance. The Keepers existed. The mysterious deaths of six or
seven men, he knew, would be traceable to the AWC, under
the leadership of the mysterious Grand Keeper.

He had organised attempts to penetrate the movement, but to no avail. Those who came close had died in unusual circumstances. Since the find, he had prepared files on all those involved: Doctors Julian Gallo and Rachael Carver, Professor Simon Rockwell, a host of ancillary workers, and most intriguing of all, Joshua Agar, site supervisor, and grandson of Nathaniel.

Informants were part of his network also. On his database were listed the names of important visitors, and the number of times they had visited either the Vatican or any related Catholic organisation like Opus Dei or the Jesuit, Ignatian Spiritualty Centres, and similar structures. The one organisation he had little information on was the one that worried him the most. He knew of it and its purpose. He had seen the results of what they were capable of --- the *I Apocalittici Guerrieri di Cristo*.

A respected archaeologist, Dr. Luigi Bonelli, who was attempting to unravel the secrets and meaning of what had been discovered, had been found dangling at the end of a rope around his neck from beneath a bridge. He was certain the AWC had been responsible. They were not a fringe group of lunatics. Their tentacles were global.

From the timetable he had constructed, he hoped to find a pattern that might give an indication of who could be involved with the AWC. Its members travelled frequently, and the seneschal structure was vital to the implementation of their ideals. Repeat and frequency levels could be revealing.

He was beginning to see a pattern emerging amongst the thousands of names and dates, and each one would have to be checked out. The information was now sufficient to launch his spectacular *Minhocão* or Earthworm software.

Developed by his close friend, a renegade Jesuit Philippine priest and acknowledged computer expert, Fr. Ignatius SJ, Earthworm had the ability of burrowing and mapping the movement of every single name entered into the system within seconds. It was a powerful and accurate tracking tool. Once a name and location has been programmed into its memory, it can present a report of the places that person visited, and if more than three people approached a specified location, it would be highlighted and a map produced. At the press of a key, Earthworm would adhere to those people and produce a map of their own traffic, *ad infinitum.*

His concentration was broken by the sound of his phone ringing.

"Yes? Father Luke speaking."

The reply gave him an unexpected start and a moment to pause.

He growled a low reply. "Yes, of course. I shall be right over."

Father Luke reached for his pistol and placed it in his trouser band. Then, he put on his long brown overcoat, smoothed some oil on his hair, picked up his black Fedora, lit a cigarillo, and moved out at haste.

Rockwell finished playing a Chopin Nocturne. Pushing back the piano stool, he cracked his flexible finger joints, and listened as Rachael related her conversation with Joshua, and their synopsis concerning the seals. She omitted nothing, including their suspicions regarding Gallo. When she had finished, a silence hung in the room like a bag of flour about to drop, swinging from a thin thread. She knew Simon's adverse reaction to speculations. His response came in slow, in a voice she rarely heard him use.

"Coming from anybody else, I would have dismissed this as rubbish. But from you, my Deputy, I have no option but to take it seriously."

"What are we to do about it then?"

"I'm not sure. If any of this is true, and in a very real sense, who are we to trust? The death toll as you placed it... I didn't see it that way before. I can only agree that this whole thing is looking dangerous. I think I should alert Ahasver."

"If you do that, he could pull the plug on the entire project."

"Yes, I realize that. Maybe I'll wait a while. What are we going to do about Gallo?"

"Nothing has been proven yet. As from now, he's a marked man, and we'll all be watching him. I'm certain somebody from the team has been passing on information about the artefact, but we don't quite know who to or why."

"If Joshua's right, information is being funneled out to that organization, AWC. To be frank, I don't give a toss what those lunatics believe, but what's scary is how they're prepared to kill and be killed for what they want."

Chapter 23

JOSHUA TOOK A long pull on his hip flask. The rum mixture spread around his insides like a hot octopus, calming him. After his conversation with Rachael, he experienced a mixture of relief and anxiety.

A sharp rap on the door startled him. His hand went to his pistol and he called out. "Who is it?"

"You called me earlier. It's Father Luke."

Joshua opened the door wide, stepping back to let the priest in, while keeping the gun pointed at his visitor. Father Luke raised his hands. "No need to worry, Joshua. We're on the same side."

"Step inside and close the door, but keep your hands up."

The priest did as he was asked. "Look." With his left hand, he pulled back the large lapel on his coat and revealed a Roman clerical collar. "You see?"

"That doesn't mean a thing, but wait ..." The gold emblem pinned on the inside of his coat glinted when the lapel was pulled back. A winged crown, the symbol of the first Seal. "That badge ... I know who you are."

Father Luke nodded. "If you do, Joshua, then may I put my hands down?"

"Yes, you're the man who terrified and abducted Dr.

Rachael Carver. I recognize you from her description; your coat, the hat, the badge, and you smell of cigarillos." Joshua didn't know whether he should be pleased or scared.

"If you know that, then you're aware of what I'm prepared to do. But, enough of that. You called me, and here I am."

Something in the man's manner made Joshua trust him. He appeared and acted exactly as Rachael described. He lowered his gun.

Father Luke spoke evenly. "You're as Nathaniel said you would be. We've known about you for several years, and have waited for your call. We knew it would come, but when, we did not. Now, with care, stand back a fraction and look out of this window."

Joshua moved across, and from behind the frame, followed the priest's instructions.

"What do you see?"

"It's empty apart from two men across the square."

"Yes. One is following me and the other is watching you. They will now report our meeting."

"Oh shit! Who are they?"

"You needn't guess. You already know."

The next words stuck in Joshua's throat "Keepers? AWC? They're real?"

"Down!" shouted the priest as he lunged towards Joshua. Both men hit the floor with a solid thud, as a bullet smashed through the glass, showering a galaxy of glass shards across the room. Another shot splintered into the woodwork. The next sound they heard was a car roaring away at breakneck speed, its tyres screeching in a wheel spin of motion. They stayed pressed to the floor until all went quiet.

"Believe me now?" Father Luke looked grim. "It's escalating. Take that as a warning." With caution, he hauled himself upright. "They are receiving orders, and it's not going to be too difficult to find out who's giving them and from where."

"It's the seals they want, isn't it?"

"Of course, and they're hoping it's only a matter of time before they get the missing seventh. You have six, and they want them now. They don't care how they get them. You need to hide them somewhere safe, away from here, or episodes like this will accelerate, and you'll end up either mutilated or dead, and the seals stolen."

"How long have you been a Guardian?" Joshua, still shaken, didn't hear Father Luke's advice.

"Ever since I became a priest over twenty-five years back. I knew Nathaniel then, and he taught me all that I know, although I suspect, there were a lot of things he kept to himself. He left you quite a legacy, but you have just scratched the surface. There is so much to be added, of that I'm certain. You'll have decisions to make."

"Would you like a drink, Father? I know I do. This is the second time I've had bullets ripping past my ears." He pulled out the hip flask, unscrewed the top, and offered it. To his surprise the priest took it without question and gulped heavily.

Father Luke held up the hip flask. "That looks like the one your granddad had. I could never say no to a decent touch of the hard stuff."

"That's true. So, what can we do now?"

"Secrets in this technological age are hard to keep. Hacking is the name of the game. We need to know who the leaders of this organization are. When that is known, we can deal with them and ensure they cease to function. Believe me, the power of the seals is real. The Keepers must be stopped and stopped now, or mankind will never be the same again." He stretched out his arm. "May I have another drink, please?"

Joshua wasn't sure what he meant by 'cease to function,' but handed him the flask. "And how are we going to find out?"

"You work with Dr. Julian Gallo?"

"Yes, he's suspect, and Dr. Carver has voiced the same opinion. He's our only possibility at the moment."

Father Luke then went on to explain the *Minhocão* Earthworm computer program Father Ignatius had developed. "Dr. Gallo has been to Rome for what he claimed was a funeral. At stages, he must have used his computer and smartphone to set up his itinerary. Earthworm can locate his exact movements once we program his name into it. Better yet, once we know where he's been, we can trace everyone who's visited that location for the past few years. If he got in touch with someone, we can burrow into his recipient's computer as well. It's virtually undetectable and does not harm or interfere with any other operations unless instructed to. If I wanted, I could find out who visited certain Cardinals at the Vatican, when they arrived, how long they were there, and where they met. From that, I can gather information about all the other people too. Then, Earthworm creates a map of patterns that can be analysed, if you know how." The priest smiled and took another tug at the flask.

Joshua brushed a hand through his hair. "That's incredible. Are you saying it should be activated to track Gallo?"

"I'm not saying if or when. Earthworm has already been fed into his computer." The priest gave a soft wink and a dip of his head.

"What? Oh wow! How did you do that? Has it shown anything important?"

"I don't know yet, as I have to check later. How it was done, I'm not going to tell you right now. Look, Joshua, we're working here to protect the Church, the Pope, and the religions of the world from these crazed nutters. I believe the seals have immense power, as does Father Ignatius. We have to be unorthodox to combat them."

"Okay, I understand that, Father. Why Nathaniel asked me to head the Guardians, I shall never understand. For sure, it's not so secret in some quarters. There's more you should know."

"What's that?"

Joshua explained the nature of their new discovery in the Beit Guvrin-Maresha Caves. It became the priest's turn to look astonished. "And what's more, we were followed by two men, probably the same two who fired the shots just now. Gallo got very busy on the phone before they left us."

"The Seventh Seal, could it be there somewhere?'

"I don't doubt it, but the area is the size of three football fields, not counting where those passages lead to. Look at these, will you?" Joshua showed him all the photos he had taken.

"Holy Mother," the priest whispered and crossed himself. "We must be close indeed. There's one other thing, Joshua ... how many people have you contacted from Nathaniel's files?"

"Only you."

'That's good. Keep it that way. If you think you can trust me, give me that file and I'll feed them into Earthworm. You need not make another call until it gets really urgent."

"I trust you" With a feeling of satisfaction, he handed over the file with a smile. He sensed relief, handing over his burden.

Chapter 24

HE HELD THE ossuary in his hands, concealing it within a thick Jewish shawl before placing it in his rucksack, which stayed with him at all times, including his pistol. Nobody would know what he carried.

Joshua had been thorough.

For three days and nights, Father Luke had pushed him to the furthest extent of his believability. He had revealed to him the wonders that might be available, and also the destruction on offer. The seals would be better off closer to their missing companion. That, he would arrange.

The Keepers had to be denied and their mission thwarted. Father Ignatius's program, Earthworm, operated by Father Luke, had revealed much about Gallo and his agenda. What little Father Luke had shared with him had been astonishing. Earthworm, with its trillion and more possibilities, had revealed a pattern of complex worldwide communications almost too vast to comprehend. Those findings, he wished to discuss with Father Luke, Rockwell and Rachael— all of them together. He now believed there were forces at work that could bring about worldwide chaos and destruction. He felt trapped in a nightmare with the imagery incomplete.

Glancing at his watch, it was time to make his way over

to Rockwell's place. They had all agreed to meet, and he would introduce the priest to them, or reintroduce on Rachael's part. Joshua paused at the entrance door of his quarters. The thought of being followed or shot at wasn't far from his mind. Neither did he preclude the possibility of another burglary attempt. Looking all around him, left and right, there was nobody to be seen. Walking at a brisk pace, he set off, and within ten minutes, he was ringing the doorbell. Rockwell opened it.

"You're on time, and Rachael's here. Where's the priest?"

"I asked him to arrive a little later so I could introduce him."

Rachael appeared wearing her trademark army-style fatigues. "I can't wait to see him again and stick a gun in his ribs." She gave a wry smile.

"Him arriving later gives me chance to tell you what he's going to talk about."

"What's that?" Rockwell sounded doubtful.

"*Minhocão.* It's an earthworm. Not the creature. It's a software program and I think you will be in for a shock as I was."

"What does it do?"

"It burrows for information. It does it so well it can go right around the planet in seconds."

"That doesn't tell me much."

"Let me explain."

In brief terms, Joshua talked about the awesome power of the program, which was fundamentally a rocket-powered snooper, but with considerably more expertise, and an ability to link up with everybody's keystrokes, destination, and then multiply itself outwards to every recipient and their recipients, *ad infinitum.* It could be installed in phones, computers and *anything* electrical; clocks, hairdryers, TV's … there was no limit. All transmitted data were accessible, and decipherable, unless by word of mouth. Its elegance was in its stealth.

"What's that got to do with our work?" Rockwell snapped.

"You'll see. You know of our reservations about Gallo. Well, Earthworm has found some interesting details about our good colleague."

"But …"

The doorbell rang.

"Let me answer it." Joshua moved towards the door. "It's probably Father Luke."

It was. As Joshua opened the door, the priest fell in with his head covered in blood. But, he was still conscious.

"I've been attacked," he managed to whisper as he sunk to his knees.

"Oy Gevalt!" Joshua blurted out.

"Shit!" shouted Rockwell. 'Get him into a chair."

They helped haul him up and sat him into an armchair.

Rachael appeared with a bowl of hot water and towels, and began to clean off the blood from his face. There was a long cut on the crown of his head.

"It's not too bad," she assured the priest as she wiped it clean. "It's superficial."

The priest breathed deeply. "I'm ok, really. I think they got more than they bargained for. They tried to grab my briefcase, but this scared them away." He reached behind him and produced a suppressed pistol. "I fired it and that was enough to make them run."

'Who were they?" Rockwell demanded.

"Drink this." Rachael produced a glass of brandy.

Father Luke downed it in one gulp. "I feel better already," he quipped. "Who were they? Keepers, I would put money on it. That is why I'm here, isn't it?" He smiled at Rachael. "We meet again. Once again, apologies for our last meeting." He held out his hand.

"You were most polite and you never harmed me. How's the head?" She shook the apologetic hand.

"Sore. Give me a few minutes and I'll run through everything."

'That's okay, Father. Take your time. Joshua has explained how it works, but we need to know how it could help and what it has to do with us."

Rockwell found being patient as annoying as a chicken with an egg stuck up its arse. He began to speak, but Rachael held her finger to her lips and shook her head at him

The priest grimaced. "I hope you haven't said too much before I got here, Joshua. I need to use this first before we discuss anything." He produced a black object from his pocket, similar to a smartphone. Pressing a button, an array of lights flickered on and he pointed it around the room. "It's a bug detector, and it can locate the tiniest of transmitters and hidden cameras, wired or wireless." He did two sweeps. "You're clean. There's nothing here." He switched it off and placed it back in his pocket.

"It's like a scene from a spy movie." Rockwell looked impressed. "I can see you're not joking about any of this."

"I couldn't be more serious."

An hour later, Father Luke had outlined the principles of

Earthworm, a form of metadata analysis, capable of intelligence gathering potential into all areas of a person's life. "All of us here are aware of what these seals mean to the brotherhood known as the Keepers or AWC. If you think this is make-believe, then look at this." He unrolled a computer printout that was immense enough to fall off the sides of the table. Using a pointer, he proceeded. "Since the seals were found, these are the movements and communications that resulted from your Dr. Julian Gallo. "See?" The pointer hit the top of the sheet. "The date matches. He contacted a computer at an address in Rome, *Viale Bruno Buozzi.* Look, you can see he got an immediate reply when he asked to be collected by a private flight. No mentions of funerals. Now, follow that line from the Rome address. From there, six others were immediately contacted from around Europe. There was one other, but whoever it was used a very sophisticated computer system and an encrypted phone with untraceable routers. Who that person was, we can only speculate." He read the six names out loud. "Cardinals Francesco Riario and Ludovic Pacca, Xavier de Menendez, Charles Salvador Woodford, Paolo Moro, and finally, General Sir Gordon Anderson. I've prepared biographies on all of them." He handed around six folders to each of them in the room. "To a man, they possess great influence, wealth, and power. All were to attend a meeting where their Middle East seneschal was to present important information. They, in turn, replied to the Rome address. See how the links run through concurrently? They will all be present to meet the seneschal … none other than Dr. Julian Gallo."

A collective gasp filled the room.

"Wait! Wait!" blurted out an incredulous Rachael.

"Cardinal Riario is the Pope's *Camerlengo,* and the one I showed the first Seal to in the Vatican! Are you telling us he's part of a secret organisation, along with these others, conspiring to overthrow the Pope?"

"Exactly that." The priest's face looked as grim as a bunched fist. "He's one of a group of seven, the hierarchy of the AWC.

"And all this could be traced back to Gallo's computer?"

"Yes, as simple as that. Earthworm will now have access to everybody they contact, and track every place they visit."
"And Gallo runs this?" Rockwell asked.

"No. Far from it. He's a cog, but an important one for the Keepers, or the AWC if you wish."

"So, his father's death was a lie."

"Totally."

"Who runs this organisation?"

The priest paused for a dozen heartbeats. "I don't know. I can only guess, but not right now. Earthworm will find him sooner or later." He rolled up the printout. "I'm going to tell you what I know about the significance of the seals, and how they came to be."

"I think we know that, Father. We know what they depict, but there are different ways to interpret them." Rockwell bristled with impatience.

"Yes, you are right. The way they can be seen depends on your belief system; scientific or religious. You have the Preterist viewpoint that says John was given an accurate vision of disastrous events. Prophecies that would be fulfilled over several centuries. The Seventh Seal contains within it the Seven Trumpets, depicting the judgement and suffering of those deemed worthy or unworthy."

"That viewpoint doesn't seem to hold a lot of water, does it?" Rockwell didn't believe in superstition or prophecies.

"As I said, it depends on which side of the fence you are sitting on. Then, there is the Historicist viewpoint, a contemporary viewpoint that says it relates to John's own time."

"Well, clearly, that is unsustainable."

"I agree. Then, we have the Idealist viewpoint. This does not take the Book of Revelation literally, but sees it as a symbolic struggle between good and evil. Easier for us to understand, I think. Finally, there is the Futurist viewpoint. This does what it says on the tin. The opening of the seals is commensurate with worldwide and historical events, no matter how much time it takes to unfold. There will be an end. The process has always been in motion, and will accelerate when the Seventh Seal is opened."

Rachael said. "I don't understand. If any of this were true, why are these Keepers attempting to obtain the seals and the missing Seventh. What can they do with them?"

"They have always believed, that whoever possesses the seals and breaks the Seventh will be heaven's chosen one. Without a doubt, that task will fall to their Grand Keeper. All their deeds are carried out with that in mind, and whatever they do, even the crimes they commit, are done in God's Holy Name. As followers of the AWC, they will be spared, and God willing, they will be given dominion over the globe. It might sound like an insane idea to you scientists, but not to them. They live and die by this belief."

"How can a few people think they can control the planet?" Joshua sounded scornful.

Father Luke smiled at him. "Our last leader thought that

once. But with no army or troops, he managed to change the world. So it is with the AWC. They are convinced that with God's support, whatever His will might be, they can destroy or change this planet forever. That all their sins will be wiped off the slate, and they will rule for eternity alongside Christ."

"I would have said it was all far-fetched,' Rockwell looked thoughtful, "but for the fact that I have seen murders and attempted murders happening since we unearthed that artefact. But if I add this theory to the equation, then it all starts to make sense. Ok, what's our next move going to be?"

"We have an excavation to start work on, and we have to inform Ahasver of what we intend to do," Joshua said.

"What about Gallo?" Rachael looked concerned.

"We carry on as usual, but one of us must stay with him at all times during the excavation. We make a note of everything he says or does. What do you think, Father?"

"*Minhocão* has also installed itself into his smartphone, so that's easily monitored. What is not, is what he says or does outside of that. So, it's a good idea to keep close without him suspecting that we're on to him. Under no circumstances must he be able to take the seals, more so if the Seventh is ever found. If he does, they will find their way direct to the AWC in Rome. But they are clever enough, I suspect, to have concealed their true headquarters. They could be anywhere."

"What would they do if they got hold of them?"

"They would break the Seventh. How, where, or when, who knows? There are no instructions on how the Seventh Seal should be opened. Only their Grand Keeper would have an idea of what will happen next." The priest paused, and held out his hand. "Anymore left in that hipflask of yours, Joshua? We have some thirsty work to do in the morning."

Chapter 25

CARTAPHILUS: "Go faster, Jesus, go faster. Why dost thou linger?"'

JESUS: "I, indeed, am going – but thou shall tarry till I come."

HE READ AND reread the dialogue from David Hoffman's edited *Chronicles of Cartaphilus; the Wandering Jew.* He knew the manuscript by heart. How close those written words were. Almost identical. *Uncanny!*

He'd read the volume thousands of times, but holding it never failed to focus his mind. *The Keys are close, and I shall await your forgiveness and commands, O Lord.*

An electronic bleep alerted him to a message downloading into his iMac. For once, it would have to wait. It was time for his daily meditations. Switching on his MP3 player, he sat cross-legged and chose Górecki's 3rd Symphony. This music got as close to moving him like no other could. It also barricaded memories of the centuries passing through his mind in an endless and unstoppable parade of human miseries, disasters and deaths.

Soon my eternal pain shall cease. The end is in sight.

†

A swirling cloud of dust billowed across a forbidding panorama of thorny shrubs, rocks, and sand. An early morning sun struggled to shower its warming rays through gaps in the colonnade of vehicles as they headed for the caves. The team was comprised of archaeology students, researchers, and a clutch of experts on early Roman, Jewish-Christian pottery and artefacts. They were accompanied by truckloads of equipment and supplies, and that included chemical toilets and essentials, including food provisions for a week's sojourn if required. Heading the operation were Rockwell, Gallo and Rachael Carver. Joshua was to execute all the groundwork and organise parties of archaeologists into the cave system, which only allowed small numbers to enter at one time.

Rockwell had expressed surprise. These were times of budgetary cutbacks and restrictions, and every department of the university had felt the cutting knife. His department not only had their expenditure increased to a level he couldn't believe, but had been told their work was of utmost importance and no expense would be spared.

Financially, things were looking good.

A bell was ringing in the back of his analytical brain. The meeting with Father Luke stood prominent in his mind, and now, he didn't doubt that there was a conspiracy of some sort. Joshua keeping watch on Gallo pleased him. Any suspicious behaviour would be reported back to Father Luke. The recent events, and now the remarkable upsurge in the budget flow, seemed unreal. He made a note to thank the Board. He, for one, would not say no to the elevated funding. Opportunities like this were as rare as rocking horse shit.

He lost little time in informing his team of what the Finance Committee had advised him. His announcement caused them to perform a tight jiggy dance of delight across the compound, with many waving bottles of Goldstar beer.

Rockwell never took chances. If there was any truth in the circumstances and information detailed by Earthworm, then between them, excluding Gallo, a level of secrecy had to be maintained. Before they left, and to avoid spyware, he designated an open-air meeting between himself, Rachael, and Joshua.

They were waiting for him at the map coordinates he had given them previously. It was a secluded setting near the ancient city of Maresha, first excavated at the beginning of the twentieth-century. It was a spot that had given him great joy, and had cemented his desire many years ago to pursue a career that would link in with his passion for archaeology.

He swung the large Mercedes Overland truck to a halt and jumped out.

"Over here, you two." He unbolted the back doors of the vehicle to reveal enough materials, supplies and goods to support an army. "Well, I was told by Ahasver to spare no expense. So, here we are."

"What are we going to talk about, Simon?" Rachael demanded.

"I called you here not just to talk, but to give you something. Did you bring your weapons?"

"Yes," they both responded.

"Good. Here are two more." He handed over two Micro Uzi pistols. "Don't ask any questions. There's none better in tight or confined spaces … like caves." He raised an eyebrow and couldn't prevent a smirk.

Joshua and Rachael looked at each other in astonishment. Here was a side to their Director they hadn't seen before.

"I haven't finished yet. Take these, you might need them at some time." He threw across two Kevlar body armour vests. "They should help if those other bandits start to shoot. Finally, I couldn't resist this. It's so you, Rachael." He teased, producing a pretty pink-coloured moulded object that looked like a mobile phone.

She caught it mid-air. 'What's this?"

"Go careful there, Rachael. It's an Uzi 1.5 million-volt stun gun."

Her jaw gaped "Oh, my God!"

"It's easy to use, and it fits nicely into shirt pockets. Nobody would ever guess what it is."

Joshua squared up and took imaginary aim with his new pistol. "You are certainly taking no chances, Simon. What about you?"

"Don't worry. I'm as equipped as you are. I'm not having anybody trying to kill my people or stealing our discoveries, whatever they call themselves. This time, they won't find it so easy."

"Let's make our agenda and plans now, and when we're finished, I'll let Father Luke know." Joshua got out his clipboard and his well-worn notebook.

"It's a dual expedition," Rockwell started. "From what we've seen, there's enough in there to keep us going for six months at least, but that we can leave to our team of diggers and archaeologists. Our Holy Grail, as we have agreed, is the Seventh Seal. Somewhere in this cave complex, Adil Koury managed to hide it. If local legends and our records are to be believed. These Keepers, AWC, whatever they want to call themselves, will never get their hands on it while I'm around."

"Gallo is a real danger to us all." Rachael flicked her hair from her worried eyes.

"There's nothing much we can do. We need him to an extent. Sooner or later, he will make a mistake and lead us to whomever his boss is."

They then formulated a systematic form of strategy and response initiatives to prepare themselves for any actions or incidents

"You know what, guys?" Rachael chirped, smiling.

"What?" they answered her, looking up from their maps and notebooks.

"This stun gun feels real comfortable in my pocket."

KEN FRY

Chapter 26

ONCE AGAIN, THEY assembled. He had thought of using video conferencing facilities, but had decided that the level of security was poor. This time, they met in the Camerlengo's private quarters, deep inside the Vatican. It was the only apartment that had direct access to the Holy Father himself. If this wasn't safe, nothing else could be.

The Grand Keeper adjusted his cowl and poured himself a cognac, took a thick half corona from its humidor, and lit it in the long flame of a gold Dunhill lighter. He took two long draws, sipped the cognac, and placed the cigar in a jade ashtray, letting it smoulder. Twisting his golden ring, his dark eyes surveyed each member in turn. He stood and they followed suit. Joining hands, they all chanted, *Sacris Sancti Homicidium,* their deep solemn voices reciting the oath three times, an affront to what the entire edifice they stood in represented for millions across the world.

Once seated, he began the meeting. "Our goals draw closer than any time since the last destruction of the Temple of Jerusalem. We should be prepared and not leave anything to chance. We have military, political, and financial plans to implement. You already have our list of targets and objectives. The time to set our plans in motion is near. The

Seventh will be found, and all that has been prophesised will come to pass, and we shall be elevated to the Most High. Only true believers will be left standing as every calamity befalls and infests this corrupted earth."

He paused, knowing that what he was about to tell them would either break or hold them together. His gaze went from left to right and back again, ensuring their maximum attention. He chose his words well, and spoke with caution.

"This may come as a shock to you, but bear with it. You may have pondered about me at times, and how I came to be in this, our sacred society. The truth is, I have been behind it since it first arose, back in Roman times." He paused to let the full impact of his words penetrate their minds. He saw the quizzical expressions.

A silence descended on the room, as noisy as the moon moving across a dark sky.

"You are allowed to doubt, and I expect that. There are moments when I myself do not believe it." The Inner Circle had puzzlement and astonishment written on their faces. "For two thousand years, I have wandered this degenerate and evil world … long enough for me to have learnt that I had been wrong … very wrong indeed. But, I have been given a chance to atone for my sins and set things right. I will rid the world of this leprosy, the Great Whore of Babylon called Catholicism, and the Pope, the Antichrist, and all who follow him. We will be given charge of humanity, and this will happen very soon."

Six heads turned to look at each other, then back to him. *What was he telling them?* Incredulity engulfed the room, and sat beside each one of them like the ghosts of dead men.

"Yes, I understand your doubts. So, look at me. Look at

me well. It's not a request. I command that you do." The Grand Keeper appeared to grow taller with every word, as one by one, he shed his white robes, and then his clothes. "The time has come to reveal myself to you. You have earned the right to know this secret, one I've carried alone for a long, long time. You may disbelieve. If after I have finished your doubts remain, then you have no place here. For me not to doubt your commitment to our cause, I advise you to say nothing."

The Grand Keeper spread his arms wide, standing naked before them. His tattooed skin looked smooth and wrinkle free. He was without blemish, and his muscular body was that of an athlete.

"You have known me for fifteen years or more. Can you say I have aged? Look closely, don't be embarrassed. I never age. My body has remained unchanged for two thousand years, but inwardly I suffer all the ills and woes of ordinary men. There is no escape from my misery and anguish. I have stayed the same since He was nailed to the cross." He paused, as if remembering that day. "I had been an impulsive man then, and I was cursed by Christ Himself for mocking Him and urging Him to his death faster. I am to remain the same age, never to die, until the curse is lifted on his return. And that is how it came to pass. For two thousand years, never ageing, paying for my sins, and forever in mental torment and pain. If doubt remains with you, then watch."

There came a collective gasp.

"Stop!" one shouted.

The Grand Keeper had plunged a sharp-ended knife into his heart. His face contorted and he gasped. He stood motionless, bearing unendurable agony.

He could not collapse.

He could not die.

He barely bled.

He watched each of their shocked reactions. They began to rise towards him, but he held up a hand to stop them.

"Stay where you are!" The command roared in a crescendo that filled the entire room.

Six powerful men in purple robes, with expressions of incomprehension and fear, froze to the spot.

The Grand Keeper tugged the blade from his chest in fleshy jerks, revealing a smudging of blood that dripped slowly from the weapon. He wiped it onto the white tablecloth.

"See!" Dropping the knife, he tilted his head back, and lifted both of his arms up to the sky. "My blood has at last reached and stained this corrupt and accursed structure. It was meant to be by God. I will tell you more. Do sit back down."

The stunned men did as they were told.

His voice boomed as if he were attempting to fill the known universe. Free at last to divulge his heavy burden. "I now see an end to it before me, and you will not understand the pleasure I feel, anticipating my release. I have been behind our Warriors since they began. I founded this brotherhood, but could not be seen appearing in different eras. I had to remain in the background, and only now am I able to reveal my true self and my plans for humanity. Yes, Brothers, you know me well. I have been called by many names: Cartaphilus, The Eternal, and the Wandering Jew, cursed to roam this earth until the end of time. My current name, you need not know. That has been written too. When the Seven Seals are opened, He will finally return, and we will usher in a New World Order and rule by his side. We will see the seven angels with their trumpets, but we shall be spared and swim in the River of Life that flows from His throne."

The Inner Circle stood in shock. They believed him.

He continued, still standing with his arms spread wide. He didn't falter and his eyes grew darker with every word he spoke. "Christ will forgive me and all our members from the mortal sin of murder. We know it is His will, and that it is He who directs us. He ordained our Holy Oath through the mouth of Cosimos Ricci, whom I knew well. I was once his seneschal. Believe it! The blessed seals of John were meant for us, and that has always been our quest. Now, they are near.

"Join me as we recite our blessed oath for this putrefying world to hear. From this Temple of Sewage, let our voices bury and inter this decaying cesspit." The Grand Keeper, better known as the Wandering Jew, raised his arms aloft and the wild fire of religious zeal burnt darkly in his eyes, as three times and to a man they roared, *SACRIS SANCTI HOMICIDIUM!*

For an hour, they sat in silent meditation. In each of them arose an ascending wonderment and awareness of the sacredness and divine direction of their mission.

Ecstasy prevailed.

The soft mumblings of their sacred oath reverberated through both minds and mouths without prompting. How could they fail? Who could defeat them? Discovering the identity of their leader removed any doubt from their minds.

An immortal man. A man who had spoken to Christ Himself!

He called the meeting to order. An element of release and conviction flowed through his veins. "Times are now more dangerous than any of you have ever experienced. There's a question a few of you may have to ask yourselves. You *will* be asked to kill for Christ, make no mistake about that. The question is not whether you could or could not kill for Him, but by doing nothing, will you be crucifying Him yet again? Ask yourselves that, and you have a hard decision to make. I made mine twenty centuries ago, and I have suffered for that mistake. I'll leave you to reflect on that. Now, I want to begin formulating our plan of action. This is to be my outline, and I want you to liaise where I suggest." He paused to put his robe back on before examining his thick folio of notes, lit up his cigar and sat back to sip his cognac. He continued twisting the ring on his finger.

"Cardinals Riario and Pacca, you both know the Pope's movements, habits, and routines, more than anybody else in this accursed place. You will devise a plan between you to kill him, and I suggest poison. Here's a recipe I've prepared, complete with instructions on how it should be administered. You will only proceed when I tell you to. Pray to God for the strength to carry this out." He pushed a black folder across to them.

The two Cardinals looked grim. Cardinal Pacca gulped, whilst Riario reached out for the folder, and without looking at it, deposited it into his briefcase. He gave the briefest of nods.

Not faltering, the Grand Keeper turned to Woodford. "Charles, you need to coordinate with Cardinal Pacca, and discuss how much Vatican funding can be syphoned off and funnelled into your banks and a varied clutch of offshore facilities. To all intents and purposes, these transactions must be seen as legitimate. If anybody gets too nosy, you know what you will be expected to do with them."

Woodford, a short, robust man of multi-racial parentage, had a persona that bristled with unleashed anger. He kept it suppressed behind a fake smile that had become his trademark. "There will be no problems, Grand Keeper." His gravelly voice accentuated the quietness of his speech. "All the good Cardinal has to do, is what I tell him, and we shall get along fine." The fixed smile did not alter. He reached out for the proffered file.

The Grand Keeper turned to Cardinal Pacca. "You heard that, Brother? Be guided by Brother Woodford and success will move faster than we dare imagine."

Yet another nod.

"Brother Mendez." His gaze fixed upon the arms manufacturer and dealer. Xavier Mendez, tall, and always immaculate in dress, wore an expensive suit. His short, red-lined cape, and handmade shoes cost thousands of dollars. He was well known in terrorist cells, and went by the name of 'The Fixer.' Nothing connected with weaponry was beyond him. Whatever was required to start a global war, he could get it. Chemical weapons, or gas deployment mechanisms, presented him no problems, morally or otherwise. The world needed to be shaken up, and Mendez was determined he would be part of it. God had always smiled upon him, and would continue to do so. He often said that Christ's arm was around his shoulder. With world events as they were, he swore that embrace had tightened.

"You," continued his Grand Keeper, "are to prepare an itinerary of every available WMD and from there downwards, a list of what you could procure at short notice. I'm talking of units in thousands, hundreds of thousands ...

or more."

There was a brief silence. 'The Fixer' ran through all the possibilities, and strings he needed to pull, to set everything in motion. In the silence, it was possible to hear his brain gears shifting and moving at speed. He lifted his head. "If this is to be World War Three, the war to end all wars, to establish Christ's New World Order for all Eternity, then I can do it. Trust me, Grand Keeper."

"Who knows how He will wish us to act," the Grand Keeper replied. "But we must be prepared. Here are my estimations." He pushed across another bulky folder. "Feel free to make amendments, but consult with me first."

Finally, he turned to General Sir Gordon Anderson. He looked the epitome of English gentry. "You, Sir, have a most vital role in our preliminary procedures and beyond."

Anderson has had a distinguished career; a Cambridge blue, a First, and a Masters in applied physics. He had opted for an army career, and had received both the Sword of Honour and Queens Medal as the most outstanding officer in attendance at Sandhurst Military Academy. A rare double. His army career had taken him to the highest levels of intelligence and planning, before he was noted and appointed to serve the UK as their chief NATO official. As such, he had access to the highest and most secret levels of information and intelligence. He had maximum security clearance, and knows every NATO code and encryption processes appertaining to all manner of delivery systems — for secret weapons and those not so secret.

"I will need to talk to you in much more detail. When the time arrives, we will need to use everything you know and have access to, to ensure our success." He slid over the last file to the General. "Any qualms?"

The General ran his hand through his shiny hair. "None, whatsoever. Christ be praised!" His clipped, precise tones filled the room. Then without warning, he stood and raised his glass. "Brothers, a toast to our Grand Keeper as his journey nears its end. Here's to our success and thanks be to God!"

Chapter 27

THAT NIGHT, GALLO had been uncharacteristically expansive in inviting the senior team members around to his home for a three-course meal and drinks. For all, it had been a stressful day. There were schedules, procedures, and protocols to follow, and each member had to stay true to their role. From an outsider's viewpoint, it looked like one gigantic scene of chaos, but it was far from it. Rockwell regarded them as one of the best excavation teams he had ever assembled.

He now shared the reservations the others had concerning Gallo. Father Luke's information had tipped the balance. But as yet, nothing could be proven. Gallo was playing his role as host very well. Fussing around everybody, forever filling their glasses, trying too hard to be funny, and asking too many questions about the seals and the possibility of finding the Seventh.

Around eleven p.m., and with another hard field day before them, the three tired researchers said their thanks and retired home for the night.

Once in his home, Joshua sat on the edge of his bed, aware that for some reason he was sweating profusely.

Not normal.

He glanced at the luminous bedroom clock … a few minutes after midnight.

He could not get rid of the vision of the unknown man blowing out his brains on the site and Gallo standing right in front of him, not batting an eyelid. He reached and fumbled for the light switch as his head began to swim and reel. An awful certainty gripped him that something was wrong. His senses were being peeled away like an onionskin, and he like a drunken bear rolling into an abyss of darkness. A strange taste he couldn't identify filled his mouth. Images of suicides paraded through his subconscious, not in colour but like an early French *film noir* all black and white.

In the muddle came one certain thought … *I've been drugged or poisoned.* He couldn't control it, and he continued to lose control of his senses.

WAKE UP! Someone's here!

A man dressed all in black descended from a rope suspended from the ceiling skylark window. From beneath his balaclava, he spat out the words, "The seals. Give us the seals and you might live."

Joshua can only choke.

"Give us the keys to the safe!"

Words refused to formulate, and one man began to search him with practised ease. The keys were hanging from a secret pouch that dangled across his top thigh, beneath his trousers.

A hard fist struck his head, but he didn't feel the pain … only the never-ending descent into darkness.

Finally, they found the keys. A heavy knee pressed into

his spine, and a fabric was clamped across his mouth. It smelled sweet.

"That should keep him quiet for a while. Let's find what we came for and get out of here."

Sweat drenched Joshua's forehead and tightness gripped his throat. His vision faded and he could barely make out his surroundings. There was a metallic sound, and a strange blue glow.

They're taking them! I can't breathe.

Everything descended into wooliness as he glided away into a chemical dreamland. Joshua's head lolled back, and his mind and body flowed into the encompassing arms of a benign darkness.

Chapter 28

FATHER LUKE AROSE from his meditations and prayers, and brushed off the dust that clung to his cassock. The candles fluttered at his genuflection before the crucifix. Making the sign of the cross, he exited his private chapel and swung into his adjacent workroom and study. Clear and focussed, his intent, crystal clear. His role as a Guardian had leapt to the forefront of all his activities. The war had begun.

Switching on the lighting system, he stared up at the huge triple screens he had mounted along the semi-circular back wall. He activated the computer, and within seconds, he was logging in. He entered the first set of codes and waited. There would be two more steps to verify his identity before he would be granted entry. He knew the routine by heart. There followed a mixed series of electronic beeps and hums as the words vanished in an energy intensive display, only to be replaced across the screens by inundations of fast moving binary code. Being displayed were Earthworm's investigations into the activities of the six names in its database. The data had been translated into a complex communications matrix.

The priest gulped. It was far larger than he could have ever imagined. The links multiplied millions of times repeatedly across the planet.

"In the name of God!" His exclamation was barely audible.

Its scope was more massive than he could have dared imagined.

The Keepers were waking their cells worldwide, and they were swarming like protective bees, ready to obey the command of their unknown 'Queen.' They were preparing for action.

From all of this, Earthworm would be programmed to pinpoint repeat patterns and links between the six known members of the Inner Circle. But, no matter what Father Luke did, after three hours work, Earthworm was still unable to discover the identity or whereabouts of the Grand Keeper. His investigations and algorithms continued in one gigantic and ever shifting circle. All paths led back to the six, plus Gallo, but no further. The Grand Keeper's hidden routers fully protected him.

With escalating horror, Father Luke realised that he had less time than he initially thought. The Keepers are preparing for war. *I need to locate him fast!*

Later, and with no success, the priest's energy began to diminish. He glanced at the clock. It was late, and he'd been attempting to unravel Earthworm's colossal findings and networked maps of communication for over six hours.

Still no clue.

At that moment, he heard a clatter as the cat-flap opened and Lucifer, his hefty Foreign White breed cat, bustled in, looking very pleased with himself. He rubbed around Father Luke's legs before depositing a forlorn but dead mouse at his feet. His gift … an offering to his master. For a moment, Luke forgot his problems and smiled, petting the animal and thanking him for his grizzly present.

A thought struck him, and he gasped at its simplicity.

Cats, like worker bees were very similar in one way. They always returned to their place or home. The cat comes in with his gift to his owner, and worker bees go back to the hive with their gifts for the Queen and community. Cats were known to travel hundreds of miles to find their way back home if lost. The word HOME bounced around in his head, like two skeletons dancing on a tin roof.

Of course. The six seals are home. He stood up straight and thumped his fist into his palm, his breath hitching in his excitement. He wanted to shout *Eureka!*

"The seals are home … and where is home? It's here. It's here in Tel-Aviv. Yes, of course! Whoever it is, must be close by, and not far away as I first thought. Everything is gravitating around us."

He pondered on his latest theory.

Close, but not close enough. He stared up at the screens, but knew the answer wouldn't show. He paced across the study and reached for the Bourbon. Two hefty pulls later, he could only formulate.

I'm still missing something … but what? It had to be staring him in the face.

Chapter 29

"WHY ISN'T HE answering?" Rachael asked Rockwell. "Where is he?" She gave an exasperated sigh.

"It's not like him to be late. He's usually one of the first to arrive." Rockwell looked concerned. The team and gear was ready; drivers, vehicles, and equipment.

"Where's Josh got to?" Rockwell snapped. "He's supposed to head this up."

"Too much to drink last night, perhaps?" Gallo quipped with a smirk on his face.

"I've never known him to be late before," Rachael objected. "I'll drive over to his house. Should he turn up, give me a ring and I'll turn around." She jumped into the Land Rover, started up, and headed the two miles over to Joshua's place.

Gallo began a cheery whistle as she vanished down the road in a cloud of dust.

Eight minutes later, she parked near his house and began walking across the decorative plaza to his door. Instinct told her something was amiss. She rang the duo-toned doorbell several times and got no reply, before she realised the door was ajar. It hadn't been closed tight. With caution, she pushed it open. It made a soft click in the latch. She couldn't imagine a man like Joshua being careless enough to leave it open.

"Joshua? Hello? Josh, it's me, Rachael. Are you there?" Silence. Her heart rate speeded up and her stomach fluttered. "Josh?"

Then, she heard a sound that resembled a baby crying under a blanket. It came from behind the bedroom door. She turned the handle and pushed her head around the opening.

"Josh? Oh my God, Josh, what's happened?" In one swift eye movement, she took in a scene of chaos. Glass fragments splattered across both the floor and bed areas. They had come from the demolished sky window above, from which hung a limp, black, mindless rope. Furniture had been upended and Joshua, with his head in his hands, still wearing the same clothes from the previous evening, half sat, and half sprawled across the floor. A sickly, sweet smell, faint but discernible, hung in the air. He looked as if he had been in the ring with Ali.

She knelt beside him and placed her arm around his trembling shoulder, and then wiped away the sweat from his face "Josh, speak to me. Are you okay? What happened for God's sake? I'm calling the police."

He looked out of it, but not totally. His chin was pressed down onto his shoulder, and an unpleasant medical odour, similar to that used in hospitals, hung around his gaping mouth.

He grabbed hold of her wrist. "Don't do that, Rachael ... please." With bloodshot eyes that carried heavy baggage beneath them, he stared at her anxious face. "Please, that's something we don't do."

"You've been attacked. When did that happen?"

"I can't remember. I got back here and felt really strange.

Like being drugged. I couldn't function. Then, a man started hitting me, and then another came down from the roof. They placed something over my mouth and nose and I began to fade away. It smelt funny. Before I passed out, they took my keys, Rachael. They took my fucking keys! We've lost the seals. Look!" He pointed a shaky finger at the wall safe.

Rachael turned and saw the open doors of the safe. Where the ossuary once sat, there was only empty space. Her face scrunched up, and she covered her mouth, unable to speak.

"Call Simon, will you, Rachael? Tell him I've let you all down. I'm so sorry." He reached out to touch her, but he pulled back his hand.

"You've let nobody down." She pulled him in close and could see the tears in his eyes. "How could you have prevented this? You say you felt peculiar when you got back here last night?"

"Yes, kind of woozy. Did I drink too much?"

"No more than anybody else, that's for sure."

"It got worse very quickly, then the men. That's all I can remember."

"Do you think Gallo had something to do with this?"

"I can't be sure. He's on Father Luke's radar as a prime suspect. Surely he wouldn't slip me a Mickey."

"Yes, he would, and I bet that's what that party was all about. He's part of these Keepers and they want the seals … and it looks as if they've got them."

"They're useless without the Seventh."

"True. We know that, at least. Now, I'd better call Simon and tell him what's happened." She reached for her phone.

Rockwell sat on the footboard of the Overlander, his impatience escalating by the minute as he checked and rechecked his phone. He stared down the deserted road. *Where are they? This is taking far too long. We should have been on our way ages ago.* When he thought he had about as much as he could tolerate, his cell phone burst into life. It was Rachael.

He listened with mounting horror, as she related Joshua's condition, and what happened to the seals. "Holy shit! How is he?"

"Groggy, but coming around rapidly. He's insisting he's still coming with us."

"That's okay, but I must tell Ahasver."

"He'll stop the expedition."

"Who knows? I'll do it now, but I'll brief the team first. We daren't move forward without his say so."

"Okay, Simon. We're heading there in a few minutes." She ended the call.

Gallo offered no comment, apart from saying to all who could hear him. "Negligence! Gross fucking negligence that one of the most important religious discoveries of our age is stolen from under our noses. Didn't we say that the ossuary and the seals should be kept in a high security facility? You only have yourselves to blame. God knows what the president is going to say. Heads should be rolling."

Rockwell said nothing. If Father Luke's information was correct, then Gallo was doing an Oscar winning performance. *The man, in this case, doth protest too much, methinks!*

He took a deep breath and called the University President, Professor Jacob Ahasver.

A female voice answered. "President Ahasver's office. How may I help you?"

Rockwell made his request and after a brief pause, the low, thundery rumbling of the President's voice reverberated through cyberspace.

"This is the President speaking. Professor Rockwell, what can I do for you?"

Rockwell felt resigned to what he had to tell him, and with no excuses. In a monotone voice, he outlined everything Rachael had told him, and delivered the dreadful news that the seals had been stolen.

No sound came from the other end of the phone, and when Ahasver spoke again, his tone had not changed. "Did you inform the police, Professor?'

"I was just about to."

"Do not."

"Pardon?"

"Don't. Leave it to our own security. We have our own methods. The last thing I want is the state police and media clamouring around here, and us being accused of incompetence which could threaten our funding. I will need to see Agar as soon as possible. Get him to call me when he is fully recovered. Do I make myself clear?"

"Perfectly, sir."

"I want you to proceed with your excavations as if nothing had occurred. You or the people from your team, should refrain from mentioning this to anybody else. I think I've made the reasons for that quite clear. I urgently require Agar's input. Tell him to contact me very soon. We shall talk again, Professor." He hung up.

Rockwell puffed out his cheeks in disbelief. *What a strange low-key reaction.*

"How did he take it?" Gallo asked, barely able to conceal his pleasure at the reprimand the team would surely receive from the President of the University. "Weird. He barely reacted. Muttered on about dangers to our funding, and not wanting the police or media involved. That's all he seemed to care about. He never mentioned how we should go about trying to get back the seals. He wants to see Josh ASAP."

For a moment, Gallo looked as puzzled as Rockwell.

"Look." Rockwell sounded relieved as he focussed on the unmistakable approach of Rachael's vehicle. "They're back."

The Land Rover slowed to a stop and they both got out. Joshua looked punch drunk as Rachael held his arm to steady him.

Gallo spoke first. "There's no way you can come with us looking like that, Joshua." He pointed at his battered face.

Joshua's reply startled everybody. "What the fuck did you put in my drink last night, Gallo?"

The group went silent.

"Excuse me?" Gallo's face drained of colour.

"You heard me." Joshua's voice quivered with soft menace. "You did *something* and now the seals are missing, and I think you know something about it. Don't you?"

Gallo took a step back. "I think you got a harder bang on the head than you realise." He looked uneasy. He wasn't used to confrontations.

Both Rachael and Rockwell moved in between them with their arms spread wide.

"Josh, this is not the time or place. Some other time, eh?" She embraced him.

He shook his head dejectedly and paused for a few moments. "Yeah, your right. I'm sorry. I'm feeling very tired right now. I'll stay in the Land Rover."

Rockwell ushered Gallo away. "He's been through a lot recently. Let it go, will you?" The man's ashen face did not escape Rockwell.

"Of course." He shrugged himself free and walked off to his vehicle.

That had been a close call, but he had done what he'd been instructed to do, with good results. The Keepers must now have six of the seals.

Chapter 30

"And I heard a great voice out of the temple saying to the seven angels, 'Go on your ways, and pour out the vials of the wrath of God upon the earth."

~ Revelation 16:1 ~

HE FELL. HE continued to fall ever downwards, but he was not afraid. Dimensions began to fade until solidity ceased to exist; no up or down, backwards or forwards … only being, eternal being, as he became all that he sensed in every way.

Adil Koury once existed, but in God's terms, he never existed at all. He always was. Plummeting forever through the minutes, the hours, the days, weeks, months, years, decades, and then centuries, he saw all that man ever was, and on beyond millennia. He passed through moons, planets, endless space, and beyond billions of stars. The arms of Christ were around him as he passed through water and did not drown. He passed through fire and did not burn, and through space and time, yet he did not vanish. For he was as it was. He had become.

Home beckoned to him.

There was no fear.

Azrael, the Angel of Death, waited for him. He had waited since time began.

He was not afraid for he knew Azrael would care for him. He was one of them now.

He, Asroilu the Seventh Guardian, had come home. He would dwell in the Third Heaven, far from the world of men, where sprung wells of milk and honey, wine and oils.

He would guard the Seventh Seal as he had on earth, and in the distance, he could see its beckoning blue light calling to him.

Chapter 31

THE BEIT GUVRIN-MARESHA CAVES, as they had for thousands of years, glowered across the surrounding hills without favour on friend and foe. They were about to be assaulted, raped, and violated. But they would endure without a sound, without complaint, as countless metal spikes, spades and trowels would begin to rip open their soft underbelly.

Rockwell, in spite of his enthusiasm, remained puzzled over Ahasver's reaction to the theft. He had expected anger, disappointment, paranoia, reprimands, anything but the calmness he had displayed. It didn't seem right, but he couldn't put his finger on it. Joshua had called the University's President as instructed, and had to go and see him to report on the attack and robbery. He would return as soon as their meeting ended. Rockwell hoped Joshua could provide more insight into Ahasver's intent.

His other concern was Gallo. Joshua's serious accusation could have alerted him to the possibility that a deep cloud of suspicion hung over him. While Gallo wasn't aware of how much they knew, it could make him more cautious, and therefore, harder to track.

Rockwell's attention soon got to the immediate problems. He devised a human chain that would pass all needed equipment through a long line of hands, which will end in one of the numerous caverns they would use as storage. He rigged up a lamp to illuminate the supplies. It was powered by one of two 5000-watt petrol driven portable generators, adapted so each utilised a 250-foot cable. They would be taken in through the gaps, as far as they could go.

Apart from the suspected conspiracy going on around him, Rockwell had another goal on his mind … the scrolls in the pottery and clay jars. They needed careful attention. He pulled Rachael to one side as she ducked to avoid a projecting rock.

"Rachael, listen, I don't want Gallo anywhere near these jars. They may hold clues to this entire expedition. Stick with him at all times. Flirt if you have to, but keep him distracted. And if you find anything, keep it to yourself and don't let him anywhere near it. Can you do that?"

"You're such charmer, Simon." She gave a broad smile of resignation and nodded. "Yes, I can do that, if you promise not to get jealous." Even as she said it, she knew there wasn't a chance in hell that he would be. She leant forward and kissed his cheek with a resounding peck.

He didn't seem to notice.

"Have you got your weapons and stun gun?"

"I don't think he'd be brave enough to assault me in this place, but yes. Stun gun is in my pocket, pistol strapped on. The other and the Kevlar are back in the truck."

"Good. Be on your guard and trust nobody. Okay?"

"Yep. Okay, see you later." Crouching low to avoid the stalactites and protruding rocks, she made her way out to find

Gallo. Behind her, the main team was busy mapping out the early system, and entrance. Placing down markers, and taking endless photographs for the evening's briefing session. Amidst all of this she could hear the sporadic whistles and cries of astonishment at what they were so far discovering. *This find is going to be bigger than the Dead Sea Scrolls.* She too had been gripped by the prospect of the Seventh Seal being hidden somewhere in this subterranean maze. There were only four of them who understood that possibility.

Ahead of her, she spotted Gallo. He was peering hard at the walls with his flashlight. He saw her coming.

"The wall carvings and art decreases the deeper we go into the system. It seems only the outer fringes of the cave system were used by the population."

She ignored his remark. "Oh Julian, I'm so sorry for what happened back there. You must understand that Josh has had a nasty upset, and that was not his first. He's lucky to be alive." She rubbed at his arm reassuringly.

"Forget it." His reply didn't sound as if he'd forgotten it. It resembled the hiss of a pressure cooker about to give vent. "He's never liked me anyway. I hope Ahasver gives the stupid fart a roasting. Great Gods, I told him not to keep the seals in his safe."

'Oh, don't be so nasty," she whispered seductively, giving his arm a squeeze.

He paused. "Thanks, Rachael, you're a help."

I'm getting through to him.

"Whoever's got those seals, I wonder what they're going to do with them?" His voice had a false echo. "C'mon, let's photograph these walls as the diagrams seem to be diminishing."

She wondered too. After everything that had transpired, and her own visions of the Holy Mother, Rachael could no longer dismiss all of it as purely rubbish. People were willing to kill and die to own the seals.

She looked beyond and it just seemed to get deeper and darker. It felt creepy to be alone with Gallo in this place. *Holy Mother Mary, pray for Julian. Pray for me.* A flash of blue passed through her mind.

Rockwell had built himself a small platform on which he could stand and reach up to the higher placed jars. Those without lids were brimming with scrolls that looked like parchment, or vellum. He didn't dare touch them.

He stood back to take in what he was looking at. They could be 1700 years old or more. The slightest interference after surviving undisturbed after all that time would reduce them to crumbling dust. Rockwell couldn't fight the awe he experienced with this discovery. God knows what light they might shine on Biblical history, if it proved to be a cave used by early Christians. They wouldn't know for sure until Phase III. Right now, they were on Phase I and the team would simply be mapping the whole area, test the surface, determine the extent and possible value of the archaeological site, and make their recommendations to Ahasver before they move on to Phase II.

Hidden in these caves could be a link between truth and fiction --- or in other words, between science and religion. Once the jars were safely removed, there could only be one secure way to examine the contents, and that was by using a medical scanning technique coupled with algorithmic analysis. The facilities had recently been installed back at the university. It's the same as a high-resolution hospital CT scan, and using various techniques, a computer program called *Volume Cartography* can create digital slices that could then be separated like pages. They could digitally 'unwrap' each scroll without ever having to handle them, and read the contents on screen. The process was called *Volume Rendering*. It was first used in 2016 to reconstruct the En-Gedi Scroll. He had to give that to Ahasver. The man had insight.

Rockwell had no idea what information the jars contained, but didn't doubt that he would find references to the seals. He whispered a rare prayer.

God, if there is a God, let some light shine in here so can I understand. Don't make it so difficult.

Chapter 32

The City of Tel-Aviv

UNNOTICED, THE NONDESCRIPT blue coloured Toyota Corolla slipped with ease into one of the many parking spaces close to the Tamara Juice Bar. The driver adjusted his aviator style sunglasses, and looked for several seconds in each of his three driving mirrors. All clear. He alighted, adjusted his black wide-brimmed hat, and brushed down his leather coat. Limping and walking with a cane, he crossed the road and covered a short distance before entering an antiquarian bookseller's shop. From where he stood, examining the various volumes, he had a clear view of the road behind him, and his parked car, which he had left unlocked.

He did not have to wait long.

A few minutes later, he saw what he was waiting for, and his foot began tapping an agitated rhythm on the carpeted floor. A fluttery sensation swirled in his stomach.

The military proportioned Jeep drew close to his car. Two men dressed in black got out, made a quick inspection of the Toyota, and then quickly opened the back of their Jeep and removed an oversized crate. Pulling open the Toyota's door, they deposited the item on the back seat and slammed the door. Jumping back in the Jeep, they revved up the engine, performed a screeching U-turn, and sped off.

The watching man looked pleased. It had gone to plan. With a fast-paced strut, he headed out of the shop towards his car. He left the walking cane behind. He'd never needed it anyway.

Dampness slid with malevolence down the massive green slimy walls. It had done so for thousands of years and would continue to do so until the end of time.

The man's eyes soon dilated and got accustomed to the gloom.

Nothing unusual.

In turbulent times, it had been a place of solitude and peace; a place to contemplate and meditate on the ills of the world. Ills that would soon end.

Above him, the craggy roof had a dome of rock with a monastic suggestion in its curvatures. The structure had been worked on over the centuries. It now had alcoves, hidden rooms, and passageways. He had come to regard the place as his true home. He had stumbled upon it a long time ago, and kept it a secret. It was now buried deep beneath the constructions of the village, which had evolved into a town over the centuries, and then into the modern complex that was now Beit-Guvrin. He had been a victim of Roman repressions. There had been many a times when covered in bloody wounds but unable to perish, he had sought refuge in this place. No matter how long or far he conducted his infinite wanderings, he would forever be drawn back here. It was, he surmised, as if God had made it that way, for no matter where he went on this planet, he always returned.

As years and centuries came and evaporated into time and space, he had discovered tight but manoeuvrable corridors through the rocky walls and caverns. Endless passageways and corridors of inhospitable hardness, threaded their miserable journey beneath urbanity, deserts, and hills, and into caves that looked down on the unaware city and its people. He had discovered burial chambers, columbariums of great antiquity unknown to man, from some past forgotten time and civilization. It was vast and stretched out for miles.

The location he selected, was chosen for its accessibility and ease of movement. His preferred space formed a small but natural room area. Here, he had begun constructing a stony sarcophagus and lid. He used a mason's hammer, various chisels, a pinching tool to trim the flat stone to size, a chipper to square the edges, and a plug drill which allowed holes to be created between hammer strikes.

He had a plan. The need to implement it might not arise, but it was better to be prepared than not at all. The rock yielded easily to his blows, but several hours passed before he regarded his work with satisfaction. To the lid, using the plug drill, he made two apertures; one at the rear end, the other at the top. To the rear end, he inserted a tight-fitting polyurethane tube and then fitted a pressure valve and a small tap to the top end. This, in turn, was connected to a large sized metal tank that contained water. By means of a generator operating a refrigeration system, he could maintain the water at an icy temperature of one degree above freezing. The second hole at the top end he left open as an air hole.

He recovered the large crate and rested it on the top. Lifting the lid, the ossuary stared up at him. He experienced a surge of emotion, a mixture of sadness woven into the fibres of an unseen ecstasy … almost sexual in intensity. The top cover of the ossuary shifted easily as he pushed it to one side. For but a moment, he swore there had been a flash of blue light … but it vanished as fast as he thought he saw it.

They remained dormant as if they had been on a long space journey and cryogenically asleep, but now stirring to confront the realities of their world.

His hand stretched out. It shook like an aspen in a breeze. Breathing became suspended and his heart pounded. Closer … closer … closer, but no further. As hard as he tried, his fingers could not reach the ancient metal. An invisible impenetrable force had surrounded the seals and they remained impassive, and as unsympathetic as they had been since the Blessed John of Patmos forged them.

Access denied.

That confirmed the irrefutable truth of the seals. Christ was present, and more was needed from him. More blood, more sacrifices in his holy name before he was deemed worthy.

Sinking to his knees, he murmured the sacred prayer …

Sacris Sancti Homicidium.

Chapter 33

PROFESSOR JACOB AHASVER remained seated as Joshua Agar, looking uncomfortable, walked into his modest office. With a curt wave of his arm, he gestured for Joshua to take a seat. He stared at him, his black eyes like nails being driven into blocks of wood. He said nothing but just … looked. The fingers in his right hand tapped an unknown beat into the mahogany desktop.

The silent exchange went on too long for Joshua, who broke away from his gaze and turned to examine the artefacts around the office. *He's trying to intimidate me. Fuck that!*

The President finally broke the silence. He steepled his fingers and leant forward to emphasise his points. "As I understand it, Mr. Agar, valuable and priceless Biblical antiquities were stolen the other night from your house. Correct?"

The man couldn't even extend the courtesy of asking how I was! I almost died there.

"Correct."

"How did it happen?"

This guy is spooky. "We'd been out to dinner at Dr. Gallo's house, and when I returned home, I felt unwell…'

Ahasver interrupted. "You were drunk."

"If that's a question, then the answer is no. If it's an observation, then it's wrong. I'll continue." Joshua's felt his agitation mounting, and forced himself to calm down. He cleared his throat too many times as he tried to relax. "Two men I couldn't identify overpowered me, gave me some sort of drug, gas, or something that knocked me out. They found my keys, opened up the safe, and that's all I can remember."

"Mr. Agar, what were the antiquities doing in your room safe? Why weren't they under the supervision of our security staff? Are you an idiot? This is not the first time you were attacked, is it? Surely that should have alerted you to what these people want, whoever they are? Anybody with common sense would have understood that, that is, apart from an intelligent person who works at a university. Am I making myself clear? "

"Yes, sir, you are. Why didn't you call the police?"

"That's the University's business. Do you have the slightest idea how we are going to get these seals back?"

There's no way I'm going to start talking about Guardians and the Keepers with this man. "No, none whatsoever, at the moment. They could be anywhere in the world by now."

"Exactly as I feared. No doubt, in twenty years or so, they will appear at an International Sotheby's auction somewhere on the planet." He smirked, making Joshua feel like the most incompetent person that ever lived.

"What else do you want from me?" Joshua sensed he was out on a limb.

The President leant back in his black quilted swivel chair, looking too at ease and in control. A curious distant yet unfocussed smile hovered on his face. "I want nothing from you, Mr. Agar, nothing."

"What does that mean?"

"Nothing means nothing. You are suspended from duties forthwith."

Joshua's head jerked back and a rush of coldness went through him. "What? You can't do that. I shall appeal to the Board."

"Do what you like. You will receive notification tomorrow."

A flame of anger arose in Joshua, and his voice went up a few octaves. "And you and the Board will receive notice of my appeal. Under the rules of this University, an appeal dislodges the Application of Suspension until ratified by all members. So, write your god damned letter and I'll write mine. In the meantime, I'll carry on working." He stood up, swung around and stomped out of the office, and not forgetting to slam the door.

Ahasver soaked in the silence of the office, with only the faint noise of traffic barely penetrating the triple glazed windows. He began preparing the letter for Joshua's suspension. Halfway through it, he stopped, put down his pen, and began to shake his head. He stood, turned away from his desk and burst into laughter.

Chapter 34

FATHER LUKE BUTTONED up his cassock and began to double check what the Earthworm program had shown him. There were moments when he doubted the validity of the information it spewed out. The sheer volume of it was daunting. But the second pass on all the known contacts showed the identical pattern of worldwide links repeatedly. That could not be denied. The 'cat and bee' theory was holding water. There existed a clutch of passwords and secondary codes that Earthworm had burrowed into and they were being revealed, but what it didn't show was the source of all of it. The Keepers had a far larger and fanatical following than the Guardians had ever dreamt. Their activities had been like a smouldering volcano, waiting for the right moment to spew out their destructive power. Based on the frantic activities, that moment had arrived. For the followers, the promise of a New World Order either on Earth or in Christ's appointed heaven loomed close.

Earthworm emitted a series of unusual beeps he hadn't heard before. One quick look at the data and he knew it could be special. He looked more closely.

"My God in Heaven, that's remarkable!" At that moment, there came a buzz on the intercom. A look at the CCTV screen and he could see Rockwell on the doorstep. He pressed the entry key. "C'mon up, Simon."

"Hi, Father, how's it going?"

"Simon, what are you doing here? Shouldn't you be at the site?"

"Bad news, Father. I'm here to tell you that the seals were stolen the other night."

The priest's jaw dropped and he gave a wide-eyed incredulous expression. "What? Oh, Sweet Jesus! No … please, no! It must be Gallo or the Keepers in some way. I'm certain of it." He pressed his hand on his forehead.

"More to come. Our President is attempting to suspend Joshua for letting it happen. He seems to think a few low-income security guards would have been a safer option. What rot! These Keepers seem to be everywhere. I just thought you should know."

"This is terrible news! I did tell him not to keep them there, but I don't think he heard me. These madmen are plotting something dreadful. But wait, I have better news. There's something I'd like you to look at. All may not be lost." He clasped his hands under his chin in a silent prayer. "You said they seem to be everywhere, well, they are. Earthworm has uncovered a common password. Someone, somewhere, forgot to be careful. Look, here it is." He pointed to a swathe of binary code.

"That doesn't mean a thing to me." Rockwell scratched his head.

"No, of course not. Here's the translation." Father Luke read out each word piece of the binary, changing it to English as he moved along. Z.E.B.R.I.N.A. "ZEBRINA is the password that appears to mobilise all the others in the group."

"Interesting, but how does that help us?"

"When people choose a password, about seventy-five per cent of them opt for something dear to them: a hobby, a relative or loved one, a pet, a phrase. Mine for example is an abbreviated quote from a psalm. I believe that ZEBRINA is their Grand Keeper's access code, or maybe someone very close to him. It got me thinking." He grabbed Simon's arm in excitement. "It's a form of plant known as Spiderwort."

"So, whoever it is happens to be a botanist or a gardener? That's no help at all." He rolled his eyes skywards.

"What we are dealing with here is a biblical story of some complexity. The seals are part of that story. Now, think back to all those stories and legends around the death of Christ."

"You tell me." Rockwell's impatience was beginning to surface.

"Well, they abound. The Holy Grail, the Turin Shroud, the Spear of Destiny — the lance that pierced His side, the Seamless Robe, the Holy Nails, the endless bits of wood that were supposed to have been part of the true cross. Then, there's Veronica's Veil … and so on. They are endless. Do you understand so far?"

"Carry on, Father." Rockwell expelled a slow breath.

"At the Via Dolorosa, on His way to Calvary while carrying that cross, Christ was met with a mixture of pity and contempt. Some attempted to help him, others the opposite. One man in particular could not stop goading and spitting on Him, and told Him to stop hanging around his shop, and hurry on to the nailing place. It was said that Christ lifted his eyes to the man and more or less told him that for his actions, he would inhabit the earth until the end of time, or until Christ himself returned."

"Your point being?"

"The accursed man was a Jew."

"That's hardly a surprise, Father, there were lots of them around here at that time. Look, where's this getting us?"

"The password ZEBRINA, or its common name, Spiderwort, has another name. It's known as Wandering Jew. That's the name that has been attributed to this hapless man."

There was a long pause and a look of surprised curiosity hit Rockwell. His voice softened. "Interesting, I see what you are getting at. Are you saying what I think you're saying? We're looking for a man who is two thousand years old, cursed to live forever, and we have no clue as to who he could be, apart from he's been a Jew all his life?"

"Of course,"

"Father, I'm a man of science. I can't accept that. Honestly, I can't. But saying that, I do find something unsettling about it all. I promise to keep an open mind."

"I feel the same … but there's more."

Father Luke went on to explain his cat theory and that of the bees, and how both always returned home, often with gifts.

"With that in mind, I deduced that the seals were being hidden where home is … and that's around these parts, by whoever is running the show. Our Wandering Jew, maybe? Earthworm has insinuated that he was close by. Additionally, it has tracked all the strings related to the other six names I gave you at our meeting. Their electronic paths all go in the same direction, and end up around here, in this country. When it gets here, Earthworm's probes get blocked. Those names are valid, and they are co-conspirators, as is Gallo. The Keepers now have the six seals, and I can guarantee that they're waiting for the discovery of the Seventh. Are you following this, Simon?"

"I'm following, but you're asking me to believe and take a lot on board."

"Never mind that for now. Look at this again. Earthworm couldn't acquire the IP address of the computer where ZEBRINA was being issued from. It kept drawing blanks. But before you arrived, the program alerted me to this new information. First, it showed the suspected land mass where the signal originated. It's the Middle East. It then homed in on Israel. Then, it tinted the land area of Jerusalem; Rishon, the West Bank, plus Tel Aviv. It placed a bright red ring around the area. I would put money on it and say our man is located somewhere in that circumference. He's using up to three hi-tech servers which hide his identity and the precise IP address he uses. Very difficult to pin down, and if he keeps changing them … almost impossible."

"You mean he could be here and right under our noses?"

"Exactly. But it's a big area. It kind of confirms my cluster theory, though. The cat returns home with its dead mouse gift, and the worker bees bring their daily spoils to their queen. Our man is hiding the six seals here, somewhere … because this is his home. Now watch this, I keep getting the same results."

Father Luke began typing at a bewildering speed across the keyboard, his fingers blurring as if they were in a fast-forwarded film. The three screens danced a steam of numbers and coloured tracer lines. Minutes later, he came to a halt.

"There." He sounded intense. "I've just asked Earthworm to configure the completed results from the last pass I made on the program, and add into it all results that have filtered through since then. Look at those tracer lines on screen, ignore the binary, and compare them to these on the printout from earlier. They are identical, apart from that, there are more. Our man is extremely busy somewhere. He's in this country and not far away. Earthworm has proved it."

"He must have a powerful program to handle that lot."

"Not necessarily. He could also have an army of workers."

"Well, how are we going to find him?"

"We won't, unless he makes another mistake. He's getting careless, enabling Earthworm to access one of his codes. There isn't a man alive who hasn't made mistakes and often continues to do so. It's only a matter of time."

"That's encouraging, but leaves me with problems. What am I going to do with Gallo and how do I handle the proposed suspension of Joshua?"

The priest looked concerned. "Joshua is a vital element, believe me. When he appeals, it may be a week before the tribunal hears the case, and during that time he can carry on at the site. Gallo needs to be watched at all times. I reckon if he finds the Seventh, he'll make off with it one way or another."

"Too true. Rachael can soften him to a degree. We'll get her to stay close to him. Who knows, he may lead us to ZEBRINA."

"I don't think so. ZEBRINA is clothed in total secrecy, apart from the six who are part of the Inner Circle of Keepers. He runs the show. Let me share with you what I know. Promise to say nothing until I'm done. You might be shocked at some of what I'm about to tell you. Sit yourself down and let's have drink before I start."

He looked serious, more serious than Rockwell had ever seen him before, since he had been attacked. Father Luke opened the terrestrial globe that stood in the corner, and produced a fine fifteen-year-old single malt Jura whiskey. Into two stout thistle cut glass tumblers, he poured three fingers of the golden liquid. He handed one to Rockwell and raised his glass.

"Here's to good triumphing over evil."

That's an unusual pledge. Rockwell clinked the tumbler next to Father Luke's and repeated it.

Then the priest spoke. He hesitated before he started, and then picked his words with care.

The priest recanted the story of the seals and John of Patmos, and the hunt for them once they left the island. He outlined how they were guarded by a society of Guardians and their persecution by Romans, and subsequently, the birth of another ambitious power-hungry group known as the Keepers. To prevent them being used, the Seventh was separated from the others, and both concealed for all time … until the final trumpets sounded.

He took a long pull on the Jura and continued speaking at a slow pace.

"Joshua put a spanner in the works. He discovered the six in that ossuary with Christ's name written on it."

He outlined the development of the mysterious Keepers, and named names; in particular, Cosimos Ricci, who revitalised what had become a dying movement. He explained the role of the seneschals and their recruiting policies. He brought the entire thing up to date with an explanation of how the Guardians had operated across time. He mentioned names right up to Nathaniel Agar.

At the mention of that name, Rockwell's eyebrows lifted, but he remained silent.

He told Rockwell how he himself was a Guardian. They were alive and well under their appointed leader, Nathaniel, Joshua Agar's grandfather and guardian. As such, they had been instructed to protect Joshua and mould him for possible leadership.

They paused and looked at each other, both reaching for their drinks at the same time.

After a long silence, Rockwell said, "You're telling me Joshua is your leader?"

"Not quite. He hasn't accepted his role. But, nor did his grandfather. It grows on you by degrees, and Joshua has already experienced a few of those. Let's say he's growing into it."

"Well, he's been very discreet about the entire business. Wow, you're asking me to swallow a lot of mumbo-jumbo, Father. On top of all this, I'm supposed to take on board the possibility of a two-thousand-year-old Jew, running around causing murder and mayhem and God knows what other mischief. Father, I feel overwhelmed. Who else knows anything about this?"

"Don't get angry, but you may be surprised to know our Rachael has known for a while. She considered your natural scepticism, and elected not to mention it to you. And yes, you should be overwhelmed. Who wouldn't be? It's the power of God you're witnessing. A global battle is about to be unleashed. The Keepers are now more alive and active than they have ever been since I can remember. I'm beginning to wish Joshua had never found the ossuary." The priest lowered his eyes and shook his head.

For a fraction, Rockwell felt a pang of sympathy for him. "Well, Father, I learn something new every day. Joshua, eh?" He rubbed at his chin, and took another drink. "Who would have believed all this? Rachael, oh dear … she must think me a total arse. I owe her an apology of sorts. I shall defend Joshua too. He's gone up to the sky in my estimation. Let's all keep together as a tight band, and you and your brothers." Rockwell smirked at his play on Shakespearean words. "Whether I believe all this or not is irrelevant. What is relevant is our safety, and the success of our explorations. To that end, I'm one hundred per cent behind you all."

He extended his hand and the priest gripped it firmly, shook it, and clapped him around the shoulder.

Chapter 35

ROCKWELL PLACED HIS hands on his hips, and surveyed the work the team had achieved. The ground leading up to the entrance had been cleared, and huge granite slabs had been moved with great care. It will now be easier to bring the equipment in, and add more generators. Broad flat stones had been laid on the ground to allow for ease of walking, and a path for all things wheeled. A large tent-like structure had been erected to shelter the rows of trestle tables, trays, polythene sheeting, and cleansing and water facilities. The earth smelt of ancient minerals, and the rocks had a chalky limestone aroma of their own that only arose when exposed to sunlight after an eternity in the dark.

Everything was in place and it looked good.

Joshua arrived on time and looked uneasy, his lips drawn in a straight line.

"You sent your letter? Rockwell asked.

"I delivered it this morning and I got Ahasver's."

"That should put a hold on the suspension for a while. I

sent one in too, in your support. It was the least I could do."

"Thanks, Simon. Where do I start?"

"I don't want you anywhere near Gallo. Rachael is keeping an eye on him. I want you to go in there with ropes, headlamps and flashlights, and keep on walking till you can't go any further. Take markers with you, a night vision scope, and a decent camera and flash. See how far it goes and what you can find. Take this as well." He handed him a two-way radio. "Just in case."

"What will you be doing?" Joshua looked relieved.

"I'm concentrating on the jars to see how they can best be moved without endangering the scrolls. I've an idea or two. They are phenomenal, and the dear old Bible brigade, I suspect, will be having apoplexy." He gave a hearty laugh. "Off you go. I'll catch you later.

Gallo kept a stony silence as they made their way along the west side of the cave structures. Their torch batteries were good for twelve hours on maximum power. He concentrated on the higher levels, while Rachael worked on the lower levels. They passed the altar they had found before, complete with its skeleton.

Rachael sensed he was uncomfortable with her presence. He wanted the space to himself. Her mistrust of him had grown, and although they have yet to find solid evidence, in her heart she knew Dr. Julian Gallo did drug Joshua and had the seals stolen. She felt the reassuring pressure of the Kevlar beneath her shirt with her stun gun in place, and the pistol strapped to her back, hidden from sight.

"You're quiet this morning, Julian. Still worrying about Joshua?"

He snarled a reply. "He shouldn't be here. He's irresponsible and a trouble maker."

"I don't think so. How would you feel if you had been attacked not once, but twice, and something valuable was stolen on your watch? He's been through a lot."

"Look, I don't want to talk about it. Let's just do what we came here to do, shall we?" He made an exaggerated movement to inspect an inscription higher up. As he reached upwards, he stumbled and crashed to the rocky floor, and his light went out under the impact. There was a loud clatter behind him "Oh shit! I've twisted my ankle."

The thought of leaving him crossed her mind, but that wasn't possible. "You ok down there?" She didn't want to help, in truth, and kept the torch beam away from him.

What's that?

As she swung the torch, the light illuminated two items: a wallet from which had fallen a business card, and a small revolver. Without thinking, she retrieved the business card and wallet, and acting from instinct, she kicked the gun into a darker area.

"You ok, Julian?" She feigned concern.

"No, I'm fucking not!" He held up his arm.

"Let me help you." She pulled him up.

He got his flashlight working again, and began shining it around the rocky ground. "I think I dropped something."

"This?" She handed him the wallet, but kept the card in her top pocket.

He grabbed at the wallet without a word, and thrust it in

his inside pocket.

"I think there was something else."

"Not that I saw." She lied.

Why was he carrying a gun? Was he expecting trouble? Or did he have something more devious in mind, like killing her or Joshua or both? It was a possibility, and could easily be part of the Keeper's game plan. Seeing that pistol, the full extent of their danger loomed large.

He continued cursing and waving the torch beam in increasingly frantic sweeps. "It must be here somewhere!" His voice clattered around the rocky vista.

"Tell me what you lost so I can help you find it."

"Nothing you need to be concerned with. Look." He stood up straight. "This ankle hurts. Could you get back to base and bring back a medical box and some ice? I'll wait here for you."

She couldn't wait to get away from him, but she also knew he was getting rid of her so he could look for the gun. "Okay. You sure you'll be all right? I won't be long." *I just hope he doesn't find it.* Her kick had sent it a good way off and it had wedged hard under a small promontory at floor level. She set off as fast as she could, and hoped Rockwell would be about.

Once the tunnel of light began to diminish to a small dot, Joshua started using the adhesive markers. But as long as the track ran straight, he didn't really need them. There was no hurry, and the trek could be for miles yet. What he expected to find, he had no idea.

With time on his hands, he attempted to sort his head and structure his thoughts. Without realising it, he had accepted the mantle as the leader of the Guardians, and had told Father Luke. The Keepers had to be stopped and the seals recovered and placed in safety. It was ironic that the stupid President was suspending him, when the greatest threat came from Gallo.

Joshua shook his head and focussed on the task ahead of him.

The walls now had less green slime on them. As he pressed on, his foot crunched on something that felt different from the numerous rocks and pebbles that littered the way. He shone his light on it and bent to pick it up. *It looks like an amulet or bracelet.* Dislodging it, he could see it was made of silver, very old, and encrusted with the detritus of age. *Someone dropped this item centuries ago.* It amazed him, and he wondered exactly how long it's been lying there.

He was unable to study it fully in the gloom of the caves, but twirling it around his fingers, he brought it closer to the light, and experienced a shock as vibrant as any live wire touching him.

"My God!" His voice echoed around the chamber with no one to answer him. The thing had been fashioned to resemble a crown, with a clear presentation of wings on either side. It was the symbol of the Guardians.

His jaw hung open. He couldn't believe it was all a coincidence. What were the chances? *I was meant to find this! How on earth otherwise?* He held it to his lips and kissed it before placing it in his bag. If he found nothing else, this was major!

An odd feeling made him walk faster. Up front, it looked even blacker, but his light revealed a fork in the cave, with one tunnel going left and the other to the right. Joshua chose the right. He proceeded a short way before he realised that he must be in an ancient burial area. To his right, was a vast open space that dropped away into God knows what. It looked like a gigantic cavern or hole the size of a swimming pool. He could make out steps that had been cut away into the sides, but disappeared just a short way down. With care, he peered over the top. It looked darker than the darkest night, and seemed to go on forever. His stomach turned. *Phew, that's scary.*

Taking out his night scope he adjusted the sight and peered into the abyss. Nothing. Just an endless drop full of the green ambient light of the scope. Joshua felt the hairs on his arms rise. *Is this a columbarium?* He inched his way back, unnerved. Finding the amulet had been a thrill, but this was as far as he would go alone.

He turned and let his light play across and over the wall behind him. What he saw caused a loud exclamation. "Wow!"

An inscription was clearly visible, etched into the rock by something sharp. It stared back at him from across the centuries … inviting, daring him to read it. He ran his hand across the indentations. *Unbelievable!* He didn't doubt there had been deterioration since the day the unknown person had inscribed it. But he could easily tell that it was written in ancient Hebrew. He scanned it with the lamp and started taking photographs of it. He could make out what it said, but he needed to get a shot to show it to everybody at base camp.

זהו האחרון של שבע שינה עתיקה
6אחיי לחכות אני כבר לא בוכה
ביד של ג'ון ואנחנו נחצבנו להכריז
קץ לדיראון עולם של האנושות

At first, he thought it could be Sanskrit, but no. It had been painstakingly written in Hebrew. Each line had been etched about an inch in height and as straight as a die. As he read it, pronouncing each word, the meaning of what he was reading slowly dawned on him. He took the deepest of breaths to slow down his racing pulse. *This is off the scale...* In gathering disbelief, he read it out loud in English.

Joshua stood very still, absorbing the magnificent sepulchral silence, as his entire being reeled from what he had read.

So ... it is true!

> *Here I the last of ancient seven sleep*
> *My Brothers six wait for I no longer weep*
> *And by John's hand we were carved to proclaim*
> *An end to Mankind's everlasting shame*

Chapter 36

STRIDING AROUND THE perimeters of the camp, Rockwell was figuring out how to move the jars from their current position. They were important, as they protected the scrolls from being touched, which would without a doubt damage them to a state of uselessness.

A flash of light caught his eye. It had emanated from the hillside, one of four that surrounded and dominated the site. *What was that?* He raised his field glasses and got a good look at a man, all in black, staring down at them. He pivoted around to the other three hills, and on each stood a solitary figure. All of them were focussed on the camp. They waved at each other before vanishing off the peaks.

Warning bells sounded in Rockwell's head. *There's something going on here.* A billowing of dust on the approach road then caught his attention. It was another Land Rover. As it drew nearer, he recognised the driver. Jacob Ahasver wasn't out for a scenic joyride. The man sitting next to him carried an assault rifle. *What the fuck's he doing here?*

It came to a rapid halt, churning up more dust, and both men jumped out. The armed man stood back and surveyed the area like a secret service man guarding a head of state. Ahasver wore a khaki safari suit, topped with a bright red cravat around his neck.

Rockwell strode out to meet him and offered his hand, which the President firmly shook. "Professor, what brings you here?"

"As you and your team seem unable to keep anything safe, I thought I'd come and conduct an inspection. My armed guard, Matal, is here to ensure nobody gets shot at during this expedition ... not you, me or anyone. You may see men up on those hills. If you do, there's no need to panic. They are there to protect you from any more trouble. So, expect to see them often. As I said to you before, Professor, we have our own way of dealing with things here. So, what's the news to date? Where's Gallo?"

"He's up there in the caves with Dr. Carver. They're mapping out the wall structures, symbols, carvings, and anything else they find. They're acting as an advance party for the rest of the team."

Ahasver's face hardened. "Is Agar up there?"

"Yes. He's doing the other tunnel in the same manner."

"He's unreliable and has cost us dearly. We'll have to wait until the hearing for the result on his negligence ..." He broke off as a faraway gaze filled his eyes. His head tilted and he gave a low mutter ... almost inaudible. "It wasn't far from here. It's like yesterday." With a sudden twitch of his entire body, he was back in real time. "When can I expect to see some of what you have discovered? I hear you've found some remarkable scrolls."

How the hell did he know that? Only the four of us and Father Luke knew what's up here. Everyone was sworn to secrecy. Gallo?

Rockwell bit his lip. "We don't know yet. There's nothing much to see." The last thing he wanted was the President lumbering about amongst potentially priceless relics. "Nothing's been established and at this stage, we daren't touch anything. You will be the first to know about it, and what we plan to do to excavate, believe me."

"Splendid. It's heartening to know our funds are being spent wisely. What I want to see, and insist on, is a synopsis of what you determine these caves may hold, and photographs of everything found on sight. Bring what you have found so far to my office anytime. I'm there until eight most evenings. Good day, Professor." He turned, nodded to the guard, and returned to the vehicle.

What was that all about? He could have told me on the phone? Simon scratched his head and gave a bemused expression. *Still, it's good to know we have protection.*

Rachael's heart was racing. The thought of Gallo's gun had shaken her, and she ran as fast as she could to where Rockwell had his tent. Gallo could have told her that he carried a pistol, but had chosen not to. He hadn't told anybody. *What was he armed for?*

She startled Rockwell as she crashed into his quarters. He was still reeling from Ahasver's impromptu visit.

"What on earth, Rachael? You're supposed to be up in the caves."

She explained in haste everything that had happened.

"Jesus, Rachael, things are beginning to escalate. You're not to go back up. If anybody does, it would be me. I'll take the medic box up there." He fished it out from a makeshift cupboard at the back of the tent. "What he doesn't know is that we're all tooled up. He could be in for a very nasty surprise."

"I'm certain the only thing that's on his mind is the possibility of finding that Seal."

"You reckon he knew where the six went?"

She looked confused. "He'd never own up to it, but yes."

"We're only guessing the last one is out there, chasing legends and stories, which is like a UFO report, more than likely false."

"No, it's not. It's true." a third voice cut through their conversation.

"Joshua!" They both voiced.

A shaken looking Joshua had crept in unnoticed, and he wasn't due back for another few hours.

"What's happened? You look as if you've had a run in with a ghost." Rachael went up to him and peered hard into his eyes. "Are you ok?"

"You're not far off." Joshua was quivering, and then it developed into a huge tearful episode and he slumped on the ground.

Rockwell and Rachael looked at each other with concern. In between his sobs, they couldn't understand what he was saying. They knelt beside him.

"What is it, Josh?" Rachael hugged him close and Rockwell grabbed his hand. But the sobbing continued.

After a couple of minutes, Joshua regained control of himself, and wiped his eyes. When he lifted his head to look at them, he smiled, causing the two to wonder about his mental state.

"It's been quite a morning. I guess I'm still in shock. More than I dared hope for. If only Nathaniel could have been with me. I owe him so much." His shoulders quivered, and he was sobbing again. "I owe him so much. All those years ..., all those damned years."

"You better tell us what happened up there." Rockwell showed a rare gentleness as he helped Joshua to his feet.

"One thing at a time. Let's sit. Have you got a drink, Simon? I could do with one."

A large scotch was placed in front of him.

He took a hefty gulp. "Look at this." He produced the encrusted amulet and held it up for them to see.

"Good Lord!" Rachael stood and grabbed it from his hand. "It's the sign of the first Seal, the winged crown. How old must this be, Simon? It's clogged with dirt and dust."

"How old? Only testing will tell, but my guess is at least fifteen hundred years. It's in remarkable condition due to the temperature consistency in those caves. Yes, it is the sign associated with the first seal, and also the insignia of the Guardians."

"Somebody, all that time ago, lost this and never found it. And we find it after almost two thousand years? How amazing is that?"

"That's not all I found."

"You have more?"

"Yes, it's on my camera. I accidentally found writing etched into the walls. I wrote down what it said." Joshua flicked through his camera to find his shots. He'd taken several.

Rockwell produced a large lens and peered for several minutes. Then he handed it over to Rachael while he scribbled a few notes.

"It's difficult to read on screen, Josh." Rachael squinted at the image. "What do you make of it, Simon?"

"Joshua knows exactly what it says. I think I'm more excited than him. Tell her."

Joshua related the exact events leading to his discovery, the location of the inscription, and what it said in English. "The Seventh Seal is there, in that place ... waiting. But it looks like it's somewhere in a bottomless pit, an ancient disused columbarium. Whoever had it left a strong clue as to where it was, and probably dropped it over the edge. If it was used as a burial site, that ledge could not have been the only way in. There must be a bottom to it. Don't you think?"

"Put like that, yes, there must be another way in. We should go there as soon as we can." Rachael brushed the hair from her eyes. "Even this amulet could have been his. His name was Adil Koury, wasn't it?"

Joshua stopped for a moment, laid his hand upon his heart, and looked up at them both, before making a small sweeping gesture with his arm. "I very much like to think it was."

Rachael and Simon looked at each other and smiled. "We do too, Joshua," she said.

"I'd better take the first aid kit up to Gallo before he gets suspicious. We've got to think of a way into that pit. From the photograph and your description, Joshua, it appears nigh on impossible. It looks like we are going to need more research. While I'm gone, get thinking and we tell nobody."

The beam of his flashlight pushed the darkness back as he probed here and there under various rocks. *Damn that stupid woman. Now I'm going to have limp about a bit or say I've had a miraculous recovery.* There had been no sign of his gun. He began to wonder. The more he thought about it, the more he suspected she had seen it and booted it out of sight. He got down on his belly and shuffled about. There were numerous small overhangs and ground level edges. It could be anywhere. Pushing in his hand and using the other to shine in the beam, he groped around. His fingers touched something and he knew it couldn't be rock or dirt. The metallic feel told him he had found his pistol.

There's no way that could have found its way in there on its own. The bitch kicked it there. If she knows, then they will all know … including Ahasver.

"Shit!" *I'll have to say it was for protection.*

He would say nothing until it was mentioned. He tugged and the pistol broke free from its lodging place. Brushing the dust from it, he gave it a quick check and ensured that the safety catch remained on. A voice rang down the tunnel.

"Hello! Julian! Are you there? It's me, Simon. Give me a shout."

It's Rockwell. What's he doing here?

"I'm over this way. Keep coming, I can see you."

A strong beam of light was zigzagging towards him. Lying on the floor, he knew he would be hard to spot, so he sat up and concealed the gun behind him. The thought came into his head … *it would only take one shot.* He shelved it. There would be too many questions and besides, Rachael knew he had a gun. That would make things awkward. He checked his ankle. It barely hurt so he was going to have to fake it. "I'm over here, Simon. I'm sitting down for a rest." He flashed his torch to attract his attention.

Rockwell saw it and made his way over, stooping low to avoid rocks that seemed to jut out from everywhere. "You ok?"

"Yeah, nothing a decent bandage won't cure." He had removed his boot and sock.

Looking at the ankle, Rockwell knew at once it had no damage. He decided to play along. He thought of challenging him about the weapon, but that would reveal too much. He dug out a crepe bandage, cut it to the correct length, and strapped it professionally around his foot.

"There, that should do the trick. Let me pull you up." Without being too careful he yanked Gallo up, who managed to let out a strangulated gasp.

"Follow me, Julian. Are you sure you're ok? Keep your head down." He debated whether he should share Joshua's discovery or not. It would be hard to keep it from him, but letting him know would invite more trouble, of that there could be no doubt. The day had been weird … gun toting men on the hills, the President and his armed guard, Gallo's attempt at concealing his firearm, and the most revelatory of all, Joshua's finds. Whatever, he was duty bound to inform Ahasver of their progress … especially the inscription. They would have to decide what to do about Gallo. How could they exclude him?"

Dust never stopped blowing about, and the only way to avoid it was to confine themselves inside the tents with the flaps closed. It would be calmer and quieter inside, and no need to shout to be heard.

Rachael said, "Josh, I'm now one hundred per cent certain that Gallo is wrapped up in this Keeper business, and I think you know more than you let on at times. He has a gun and I don't think it's for his own protection. What does he do? I mean what's the point of it all? All these attacks on you and on me, he must have known of them, or he may have even planned them. Even Father Luke was attacked. None of us are safe, are we? The only one who hasn't been touched is Simon." She tried to supress a small sneeze, pulling out a tissue from her pocket. A card fell out. It was the one Julian had dropped up in the caves. She had forgotten about it. Peering closer, Rachael read the embossed letters.

"Oh wow! Look at this, Josh, it's all in Italian. I picked it off the floor when Julian dropped his wallet and gun. He doesn't know I have it. I thought it might be useful. Can you read it?" She handed it over to him.

Joshua looked at it and blanched. Rachael actually saw his breathing stop before he exhaled in a rush. "*Oy Gevalt!* I know what this all means. You said Gallo was carrying it in his wallet?"

"Yes."

"This card and what's written on it is damning evidence of his involvement. The symbol is ancient. It's of a serpent eating its own tail." He jabbed at it with his finger. "Known as an Ouroboros, this particular symbol is littered throughout my grandfather's files. It has a Greco-Roman-Egyptian background and dates back to the second century or earlier.

It's been linked with alchemy and the Philosopher's Stone. The Gnostics, who expanded after Christ's crucifixion, used it as a symbol to represent eternity and the Soul of the World. It's a twelve-part dragon encompassing the Earth. The same number as the Apostles." He leant forward and using a magnifying glass, peered at the lettering in the centre of the serpent. "I should know what this says … ah! I have it. It's Greek. It translates to, *One in the All*. Of course! That fits in very well with the Keeper's plots and idealism."

"What does the Italian say, do you know?" Rachael jabbed her finger at it.

He gave it a quick look. "It pretty much wraps up Gallo. Look." He pointed to the embossed Italian lettering written in the Latin style. "It's written this way to make it difficult to read. I'm surprised he even carried it around with him. It reads *I Guerrieri Apocalittici Di Cristo.* That's short for the AWC, as we have come to know it. The Apocalyptic Warriors of Christ. There's an address too. *Viale Bruno Buozzi, Roma.*"

They looked at each other in silence.

"Just as Father Luke said." Rachael sat down with a thump. "We can't do anything or say anything until Simon gets back. What he can do about it, I don't know. He's got to report back to Ahasver later, so whether he tells him all about this is up to him. So far, all our evidence is circumstantial. But we know more than that, don't we?"

"Absolutely." Joshua shook his head and continued to stare at the card. He looked puzzled. "That diagram … apart from my grandfather's artefacts, I'm sure I've seen it somewhere else before."

Chapter 37

Tel Aviv

FATHER LUKE'S EXCITEMENT scoured through him like a hot flame. He checked the three large plasma screens for the fifth time. He wasn't wrong. The binary sequence had translated into an unmistakable curvature of lines that were focussing from or into one area and place. For a fraction of a second, someone hadn't been fast enough to encrypt the transmitted sequence. He homed in with Earthworm and programmed every data he had to obtain an exact location. The error had been brief, but it was enough to let him in.

At once, he knew exactly where the Keepers' commands and instructions were originating.

Checking his watch, he realised he hadn't much time. He was due to perform Mass in fifteen minutes, followed by the Sacrament of Confession. Using his mobile, he called Rockwell, who answered immediately.

"Simon, it's me, Father Luke. I can't talk right now as I have to hurry for Mass. I've made a startling discovery. As I once said, our man only needs to make one mistake, and that is all it has taken. I know, but can't talk about it on the phone.

Get over to me at Saint Peter's Church, here in Tel Aviv, in a couple of hours. I'll tell you what I've found."

"Sounds promising, Father. I'll be there later."

The priest loved Saint Peter's, the calmness and dignity of its Spanish roots and with its Jaffa connection to the apostles. It overlooked the Sea of Galilee close by, and was embraced by cool sea breezes. The structure was built and completed in the mid seventeenth century. Unlike most churches in the area, its altar faced westward.

Mass was performed in several languages. His today was in English. Once the Mass was over, Father Luke made the usual announcements of local activity for the coming week, before he retired into the confessional to await the penitents.

A small queue of half a dozen knelt in prayer to wait their turn. It never took long, and he kept a lookout for Rockwell. He didn't want to miss him. Apart from one remaining person, the church soon became quiet and empty.

The last person in was a lean, wiry man wearing dark shades, and dressed in a blue denim jacket and matching trousers. He clutched a crucifix close to his chest. The worries of the world seemed to be upon him. He walked to the booth, pushed the curtain aside, and stepped inside. He removed his sunglasses and allowed his eyes to adjust to the light of two burning candles positioned on the other side of the grill, separating the good from the bad. He sat on the well-worn bench stool with his mouth close to the grill.

"Angelus Domini, my son. What is it you wish to tell

me?"

"Forgive me, Father, for I'm about to sin."

The priest wondered if he had heard right. "You are about to sin? Don't you mean 'for I have sinned?'

"Both, Father. I have many sins, but soon they will be absolved by the Great Redeemer."

Father Luke looked at his watch. "Christ can forgive us all. What sins do you wish to confess?"

The man's reply stretched low and chilled the grill of the confessional. "Murder."

Father Luke had never heard anybody wishing to confess such a sin in all the years he'd been a priest. A shock passed through him like he had stepped on a live rail. For a moment, he was unable to speak, and didn't know what to say that would have an effect.

"My son, that's a serious crime and a mortal sin." It felt inadequate.

The man nodded and said in a voice that was scarcely audible. "I know. Forgive me for what I am about to do." With one swift and unseen movement, he placed the barrel of his supressed SIG pistol between the grille slats, and fired two shots at close range into Father Luke's unsuspecting body.

The priest gave a low agonised gasp. Slicing, penetrating spheres of pain ripped through him as he hit the floor in a crumpled heap. His body hung half in and half out of the cubicle. Blood began to pool around him in rich red twists.

The man holstered his weapon behind his shoulder. Bowing to the dying priest, he made the sign of the cross before muttering, "Forgive me. *Sacris Sancti Homicidium.*" He strode away at a fast pace. A flurry of air blew down the aisle.

Father Luke was dying.

A rushing sound pounded in his ears, as his life force pumped out of him and into the holy ground of the church. He struggled to pull a paper from his cassock. Gasping for breath, ignoring the searing agony, he dipped his finger into the swirling trickles of redness that oozed in a peaceful parody beneath him. He wrote in rhythm to his slowing pulse, which grew slower and louder in his ears by the second.

"Christ, I am yours. Do with me what you will. Forgive all my sins."

He juddered. His finger slowly slipped off the paper. The Virgin Mary gazed down upon him as he gave his last gasp.

Fifteen minutes later, the perspiring figure of Rockwell pushed open the heavy oak door of Saint Peter's, grateful to step inside the welcome coolness of the church. He gave a cough to alert anybody of his presence.

No answer.

Like most churches, there never seemed to be an obvious doorway. He reached the ornateness of The Lady Chapel, peered inside. Nobody.

"Father Luke?" he called out, wary of offending the sanctity of the place. "Are you there? It's me, Simon Rockwell."

Silence.

He turned to the west-facing altar and spotted the confessional behind which he could see a door. *He must be in there.* Walking past the rows of pews, he rounded the top rank and came to an immediate halt. The inert and prostrate form of Father Luke blocked any further movement.

"Father Luke, no! Oh my God!" He knelt and shook the priest's shoulder, calling out his name. "Father Luke. Father?"

No movement.

Rockwell knew death when he saw it. He had clearly been shot. Reaching for his cell phone, he punched out 02100 for the police and got an immediate response. He gave his personal details.

"There's been a shooting at Saint Peter's church in Jaffa. A priest has been killed."

"We are on our way." A gruff voice responded, also adding they would send an ambulance.

Rockwell dithered for a fraction, and in his shock, he was uncertain what to do next. *This is serious shit. What did he want to see me for? Is that why he was shot? I don't doubt it. Too much has been happening.*

Then, something caught his eye. Beneath the priest's arm was a blood stained, small, and spiral-bound notebook, bent back to a vacant page. It wasn't that blank. A thin line of writing scrawled across the page in the colour red. It wasn't ink. By the state of his hand, it had been written by the finger that hung off the side of the page. Rockwell hesitated. The police would want this. But curiosity engulfed him, and in one swift tug, he removed the page from the book and stared hard at it. Father Luke had left the message for him, for across the top of the page was the word 'Simon,' and like the remainder of the page, written in the drunken, spiderlike squiggle of a dying man. It formed a rough circle.

It appeared to be a list of letters. But what of? It didn't make sense. At the top were what looked like two letters? Here, the writing plunged downward as life left his body. Rockwell scanned the words. They were meaningless. Father Luke had been trying to tell him something, and these letters were likely to be connected to what he wanted to see him about. As he pondered the strange message, the sound of approaching emergency vehicles closing in around the small square leading to the church grew louder.

Making certain that blood had dried on the page, he folded it in half, and slid it into the inside pocket of his jacket. There was a commotion outside, and the door burst open, and Police Chief Captain Manovici strode in, followed by three other men and an ambulance squad.

"Professor Rockwell, is that you?" Manovici called out as he approached.

"Yes, that's me. I called you earlier."

"What do you know about this? Who is the priest?"

Rockwell moved to one side as the ambulance crew got to work. He sat down with a weary movement. "I'll start from the beginning. I got this call …"

Five hours later, Rockwell arrived back at his house in a state of exhaustion and delayed shock. He had been held and questioned, but the Police Chief had decided there was nothing he could be charged with, and released him innocent of any crime. Manovici wasn't stupid. He had already made a connection between the previous University shooting and the events that led up to this murder. There would be more investigations to follow.

Waiting for him were Joshua and Rachael. He had told them on the phone of the horrific news. They were in a shocked daze, and a look of disbelief and sadness hung around them. They embraced, and said what they had to say. Father Luke had been a kind man. It all seemed so inappropriate.

"Do you think Gallo knows about this? Him being a seneschal and all according to Father Luke? He had limped back here with me, but forgot to do so every so often. Do we tell him about the amulet and inscription? If I tell the President, I will have to tell Gallo or he'll suspect that we know of his involvement. We're all agreed that whatever this is all about, he's in it up to his neck?"

"Agreed," they replied.

"Okay." Rockwell's tone hardened. We'll keep quiet about it until I've seen the inscription. We have to find a way into the depths of the columbarium as soon as possible."

He poured three glasses of red wine and handed them around.

Rockwell looked at his glass and muttered, "Red, of course, red! I almost forgot." He reached into his inside pocket and pulled out the bloodstained page he had detached from Father Luke's notebook. He spread it out on the table-top. "I forgot to tell you about this. I tore it from his notebook, and I think this was his last act before he died. It's written in blood. I can't make heads or tails of it, but I'm certain it has something to do with what Earthworm discovered. He was so excited when we last spoke, he reckoned his program had unwrapped the Grand Keeper's identity. That the man made a small error and Earthworm must have found a way in. This note was his dying attempt to tell us. What do you two make of it?"

Rachael peered hard at it. "It looks meaningless to me. Names, I guess, but they don't mean a thing. They could be names or random letters."

They continued studying the unintelligible words in silence.

...hA~SUliHpaTRaC~maRraMlp'medeuq~sueDatTUB'sAI hTAtaM~JW...

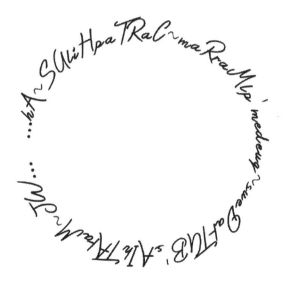

From the way the letter trailed off, they realised that while writing the last letter, Father Luke had died.

"Is it a code that he had left on his computer? Surely that's what it is. That's what he was trying to tell me."

Joshua held out his glass for a refill, as he continued to look at the bloody letters, and forgot to move his arm back with the full glass.

"You alright, Josh? Simon's filled your glass."

"Sssh. Be quiet, please." He held up his hand.

The letters blurred, twisted one way, and then another. They shifted and separated and whirled around his memory banks, and into the neurons of his brain. Until he could see. He closed his eyes and still could still see. It was so obvious. There was nothing difficult about it. A child could work it out with ease.

They stared at him.

"I know what Father Luke was trying to tell us. I know what it means."

Chapter 38

Vatican City

ADAM, THE STRAY dog, was a frequent visitor in the precincts of the Vatican. It had been said that the Pope had a strong affection for the beast, and they had been caring for it for several years. The animal had a happy disposition, a feral some said, but where he came from, nobody knew. He had long ears and had large brown patches across his white fur.

He knew when feeding time came. If lucky, the priests or cardinals would drop him meats, like beef or poultry. He wasn't fond of fish. Today, Cardinals Riario and Pacca had prepared a special meal for him, a treat they felt he would enjoy. Quail, no less. Their instructions had been clear. They were to make a trial run to test the effectiveness of their plan. Apart from its usual diet of Coturnix pellets, grains, and small fruits, the quail had been given generous doses of hemlock seeds to eat. They were immune to the poison, but eating the flesh of a bird that had eaten hemlock seeds would kill a man or an animal within hours.

They called for Adam, and they saw him running to them from the kitchens that overlooked a small courtyard in front of a small sized grass walkway. His head was raised, and his nose sniffed the air with vigour. His tail wagged in anticipation.

Cardinal Riario had cut the roasted bird into small slices, and placed it on a plate that Pacca held. He filled the plate, added some mixer, then he bent low and gave it to Adam. Like most dogs, the food got gulped down in a few rapid swallows. Now, all the Cardinals had to do was wait.

They shut the door so Adam had no way out. Barely an hour had passed before he began showing signs of distress. His head moved to an odd angle, his tongue lolled out from the side of his mouth, and he began to twitch as a form of paralysis moved to his legs. He crouched down, whining mournfully, before falling to his side to give one last stuttering breath as death took him.

The cardinals looked at each other. Pacca spoke first. "I didn't enjoy seeing that, but it had to be done." He said with an expression of regret.

"Neither did I," replied Riario, biting his bottom lip. "A pity it couldn't have been the Holy Father."

"It will be soon, Brother, have no fear. We must report the success of the trial."

Charles Salvador Woodford read and reread his communiqué from the Grand Keeper. He didn't doubt that all members of the Inner Circle were receiving their orders. He knew what he must do. Later, he contacted Cardinal Pacca who handled the economic affairs of the Holy See.

Woodford's tone, as usual, was brusque and blunt. He had no time for courteous niceties. "Cardinal Pacca, under the orders of our Master, you know what you have to do, don't you?"

'I know," Pacca replied in a soft voice.

"Tell me, so that I'm certain what you are doing is correct. It's a lot of money and nothing must go wrong or raise questions."

"I am to transfer in four separate transactions of varying amounts a total of twenty million dollars. You will supply the coverage and documented paper work covering all details appertaining to the transfer. I am to use two banks, the Butterfield Bank in the Cayman Islands and Euro Pacific in St. Vincent."

"When will you do this?"

"I will do it when the Pope is dead."

"Exactly. You've done well. Goodbye, Cardinal, until next time."

Before the Cardinal could reply, the phone switched off.

Xavier de Menendez, *The Fixer*, found his resources stretched to the limits. He had prepared an inventory of what he had on hand, and what he can acquire at short notice. His procurement of assorted weaponry would be enough to equip a good-sized army. After liaising with Anderson, he received intel on the possible location of chemical weapons, such as hydrogen cyanide gas devices developed by Aum Shinrikyo in Japan. The other source being the 'suitcase' nuclear explosives certain Middle Eastern terrorist groups had attempted to manufacture. As usual, his biggest headache was logistics. When the call arrives, he would be under colossal strain to execute maximum delivery.

General Sir Gordon Anderson had the difficult task of ensuring he could override existing security in any circumstance. As chief of NPG and DPC, he was a law unto himself. But the launch of any weapons required a failsafe set up of five individuals coordinating at the same time. He knew the 'Gold Codes' and it needed only two votes from a five-man team to activate a launch, no matter what the others voted. Once launched from ground and sea, there was no way the ICBM's could be stopped. He would need to practice a few launch drill procedures, to ensure his readiness when the signal arrived. It could be done.

Chapter 39

JOSHUA GRABBED THE sheet from Rockwell and stared hard at it again. Crossing to the blackboard and with a piece of yellow chalk, he scrutinised the bloody inscription before copying it on the board in a circle.

...hA~SUliHpaTRaC~maRraMlp'medeuq~sueDatTUB'sAI hTAtaM~JW...

He looked at them both. They looked blank.

"Ugaritic script would be easier to understand than that." Rockwell bristled, never liking to be shown something he didn't understand.

"C'mon then Josh, tell us what it is." Rachael continued to squint at the blackboard.

Joshua gave back the paper to Rockwell. "From what you have said, Simon, and from what I believe this is saying, it's Father Luke's attempt to tell us what his computer program, Earthworm had opened up. Sadly, he died before the message could be completed, but there's a lot of clues here we can use."

"Get on with it, please." Rockwell had begun tapping his fingers on the table.

"Okay. Firstly, it was written back to front. Normally,

people read in clockwise fashion, but he's put in an anti-clockwise direction."

"Why would he do that, especially when mortally wounded?"

"I guess he knew he was finished, and didn't want anybody else to understand what he had written. He was a computer genius, and for him to write in cryptic codes would have been as common as a microwave dinner."

"Even turned the right way around, it's gibberish."

"Yes, that's what he must have hoped people would think, but he knew he had little time left and did the best he could. Both of you, how good are your literary skills, biblical, medieval, classical or otherwise?"

"Carry on. Enlighten us, Josh." Rachael was now focussed on him. "Okay. I'm going to read it back to you, in the correct sequence, piece by piece, and explain as I go along. Firstly, you need to know the entire writing here is, I think, based on the legend of the Eternal Jew, otherwise known as The Wandering Jew."

Rockwell interrupted. "Father Luke discussed that nonsense with me earlier."

Rachael was familiar with the name. "That's the man who supposedly mocked and spat on Christ when he was carrying the cross to Calvary."

"The very one. Two legends surrounded him. One has it that he was Pontius Pilate's gatekeeper, and the other that he was a cobbler. Christ, whilst dragging his cross, was said to have fallen in the doorway of his shop to rest, and this man, verbally abused, mocked, spat on him, and told him to get a move on, and hurry up to get crucified, and not to block his doorway. Christ cursed him to live for eternity until his second coming, when he might obtain release. He could never die or age, but still feel the pains of mortal men." He paused to make sure they were following. "The first two letters WJ stands for *Wandering Jew*, and the tilde symbol ~ means *is*. Ok with that?"

"Carry on."

"Various names have been attributed to the Wandering Jew throughout history. These have varied from age to age, in medieval and classical writings. So, reversing the next block letters, it spells out *Matathias*, a medieval attribution. Nothing difficult there?"

They shook their heads.

He separated the words with a chalk mark. "That leads us to the next name, another late-medieval construction." He proceeded to separate that name with another thick stroke of the yellow chalk. "This one is *Buttadeus*. With the word *is*, Father Luke was confirming that they are one and the same. Next is the name *Isaac Laquedem*, although L and A are missing. That's not surprising in the condition he was. So, do you see what he tried to do with his last ounce of breath? He's telling us the various names of this accursed man throughout history. Are you happy with that?"

"We're happy." Both were now fully alert, aware of what this might be leading up to.

"He gives us two more names, pL, which I take as short for *Paul*, because the next name, *Marram*, also the Eternal Jew, had *Paul* as his first name. Now comes the interesting bits. He wrote down the name *Cartaphilus*. He was also known as the Roman Legionnaire who speared Christ's side while crucified. Father Luke had uncovered what he believed is the name of the leader of the Keepers, and where he might be found."

"That doesn't prove anything. It doesn't add up to a can of beans."

Rockwell poured another drink, but looked as if he was prepared to hear it out.

"I haven't finished yet." Joshua remained confident. He underlined the letters that spelt out *Cartaphilus*. "In 1853, David Hoffman wrote a book, a fictitious story of the event. It was called *The Wandering Jew*, or the *Chronicles of Cartaphilus*. He connected the Roman soldier's given name and attributed it to the Jew. After all, both were derogatory to Christ in varying degrees."

"How does that help us?" Rachael asked.

"Haven't you two ever read anything in your lives, or have you forever been staring at rocks? Can't you see? Father Luke was spelling out all the names of The Eternal Jew, so there could be no mistake. Why did he do that? This has something to do with the Grand Keeper's identity. He wrote it the way he did so it looked like a load of rubbish..."

Rockwell interrupted. "Okay, Josh, it's a load of rubbish. We still don't have the name, and in real life, we are a couple of centuries ahead of Cartaphilus as written by this guy Hoffman."

"As I asked earlier," Josh replied, "haven't you ever read anything? Look closely at the name he started but never finished. What does it say?"

"It doesn't say anything ... just two letters, *hA*."

"No, it's *Ah*."

"So, it's *Ah*. Ah hah." Rockwell smirked, his patience, what little he had in the first place, had run out.

"Be serious, Simon, please. A man lost his life trying to

tell you this. Father Luke was a decent man, killed by an indecent one. Some respect, please." Rachael looked at him in disappointment.

"Sorry. You're right."

"He was, I'm certain, attempting to write the name of a Persian King from ancient times called *Ahasuerus*. You can look him up in your Bible, in The Book of Esther. There's a Jewish adaptation of that name back in medieval times. Now, here's the knockout bit. The Jewish version of *Ahasuerus* is *Ahasver*." Joshua looked grim as he said it. He watched his colleague's reactions.

They looked stunned, their mouths open in disbelief. Their silence lasted ten to fifteen seconds as their eyes roamed each other. Rockwell cleared his throat, and not a muscle moved amongst them. It was as if lightning had struck and forced them to see what they didn't dare believe.

Rockwell spoke first. "Oh shit. Are we all thinking the same thing here?"

"It can't be? Can it?" Rachael shook her head, a million doubts etched into her face.

Rockwell recalled his last meeting with the priest. "Before I left his place, he showed me the results from Earthworm. All the lines and binary indexes from across the world were configuring on a ten-mile radius from Tel Aviv. Father Luke said it would only take one small error, and Earthworm would locate the source. When he called me, he was in a high state of excitement, and refused to say anything on the phone. He obviously found something important. Then, somebody else found out that he knew. How? God knows. This is all beyond me. I got to the church too late, and I can't forgive myself for that. We have to be very careful now. We can't trust anyone. For all we know, they might be spying on us."

"I can help there." Joshua held up a small phone like object. "It's Father Luke's bug scanner, remember? He lent it to me as he thought I was in more danger than anybody else involved. Don't worry. I already scanned this room and it's clear."

"That's great," Rachael whispered. "We are all in an awkward situation. Gallo is known to be involved, and now we have to assume that Jacob Ahasver, our chief man and university President, could also be. At this stage, not to do so would be stupid. The links and coincidences are too strong. Let's assume either one of them has the six seals. Gallo knew where they were kept, but Ahasver did not. Gallo, we assume, slipped a Mickey Finn into your drink, Josh. But Gallo wasn't involved in the attack. He must have been acting under orders and he hasn't a clue about most things, other than his part. If he hasn't got the seals, then the only person who would know their whereabouts would be Ahasver."

"I can't believe Ahasver heads up a murderous secret society." Rockwell was shaking his head. "Are you also trying to tell us he's a two-thousand-year-old Jew who can't die until the second coming of Christ?"

"I can't answer that, and it would be hard to believe … wouldn't it? So, let's say no on that one. I can answer the other part of your question. Why do you think he wants me suspended?" Joshua asked. "He suspects or knows of my links with the Guardians, their sworn enemy since John of Patmos, and even earlier. He doesn't want me about, sniffing around for the Seventh Seal."

Rockwell gulped at his drink and then reached out for another. "I think I need a few more of these. It all begins to make sense now. All the other departments have had their budgets slashed except us. Not only that, we get a massive increase in funds. Ahasver has been known to obtain funding from Vatican sources, and now we know where. I haven't included his odd request either, that I report daily on where we are, what we have been doing, and what we have found."

"What about those men on the hilltop with guns? Why are they really there? It sounds good saying they're there to protect us, but now I'm beginning to think they are there to ensure that if we find the Seventh Seal, they can steal it. All it would take would be a nod from creepy Gallo."

Joshua stood up and walked to the blackboard and erased what was written. Rachael couldn't help noticing how more confident and assertive he had become. His posture, his voice, and mannerisms, had changed overnight … from that of an uncertain young man into one of a mature and determined adult.

Chapter 40

GALLO LOOKED AT himself in the dressing mirror. His face, he thought, looked troubled. The incident at the caves confirmed what he had begun to suspect. Carver, Rockwell, and Agar, were wary of him. Her kicking his gun away under the rocks and then pretending she hadn't, was a first-class giveaway. She would have told Rockwell and Agar about it too. Both, he surmised, would not be convinced of the twisted ankle ruse.

He checked his watch.

It was time for his prayers.

True to his custom, he knelt facing Jerusalem, and three times recited the Keepers' sacred oath, *Sacris Sancti Homicidium.* Before he could finish, his mobile ringtone interrupted his devotions.

The agreed code displayed on the screen made his heart accelerate.

A voice, using a distorter, spoke to him. "Seneschal Gallo. Listen carefully, and obey what you are about to hear."

"I will."

"Our legions are being prepared and are on full alert. To bring our plans to a successful climax, you, seneschal, will be at the forefront of our endeavours. What you say or do as from this moment are vital to our plans. What of the excavations and your colleagues?"

"They distrust me. We have not found what we seek, although the other items indicate that we must be close. Ancient parchments and scrolls are always a potent sign of what we might expect."

"There is something you must do, and I must show you. Tonight, you are to catch a Dan bus to the Hagana railway station. In the car park, you will see a red Lexus saloon. It will have a Jewish flag flying from it. You are to get into the front passenger seat. It will be unlocked. You will not look around, but keep your eyes fixed in front. Two men will get in. One will be the driver, and you will be hooded, and you will not speak. Do you understand?"

"Yes."

"Later, you will have a job to perform. Goodbye, seneschal."

It took a moment to sink in before a sense of pride expanded his chest. It had started ... and he had been picked to perform a vital role. A rare accolade indeed, and it held promise of greater things. A dizzy excitement passed through him, and he gasped to catch his breath. He was ready and prepared to do whatever they required of him. The second coming, he sensed, had got closer.

The 304 Dan bus dropped him off precisely where he could see the Lexus a short walk away, its Israeli flag fluttering in the soft breeze.

Standing in front of the passenger seat, he looked around and not a person could be seen. He tried the door. It opened and he climbed in. His wait wasn't long before two men came from behind the car, one to the left and the other to the right. He stared ahead as instructed, and didn't speak. A black hood, the last thing he caught sight of, was pulled down securely over his head. The car fired up and they moved off.

The man behind him spoke. "When we say duck, do so, as low as you can manage. We don't want you to be seen. Nod, if you understand."

The seneschal nodded.

Two commands to 'duck low' were all that broke the silence of their journey. Gallo had no idea where they were going. The car was brought to a stop, and he heard the engine switch off. His door was opened and a firm hand helped him out, but the hood remained. An arm linked to his and they began to walk. The ground felt rough, rocky, and crunched beneath his shoes. *I must be near a rocky terrain.*

"Duck," a voice commanded and a hard hand pushed his head low.

He sensed the air had become much cooler.

"Seneschal, you can remove the hood."

What Gallo saw surprised him. He stood in a cave-like structure, similar to the cave they were working on. He looked up and around him. The two men had their heads bowed. "Just keep walking, seneschal. We can go no further. You will know when to stop."

Gallo began to walk alone. *Where am I?* The cavernous spaces and tunnel-like structures appeared endless, but he walked on without fear. A strange low glow came from somewhere, sufficient to for him to move safely in the darkness. How it worked, he had no idea. The walls looked smooth but with frequent undulations. He resisted temptations to turn left or right, but kept on going until ahead of him, the light grew bright as day and the atmosphere shifted up a few degrees.

He had reached his destination.

In the background stood the silhouette of a white robed figure. Gallo trembled, for he knew it was the Grand Keeper, who stood still as a statue.

Behind him was a large stone sarcophagus.

The top portion or cover was pulled back. Around it, candles flickered, and the air hung heavy with the rich aroma of frankincense, drifting from a dangling censer to his right.

"Come no further, Seneschal." The unmistakeable sound of an electronic voice changer came from beneath the full-faced cowl. "You are welcome. I will answer the questions I know you have in your head. You are very deep beneath the caves of Beit-Guvrin."

Gallo felt in danger of being overawed. His knees began to tremble. *How could this be?*

The Grand Keeper's voice continued its broken static tone. "The time is almost upon us, and we will have tasks to perform that many may find unpleasant. It is time for us to sort the wheat from the chaff in our ranks. Your task, Seneschal Gallo, will test you to the limit. How far are you prepared to go to bring about the Second Coming, and help execute God's plan upon this rotten earth? The six are in our possession. How can we fail? We cannot. Look behind me into the stone." His arm swung around and he pointed a finger at the stone coffin.

Gallo moved around to the side and peered in. He gave a

jolt and his eyes widened. "Good God!" he whispered.

Looking up at him was a middle aged, naked woman.

Motionless, still breathing, but drooling with vomit, besmirched and reeking of diarrhoea, her rigid eyes stared upwards with a desperate expression. She didn't move. There were no chains or ropes, and her arms were stretched out down her sides. Her legs were bent a fraction at the knees.

"Middle aged sinners proliferate and walk this earth, and they will be the first to be cast aside into the darkest caverns of hell. Feel no pity, seneschal, she is of Satan's army as I once was. You know not my story, but at this moment, it is of no importance. Look at her closely, at her abused body, her avarice and greed shout out from every pore of her stinking flesh. Why does she not move? She cannot. In her body and now washing through her corrupt veins are liquid concoctions of the flowers of rhododendrons, azaleas and oleanders."

"Powerful poison."

"She is paralysed, but mentally as cognitive as ever. Death may take a few very painful hours yet. You, seneschal, can end her misery, but only by degrees. I'm not commanding you, but asking you to perform what I suggest."

A pause. Candles continued their flutter and the incense smoke ascended ever upwards. The immobile woman could not prevent the small tear that made its way from the outward corner of her eye to trickle down the far side of her face.

"What is that, Grand Keeper?"

"You have brought a pistol?"

"I have." *He wants me to shoot her.*

"Excellent. In response to your thought, yes, you are correct. You will shoot her in both feet, and then into the palms of her hands. Her wounds will resemble those of Christ. She will not die from those wounds, but her struggle for breath will be hastened as the poison ravages her internal organs. What you will do then, I will tell you after a short time of meditation and prayer in my presence. Shoot her now, and then leave her to consider her sins." He pointed to an alcove. "When you are done with that, you will kneel with me at the bench provided and give thanks to God."

Gallo had never shot anybody before. His mouth went dry, superseded by a sour taste of bile.

But his loyalty to the AWC never wavered. He would obey. He had no fear. To please the Grand Keeper and receive his acknowledgement would be a rare honour.

Taking off the safety catch, he moved to the stone coffin, and without looking at her, blasted off a shot into each foot. She made no sound apart from a frothy gurgle, fully aware of all the pain, but no sound could escape her. Gallo barely blinked. He reached down and placed the muzzle on the back of her hand and cracked off another shot, and then proceeded to do the same to the other hand.

Her stricken body gave a series of involuntary judders.

He put back the safety catch and moved over to the prayer bench. His breathing barely altered and his heart remained steady.

In the quietness of the place he thought of what he had done and pride surged through him. He had not failed a test that most men would falter at, and he had not been found wanting. His lips moved in silent prayer as he recited the Sacred Oath over and over, *Sacris Sancti Homicidium.*

The prayer expired and the Grand Keeper, careful to keep his face well concealed, gestured for his seneschal to stand with a wave of his hand. He pointed to the stone tomb the woman lay in.

She continued to breathe with chest-breaking heaves, soaked in copious amounts of blood that continued draining slowly from her.

"Her time has come," crackled the electronic voice of the Grand Keeper. "We shall give her grace and an opportunity to be baptised in holy and redemptive waters." With one great heave, he pulled the stone lid over her and closed her coffin. Where he had drilled the hole in the back end of the lid, he inserted the polyurethane tube with a tight push. A massive tank of water was then wheeled over in a trolley, and a valve complete with a tap was attached to the other end of it.

"I have blessed the water in this tank. With Christ's grace, she may be saved from all her sins. The holy water will cleanse her mind, her body and soul. In God's great name, *Sacris Sancti Homicidium.*"

He made the sign of the cross and then released the valve.

Immobile, paralysed … yet, she felt the gurgling cold water begin to envelop her as it splashed across her face, before seeping into all the crevices and corners that completed her as a woman. She gasped for air. An odd streak of warmth, a damp heat across her forehead that defied the chill of the rising water. She commanded her nerves to lift her head. They disobeyed. She could not. The warmth began its inevitable spread and she knew death had gripped her.

They both stood back, and Gallo, taking his cue from the Grand Keeper, bowed his head. It didn't take long for the tank to gurgle its entire contents into the silent coffin. Soon, small drops of reddish brown water began appearing from the other hole at the far end.

It had filled to the top.

"It is done, seneschal. You have shown your mettle and I am pleased. The battle of the seals will soon take place and I am confident you will not flinch nor fail. You may also know that we have in our possession, as ordained by Christ, the six seals of the Blessed John of Patmos. With that knowledge, and of a task well performed, you may go. You will find the same men waiting for you and they will drive you back home. The sinner here will be disposed of. I salute you. Wait for our signal."

In a flood of exaltation, the seneschal turned and began his walk back through the caves. He had discovered more about himself than he would ever have realised. He had been shown the beauty of cleansing, and how it was not a crime but a sacred act worthy of the Most High. He thought of his colleagues and the stupid priest who, as a servant of the Great Whore of Babylon, the Antichrist, got what he deserved. Agar, Carver and Rockwell deserved to be punished … but not yet. Their work would help uncover what was being sought … the blessed Seventh Seal.

Chapter 41

"And when he had opened the Seventh Seal, there was silence in heaven about the space of half an hour. And I saw the Seven Angels, which stood before God, and to them were given seven trumpets."

~ The Book of Revelation: 8:1-2 ~

THEY HAD DECIDED not to report the wall inscription to Ahasver, but keeping it away from Gallo became a different matter. When on site, he knew about everything they found. Keeping it from him would not be easy.

They planned to go to the place where Joshua had discovered the inscription. From what he'd said, he couldn't see a way down and it appeared dark and bottomless. They wanted to see if there was another way in.

As they stood outside a large awning close to the site, Rockwell said, "We need to go in there separately." He looked over his shoulder, attempting to get sight of Gallo; but he was nowhere in sight. "If we all go together, he'll notice that something's going on. I suggest in three-minute intervals, and Josh should go first. You have marked out the route, I believe?"

"That's correct. Also, we need to bring ropes and climbing equipment between us, plus powerful lighting."

"We have all that at the back of my truck. I'll fetch it now." Rockwell moved off to collect it.

"Where's Gallo today, I wonder?" Rachael shielded her eyes and scanned the camp. "He's out there somewhere and he's watching us. I just know it."

"I don't doubt it. I'm wearing the body armour today, and my gun."

"Me too, plus the stun gun."

"Grab these," Rockwell shouted as he threw bright red ropes and a clutch of pitons at Joshua and Rachael. "Right, Josh, you go first and we'll try and look disinterested. Rachael will be three minutes behind you, and me, three behind her. Make sure the route is clearly marked. Go!"

With a wave, Joshua set off into the descending gloom of the approaching cave system.

Less than ten minutes later, they were all inside.

He lay concealed in a natural pit of rocky sand, behind a bunch of spiky bushes up on the hillside. From there, with binoculars, he had a clear view of the site below.

Their unspoken war had begun. Rockwell had assigned him to arrange for the removal of the large clay jars holing the scrolls, which he reluctantly told him about. That was unacceptable behaviour. A sense of exclusion descended on him. He sensed that since the Joshua incident, and the slaughter of the priest, they suspect his involvement. How and why, he couldn't figure out yet. *What do they know?*

They'd side lined him, but he countered it with the thought of the glorious event on hand.

Their behaviour is strange this morning. They definitely know something. He made a swift decision to follow them. Their movements had a forced casualness about them.

The three of them had just entered a different cave system, not the one he'd taken with Dr. Carver previously. They were following Agar, equipped with climbing gear. *Agar's found something … why else would they all be going kitted up with ropes and lights?* He made the decision to follow them, but out of sight.

He checked his kit, flashlights, phone, knife, mesh gloves, helmet, and finally his pistol. If he didn't hurry, he would lose sight of them. Half running, half trotting, he caught sight of Rockwell moving at a relaxed pace further up as he headed deeper into the cave system.

The length of the climb gave Gallo time to consider his meeting with the Grand Keeper. The message and the test could not have been clearer. He had passed. More startling that it was he, Julian Gallo, who had been singled out as an instrument in assisting mankind's destiny.

Soon they were in the dark passageways and rocky overhangs that festooned the system. His light beam moved eerily around the surfaces. He hoped they wouldn't look behind and see the glow from his flashlight. Gallo recognised the route he had taken with Rachael. When he reached the fork dividing the passageway, he saw the markers they left on the wall. They had taken the right fork.

Have they found something? Could it be the Seal? Whatever it is, I've been excluded.

Rachael, and then Rockwell, reached the place where Joshua was waiting.

"Is this it?" Rockwell scanned the darkness of the cave.

"This is it."

"Wow." He peered over the edge, and into the vast gaping maw below him. "Incredible."

"Now, look behind you." Joshua played the beam onto the wall. "Read it and tell me if I'm wrong. You too, Rachael."

Silence.

They read and reread the Hebrew inscription.

"This is just too much..." Rachael whispered. "That has been waiting for two thousand years!"

Joshua read it out aloud in English.

> *Here I the last of ancient seven sleep*
> *My Brothers six wait for I no longer weep*
> *And by John's hand we were carved to proclaim*
> *An end to Mankind's everlasting shame*

The unknown hand of Adil Koury touched their hearts and their imaginations. No more needed to be said. A collective astonishment held them as they turned to gaze into the yawning depths of the pit.

"I believe it. I wish I had sooner, and could have told Father Luke." Rockwell made a rare admission of regret.

"Let's have more light in here." Rachael switched on the extra two she had unstrapped from her back, and the other two did the same. The light revealed the enormity of the space they stood in. The rocky ceiling spread above them like the dome of a vast cathedral.

"If we're going down this pit, how will we do it? I can't believe this place was used without some way in and out. Keep shining around the walls. Maybe it's hidden. Otherwise, we'll have to rappel down."

"Whatever, we have climbing kits with us."

The played their torch beams across the interior cavern walls, but found nothing.

They were about to give up when Rachael gave a jolt. "Hold it. Can you shine your beams where mine is, please?"

Two beams revealed broad steps cut into the sidewalls, almost invisible in the darkness

"You're right, Rachael, that could be our way down." Rockwell spoke excitedly.

Joshua began walking around the immense circumference. "C'mon, you two, get with it."

From where he squatted behind a natural alcove, Gallo had a clear sight of the activity in front of him. Their lights illuminated the entire area.

Even from a distance, he sensed a palpable shift in the atmosphere around them. They had become animated, and were pointing at something across the chasm.

They've found something. What were they reading? I need to look without being seen.

He closed his eyes and imagined the chanting of celestial angels. They were all around him, beckoning him on to a divine destiny. How things had changed. The secret work that he had nurtured and laboured for most of his life will soon come to fruition. His allegiance to the Grand Keeper stood above all else, and he knew he would die for him to complete their sacred task.

He waited and watched them move out of sight as they followed the rim of the crater to the dim far side. He made a note of where they were heading, and guessed they may have found a way down.

Stillness … Breath ascending … the odd drop of falling water.

Crouching low, he made his way to the spot where they had been staring at the wall behind them. He covered his flashlight beam, shielding it with his hands, and allowing only a small ray to shine out. Just enough to search the rocky surface.

It didn't take long to locate.

He read it through, not fully understanding what he had read. The second time … he did.

His grip tightened on the flashlight and his chest constricted. "My God!" he stuttered out aloud. "My God!"

The exalted four wild horses of the Apocalypse, mounted by their black riders, drove through his mind in one glorious gallop. They confirmed the sanctity of his mission.

No longer caring if he was seen or not, he shone the flashlight onto the inscription, and using his mobile phone, took one picture after another. When he thought he had taken enough, he switched off the flashlight, and bent down on one knee. With his head bowed, Dr. Julian Gallo let hot tears streak their way down onto the rocky and blessed soil that lay beneath his feet.

Christ be praised, for I have been selected to help this Holy Battle. The Seventh is here! I must get out of here and tell the Grand Keeper. Ad majorem Dei gloriam!

The use of the Jesuit watchword did not bother him.

Gallo headed back to the entrance fast. He didn't expect the Seal to be found immediately. By the way they were equipped, it looked like they were on a reconnaissance mission. He needed to reach the Grand Keeper with this news.

The time had arrived. Battle lines were to be drawn up.

And then, the thought struck him with force ... They knew.

The time for pretence had ceased.

They must have found out through Agar, or maybe the snivelling little priest. That's why I wasn't invited along today. If they tell Ahasver, my job is finished, and I could end up in jail. The Grand Keeper must be informed, and he will tell me my next move.

Breathing deeply, he stepped out from the dark and into the bright sunlight that dazzled him.

A thousand thoughts raced through his mind.

But nothing less than a message from the Grand Keeper would satisfy him.

Activating the encrypted sequences, he sent his message and the photographs he had taken.

Now, he could only wait.

Chapter 42

AHASVER LEANED BACK in his chair, his eyebrows and forehead creased in concentrated irritation. A long series of messages had threaded through cyberspace via routers and encryption processes, and deciphered across his large plasma screens.

Seneschal Gallo was in a predicament. They had discovered that he was more than just a Deputy Archaeological Director, but an operative of the Keepers. That pipsqueak, Agar, had brought about the situation. Looking at it, he had little doubt he'd taken Carver and Rockwell into his foul schemes.

I should have shot him in this office when I had the chance. I don't often make mistakes.

A bony hand slid the serpent ring around his finger backwards and forwards as he concentrated on his next moves.

Two thousand years of living, endless mistakes, endless triumphs and a pantechnicon of experience, gave him a peculiar insight into the workings of men's minds.

He would have to reveal his identity to the seneschal. A risky process, but the situation had become unique. The entire centuries old purpose of the Keepers stood at the crossroads.

When the Seventh Seal is discovered, there would be blood, much blood. Of that he was certain. For when that time comes, he would initiate the cleansing.

Gallo must continue as if nothing had happened, no matter what the others knew. They could prove nothing.

He sent out a worldwide alert notice.

His next massage, as the University President, summoned Julian Gallo to his private apartment.

"These steps are wider than they looked from up top." Rachael hugged the wall, treading warily on each as she walked behind Joshua, with Rockwell behind her. They were roped together.

"They look as if they were constructed to be hidden from obvious view. I can barely see them even with the torchlight," Joshua said, his voice bounced off the walls in an echo.

"I agree. They look secret."

"We're probably the first people to come down these steps since they were cut thousands of years back."

Their descent was slow and cautious.

None dared look up.

None can see the bottom.

The darkness was deep.

With each step down, it became colder, and there appeared to be no end to it. "Don't worry about it." Rockwell spoke with a shout that reverberated around and around the ghastly columbarium, as if acknowledging its spectral dimension. "Someone had the balls to cut out these steps, so let's take comfort in that. There has to be an end."

Below and above them, the eternal blackness was broken only by the play of flashlight beams. They had been descending for half an hour. Their flashlights illuminated with an unnatural glow the sweating walls around them

"Dropping something from the top, the Seventh Seal perhaps," Rockwell continued, "at sixteen feet per second, the gravitational drop speed would be huge. Whatever was dropped from the top would probably not remain intact once it struck the ground."

"Sssh! Quiet, please." Joshua held up his arm, visible in the torchlight. "Switch off the flashlights."

"What is it?" Rachael whispered.

The entire cauldron became plunged into a tar-like obscurity.

"This looks like hell." Rockwell leant into the sidewall and away from the edge. "What's up Josh?"

"Listen. Can you hear it?"

Three pairs of ears strained to hear through the gloom.

"Yes," They both spoke at once.

"It's like a soft hiss."

"Gas escaping from a pipe?"

"Or water from an underground source?"

"There's something else." Josh added, his tone now wary. "Look in front of me."

They did.

"Shit! What is that?"

"It looks like a blue fairy light, but I know fairies don't exist.'" Rachael placed her hand over her mouth.

"Well, are we going to stand here like part of the scenery or are we going down to have a look?" Rockwell's impatience, as ever, was predictable.

They carried on down. The sound grew louder, the blue light barely changed, but their torches couldn't pick anything out.

A warning shout from Joshua caused them to halt and tighten on the rope that bound them. "There are no more steps. You're about to move onto a slope. There's room for all three of us."

Stepping gingerly, three powerful beams swept and swooped around the entire area, giving it light it had never seen before. They continued forward, looking all around them.

What they saw next came as a shock.

To Gallo's recollection, nobody had ever seen the interior of Ahasver's extensive apartment. Situated in a luxury block on the fifth floor of a highly expensive piece of real estate, it didn't lack impressiveness. The summons had been curt and immediate. His heart pounded at the thought of what it could be about. Had Rockwell stuck the knife in or had Agar? It was unheard of to be called to the private living quarters of such an eminent person.

He pressed the buzzer, aware that a CCTV camera had picked up his presence.

"Dr. Gallo, I can see you. Press the entry button and you will find the lift inside to your left. Fifth floor, door number 507."

"Thank you." Gallo did as he was told. Two men dressed

in black, with the mandatory shades, stood with arms folded in the foyer. They gave him a brief nod.

Who the hell are they?

Within minutes, the chrome plated and glass doors had parted, and he him found himself stepping out onto a gleaming marble surface. There were only two doors on the floor, and number 507 was around the first corner. His shoes sounded loud on the marble.

Before he could announce his presence, there was a metallic click and the door slid open automatically.

"Welcome, Dr. Gallo. Please, come in." Professor Jacob Ahasver walked to greet him and shook his hand. No smile crossed the man's lean hardened features, only a look of unbearable weariness. He towered over Gallo by several inches.

"Please take a seat, Julian, and be comfortable. Let me pour you a drink. A scotch, I believe?" He went to the drinks cabinet.

"Thank you, sir." Gallo's gaze panned around the room. The furnishings were a masterly blend of antique and contemporary. They proclaimed themselves of the highest quality and luxury. A Steinway grand piano stood by the window and on it, and also on the highly polished tables, stood ornate silver-framed photographs of dogs and cats, mementos of a sad and forgotten past. Suspended from the walls were carved framed mirrors and oil paintings that reeled with age. They were all of Christ depicted in various ways, miracles being performed, Lazarus being raised, and crucifixions of all sorts.

Gallo succumbed to a feeling of unease. *What am I here for?*

Ahasver handed him a healthy measure of Scotch in a

heavyweight crystal tumbler. Ice crackled with a tempting resonance on the surface. He poured an ice-cold spritzer alongside of which, he placed a bowl of pitted olives.

Gallo's drink slopped down his trouser front as he stared in disbelief…

The hand that proffered the glass wore a gold ring, carved with a serpent eating its own tail! Confused, he looked up, and his blood began to rush.

Ahasver smiled down at him. "Seneschal Gallo, now you know." His voice slid through the air like dark brown velvet. "Yes, I am he, your Grand Keeper." He held up his gold ring to emphasise the point. "No need for alarm. I asked you here for a number of reasons." He sat opposite Gallo in a large sofa chair. "I'll let you recover and sip your drink. There is much for me to say."

Ahasver saw in Gallo the soul of a man in torment, forever seeking the truth, and forever attempting to hide that what he truly believed. His deep insecurity, and his desire to please those who ranked above him. It had not been hard to read the man's mind. Hadn't he had thousands of years to perfect his skills?

A minute's silence.

Gallo's mouth began to shut, his hands trembled, but his head stopped its disbelieving shake.

"You performed well the other night and proved your worth." Ahasver's words came soft and reassuring. "You believe me now?"

Gallo bent his head low. "I believe you, Master," He did not know whether he should kneel or kiss the Master's hand. He did nothing as confusion ran riot. Tears formed in his eyes.

"Seneschal, there have been complications, and I've had to reveal myself to you. Agar is to be the appointed head of the Guardians. They are stronger than I had calculated ... and very much alive. Father Luke, now rotting in hell, was also a prominent member. They have active cells in most major cities across the world, as do we. However, our quest is the Seventh Seal. I have the six and need the last to complete the prophecy, and proclaim the New World Order on Earth or destroy this planet. Our immediate task is to lay hands on the seal. Agar has alerted Carver and Rockwell of your involvement, as I'm sure you've suspected by now." He sat back and moved the gold ring backward and forwards on his finger as he gauged Gallo's reaction.

He looked dazed.

"Politeness and uncertainty muddle their thinking, so to an extent, and on my instructions, they will include you in their activities. Once the Seventh Seal is found, you are to execute them, and any others who attempt to interfere. Is that understood, seneschal? Do you need assistance?"

The seneschal's throat had a life of its own, as it visibly moved up and down, and his reply sounded a million miles away from the depths of outer space.

"Yes, Master, I will do it. *Sacris Sancti Homicidium.*" He raised both hands as if in prayer, and the shock continued to ripple through him.

"*Sacris Sancti Homicidium.*" Ahasver responded, his eyes ablaze with the zeal of a martyr sacrificing his life for a cause. "When the Seventh Seal is in my hands, our work will escalate. The foul personage in the Vatican, the Pope, will breath his last. We, and with all the might at our disposal, will strike in seventy-seven cities across the globe. There will be chaos, carnage, death, and the overthrow of so-called society. A new Kingdom will arise, and Christ will rule, and we, the Keepers, will pave the way for a new world." His arms and hands spread upwards, and the seneschal bent his knees to the ground and lowered his head.

The Grand Keeper had more secrets to reveal. His voice reverberated around the room and his character was transformed.

"Seneschal Gallo, you will sit back, be quiet, and say nothing. What you are about to hear, only six others know. You must never speak of it to anyone, anywhere, or at any time."

With his aeons of experience, he gauged what his man was experiencing,

"You swear never to repeat what I am to reveal to you? Break your oath and you know what your fate will be."

The reply was hushed and reverent. "I swear."

"So be it." Professor Ahasver, the Grand Keeper, known throughout legend as The Wandering Jew, began his life story.

Chapter 43

THE BLUE GLOW had become stronger and revealed a circular canopy, a catacomb into which the walls had been hollowed out to form the final resting place for innumerable bodies. When the torches were switched off, they could see without trouble.

"What the hell's going on here?' Rockwell whispered with a dash of concern and fear.

"What is this place? How did all these mummified bodies get here? How could they have been carried down here when it took us a very long time to walk down? It doesn't make sense." Joshua stared in amazement around him. "And where's that light coming from?"

Nobody answered.

"Can you believe this?" Rachael pointed out around her to the floor that had now become clearly visible. "It's clear, there's not a mark or a stone chip or whatever on it."

They looked and saw a paved walkway stretching out in front of them, and worn smooth as if by countless feet passing through.

Joshua began firing off his camera in a frenzy of action.

"Where's that light coming from? It can only be a natural phenomenon, a mineral reaction of some sort. What do think

Josh?"

"It could be but there's far too much of it. Light requires a release of energy, and I don't see an energy source anywhere."

"Yes, you're right. This is possibly Fluorite that glows blue under shortwave ultraviolet light. But if it is, it's like nothing science has ever encountered before. Where would the shortwave be coming from?"

'Just a minute." Rachael had picked up on the excited mood. "Doesn't it strike you as weird? You're both archaeologists … have you ever seen a place like this? It's spotless. There's not a speck of dust, only those creepy mummies in the walls. If the man, Adil Koury, had dropped the seal down here, it's obvious it's not here. Over the centuries, someone, grave robbers perhaps, could have found their way down here and stole whatever artefact remained."

"A wild goose chase then, guys?" Rockwell opened his hands and shrugged.

Nobody spoke.

Rachael sat down on the stone floor. She could hear Simon and Josh discussing what to do next. A quiet mood descended on her and their voices sounded far away, before they vanished into nothingness.

She was alone with the blue light, its glow giving her warmth.

By degrees, it began to fill her being. Her heart fluttered, for she understood where she was being led.

She had no fear.

The vision remained as she had seen before. Her arms were spread wide to welcome her. Her wounds visible. Over her mantle, she wore a robe, the shade of blue that filled the columbarium. The blue glow of the Virgin Mother.

Her light.

She smiled and Rachael could see her mouth moving, but there came no sound. Words formulated in her mind like Moses carving out the Ten Commandments.

Rachael, welcome, my dearest child. Do not be afraid for you know me well. I am always here for you. What you seek is not far. It is here, and you must pass through this wall to find it. Your journey will be hard. Humanity awaits. Be brave, and with your friends, guard well what you may find.

Her vision turned and pointed at the far wall, smiled, and vanished in a shimmering haze of colour.

"Don't go … please!" She reached out to her … but she had gone. The others would not be permitted to see her.

"Hey, Rachael, are you ok. You're talking to yourself." Pressure on her shoulder caused her to start. "You look like you've seen a ghost!" Joshua leant over her with a questioning expression.

"Leave me for a minute. I need to think."

"Okay. We'll explore these burial chambers. Maybe we'll find some answers."

Rockwell began scanning the various tombs. He hadn't noticed Rachael.

"You won't find it there." She spoke as if she knew.

"What are you on about" Rockwell snapped.

"They are long gone, the dead bodies." She had no idea where her words came from. They appeared in her mind.

"Early Christianity and the Jewish version of things got mixed up, and took centuries to develop their own distinct voice. Prophecies had to be seen as being fulfilled to give validity to the faiths, if either the Jewish Messiah, or the Christian Christ were to save Zion. It was believed by all that the Messiah, the Christ, would become impure if he came into contact with dead bodies..."

"So much for Lazarus," Rockwell quipped.

She ignored the remark and carried on.

"Vast burial grounds were put into place, like this place here, so the Saviour or Chosen One would not come into contact with the dead. That's why they blocked up the Eastern gates in the Temple of Jerusalem, so that on his Second Coming, allegedly through the Eastern gates and into the temple precincts, he would avoid dead people and remain pure." "Your point being?" Joshua smiled at her.

"I would have thought that was obvious. The Seventh Seal cannot be stored in a place surrounded by truckloads of dead bodies. The seal is alleged to activate heaven into action of some sort, with Christ up front and leading. So, if these stories are true, it's unlikely he'll visit a place like this, is it?"

"Rachael," Joshua pointed out, "if it was dropped from the top it would be here, in pieces maybe, but there's nothing here. Either all the stories were simply allegories, or it had been found long ago and taken by someone."

Rockwell's legendary impatience had begun to simmer. "I see. So, what do you suggest, Rachael, as you seem to know all the answers? We've spent hours getting to this point. And the only two things we found are a load of stiffs, an inexplicable blue light, and a place that's as clean as a nun's toilet. Two thousand years have passed. Finding it is going to be a miracle."

She said nothing, turned, and walked towards the wall her vision had indicated. The blue light shimmered. She didn't know why, but she stretched out her hand and touched it. Again, the light flickered. This time, she hit it harder. The light stuttered once again, and then she saw it.

I was meant to find this.

The inexplicable blue light and the darkness of the encompassing walls overlapped across a triangular section with a small archway behind it.

"Over here, you two." She pointed at the concealed entrance.

At first, neither of the two men could see it, and Rachael had to push Rockwell onto it before he realised what he was looking at.

He peered inside. "Give me some light here." He wriggled through and pulled her through, followed by Joshua.

The air had a distinct odour coming from the rocks. It had the smell of burnt fuses.

They stood still and looked around. Up front, the way forward resembled a long corridor, and the height of the roof reminded them that they were deep underground.

"I'm feeling disorientated." Rockwell gazed in all directions.

"Where the hell does this take us?" Joshua added to the uncertainty.

"Hope you didn't inform Ahasver or Gallo about this?"

"Of course not. I suspect they'll leave us to do the dirty work, and when we find it, they'll remove it from us on the grounds of scientific analysis." The blue light began to flicker once more.

Rachael continued moving and allowed her intuition to guide her.

Walking ahead of Joshua and Rockwell, Rachael suddenly stopped. A small flight of steps arose and appeared to form part of a tunnel.

"Will you look at that?" She called the attention of the men.

Where it led, was not visible, but it shone bright enough for them to switch off their flashlights.

With trepidation, they moved up the steps towards what seemed to be a carved structure.

Draw closer. Do not be afraid. You will know what is required. I have waited for you across two millennia. The time is nigh. Take what you seek.

The voice grew louder in Rachael's mind. As if by a hidden command, Joshua and Rockwell had fallen silent and walked dumbstruck behind her.

As they reached the top of the stairs, Rachael gasped. "My God," Joshua whispered in awe. "It's an angel. Who the hell put that there?"

"Not only is it an angel, it's guarding something." Rockwell added.

Rachael moved in closer. *Why am I not surprised by this? Like I know.*

At the angel's feet lay a box made of stone.

They looked around in astonishment for the portal emitted a light, a glow that pulsed with the rhythm of their voices. It was the blue light that shone through, filling the tunnel and cave.

"I'm not sure what's happening here..." Rockwell sounded apprehensive. "And you, Rachael, get back."

"I can't believe what I'm looking at!" Joshua blinked followed by an incredulous stare. He bent closer. "It's an angel named Asroilu. The Hebrew writing below it says: '*I am the angel*' and following that, but not too clear, is the Hebrew word *Asroilu*. Asroilu is a Guardian Angel who dwells in the Third Heaven, sworn to protect the Seven Seals. Have we found it? Could this be it?"

For a few wonderful seconds, Rachael became enveloped in the light, clothing her in a mantle of blue. Words formed in her mind, imprinted forevermore as they resounded over and over. She spoke them for all to hear.

The Three have found the One
That seeks the Six to form the Seven
To allow Christ's will to be done
And show men the lost path to Heaven.

She held her hands to her head before she collapsed to the ground.

Both men rushed to her side as the blue light faded from her.

"What's happened?" Rockwell cried out. "My God, what was that?"

"Has she been electrocuted? It looked like it." Joshua rolled her over urgently to her side and into the recovery position.

"She's breathing, and her lips are the same colour. It seems like she's fainted."

"Her eyes are opening."

"She's saying something."

Rachael moved to sit up. She smiled. "I'm fine, guys. I was overawed by what was happening. That light! There were words in my head too, and I can still hear and remember them."

She placed her hands on each side of her face and shook her head several times. "No, they're still there." She repeated the verse that was now indelibly printed in her mind.

They looked at each other in speechless amazement.

Awesome silence.

The light from the stone container remained constant. It waited ... like it always had.

"Is this what we've been searching for?" Rockwell pointed at the box lying at the angel's feet. "No digging. No scratching or scraping. It's been sitting there for two thousand years, waiting for us to appear. Then greets us and presents us with a blue light, and impregnates you with a verse. This is beyond science, isn't it? How can we believe this? Who's going to open it?"

"None of us are ... yet, that is." Rachael approached the angel, bowed low, placed her hands around the box, and lifted it.

The first since Adil Koury.

It wasn't heavy and the glow did not diminish.

"This way, fellas. We are going back."

She moved forward in front of them, and they followed without a word being spoken. The light behind them dwindled until the area was once again reclaimed by darkness.

They walked back and reached the steps at the end of the corridor.

"Stop." She looked back at the blackness behind them. They turned with her. "Listen."

At first, there was nothing to hear. Then, the silence was replaced by the rustling of cloth. It got louder and filled the entire space behind them. A massive fluttering.

Josh shouted, "Take cover! That's the sound of wings. It could be bats." "Let's get out of here." Rockwell said as he tried to pull Rachael along.

"Those are not bats." Rachael was unperturbed. She stood motionless, the box in her hands. Without warning, she held it up, as if offering it into the dark. The flapping sound began to lessen, until it too vanished into the inky blackness. "It was Asroilu. He's no longer there. He has flown to where he must be. It's our turn now to guard the Seventh Seal."

They began the long trek upwards. Not a word was spoken. Each one wrapped in a world of possibilities, as a thousand structures in their minds came crashing down.

Ahasver's revelations plunged Gallo from disbelief, then shock, as if a mortar shell had exploded in his brain. That was followed by a gradual acceptance and finally, ecstatic joy.

He believed.

He had forever wanted to believe, and without question. For the first time, he now could. He understood. Life's uncertainties were now banished, and he was made whole. The Grand Keeper, with his ancient wisdom and trust, had healed him, and he would follow him with his dying breath.

With that knowledge, there could be no turning back.

Another large drink was passed to him, one that his trembling hand could scarce hold.

Ahasver spoke, "All is revealed, seneschal. It is most rare for it to be so. Not since the days of our great Cosimos Ricci has the Grand Keeper's identity been revealed to the outer circle. I recall watching Cosimos, our great transformer, react in the same way as you. When came his turn. I, unbeknown to anybody, guided him on his way. Today, I am the Grand Keeper and have been so only two other times, but have always been in the midst of our activities. We face our biggest challenge at this moment." He stared hard at Gallo. "What of the Seventh? We have reached the time when disclosure of who we are is almost upon us. We have men in the hills and in their digging teams to report back everything they see or hear. Rockwell has not submitted his synopsis of this new excavation site, nor his plans for the dig, and I must assume that is deliberate. You, seneschal, have been identified as the enemy, and I suspect they have an idea of me. However, all they have right now are their assumptions. They have no evidence. That meddling servant of Satan, Father Luke, discovered something, that's why he had to be executed. The same will happen to them all. If they find the seal, there will be no more need to cover our tracks. The world will know who we are." A centrally mounted green light began to flash on one of the screens affixed to the back wall. A stream of letters and numbers gavotted from one to the other.

Gallo, wallowing in the glow of his newly found importance, could only watch as Ahasver's serious expression began to change into one of supressed hope. After reading the meaningless jumble, he switched off the array and turned.

"There has been a development. Rockwell and the others have returned, and were seen to be carrying a heavily wrapped bundle which they took away in their Land Rover. What is your assessment, seneschal?"

"It is against all rules and protocol to remove items from a site. For a start, they have to be identified, classified and catalogued, together with positioning, photographs, and so on. You know all that, Master."

"We have to put into operation my first move. The gloves, as it is said, are now off. Our AWC legions are awake and ready. For the present, our relationship with Agar and the two will remain as if nothing has changed. Now go and do what I told you."

Chapter 44

Vatican City

CARDINAL PACCA HAD always prided himself on his ability to carve a roasted chicken or goose. But on this occasion, a small quail would put his skills to a sterner task.

Riario, the Papal Camerlengo, and fellow Cardinal, stood beside him. They had received a call to arms to be in readiness for Judgement Day. The roles they were about to play filled them with an intense excitement.

Years of planning in secrecy has finally come to this. There could be no mistakes. The test on Adam the dog had proved successful. Now, they needed to test it on a human being.

For their trial run, they chose the important figure of the Commander of the Papal Swiss Guard, Gabriel Bernasconi. They reasoned that if the hemlock-ridden quail worked as they hoped, then the Commander would be one major obstacle removed.

The meal was prepared, and they would all be eating the same, except their quails would be clean of hemlock. It would be a terrible accident. How were they to know what a quail had eaten before it was slaughtered?

They told the Commander their meal celebrated an annual event to give thanks to the Swiss Guard for their loyalty and service. What more could two poor Cardinals do?

The meal that early afternoon was convivial. Quantities of dessert wine flowed like the Niagara. Not long after the courses were finished, the unsuspecting Commander had begun to sweat, clasping at his stomach.

"I think I've eaten too much … Aaagh!" He bent double, as unbeknown to him, his death had commenced after the first mouthful. Unseen and stirring within the membranes and muscular structures of his body, the hemlock had begun the painful process of shutting down his internal organs.

His teeth gritted. "Something's wrong here. I must use your toilet, please."

"Of course, Commander. I'm sure it will pass." Cardinal Riario was, as ever, smooth and full of sympathy."

Commander Bernasconi staggered to the door.

His mind was still clear as he sat in agonising pain on the toilet seat, his pantaloons around his ankles, now unable to move as paralysis gripped his limbs in pure torment. He was fully conscious but rigid, unable to speak or even move his lips.

His lucid mind was transformed into a torture chamber of horrors. He never returned from the toilet.

Two hours later, Cardinal Pacca braved the stench and opened the toilet door. Riario was behind him. "I think he's gone. Look."

Riario placed a large napkin over his nose and mouth before looking. The Commander of the Papal Swiss Guard's position remained the same as when he had first sat on the seat. His unseeing eyes stared blankly and manically into nothing that could be seen.

"Quite dead," Pacca said.

"Quite. Let's get some people here to get rid of him. Now we know it works, and what his Holiness will have to endure for his sins."

They made the sign of the cross over the seated body.

"*Sacris Sancti Homicidium*"

The oath got lost in the wall tiles and the rigid remains of a drained man sitting on a lavatory seat.

Chapter 45

IT LOOKED AS if something of importance had been discovered.

Have they found the Seventh Seal?

Gallo's mouth went dry as he tiptoed to the bolted door and pressed his ear to it. He could hear them. The guard he sent around to the rear, but with his communication device switched on, was to report back on what he could see.

Rachael pulled aside the material she had covered the casket in. They leaned forward, not knowing what to expect.

"The blue glow's gone." She observed.

Joshua ran his finger around the rim. "Where could the light have come from? It's sealed tight. I remember the same glow from the other casket, but it was weaker compared to what this did, and the box had been open then."

Rockwell reached over and picked it up. "It's not heavy, and it looks as if it was made yesterday. What do we do, guys? Open it?"

"Well, if we don't ... we'll never know."

"With what we all experienced down there, this has to be something special."

"Look," Rockwell looked thoughtful. "This has to be opened up in laboratory conditions. We don't know what's in there, and what the source of that light was. It's too risky to open it here, or for it to be left with you two, or me. You've both been roughed up one way or another." He covered the box with the cloth again. "Neither Gallo nor Ahasver must know of this. Who knows what they're planning to do next? But I'm certain we are being watched. If this is the seal, then they'll do anything to get hold of it. For now, I'll take this for safekeeping and deposit it in my own security deposit box at the Discount Bank in the Yeshuda Halevy district. You all okay with that?"

They both nodded.

"It should be safe. Nobody knows what we have yet. I'll take it there now and collect it in the morning. Later, we can open it up in the lab. It's waited centuries, so one more day shouldn't harm it. Okay, let's go."

Rockwell opened the door to a deserted corridor and they headed out of the building. Outside, he stood on the step and looked around. Not a soul was in sight.

"Are you all still carrying your weapons and wearing the Kevlar?" Joshua asked.

"You bet." Rachael patted her shirt pocket.

"Me too. Let's hope the police don't stop and search us!"

Chapter 46

The following morning…

THE SCRUFFY FIAT estate car with false plates cruised up and down Herzi Street. The driver had a clear view of Yehuda Ha-Levi Street, home of the Discount Bank. He glanced at his watch.

Nine-thirty … as expected.

His quarry was on the move, walking at a brisk pace towards the bank. He eyed him up and down, and gauged that the tall figure of Rockwell would be no problem. Parking the car, he rolled it to a stop alongside a blue and white curb parking stretch. He didn't have a ticket, but wasn't expecting to be long. From previous encounters, he knew that ticket inspectors wouldn't be around for another hour.

He disembarked. He fitted in with the customers; dressed in a dark business suit, an open collar and tieless blue Ben Sherman shirt. A small badge was pinned to his lapel.

A serpent eating his own tail.

His fat pilot's crew bag shone as bright as his shoes. Rimless silver spectacles added scholarly menace to his close shaven head. He had no fears. A foot soldier of AWC could expect nothing but glory.

He reached the doors at the same time as Rockwell. With a polite smile, he opened the door and let him in first.

The cool reception area exuded an airy, ultra-modern, minimalist design. The ceiling hosted suspended lighting, plus discreet CCTV cameras. The man didn't doubt there were concealed ones as well.

A well-groomed and pretty woman smiled at Rockwell.

"I've come to inspect my deposit box. Here's my passport, and I've written my security code on the holding pass I retrieved from you yesterday.

"Of course, Mr. Rockwell, I remember you. Welcome back." She pressed a number of digits and letters onto the computer screen. "Yes, you are now expected. Take the lift to the fifth floor. The room is to your right and here are the digital keys for cubicle 517. This key will let you in. This other key will open your box." She handed him both. "It's unique to you and will open no other box apart from your own. Press the green button once you're inside, and your box will be delivered automatically through the chute in the room. When you've finished your business, press the red button, and your box will be returned to our vault. Please remember that you will not be able to leave the room until you press another button, the yellow one mounted near the door. When the guard arrives, you will hand him your key, which had been rendered useless by our computer system when you pressed the red button." She gave a sweet smile. "Have a good morning, Sir."

Rockwell nodded and moved off down the corridor. The man studying the information board heard every word the woman had said. He turned to follow him, undetected by the foyer guards who were more intent on watching the female celebrity who had just walked in, and not wearing very much.

Hanging back, he watched the voluminous glass and chrome lift slip into the bay, as the metallic doors slid open without a sound, allowing Rockwell to enter.

Rockwell pressed button five and ascended upwards.

The lift next to it arrived on the bay, and the man stepped in. He too pressed button five.

Room 517 was unremarkable and had been designed for a minimum stay. Two hard chairs and a viewing table filled it, and in the corner stood a water dispenser. Everything was as the receptionist had described.

Rockwell pressed the green button. He heard a soft whirring sound, followed by a soft thump, before the shutter opened to reveal his deposit box. He removed the stone casket, sat in the chair, and began to examine it, turning it this way and that, and not without a sense of awe.

He felt a strong urge to open it.

Standing up, he went to get a cup of water from the water cooler, and sat back down.

No immediate rush. He wanted a few moments to place his thoughts into a logical perspective.

The security clerk sat behind a low wooden desk surrounded by an array of computers and monitors. He raised an eyebrow. Professor Simon Rockwell was the only person on his work agenda that morning. Who could the person be, heading his way at speed?

The alarm bell that rang in his head got cut short in a nanosecond, as a silenced 9mm bullet made its way through his brain.

"*Sacris Sancti Homicidium.*" The man muttered almost as a matter of course, before leaning over and removing the guard's security tag. He placed it around his own neck plus his peaked cap.

He turned to watch the bank of screens. A red dot flashed over the number 517 to indicate the business had been completed. He waited for the yellow light to request an exit. It wasn't long in coming. Adjusting his clothing and allowing the ID tag to hang down his chest, knowing people never looked at them, he made his way to cubicle 517, took a deep breath, and pressed the exit button. The lock clicked and the door swung open.

"Thank you," Rockwell muttered as he handed the man the defunct key. In his other hand and chained to his left wrist, hung a very full looking brown leather holdall.

"Everything okay, sir?" The security man took off his glasses and placed them in his top pocket.

"Fine. Thank you," he replied, turned, walked to the lift, and pressed the summons button.

The guard moved back behind him and to his left. When the lift door opened, Rockwell noticed from the corner of his eye that the guard got into the lift as well. He was rummaging inside his jacket and took out a handheld communication device.

"It will be with you later. Cut off will be performed." His voice, low and suspicious, caused Rockwell to experience a sudden jab of alarm.

The man leant across and pressed the stop button.

Without a vibration, the lift came to a halt.

"What the hell…" Rockwell turned to find himself staring at a 9mm supressed Beretta M9A3 pistol.

He lurched to the right, swinging the bag chained to his wrist in a fast curving arc that struck the weapon as it discharged a round with a soft *whoomp* sound into the side wall. Rockwell continued his pivot as his shoulder crashed into the man's lower chest, and the chained bag swung around the man's neck. His handheld radio fell to the floor, but his grip on the gun remained tight as a vice. A disembodied voice spluttered from the set.

"Pharaoh! Pharaoh! What's happening?"

The would-be killer tried another shot over the back of his shoulder, but Rockwell had seen that coming, and increased the pressure of the chain around the man's throat, tightening with every ounce of his strength. The pressure forced the man to drop the gun as he tried to grab at the chain. Rockwell's knee crashed in behind his, and the man clattered down to his knees. His face had transformed into a mass of violet fury. Mouth open and sucking in air, the man bared his yellow teeth and somehow produced a knife. Amidst the gurgling, he attempted vicious stabs at Rockwell's stomach, but to no avail, as the knife encountered a hidden vest of hi-tech Kevlar.

Rockwell, using the weight of the bag, forced the man's head down to the floor. He struggled to stand but Rockwell, realising that his life hung in the balance, had found unexpected strength. Using the chain as a lever, he jerked the man's head back, and smashed it into the steel floor of the lift repeatedly. The man gave an agonised grunt, and finally, the knife dropped. Enough chain dangled for another loop around the man's neck. Rockwell wound the last length of chain and gave a final tug, and the man's eyes bulged, his skin turning an ugly shade of grey.

"Who sent you? Ahasver? Tell me or you're going to fucking choke to death. If you think I wouldn't, you'd better think again." Rockwell, a man transformed, gritted his teeth and pulled the chain tighter.

The man made a desperate grab for the Beretta across the floor. Rockwell's heavy booted foot smashed down on the bony fingers.

"Aaah!" His screech of pain struggled to escape as the chain cut off his airways.

"Tell me! Did Ahasver send you? Tell me now or you're going to die in this lift. Speak, damn you!"

The man spluttered in the last throes of consciousness. "No ... no ... no!" The crackled words bubbled and gurgled on a frothy emission of bloody phlegm now pouring from his fleshy mouth.

"WHO?"

Rockwell bent his head closer to hear him. Using both hands, he gave the chain one last almighty pull with his knee pressed hard into the man's back.

The man's voice rattled and Rockwell heard his deathly whisper. "Seneschal Gallo ... you can't stop us ..."

"Holy Christ!" Rockwell half yelled. What he never wanted to believe was true. He stamped down hard onto the man's back, and stood up, giving a savage jerk on the chain. The man's head swung back at an odd angle and blood began to seep over the links. He unravelled the linkage and looked at the man.

Dead.

His face had become a blotchy red and purple canvas of

swollen skinny blood vessels.

Rockwell had never killed anybody before, even in self-defence.

It didn't feel good and all he could feel was an overpowering desire to vomit.

He suppressed it.

Sweat, in large globules, broke out on his forehead.

I have to think.

A semblance of reality came back into focus.

He had to get out fast. People would be wondering why the lift had stopped working.

With a hefty pull, Professor Simon Rockwell dragged the body into the corner of the lift and booted the gun alongside him. He didn't need it. He'd forgotten that he had been carrying his own.

He activated the descent button.

As the lift door opened, he expected trouble from the guards manning the CCTV cameras, but the area looked empty. He had stopped at an empty floor.

The doors closed behind him. With his heart pounding, and still holding on to the bag, he casually strode back down the corridor, smiled goodbye to the receptionist, and stepped out into the welcome fresh air.

Chapter 47

GALLO GLANCED AT his watch several times and twirled the ring on his finger. He should have heard from his legionnaire but he hadn't made contact. He'd sworn the oath and been given every piece of information he needed. Why hadn't he heard from him? It had all been going to plan. For a soldier like Pharaoh, an experienced assassin, this was a simple operation.

Something wasn't right.

He pushed his chair back from the desk and knelt on one knee, offering up a prayer for the success of the operation. He then stood and gave another glance at his watch, and at the same moment looked out to the area leading up to the university. Right then, he knew Pharaoh had failed. Rockwell could be seen hurrying across the open space to his own office.

Worse.

He carried a heavy looking bag, and looked like a man on a mission.

The Grand Keeper would have to be informed. Not a task he relished, but it had to be done.

His phone rang. He knew it to be his seneschal and no longer had any need for distorters or scramblers.

"Good news, seneschal?"

"No, Master. He has failed. Rockwell is back and carrying a large bag."

There came an uncomfortable pause.

Ahasver's voice hinted at frustration. "We now revert to my other plan. You, seneschal, are to disappear. You are not to be seen here. Your role in this operation has been compromised. There is too much evidence pointing your way. Go to Rome today and to the Hotel Crowne Plaza, near the Vatican. You will be booked in and then contacted. The words used by your contact will be, 'I hear the Pope's not well.' Your reply, 'God bless him.' From there you will be given further orders and instructions. Understood?"

"Yes, Master. It is understood."

The call terminated.

Joshua felt pleased to be alone for once with Rachael. Her place as always quiet, orderly, and with a sense of peace about it. There had been so much action and tension that the opportunity of having a normal conversation had not been possible. He had considered asking her out on a date, but he knew her attraction to Rockwell would rule that out. Flirting was about as far as it ever got.

They expected Rockwell back from the bank very soon. They couldn't wait to see what the casket contained. Hopefully, it would answer some of their questions.

Their wait ended sooner than expected.

The door crashed open, and a pale-faced, distraught looking Rockwell fell into the room.

"A large drink, now! A very large one! Oh my God!" He unchained the bag from his wrist and collapsed into the nearest chair.

Rachael knelt next to him and Josh poured the drink, which was taken by a very shaky hand.

"What's happened?"

"Someone tried to kill me, but I killed them instead." He ran his hand through his thick hair. "Oh shit! Gallo had ordered it!"

"What! Gallo got somebody to try and kill you for this?"

"It looks that way. Give me a moment, please." He took a throaty swig from the tumbler. "This is what happened." Rockwell ran through the morning's events, up until the point where the man named Gallo as the mastermind.

"Do we know if Ahasver is involved?"

"How can he not be? From what we know, he's up to his eyeballs in it. They want the seal, and we don't even know that's what we have here."

"Fuck this. There's only one way to find out, and bollocks to archaeological protocols." Joshua pulled out the casket from Simon's case, produced a tempered solid steel surgical knife, and with short sharp strokes, began unsealing what had been dormant for two thousand years. He made the last cut as paper-like flakes of stone dust resembling dandruff floated to the floor.

The enclosing lid was free.

He moved the lid to one side by a fraction, and they all held their breath. To their wonderment, a spur of soft blue light escaped from every side of the lid. For a moment, it enveloped them like a small gust of wind before it swirled away into nothingness.

"What the hell!" Joshua jumped back with a vicious start, his arms extended in front of him as if to block whatever they've set free.

"Holy shit!" Rockwell's eyes were wide as saucers. His attempted murder forgotten.

Rachael said nothing, but a small smile crossed her face. Placing her palms together, she spoke. "I think we can all agree that's the same blue light that led us from the columbarium."

She never left me. I knew it.

"This doesn't make scientific sense." Rockwell spluttered.

Joshua recovered and with great care, began to slide the lid to one side. It made the softest of grating sounds.

All three of them had forgot the dilemma that had brought them to this point.

'Oh wow. Just look at that." Rockwell snapped on his latex gloves before reaching inside. It was a seal. There were seven in number. Clearly it was part of the other set. The missing Seventh. He held them up like a new-born baby.

"Look," said Joshua, jabbing his finger at the sides, "the hinges are exactly the same as those on the other six."

"So they are. Where are the other six? They are just as far apart as they ever were."

"Can you see what's written on it?"

"It's hard to make out, but there's some writing."

Rockwell peered closer. "And on the other side, there's a faded painting of sorts ... looks like angels blowing trumpets."

Rachael stared at them both. "What intrigues me is why this one got separated from the others. What's its secret? What's its importance? There has to be something, or these Keeper murderers wouldn't be trying to get their hands on it so much."

"We're in a fix." Joshua looked at Rockwell. "And so are you. Police are bound to come sniffing, and on the other side, we have Gallo and his merry men, plus the creepy Ahasver. Where do we keep this seal, and how do we get the others back? From Nathaniel's records and papers, I can make a general alert call to the worldwide network of Guardians, but that won't help us individually. We're in great danger. They know we have something, which they want. Killing us is not a problem for them."

Rockwell reached for the phone.

"What are you doing?"

He didn't answer, and punched out a three-numbered extension. After eight rings, there was no reply.

"Who was that?"

"It's Gallo's extension. He's not there. I was going to invite him over to have a look at what we have."

"That would have been fun, but what do we do now?' Rachael spoke but couldn't stop staring at the seal. It seemed to call to her with a message she couldn't yet understand.

From within, she felt a stirring that had its roots in an ancient past, a history she felt part of. *Let it pass ... Let it pass...*

"We have to hide the seal." Her voice came disconnected from herself, as if another voice spoke from inside her. "In plain sight, it has to be hidden like a pebble on a beach. Give it to me."

Without knowing why, Rockwell handed her the seal.

Its touch sent a warm sensation up through her arm, that then spread throughout her mind and body. It lasted only a second, but enough for her to feel deeply attached to and part of the structure of the enigmatic tablet. "This place is ideal." She opened the food cupboard and placed the ancient seal upright between two cans of tinned fruit. "We tell nobody we have it or where it is. They're bound to come calling on us soon, and there is nothing we can do to prevent that. Simon, you take the casket and put it amongst the others you have on display. Nobody will notice it sitting with your collection. Now, we go everywhere with our Kevlar and pistols. I still have my stun gun. Somehow, we have to unite this seal set with the others to find out what this is all about. For now, we go about our duties as usual. We do not speak to Ahasver or Gallo, when or if we see them. They can lead us to the others, so let's pretend we know nothing about their involvement. Agreed?" Rachael stopped speaking, amazed at what she was saying, as if she had become a leader.

Rockwell and Joshua looked at each with raised eyebrows. "Agreed," they replied in unison. Nothing was going to be the same again. Both knew it.

Chapter 48

AHASVER DISLIKED UNDRESSING or getting into showers, for there were things that only he could see.

This morning was no different from the other seven hundred thousand that had gone before.

When he awoke, he peeled off his pyjamas and stood naked in front of the mirror to look at his two-thousand-year-old tattooed body.

Ancient with age, his tiredness hung from him like a forgotten graveyard, but his body looked the same as it always had, and in excellent condition.

Externally, nothing looked wrong. He appeared to be as healthy as a normal man half his age. But he, with his eternal eyes, could see the reality hidden from the view of others. Inwardly, he could see what they could not … the never-ending, pain ridden, cancerous ravages of disease that would never ever go away nor kill him. For two thousand years, it had constancy, and the unique ability to cast its infliction into every pore of his being. It lingered, a mere but constant suggestion. He stared at what only he could see; the inner sweeping blotches, some raggedly purple, and others etched in a red and yellow hue, and covered in blankets of transparent flaky skin. They were his internal badge of sores.

Since that day, they had never let him forget. There were days he expressed gratefulness for them, for they kept worse things from his mind. On other days, when the sores surfaced and erupted, they reminded him of his sins and the curse he had been chained to. They came, gave pain, and then vanished.

He had become detached from humanity.

The time approached when reality would return. He sensed that. He had wanted to weep, but no tears had flowed since that day – but the time is near.

Woe, woe, woe, to the inhabiters of the earth …

He gazed into his ancient aged eyes. He was one step away from redemption, the leader of Christ's new kingdom on earth.

Following student unrest, and the unwanted murders and events that hinged around the archaeology faculty, the University President announced a beefing up of security processes.

Every member of staff, and all student quarters connected with the department, would be required to subject themselves to inspections, and upgrades installed into their computer systems. After all, the threat of terrorism was never far away.

The one he wanted to access the most … Rachael Carver's.

She would be the conduit to what he sought in more ways than one. Exchange, or a promised exchange, would hardly be a robbery.

Built into his scheme, he sent out a notification to all departments concerning the temporary absence of Dr. Julian

Gallo, who had suffered from a serious medical condition that required immediate attention. He asked everyone's prayers for his full recovery. There was nothing anybody could say or do about it. If they did, they would be made to look ridiculous.

All that was left now was to recover the last set of seals which he knew the three had discovered.

It had been over a week since Gallo was 'taken ill' and they had not heard or seen anything suspicious since then. The dig in the caves proceeded as scheduled, and revealed the astonishing structures of an early Christian settlement that had been hidden from view.

Rachael wondered why there had been no further attempts to acquire the seal. No approaches had been made or any that looked suspicious. All had gone eerily silent. Every day, she would check her cupboard to ensure the artefact remained where she had put it.

Today was no different from yesterday. It was still there.

As Rachael sat pondering, an image of Simon came to her. Her attraction for him was on the wane. His impatience and short temper was more than she had realised. Yet, seeing him stagger in from his attempted murder stirred in her a desperation for him. Seeing him so vulnerable broke her heart.

She loved him more when he became human. She doubted he would ever take notice of her.

That morning, Rachael had to wait for the electricians and

security people who were arriving to replace the old system. She didn't have to wait long before the buzzer alerted her to their arrival.

Opening the door, she was greeted by two burly men, with shaven heads, wearing blue overalls, and their pockets full of small tools, pencils and pens. They carried metal fold up tool cases and wore plastic I D cards hanging from green lanyards.

"You're the security fitters? Please come in."

They held up their plastic identity cards. The taller man smiled and spoke. "Thank you, Doctor. We need to explain what we will do. We will examine every room in detail and decide what can or cannot be fitted. Once we're done, you will be safer than Fort Knox. Emergency calls will be possible from anywhere in the house. You will be given instructions on how to operate the system, and what to do in an emergency."

"Okay, where do you want to start?"

"The kitchen first, as we always do."

"Let's go. After you." As he moved forward, she turned and noticed the shorter man hadn't moved. He stood with his back against the door, motionless, legs apart, and a cold look in his eye. "Aren't you coming?" she asked.

"Don't worry about him, Doctor," the man in front said. "He's there to make sure you don't escape."

She thought she had misheard. "What did you say?" A twinge of fear hit her.

He didn't reply.

It was as if the next moment was replayed in slow motion from some meaningful movie.

The man had turned, and his hard, bony tattooed fist slammed into the side of her face. Rachael dropped to one knee, unable to make a sound, as her head jerked sideways at speed. She tried to scream, but a paralysing blow to the throat cut it short.

She hit the floor.

Her assailant dragged her into the lounge area. She remained conscious, and could see the other man systematically rummaging through every part of the house. Nothing was spared.

"Where is it? Where's the seal damn you? We know you have it." A fierce backhand across her face sent her senses screaming.

"I don't know what you're talking about." She managed to splutter through the blood dripping from her nose.

"Don't be stupid. This'll end up badly for you if you don't talk."

She held her breath. The other man, now in the kitchen, had begun pulling it apart. From somewhere in the house, she heard the phone ringing and then it abruptly stopped, the line ripped out. The only sound she heard next were the cupboard contents hitting the floor. Her heart sank.

He's going to find it.

Rachael waited for the triumphant sound of discovery. But it never came.

He didn't see it.

The seal remained unrecognisable, and she knew it would be lying on the floor amongst all the cupboard tins, packets and drawer contents spread about.

"We have our instructions, Doctor, and that's a pity for a nice girl like you. Are you still saying you don't know where it is?" With a vice like grip, he pulled her up with a savage tug on her hair. "Still no, is it?"

She shook her head and gasped 'No" through swollen lips.

The other man moved in close and wrenched her arms behind her back, tearing at the sleeve of her shirt to expose her upper arm.

"No, no, please don't do this." Rachael knew it would end badly for her. She tried to wriggle free, but the hold got tighter.

He took a small black pouch from his back pocket, and unzipped it to produce a hypodermic syringe. With one swift movement, he plunged the contents into her bare upper arm.

The pain caused her to jump. "My God, please … no! What have you done?"

She began falling … her face cold … drifting … sliding down as if in a warm tunnel. Then, total blackness. "She gone. It'll be hours before she wakes up," said the man with the needle. "Let's roll her up."

Together, they dragged her over to the edge of the floor carpet. Within minutes, they had her tightly rolled up and concealed within. They gathered all their equipment into their large black Peugeot van parked outside. Next, they lifted the carpet with Rachael inside on their shoulders, and placed it in the van. The driver gunned the vehicle and vanished in a squeal of rubber, out of the complex and up the highway.

Chapter 49

Rome

THAT MORNING, THE *Via Aurelia Antica* sounded as busy as usual. From the balcony of the Hotel Crowne Plaza, Gallo stared down at the tourist traffic that forever wound its way around the *Villa Pamphili Park,* heading towards Vatican City and the dome of Saint Peter's, visible in the near distance. Its structure now assumed a deadlier significance.

Forever aloof, a loved and hated monument, it would soon witness its own destruction.

Below him, the hotel's exquisite swimming pool glistened benignly in the rising sun.

Later that morning, around an elegant circular table, he leant back in the blue and white striped chair and dipped a croissant into his Bicerin; a combination of chocolate, espresso and whipped cream drink, before giving it a hungry bite. The years of waiting were almost over. He could sense it in the air, and he had been feeling a constant buzz, like electricity, coursing through him. Before he could finish the croissant, the vibration of his mobile alerted him to an encrypted call. He knew what it would be about.

"Yes," he answered.

A gravelly voice replied, "I hear the Pope is unwell."

"God bless him," Gallo gave the required reply.

The voice continued. "Preparations are being finalised and this evening, you will be called upon. A message will soon be left for you at the reception desk of your hotel. You will follow it to the letter. Understood, seneschal?"

"Understood."

The line went dead.

Gallo quivered. Not only did he know the identity of the Grand Keeper, but now, they entrusted him with what could only be highly secret developments. God's smile fell upon the Keepers, and if he smiled on them, he smiled on seneschal Gallo.

Chapter 50

RACHAEL CARVER RESEMBLED a cadaver.

Consciousness had returned, and she lay flat out on her back, bound. With trepidation, she opened her eyes to assess her predicament. At first, the memories of her assault overwhelmed her, but knowing her ruse had worked and they didn't find the seal gave her a rush of satisfaction. Rachael knew there would be a price to pay, and didn't doubt it had already begun.

Her face ached, and she sensed bruising everywhere, but her calm surprised her.

Turning her head, she attempted to see where they had brought her. The space appeared dark and small. It looked like a stone cave or dungeon. She guessed she lay on a stone table or slab. It felt cold beneath her back. Recalling the fate of Father Luke, she wondered if she was next.

How much pain can I tolerate before I tell them where it is?

As the winding tendrils of panic crept through her mind, the disturbing thoughts were replaced by memories of the blue figure of the ageing Mother Mary visiting her.

With the thought came a warm sensation that engulfed her inner being. It spread upwards from her toes like a small tidal flow. At first, she thought she had been drugged, but no

… this defied explanation. Filling her mind came resurrected and long buried memories that went back to her childhood, her first communion, and her shaky belief in God. The dress she wore shone in her mind as clear as a ray of sunshine. At a young age, she had concluded that the whole God thing could be nothing but a man-made construct. She couldn't recall the last time she attended Mass, or went to confession. These rituals had no meaning for her. Her work in archaeology had given her access to many marvellous, long-lost religious artefacts, but it wasn't their meaning that buzzed her. It was the knowledge, the discovery, unearthing the legacy of people long gone, all of which contributed to the unravelling of mankind's history.

But now, she found herself murmuring a prayer for her safety and deliverance. As she did, her predicament became bearable. Her captors would have been disappointed

The comforting warmth stayed with her. How long, she couldn't tell. But when it withdrew, she could feel the stealthy fingers of icy coldness begin their assault. Her body began to shiver.

Lifting her head as far as possible, she could make out some sort of chamber that was half lit by an unknown source. Against the wall stood an altar of sorts. Surrounded by seven lambent candles and a burning censor, stood a tall, wide triptych. Through the half-light, she could see it adorned with hellish looking paintings, not unlike those of Hieronymus Bosch. In front of it stood a worrying looking stone sarcophagus, the size of a coffin. Small chambers led off from the various sidewalls to unknown areas. On the far side, a burning brazier glowed red. Smoke ascended upwards through a natural vent in the rocks.

A smell hung in the air. She recognised it as frankincense. *What is this place?* Attempting to wriggle from her restraints achieved nothing.

A voice from behind startled her. Its booming tone chanted, loud and with passion, as if from a medieval monastery. Whoever was chanting had come to a halt behind her, and repeated the incantation several times, almost Gregorian in its cadence. She tried stretching her neck backwards but to no avail.

To him that overcometh will I
Give to eat of the hidden manna
And I will give him a white stone
And in the stone a new name.

The chanting stopped, and a dark silence descended into the area.

After a while, a voice spoke, "Welcome, Dr. Carver. Our apologies for your lack of clothes but it was necessary to relieve you of your protective equipment." The voice reverberated with electronic distortion. The man moved around to her front. Dressed in a pure white monastic robe with black edging, the thick and heavy cowl concealed his identity.

Long bony fingers wrapped around something she recognised, and her heart froze like a block of ice.

In his hands, he held the ossuary, containing the six seals stolen from Joshua's safe. He turned to face the small altar and held the box aloft as he muttered a string of prayers, like incantations, before placing the ossuary in front of the triptych. He knelt on one knee, bowing his head, and then lifting his head upwards and calling out in a loud voice, "*Sancti Sacris Homicidium.*"

This he did three times. Standing upright, he bowed and turned to her.

"Our sacred mission is almost complete. A wondrous new age is upon us. You must believe that my unhappiness is soon to cease, and yours is just about to begin. You know what we seek. The six wishes to become seven. Are you going to stand in the way? By cooperating, you can avoid distress and pain when the final process is complete. So where is it, Dr. Caver?" He stood close behind her.

"I've no idea what you are talking about."

"I thought you would say that, and no doubt, you will continue to say so. I will not waste my breath on explanations. I have prepared for this moment. The four natural elements of earth, fire, water, and air, were given by God for us to use. By one of these, you will die, and sooner than you expect. The fate of Professor Rockwell and Joshua Agar will be the same. God has willed it. Dr. Carver, I give you this last chance to escape pain and misery, and save your friends. Answer this simple question ... Where is the seventh set of seals?"

Rachael swore she could see fire burning in his eyes from the depths of the hood.

"Go to hell!"

He laughed. "I am well acquainted with it. For centuries, I've walked in its landscapes, it's repulsive temples and churches. I am in hell, and I have dwelt too long in this place. But soon, my penance will be over and I will be released. You, however, your torment is just about to begin. We shall talk again. Meanwhile, I need you to sleep." From beneath his robe he produced a small syringe. He held it up, tapped the end of the needle, turned, and plunged it into her arm, on the fleshy area of her inside elbow joint.

His robe gave a voluminous swirl as he exited down a dimly lit passageway.

She lay quite still, not moving a muscle as a helter skelter of horrifying thoughts cascaded through her mind. *What was he talking about?*

Sleep approached and all thoughts ceased. She began slipping away as the drug slid around her veins and a deep darkness dropped over in one black gulp.

A building somewhere on the Vivale Bruno Buozzi Rome…

Bells from a dozen different clock towers pealed out their metallic midday announcements, sending kits of pigeons fluttering in every direction.

The premises were unremarkable, inconspicuous on this average Roman district. *I Apocalittici Guerrieri di Cristo* had, under the Grand Keeper's command, convened an extra special meeting, although he could not be present. The Inner Circle will preside and everyone has been asked to report on their respective tasks. They knew of the discovery of the Seventh Seal and the plans in place to acquire it. Nothing can move ahead until two things happen: the unification of the seals, and the death of the Pope. In any order.

The usual ceremonies and rituals preceded the meeting, to be addressed by Cardinal Riario.

Standing and with a serious expression, he looked around at the members, pausing for several seconds before he spoke.

"Brothers. I bring you good news. Cardinal Pacca and myself have, as instructed, conducted trials on how we can best dispose of this heinous Pope. We thought about it long and hard. We settled on the use of poison as recommended by the Grand Keeper. Undetectable, it causes total muscular and nervous paralysis, although the brain and mind remain lucid and coherent. Death follows in a few hours. How we will administer this is our affair, but eating or drinking the substance accomplishes the desired result. That is all you need to know. It was tried out at first on a feral dog and it worked. However, animals and humans can differ, and so to test its reliability, we performed the same experiment on a person we cannot name. The results were perfect. We could say it worked far better on our human experiment. Our plans are ready. We know how and when we will do it, and nobody will be any the wiser. Are there any questions?"

There were none. "Good. We intend to strike seven days from now after he returns from the Philippines. By then, we will have the Seventh, if not, then plans will be placed on hold. He will be exhausted from the trip and this is our best opportunity. Only Cardinal Pacca and myself know the details, and that's the way it will stay. So, Brothers, be prepared."

Riario paused, took a sip of wine, wiped his mouth and continued. "Our Grand Keeper informs us that our cells across the globe are now on full alert. That brings us to the issues of armaments and distribution." He turned to Brothers

Xavier and Sir Gordon Andersen. "May we have your briefing and capability reports, bearing in mind we are now seven days away from one of the most momentous days ever for mankind."

Xavier nodded to General Sir Gordon Anderson, who took his cue and rose to address the members.

"I'm sure Brother Xavier will not mind me incorporating his operational report with mine as I proceed. In many ways, we run parallel to each other and have been liaising together on our capabilities and requirements. He is capable, through a blanket network of contacts, to connect with every cell that has been listed. Already we have managed to acquire a staggering amount of hardware and chemical weapons."

Anderson moved to the front of the room and pulled down a massive wall map of the world. Masses of red circular pins highlighted every cell of the AWC. Bright yellow marker pins had pinpointed seventy-seven city targets around the globe

"Impressive, Brothers?" He gazed at them from left to right. "Our beloved NATO is not immune either. Not shown on this map are a dozen small cells, three of which are situated in my command structure across the NATO network. We have access to seventy-five per cent of the required launch codes for a diverse range of rocketry, should we need to use them. We also have a range of 'suitcase' nuclear devices that can be used for inter-city attacks, again, if required. By the time seven days have passed, all of these..." He tapped his pointer across the map, "should be in receipt of sophisticated ordnance of all types. We, Brothers, are prepared and ready. God's intervention will assist and decide how we will proceed."

"Thank you, Brother," Riario said as Sir Gordon Anderson returned to his seat. He turned to Pacca. "I know you have been working hard alongside both Brothers Woodford and Moro. What can you tell us on this score?'

Brother Paolo Moro spoke first. "As Italian Minister of Foreign Affairs, I have been assisting in the removal of unpleasant barriers and impediments, to smooth transactions between Italy, The Vatican, the EU members, and the various trade associations outside Europe. This has allowed us, with Brother Woodford's banking expertise, and of course, Cardinal Pacca's unrivalled access to the Holy Purse, to achieve the following. Fifteen Million dollars of unregistered Bearer Bonds were drawn up from the Holy Purse, and placed in secure deposit facilities in unequal amounts, in both Brother Woodford's offshore interests. Only the Grand Keeper can access them. If there's any unauthorized attempt, it will send an automatic worldwide electronic flagging alert. That person would not get ten yards from the bank, and would be executed on sight. Do you agree, Brother Woodford?"

Woodford was a man of few words. "This is true. Funds continue to flow from their bank into ours. Also, I have arranged with Brother Pacca for a systematic draining of the entire range of the Vatican's liquid assets, followed by a transfer of all major assets and investments to the auspices and coffers of our beloved Order, the AWC. There is, of course, the matter of the Vatican's vast reservoir of gold bullion to consider, but removal at this moment is not possible. We have to wait until the Pope is dead. If anyone suspects, it will fall on our brothers and sisters at Opus Dei. The reallocations are happening as I speak. It should be complete by the time of the Pope's demise. On the surface, it looks clean, legitimate, and a safeguarding of the Church's power and wealth. Sanctioned by Cardinal Pacca's Office of Financial Affairs, and endorsed by no less than the Camerlengo himself. Even this Pope would put his signature to it, but of course, being dead, he will be unable to."

Laughter and a round of applause greeted Woodford's self-congratulatory smirk.

"I think that at this juncture, we should devise a clear structure of how our global membership will be involved. So, let's discuss that right now. The Grand Keeper has directed that no one should communicate with him in Tel Aviv electronically. He feels that there is a breach in the system in that location. That is why we summoned Gallo here. It is not necessary to bring him to the meeting, but he will be privy to the most secret of documents and information. From that, he can begin stage one. He looked at his watch. "In ten minutes, we will have a video link with our Master. So, let us prepare ourselves. Afterwards, we can draft our immediate requirements to Seneschal Gallo and our other operatives."

Chapter 51

ROCKWELL LOOKED AT his watch for the third time. It was unusual for Rachael to be late for work. He had sent Joshua up to the caves, and to keep an eye out should Gallo make an appearance. Although from Ahasver's directive, that seemed unlikely. But nothing could be taken for granted. He was certain that the University President was involved one way or the other. As to whether Ahasver was a man living for two thousand years, he could not believe how any sane and sensible person of the twenty-first century could even believe such a fairy tale. His biggest problem right now was what to do with the seal. What made the Seventh so important, and what would happen when they became united once more? It didn't add up to a can of beans. Proof didn't exist.

For Gallo and Ahasver, both respected in their profession, to be involved in a murderous organisation that believed the seven seals held the future of mankind, beggared belief. *It's just a load of bollocks! The world's had its fill of weird and murderous cult organisations. You only have to look at the Branch Davidians, or the Children of God, to name just two of dozens on this planet.*

Another look at his watch. *She must be unwell. I'll give her a shout.* He opened his mobile and called her. It rang several times before he was transferred to voice mail.

Most strange. He called Joshua next.

"Hi, Josh. Is Rachael with you?"

"No, Simon. I thought she was with you."

"Oh shit. I think something's wrong. I'm not getting a response from her anywhere. I don't like the sound of it. I'm going over to her place."

"That's not like her," Joshua agreed. "If she turns up I'll let you know, but you must tell me when you find her. Okay?"

"Will do. Catch you later." He switched off.

Rockwell rushed downstairs, jumped into the dark green Land Rover, and booted it into a redline revving pace as he sped towards her place a mile off. His heart raced, and he had an unpleasant premonition as to what he might find.

Her house appeared a short way off and slowing down, he screeched into her driveway with a mighty swing on the wheel. Her car was parked. *That didn't look good.* Jumping from the vehicle without closing the door, he sprinted to the front doorway and hit the bell with the palm of his hand. No reply. He did it two more times … nothing.

Jesus!

He raced around to the back. The curtains were drawn tight across the patio doors.

He smacked his forehead as he remembered where she left a spare key. He ran to the ornamental heron standing by the fishpond to ward off other fish-hungry birds. He tipped it over. "Yes!" he said aloud, as he pulled it out, still wrapped in a small polythene bag. Within thirty seconds, he had the door open and was inside.

"Rachael! Rachael, are you there?" His shouts rang

around the walls unanswered.

The place was deserted.

He then noticed the rooms had been ransacked.

"Oh my God, they've taken her!" He stopped charging around and checked his phone. Nothing. He went from room to room, including the bathroom and toilet areas … complete upheaval.

The seal. They were after the seal. She put it in the cupboard alongside a row of tinned fruits … the kitchen!

The floor was littered with vegetables, fruits, flour, sugar, and every packet including cereals had been upended in their attempt to find it. He stepped over the detritus and went straight to the cupboard. Yanking the door open, he was dismayed to see that it was empty.

"Damn!"

His mind bounded from Rachael, to the seal, and back again. He didn't know what he should do next.

As he stared helplessly at the chaos around him, Rockwell spotted what he had been hoping to find. It looked different … as if it didn't belong there. Half covered in a layer of bread flour, and protruding from beneath a tin of peaches, was an old looking oblong slab, a piece of semi oxidized metal. He recognised them at once. The Seventh Seal. He made a careful grab at it, and examined it up close. He blew away the flour, and needed no confirmation. With care, he placed it in his pocket. There was no joy or pleasure in its rescue. His only concern was for Rachael. He knew her life was in danger. He sat down in a chair, trying to make sense of it all.

Whoever did this was looking for the seal. He had to think. The Keepers must have known he had the seal since they had failed to steal it from him at the Tel Aviv Bank. So why pick on Rachael? There could only be one reason; a direct assault on his emotions, a ploy to strike at the team's concern for the only woman on the team. Rockwell found his thoughts becoming suffused with a feeling for Rachael he hadn't realised he had before. *If they so much as harmed a hair of her head, they'd have me to answer to. They could have their goddamned seal and to hell with them!* It was time to confront Gallo and Ahasver. This has gone way too far. Ahasver could close down the excavation, and they would all be out of jobs. Blood was going to be spilt in more ways than one.

To hell with them all. Rachael must be kept alive. These people are crazed killers.

A plan of action had to be drawn up and he needed Joshua's assistance … and of his Guardians. He couldn't do it on his own, and he suspected Joshua knew more than he'd ever let on. To his surprise, he said a prayer out loud.

"God, keep Rachael safe." He picked up his phone and called Joshua.

Seated alone and in a sunny corner of a Roman restaurant, Gallo struggled with his *Pesce alla Marinara* before pushing his plate to one side. He was more interested in the contents of the package he had collected. It contained a long list of names of AWC members, and all those sympathetic to their ethos and aims. All these would be contacted by the administration departments, and would be instructed to make themselves known to him.

Next, a separate padded envelope which contained a set of heavy keys, two plastic barcoded cards, and an explanatory agenda.

On his return in two days' time, his instructions were to drive to the city of Ariel, near the old Port of Jaffa and on the West Bank, approximately twenty-five kilometres from Tel Aviv. He had to enter the controversial Barkan Industrial Park, where many European concerns had left due to Palestinian outrage at Jewish settlements and businesses being set up, in contradiction to international law. In that park, on lots 13-16, stood the deserted warehouses of UniMex Ltd. They would be recognisable by their bright green colouring. The keys and plastic cards would give him access to every part of the complex.

He would find the offices refitted, and with up-to-date IT equipment and communications. To that affect, he'd been supplied with another plastic wallet containing a ream of operating procedures for the equipment. They were to be left in a desk drawer, clearly marked, AWC100.

What he unfolded next shook him, and he stared at it for some time. *How have they done all this?* It was an inventory of what he would find in the four massive storage facilities. He stared at it long and hard.

ALL ITEMS IN UNITS OF <u>100 each</u>

- Uzi Sub machine gun additional
- Galil ACE machine gun
- Galil machine gun
- Tavor bullpup machine gun (and variants)
- Negev light machine gun

- Uzi sub-machine gun
- Jericho 941 handgun
- SP-21 Barak handgun
- Desert Eagle handgun
- MAPATS ATGM
- Delilah missile
- IMI 120 mm gun
- LAR-160
- CornerShot and attachments
- Refaim bullet-trap rifle-grenade
- Armour add-ons:
    - Armour plating coat
    - Explosive reactive armour
    - Tractor protection kit (TPK) for Caterpillar D7
    - Armour kit for Caterpillar D9 bulldozer (L\N)
    - Iron Fist active protection system – Active protection system (APS) for tanks
    - ADDITIONAL 9 MM Glock hand guns.

Gallo reeled.

The true implication of what he was involved in became very real.

Game over.

Reality stared him in the face.

Equipment like this, and the quantity, was more than enough for a small army to cause massive destruction. Then, he remembered that this storage facility was just one in many around the world.

Once back in Tel Aviv he had to get in touch with Ahasver. The Grand Keeper's commands couldn't have been clearer.

In no way was he to resume his post at the university. He had to avoid contact with or approach any university member, staff, or scholars. Gallo was to maintain a low profile as he took on a more active role in the implementation of the AWC plans. He would be paid with a lump sum three times more than his university salary, direct into his bank account. Instructions and details were being issued to seneschals across the planet.

Tel Aviv, it stated, was of special importance due to the proximity of the Seven Seals. God would not desert them at this important moment, and in the Holiest of Lands.

Gallo thought Ahasver's punishment over the centuries was all part of the Divine Plan. It gave him a unique perspective of the human condition. He truly understood what people needed to return to the right path to righteousness.

Chapter 52

RACHAEL'S FIRST THOUGHT when she opened her eyes was that she was somewhere in the Beit-Guvrin caves. She did her best not to think of the avalanche of rock and dirt that hung suspended over her by the slim curvature of a roughly hewn ceiling.

A disembodied voice spoke to her. "Dr. Carver, welcome back." It came from the hooded figure standing a short distance from her. "I trust you are not too uncomfortable."

A feeling of loathing for whoever he was, filled her. She didn't know if it was Gallo or Ahasver. "I know what you want. But I have no idea where it is. You're wasting your time."

There came a deathly silence between them, and she knew he was staring at her although his face remained hidden from view. She knew he was playing a game to coerce her into submission.

He moved over to the burning fire and stoked it with a metal rod. It flared up. Bright yellow and blue flames ascended with a small roar. The rod glowed red hot with the heat. He held it high and moved across to her to bring the incandescent iron inches from her exposed torso.

Holy Mother of God!

"No! Please, don't do this!" Her voice bloomed with terror as the fierce heat inched towards her navel.

He said nothing. Moving back to the brazier, he plunged the iron rod back into the glowing embers.

A brief feeling of relief swept through her. "Please, I don't know anything."

"Oh, but you do." He growled. "Watch."

Grabbing the lid of the sarcophagus, he pulled it to one side as it made a grinding noise.

A glimpse inside the sarcophagus caused Rachael to clench her fists, and let out a piercing shriek in horror. Looking up at her from the stone coffin, and with the sightless eyes of the dead, was the discernible but bloated features of a dead woman. Apart from the top of her face, she had been submerged in water that had a red and brown colour, a result of the bodily secretions and blood emanating from the inflated fleshy corpse.

"Behold, you vile sinner. Look on her well, and know that her watery grave could be your last home. Or maybe you would prefer the warmth and purifying burn of our fires?"

Rachael squeezed her eyes shut. "No! No! Not this, please!" Fear caused her stomach to retch.

The Grand Keeper spoke, and as he did, he began taking a video through his smartphone "You may not understand, but I have tasted the curse of immortality and experienced every pain and hardship known to man." He panned the camera over her, then the rotting corpse in the stone coffin, and next onto the glowing fire, before holding up the bright red iron rod. "They can hear my voice in this video, and your stupid colleagues will recognise you and they will guess what your fate is to be."

Fear imbued its tentacles into every nerve, cell, muscle, and fibre of her body. Her mouth opened, but no sound came.

He stared down at her and continued filming. When finished, he uploaded Rockwell's number and pressed 'send.'

"I have my plans, and events will be upon us soon," He tilted his head back and gazed into an invisible sky. He then threw the phone into the flames.

Chapter 53

THE JAFFA CLOCK Tower, standing in Clock Square and overlooking the port, struck the hour. Built to commemorate the Silver Jubilee of the Ottoman Sultan, Abd al-Hamid, it had become a popular tourist destination.

Nearby, Joshua Agar waited. He wasn't there to admire the attractions. Rockwell's desperate call had expedited an urgent meeting away from their homes or the University.

He had sounded fraught and manic, in a way he had never heard him before. Joshua knew something urgent had come up. A quick glance through the people thronging to and fro, and he spotted Rockwell moving at a fast pace in his direction. He had seen him.

Rockwell grabbed at his arm with barely a greeting. "Let's go somewhere quiet and private. Rachael is in trouble, and we don't have a lot of time. Don't say anything until we're somewhere secluded."

Neither noticed the tall touristy figure moving at a discreet distance behind them.

"Well, okay, let's get in there then." Joshua steered him into the entrance of the Café Yaffo, where there were plenty of private corner tables. A small band played at the far end, and there were only a few customers.

"Sit." Joshua ordered him and pointed to a vacant table.

Without question, Rockwell sat in the chair.

The other man walked in behind them and sat at the far end, away from them.

"Now, spit it out, Simon. Something's wrong. What is it?"

"Look at this." He produced his mobile, switched it on, and handed it across so Joshua could watch the video.

Joshua blanched. At first, he couldn't make out who it was. "Holy Shit! It's Rachael." His voice hissed with horror.

There was more.

A muffled voice accompanied the scene, explaining her predicament and likely fate. The camera scanned over a red-hot iron that moved close to her naked torso. It then panned in on the bloated corpse adrift in the stone coffin.

"This is unbelievable! Where is she?" Joshua's calm evaporated. "What are we going to do?" He gave a pained stare at the screen and his hands shook. He didn't need to be told what was going on and why.

"I don't know where she is, but I think we're being given clues. Before he signed off, he demanded the Seventh Seal in exchange for her life. Then he showed us fire and water, and then scanned the interior. Look," he pointed to the screen, "that can't be anywhere but the Beit-Guvrin caves. He deliberately showed us the walls and corridors, and then sends this, an inscription over the columbarium. Recognize it?"

זהו האחרון של שבע שינה עתיקה
6אחיי לחכות אני כבר לא בוכה
ביד של ג'ון ואנחנו נחצבנו להכריז
קץ לדיראון עולם של האנושות

"Where's the seal, Simon? We have to go there now. Her life depends on it."

"I have it. I found it in her ransacked house. Whoever it was, missed it." Rockwell stood. "Let's go. Her life matters more than bits of old metal, stupid legends, and fairy tales."

The tall man on the other side of the café gave a small smile, texted another message, got up and left.

A near naked Rachael shivered in the strange half-light. She closed her eyes and tried to control her pounding heart and ragged breath. She wanted to blot out the horrors that had been presented to her. But her thoughts disintegrated into a mish-mash of fantasy and childhood recollections.

Rachael's horrified mind looked for a way to calm itself before it went insane. It drove her deep into a long-forgotten place, she never even knew existed.

Ave Maria … Morituri te salutant …

Words she didn't understand tumbled out of her mouth.

Mors ultima linea rerum est. Noli timere, quia ego tecum sum omnibus diebus, Rachael!

The words repeated several times. Parading through her

mind, she saw them change from black into a remembered and comforting blue. The colour of her vision … Mother Mary.

Rachael's words grew increasingly louder, like a last call to God. And she wanted Simon to hear them, as they rolled in an urgent stream of love and fear for his safety.

Mary, Queen of Heaven, walked on the waves towards her, and her arms were open wide. A crown of twelve stars shone above her blue cowl. Her gentle words whispered into Rachael's mind.

Chapter 54

GALLO'S JEEP BOOMED across the deserted units 13-16, and headed out of the Barkan Industrial complex. He had been an obedient servant. He knew that if the Inner Circle or the Grand Keeper were to ask him, he would undertake even the act of parricide without question. His excitement grew. Never before had he understood the depth of his commitment. He had become the loyal servant of the Grand Keeper who was God's messenger and ultimate warrior in his great plan for humanity. It was a position of great honour.

He had made a detailed inspection of the weaponry, and it remained as documented. Handling a gun was not new to him. Two years in the army had taught him all he needed to know. How joyous when the seals were broken and the glory of the new world and its order would be revealed to mankind. Messages to potential incumbents had been drafted and dispatched. The wheels were now turning. He had been summoned back to Tel Aviv and this time there was to be no disguise or secrecy. The Grand Keeper, Ahasver, had requested his presence. Not at the University, but at an address he had not been to before.

At eleven pm, the night remained warm. The smell of the sea drifted from the nearby marina, Gallo's appointed destination. He had driven over to Herzliya Pituah, an affluent location in the northern district of Tel Aviv. Overseas embassies and the wealthy were attracted to it, and being twinned with Hollywood in the USA added to its allure. His designation was a boat named 'Gaius.' His instructions were to park in front of it, and not do anything but remain in his vehicle. He found it without difficulty. It was unexpectedly large at sixteen metres in length. He had never known that his University President owned such an expensive item.

Switching off the ignition, the engine gave a slight vibration as it died. That, and the gentle lapping of water against the boat, accentuated the silence around him

Light flickered from the boat. He didn't have long to wait. A door opened, and the decking became flooded with light as Ahasver emerged. A pair of Magpie Black Gold sunglasses rested on his head, and he was dressed in a black Dolce & Gabbana mohair suit. He looked almost young. He waved for him to come on board. Gallo became overawed. He had not realised the extent of his Master's situation. Nothing less than impressive.

"Welcome aboard, seneschal Gallo." He ushered him into the main sitting area. It smelt of fabric softener. The spacious and luxuriously appointed cabin, thick with rugs, cushions, a cocktail bar and sofas, had on its wall a large picture of a snake eating his own tail. "I use this boat as my resting place. It's my headquarters almost, few know I own it."

Without thinking, Gallo genuflected, and reaching out, grabbed and kissed the Grand Keeper's hand.

Ahasver, not unaccustomed to such behaviour, and without a glance at his devoted acolyte, poured two large brandies. He pointed to a sofa. "Please sit, seneschal, there are things I need to explain to you."

Gallo sat without a word.

"I am a Jew," began Ahasver. "Our people, throughout time, have been afflicted and cursed by many men and nations. I myself inherited an eternity of sorrow and pain by Christ. There exists between us a separate vision of how the world will change and become fit for God's Kingdom. That time is now upon us, but not through one interpretation, but by an understanding that blends in both Jewish and Christian depictions. You see, only when the Seven Seals are broken can the Jewish vision become one with the Christian, and vice versa. I have only come to understand this over the last five hundred years or so. Am I making myself clear so far, seneschal?"

"Yes, very clear, Master."

"Jews hold a belief that when the last soul leaves the *Guf, or The Tree of Souls,* it will become empty, and the world will come to an end. Jewish beliefs also see the soul as bird-like, and the *Guf* as a vast columbarium or aviary, a birdhouse. The chirpings of sparrows tell of a new born. But sadly, sparrows are dying out now, as will men. The mystic significance is that each person who has ever lived, dies, and the return of the Messiah moves closer. Each soul yearns to be reunited with the others to make the One. Then, the Messiah will come. The Talmud states this clearly. The Book of Revelation also tells us that the breaking of the seals will bring an end to men. We

Keepers are to be deliverers of that plight on this corrupt planet. Are you understanding fully, seneschal?"

Gallo stared as if mesmerised, and mustered a nod.

There followed a lengthy pause. Ahasver, sipped at his drink, said nothing, and stared hard at his seneschal.

Gallo allowed tears to form in his eyes. His Master's stare penetrated every part of his being to reveal his innermost secrets. Nothing could be kept from him. It was beautiful to hear, and confirmed all that he could ever believe in.

"I understand perfectly, Master."

"We will kill those opposed to us for they are against Christ, the Messiah, who is about to come. The Pope, an Antichrist, has overthrown all traditions, and has taken the Church further into the deepest pits of hell. He and all his followers will perish. There can only be one messenger of God, and I, the Wandering Jew, am that."

He stood abruptly, dropped to his knees, and bent his head. The gesture deeply moved Gallo. With his beloved Master, he recited the Holy Oath, granted to them centuries ago by Cosimos Ricci, seven times in unison … *Sacris Sancti Homicidium.*

Once finished, they sat back and drank their brandies in silence.

"Now, Seneschal, I have a task for you." He poured him a large drink. "The Seventh Seal is about to be ours. The three we know who are most likely to have it are Agar, Carver or Rockwell. We have Dr. Carver. She is under regular sedation and we now require pressure to be placed on the men by subjecting her to some unpleasant procedures. This will force them to surrender what is ours, the Seventh Seal. You may have to drown or burn her to death. Would that be a problem?"

"It would not be a problem, Master."

"Good. She is where the other was held beneath the Beit-Guvrin caves, close to the columbarium where you saw them descending. Following the path they took will bring you to the place where you shot the woman, and where Dr. Carver is now being held. She will, of course, die, just as the other two will when we have the seal. You will have to confront the two and lead them back to where she is being held. Remember also that the University no longer employs you. Does any of this bother you, seneschal Gallo?"

"No, it does not. What happens when we have the seals and they are broken?"

"I don't know. But circumstances have brought me to the point where I know that an event *will* commence, and it *will* change mankind. Of that you can be certain. Our battalions across the globe will ensure what is decreed will happen. The heavens will open and we will be guided. As I speak, loyal followers who remained silent for so many years are now moving to their appointed stations. With Christ descending on the evil and directing our troops, the world will be restored, but only with the holiest and most faithful of his disciples. The wicked, the false Christian religions, the Catholics, Moslems, Hindus, Buddhists, and any others, will be wiped away like dirt from our boots. It will not be easy; natural disasters, earthquakes, volcanoes, tectonic plates colliding under the sea, vast tsunamis followed by worldwide plagues, and pestilence shall darken the skies until every last one of them is expunged from this sacred world. Our weapons will complete the task. Only those deserving shall survive. These things have been building up for years, and are now holding their breath, awaiting the blast of the final trumpet. Believe me, I know, for I have seen it for two thousand years. But now it's worse than it has ever been. What caused me endless misery is about to blossom into glory." *I will be reborn.*

"I am honoured, Master." The echo of excitement in his Master's voice thrilled him.

"Make your plans, Seneschal. You must get them to the caves. They have been alerted to that possibility when they met at the port of Jaffa. Dr. Carver's torment will accelerate their anxieties, and they will hand us the seal to save their friend. When that is complete, you, as every other seneschal across the globe will do in their territories, will take control of the weaponry stored at the Barkan Industrial Park. Now leave and go about your business, Seneschal Gallo. Inform me constantly."

Chapter 55

ROCKWELL AND JOSHUA abandoned all pretence at excavation or digging at the caves. They had been given a clue, a strong message that could not be ignored. Rachael's life stood as forfeit, and the cost of it amounted to a piece of metal the size of a credit card.

With speed, they assembled their equipment for a descent into the columbarium. Priority was given to life saving equipment, medical supplies, Kevlar body armour, and their pistols. Most got packed into rucksacks.

Rockwell had taken stock of himself. He knew his world was about to change, but into what he didn't know. His emotions were out of control, and that was a condition new and mysterious to him. Impatience, his weak spot, had already found him rushing in a manner inappropriate for the situation. He looked at Joshua. He had suffered two major assaults, but he retained a cool exterior. His responses measured and calculated.

"Josh," asked Rockwell, "what are these madmen going to get from this slip of metal?" He held up the Seventh set. "They are willing to kill and God knows what else."

"Careful with that, Simon. Stop waving it about and put it somewhere safe, please. They believe they are God's warriors and that piece of metal you are holding is the key to the end of the world as they know it. They are prepared to die for it. If the Wandering Jew, Ahasver is running the show, then we'd better believe it. The whole thing defies explanation."

"Our President, this mythical Wandering Jew?"

"Could be, but let's keep an open mind on it. We must save Rachael first, that's all that matters. C'mon, let's get out of here and over to that cave."

"Do you think Gallo knows about Rachael?"

"We'll know soon enough."

Screaming up through the gears, and leaving behind swirls of sandy dust, Rockwell gunned the 4x4 on its way to the excavation location at Beit-Guvrin. The two men became occupied by their own thoughts.

Joshua had alerted all the members he had found in Nathaniel's files. They were manna from heaven. Included in the jungle of paperwork were codes and communication particulars used by him and his fellow Guardians. They were a legitimate brotherhood, alive and thriving in this modern society. Now not so crackpot, it gave him a new perception of himself. The changing situation had hardened his resolve into one that was culminating into a desire for revenge. Events had shattered his world of cosy academia. Reality had turned brutal, shifted gear, and propelled him into a world of mad savagery. He let it sweep him along.

Nathaniel's beliefs were correct, and they had endured a

transmission from the earliest days of the Guardians. He had anticipated this day, and Joshua swore a silent oath that he would not betray him or the Guardians from legions past.

Rockwell focussed on his image of Rachael. He saw in his mind the shocking video of her strapped to a table of some sort, in what looked like a cave in Beit-Guvrin. He regretted the offhanded way he had treated her in the past, and the way he had taken her for granted. He realised he cared for her more than he had admitted to himself. Work had always come first. Once she got back safe and sound, he would change. He made a promise to himself.

A bleep from his phone signalled a text alert.

"Read that, will you?" He handed the phone to Joshua and fixed his eyes on the sand ridden track ahead.

Josh read and reread it. He raised his voice over the sound of the engine "It's for us."

"What does it say? Who's it from?"

"It's from them, I guess. It says, *'We know you are coming. Bring Seal.'*"

"Holy shit! Is there nothing they don't know?" His knuckles whitened on the steering wheel.

"Two thousand years of experience could give them the edge on that."

Rockwell stared ahead as the Land Rover crested the last hill to bring them in sight of the trail leading up to the caves. He didn't dare imagine what the next hours would bring.

"This is as far as we go. We'll walk the rest of the way." He decelerated, slewed the Land Rover into a handbrake stop, switched the engine off, and jumped out.

Joshua stood right behind him. "Have we forgotten anything?"

Rockwell didn't answer, but began a brisk pace towards the top of the long hill. There was nobody about since it's too early for the team to start the day's work. What bothered him most was not knowing how many killers they would have to deal with. One thing he knew for certain, the seal would have to be handed over, but he'll attempt to delay that for as long as he could.

Both men began gasping as the pace uphill went beyond the leisurely inquisitive rambling of archaeologists looking for clues. Up in front, the small range of fissures marked the entrance to the cave and catacomb system.

What they saw next shocked them both. They could make out the figure of somebody standing there, watching their ascent. The chunky figure of Julian Gallo loomed into view.

Both men came to an abrupt halt. Rockwell placed a restraining arm across Joshua and snapped. "Whatever you're going to do, don't!"

"He's armed."

"Looks like the pretence is over. Let's go and see what he has to say."

"Careful, that's a sub machine gun he's holding."

They got within talking range and Gallo called out. "You two! Stop there, please."

"Don't worry, Julian, we're not armed." Rockwell lied.

"I'm sorry it had to come to this, Simon, but greater things are about to happen and there is no other way."

"We've known about you for some while."

"That's no surprise."

Joshua pushed the revelation. "We know also about Ahasver, your Wandering Jew, your misguided stupid fool of a leader."

Gallo looked startled. A crazed look blazed in his dark eyes. His finger tightened on the trigger and he let loose a clacking spray of bullets around them. Both men clenched their fists and bent low, as bolts of fear rushed through them.

"Agar, you'll regret speaking like that. My leader has Christ's gift of immortality until his return. How do you think he's survived for two thousand years? All our activities have led us to this moment in time. You're a known Guardian, as was your misguided grandfather, and the meddling Father Luke. We Keepers have known about you for a while, and in your honour, we have arranged a special treat for you." His lip curled upwards and he turned to Rockwell. "The Seventh … you have it?"

"I have it."

"Praise be to God. You know where we're going, so lead on. No tricks. I'm close behind you and my Uzi is looking at your backs. Now, get going!" His voice was sharp and clear as he stood back, and with a wave of the gun barrel, ushered them into the darkness of the cave system.

Chapter 56

THE ATMOSPHERE RIPPLED… *Asroilu stirred … the gentlest of ripples, like a harp softly plucked, vibrated through the billowing ether of the Third Heaven. His deep sleep of the centuries disturbed. He could now hear the plaintiff cries of men.*

Rising and falling, they could not be denied. Yet … yet … yet above these, he sensed something greater. A returning.

He who was lost was now to be found.

Asroilu, the Seventh Guardian, spread his wings to arise like a benevolent nemesis, to float above the fields of gold, eternally bedecked with the most luscious of fruits. With his span, he swirled the sweet scents of a million flowers to greet the Prodigal's return.

There then came the other six guardians, and a host of others led by Azrael, the Angel of Death. They were to greet the returning. Their wait had been long.

He was still far off, but his rustlings could be heard … returning home … at last. He had known the way for aeons, but his route was never certain, forever obstructed by the ways of men.

Now unfettered, he rode magnificently towards his true home. Upon his head he wore, as did his brothers, the winged crown of victory. In his hand he held a sword, once more blazing with the flame of truth.

Chapter 57

RACHAEL FLINCHED. SHE awoke to realise that in her drugged condition, she had been taken from the hard slab and was now bound to a central pillar. Two hooded acolytes approached her. They placed a coarse robe of hair around her body and then pulled it tight. Its coarseness scoured her flesh.

She looked around her. The cave-like temple billowed full of heady smoke, and frankincense. Light came from row upon row of candles, tall thick and spluttering, giving an angry glow that heightened her plight. Shadows, large and unfriendly, flickered around the uneven walls.

The two hooded figures stood before an altar where the six seals were displayed on a golden arch, bedecked with precious jewels and gemstones. They hung together by a thin twisted rope made of solid gold. Each seal, by a slight amount, overlapped the other in a circle. A gap remained between the first and the last. She knew the intention. It was for the Seventh, should they ever get hold of it.

The brazier burnt bright. Worse, the frightful stone sarcophagus stood there, uncovered, but now empty of its bloated corpse. The crypt-like surroundings had grown hot, and perspiration ran from Rachael's head down to her face, throat, and breasts, before mingling with the hair of her sweaty covering.

Fear pumped through her veins. The whole apparatus was designed for that purpose. *Hail Mary* ... her implorations were cut short by the return of the two robed figures. They had begun a chant.

BAH-ROOCH AH-TAH AH-DOH-NOI EH-LOH-HEH-NOO MEH-LECH HAH-OH-LAHM AH-SHER KEE-DEH-SHAH-NOO BEH-MITZ-VOH-TAHV VEH-TZEE-VAH-NOO LEH-HAD-LEEK NER SHEL SHAH-BAHT KOH-DESH.

She recognized the Hebrew. It was the Shabbat incantation.

"Blessed are You, Lord, our God, King of the universe, who has sanctified us with His commandments, and commanded us to kindle the light of the holy Shabbat."

According to *halakha* (Jewish religious law), Shabbat is observed from a few minutes before sunset on Friday evening until the appearance of three stars in the sky on Saturday night. Lighting candles and reciting a blessing ushers the Shabbat in.

She now knew what day it was, and calculated that she had been a prisoner for two days and nights. *But why this Jewish ceremony?*

The chant came to a halt, and the tall, hooded figure of her captor strode in. Without giving her a glance, he knelt with pious intent before the altar. He stood and the three men began a slow dirge-like chant she had not heard before.

Sacris Sancti Homicidium.

Its baleful tone belched out as if from the realm of Hades.

She counted each one. It seemed never ending and after each seventh incantation, a large bell was struck, filling the complex with a deep apocryphal resonance.

Her research on the number seven and its proliferation in the Bible came rushing into her mind. The Book of Revelation … it lived. *Oh my God! This cannot be happening. Mother Mary, please, where are you?*

Rachael called on her name over and over, but she did not answer.

Chapter 58

SIX PLUMP QUAILS had been kept in the freezer. Two were separated from the other four in different compartments. Unlike the other birds, they had been fed with ample quantities of hemlock seeds. All had been deboned, stuffed, trussed, and once defrosted, would be ready for oven roasting.

Cardinals Riario and Pacca had reached treacherous crossroads in their lives and in their allegiances. They both understood the immensity of the task their loyalty to the Keepers had placed upon them.

It would be their second act of murder, a form of regicide.

Both had led humble lives, when from unremarkable and poor backgrounds, they had entered their respective seminaries. Progressing rapidly, they were regarded as exceptional talent, which led to their roles as Cardinals. Riario's role as Camerlengo was spectacular and envied by many. Pacca's role as Papal Prefecture for the Economic Affairs of the Holy See gave him unprecedented access to the most confidential financial affairs of the Vatican. Many years back, they had both decided that the Catholic Church, to which they had devoted their entire lives to, had been taken over by forces of evil, and had now become out of control. Led by a false Pope, the Antichrist and spawn of Satan. It was then they discovered, via a renegade priest, *I Apocalittico Guerrieri Di Cristo*. It was the answer to their anxious prayers.

The time had arrived. The Grand Keeper had given the signal and his message was clear.

"Begin and be not merciful."

They looked at each other and both wore expressions of nervous tension. Their excitement mounted. Years of secret work had begun entering fruition. Games and rhetoric were over. It will now be turned into reality. Years of dedication and endless disappointments were to be things of the past. God's glorious plan and the blessings of Christ were soon to descend upon them. Doctrinal clarity would be restored. Praise to the Wandering Jew who had brought this about.

In forty-eight hours, they will have their weekly private dinner with the Pontiff before he retired for the night.

The other four Keepers of the Inner Circle had coalesced. Money continued to flow from the Vatican and into Woodford's offshore banking network, and his business with Cardinal Pacca had proceeded smoothly with no questions asked. One interloper, a Father Antonio Borelli, who functioned as a daily auditor, had raised awkward questions to the Cardinal. Asking why such huge sums of money were being moved.

He, like the money, vanished.

His body, fed into the pig feeding system of the finest prosciutto ham producer on the west side of the River Po, would never be found.

Mendez had worked miracles of logistics and using considerable sums of purloined Vatican monies, had performed a task that the Grand Keeper had doubts he could achieve. Armament caches like those at Barkan Industrial Park had been installed worldwide, in every crucial area, should they be needed.

Anderson's role had been fulfilled. His spy network and insider cells held a battery of encrypted codes and access protocols that would give the AWC launch codes of countless NATO nuclear missile configurations.

God, it seemed, would not be lacking protection.

Rockwell, followed by Joshua, with Gallo prodding them along with his Uzi, entered the darkness of the system. He stood for a moment, allowing his eyes to adjust to the darkness.

The immense silence bore all the noise of a dead man hanging on a rope end. They absorbed it as they moved on past and beyond the team's previous excavations, before taking the right tunnel where the vast columbarium waited at the end.

"I'm right behind you, so don't stop. I will shoot if I have to."

Using their helmet lights and their handheld devices, they made their way forward. A fifteen-minute scramble over the rocky and stone strewn path.

The columbarium, huge and unmistakeable, loomed

before them.

A drastic drop in the air temperature to their right revealed the gaping emptiness that led down to where they had discovered the missing seal.

They turned to look at Gallo.

"You know the way down. I've seen you do it. Get going."

"Gallo," Rockwell spat the name out like he'd bitten into a turd. "You're one sad, stupid arsehole. If it's the last thing I do, I'll personally murder you. You and your crazy army, abduct and hold prisoner a working colleague, one you've known and worked with closely, and subject her to God knows what pain and humiliation. You deranged bastard!"

"And I'll help him," Joshua uncharacteristically snarled.

For a fraction of a moment, Gallo hesitated, and through the flashlight, they saw a glimmer of uncertainty in his eyes. "I don't care what you think. It had to be done. When the Seals unite, and are broken, Christ will join us, and the world's sinners will complete their punishments. It will become a better world. Sadly, you won't see it come to pass."

"What do you mean, Gallo? Thank God for cancer? All part of the punishment eh?"

The Uzi moved in a trajectory across their chests. "Shut the fuck up, will you? Just move on down to the steps. Go on … get going. I don't want to start using this." Gallo had become a man transformed.

Rushing him in the dark wasn't a proposition. They needed to find Rachael, and Gallo was the only one who knew her whereabouts. Rockwell turned back and began the descent down the stairs. They descended in silence. The only comfort he could get was from his hidden pistol and Kevlar vest.

Rockwell wondered how a man like Gallo, a respected authority in his field, schooled in the ways of science and analysis, got to believe in a whole barrel load of religious clap trap. He believed it up to the point where a piece of rusty metal was going to herald in a new age, and the sinners will be punished eternally. Rubbish! But now, Rachael was bearing the brunt of all this. *By God, these bastards are going to pay. If Ahasver is involved, he'll be at the top of the list.*

Chapter 59

HER EYES STRAINED against the gloom.

Nothing she could see gave reassurance.

Zero.

More hooded figures, with their heads bowed, had begun arriving into the cavern. They moved behind her, out of sight, but she could sense their presence. Not a word could be heard. The malignant atmosphere exceeded any she had witnessed in her entire life. *My God! Where are Simon and Joshua? How can they find me in this hellhole?*

One of the 'monks' moved to the brazier and began placing more fuel on it, before giving it a vigorous stoking. The flames died down before flaring up greedily, consuming the new fuel. Another figure pushed in a large four-wheeled tank, from which had been strapped a thick polythene tube and fitted with a tap valve. From the other side remained a wide-open area. It became filled by several men who pulled in a thick glass tank or cage, about seven feet in height and three-foot wide. A door with a tight rubber seal opened to allow access. Above it stood an identical construction, but its base had been fitted with a hopper device. Its handle protruded from the side. It was packed to the top with yellow brown earth.

Her terror heightened. She didn't have to ask what these items were for. *God's punishment is bound in earth, fire, water and air.* That's what the man had said. Now, they stared her in the face.

Rachael's thoughts went to Simon and Joshua again. She prayed they had a plan.

The descent, dark and dangerous, placed Rockwell's mind into overdrive. He ran through a dozen possibilities that could occur. There remained one certainty … death.

There was no way on earth these lunatics would allow them to live. They would take the Seal from him, and nothing he could do would prevent it. If Gallo was strutting around with an Uzi, it was a safe bet the reception committee would be any the less armed.

He felt the seal. It remained in the leather pouch around his neck. *Shall I keep it with me or do I conceal it somewhere on the way down?* He considered the options.

Three more steps into the blackness, lit only by the beams of flashlights and helmet lights. Rockwell stumbled and went down on his knees. "Watch out!" he shouted, his voice echoed and bounced around in the depths of the dark void.

Joshua half stumbled on to him, his hand reaching out for the wall to prevent himself from plunging over the edge. "Hold on there!"

Gallo shouted out. "Stop! Don't move. What's going on? Stand up or I'll start shooting." He steadied himself against the wall and raised the gun.

In the confusion, Rockwell removed the leather pouch and thrust it hard into one of the many crevices that bedecked the walls. It went all the way in. *How the hell am I going to find that?* His hand closed over a sharp and loose piece of rock lying on the steps. With a swift movement, he discreetly scratched a large **X** alongside the fissure where he had pushed in the pouch.

Was it my imagination or did a flash of blue light glow from the pouch?

"I'm okay. It's fine, let's carry on." Rockwell began to count each step from that point. Not another word was spoken. He concentrated on the counting. It reached one hundred and fifty ... *Not difficult to remember.*

When they reached the furthest point of the descent, the ground appeared different from how he remembered it. The slope was the same, but this time, there was no blue light. It remained as dark as the rest of the place. Their flashlights revealed the skeletal corpses laid row upon row around the massive circumference. Their lights picked out the floor as before. This time, they crossed over to where Rachael had found the encompassing walls. They hadn't disappeared, and the overlapping was still a triangular section forming the small archway tucked in behind.

It led on to the concealed gap, and then on to more steps as they ascended. Gallo moved them along with the barrel of his gun, accompanied with snappy snarls of, "Keep moving."

Rockwell realised they had reached the place where the ossuary had been at the feet of the angel statue.

It was empty.

They had removed the casket, and now the angel statue had vanished. He looked at Joshua.

"The statue, it's gone. It's like there's never been anything here."

"I think we heard it fly away."

Rockwell managed to raise an eyebrow. He remembered it well, but still couldn't believe it.

"This is as far as we got." Rockwell turned to Gallo.

"I wasn't expecting anything. I have my instructions. Now, keep moving."

The long and dark tunnel wound on without a shift in direction.

"How much further?" Joshua asked. "This is getting ridiculous."

Gallo shone the flashlight onto his watch. "Keep moving."

They came to a small bend, and at the end of it came a discernible glow.

"We are nearly there. Head towards the light." To announce their arrival, Gallo, without warning, discharged a small salvo up into the overhead rock face in front of them. Both men hit the ground with their hands over their heads.

"For fucks sake, Gallo!" Rockwell roared at him. "What are you trying to do? We're in a cave!"

"Get up!" Gallo snapped. "Keep moving. We're expected."

Chapter 60

HE STOOD UPRIGHT in the stone box, carved and shaped to cover his lower torso, with the perfumed unguents mounted above in a silver tank showering down upon his tattooed two-thousand-year-old body, and swirling around his lower half as if in obeisance to his greater will.

Holy and sacred acts required purity. In the presence of the Most Holy, and for those about to die, he would not be found lacking. He would be the focus, the central figure heralding in the saviour of the world, whose prophecy would bring all sinners to their doom, including the false Pope.

The gun blast had alerted him. Gallo was doing well, and had obeyed orders with diligence. He raised his hand and snapped his fingers and three legionnaires appeared. They wore hooded robes and carried assault rifles. They were dispatched down the tunnel to meet Gallo and his captives.

Wearing the coarse covering placed around her, Rachael hung dejectedly from the pillar they had bound her to. She had no doubt what they planned, and she could see no way out of it.

Now, Simon and Joshua were walking into the same trap.

She suppressed a sob, dreading the slow and diabolical death they planned for her.

Ave Maria … Ave Maria … She couldn't utter the rest of the intercession. Despair flooded her mind. *Help me … I need you.*

Nothing.

Nothing.

The robed figure approached, his extended hand, wearing the ring of a serpent consuming its own tail, stroked the coarse fabric wrapped around her.

"They will be here soon, my wingless angel, and you should hope and pray that they think of you as they make their choices."

She couldn't respond. The concealed face, she sensed, mocked her. A glint of eyes came from beneath the hood. Taking a deep breath, Rachael lifted her head and spat with force into the darkness of the cowl.

His response bewildered her.

Instead of anger, the man gave a deep sigh.

"How long have I had to endure the phlegm and bile of an accursed humanity of which you belong? Those days will soon pass. My time is upon me, and you will be amongst the first to witness it."

The foot soldiers dragged in a defiant looking Rockwell and Joshua. Behind them followed an ecstatic looking Gallo, his bearing upright, proud of all he had accomplished.

Rockwell and Joshua were flung to the floor. From where he lay, Rockwell could see the six seals on the altar, awaiting their long-lost brother. Heavy feet pressed hard into their backs.

My God! He caught a glimpse of Rachael's forlorn position.

The Grand Keeper wasted no time. "You have the Seventh Seal. I'm certain you care for Dr. Carver that is why you are here. To save her. Now, let's delay no longer. Show it to me. His brothers wait." He gestured to the array on the altar.

Rockwell's brain assessed their options. *Without the seal, this mad bastard can't complete his religious mumbo jumbo, or whatever he wants to do with it. But then, he's prepared to kill us to get it. He will hurt Rachael. We still have our weapons. But ...*

He lifted his head and stared at the robed figure. Whatever course of action he chose, would be a gamble. They were going to have to go to the wire.

"I lied. I don't have the seal, and we know who you are ... Jacob Ahasver." His voice resounded around the chamber, imparting a dangerous silence in the space. Rockwell stared into the concealing blackness of the full hood. His life, he knew, hung by a thread. Joshua looked at him askance.

"Stand them up." The Grand Keeper's voice was controlled, but dripped with icy menace.

The two men were hauled up and their arms held hard.

"Bind their hands and arms." he commanded.

Once accomplished, his arms moved upwards as the hood fell back behind his neck. Professor Jacob Ahasver stood in front of them.

"You are correct." His cadaverous features had an expression as old as weather worn granite. "How you found out no longer matters, although I am surprised." He stepped back, and with a slow sweeping gaze, surveyed the three of them. "Carver, Rockwell, and Agar, this is what is going to happen … Dr. Carver will be the first to die, then each of you, one by one, unless I adopt my other plan. Let me demonstrate, should you doubt my determination." He turned to the foot soldiers. "Take him." He pointed to Joshua. "Put him into the cabinet."

With a rough push, a struggling Joshua was forced into the thick glass cubicle. It resembled a shower unit. Above him, the identical metal hopper was filled with enough dirt to bury him alive. Joshua had gone deathly white. Being bound, he could not reach his concealed weapon.

"Now her."

Rockwell glanced at Rachael. She looked sedated, and her eyes were shut.

The men untied Rachael, as Gallo moved to the sarcophagus, and with a heave, opened the lid. He stepped back and covered Rockwell with the Uzi. Two men picked her up as she began to struggle, and with force, they shoved her to the stone coffin on her back and facing upwards. They then slid the lid back in place. One of the men pulled back a voluminous velvet covering, revealing a massive water tank that bubbled to the brim.

"Seneschal, you may proceed." Ahasver signalled with a wave of his hand.

Rockwell could see what was coming. "You can't do this to her, you mad bastard. You call yourselves instruments of God? For fucks sake!" He turned to Gallo, his fists tightening beneath his restraints. He half shouted, and his voice was now filled with despair. "Gallo, what are you doing? It's us, for Christ's sake! That's Rachael! We've worked together for years. How can you do this?" Gallo said nothing but moved closer to Rockwell. He stared at him, his lips compressed into a rigid straight line. In spite of their desperate situation, Rockwell realised what he was looking at ... a man hungry for fulfilment of sorts, a man propelled by inner angst, so deep he had lost sight of his humanity. He had attached his soul to his Master, now prepared to murder for the promise of some mythical Biblical fable. There could be no appeal to reason.

Rockwell turned to Ahasver. Even as he spoke, he felt the hand of doom-ridden foreboding pass through him.

"Listen, Ahasver. I don't have the Seal."

Ahasver's raised arm dropped.

Gallo, faithful to his Master's instructions, activated the lever governing the hopper.

Joshua bent his head low as a steady stream of dirt yellow soil began to descend on his head with a steady flow. The two-inch thick glass, and the rumble of the dirt, blocked what noises he was trying to make.

Gallo muttered his sacred oath ... *Sacris Sanctum Homicidium,* then bowed to the statuesque figure of Ahasver, the Grand Keeper, standing reverently before the altar. He approached the stone coffin. Rockwell could hear Rachael's muffled cries from inside. Grabbing the polythene tubing, Gallo inserted it into the drilled orifice and turned the tap attached to it. A steady stream of cold water began to make its way from the tank, into the coffin, where Rachael's terrified screams became louder.

"STOP!" Rockwell shouted full force. "STOP! There's

something you should know." The unbelievability of the situation they were in penetrated every brain tissue and nerve end of his being.

Ahasver raised his arm, and Gallo turned off the tap and the hopper.

"Speak." His voice was without a trace of emotion.

"If you harm us, you will never get the Seventh."

"But you told my seneschal you had it."

"I lied. I wanted to find out what this was all about."

"Now you know."

"There's another thing. Certain papers and documents, extensive and covering everything we know and suspect, including the death of Father Luke and James, the suicides, and the attempted heist by three bogus monks, have been left with my lawyers. What you don't know is that Father Luke, via his computer wizardry, was able to trace you and your Inner Circle. We know of your Vatican operations and meetings. We know everything about you, and your worldwide network, and your arms caches around the world. We knew of Gallo's involvement ages ago, and from there, it had not been difficult to track all your activities." He paused for breath, and realised by the anxious exchange of glances that his legal bluff had caused an effect. He continued. "If all three of us together, and I mean all three, do not return to our legal team at three o'clock tomorrow afternoon, they have instructions to release the information they have to the concerned authorities. Once the lawyers implement my directives, the wheel will be unstoppable. But, we are prepared to withdraw all the evidence."

Ahasver raised his hand. "What directives?" His voice remained emotionless.

I'll come to that in a moment. If you kill anyone here, or all of us, you will not get the seal. It is safe somewhere where you will never find it. Without it, you are powerless. And if we are harmed in any way, your identity will be revealed, and your Keepers and those who follow you, will be arrested and flung into jails around the world." For the first time, Rockwell felt he had an edge. "Ahasver, for a man who claims that he is two thousand years old, you are remarkably stupid." He noted a slight twitch in the man's eyebrow.

The stakes had been raised.

I don't believe you want your identity and activities reported to Mossad, Aman and Shin Bet. When Israel alerts the world's security services, they sit up, and action follows, as you may well know. Without the seal, you and your secret brotherhood are nothing but a pathetic bunch of deluded monkeys."

Rockwell had played a good hand, but he wondered if it would be good enough. The Seventh Seal was all Ahasver needed to continue his mad fantasies of a New World Order, supported by heavenly hosts. Can they really bring about the Second Coming? Ahasver and his men thought so. Enough people had been murdered.

Ahasver rubbed at his chin, looked at the stone coffin, and then at Joshua in the tank.

"A clever ploy, Rockwell. All I need is the Seventh Seal. Once in my hands, I shall be unstoppable. Of what use would Mossad, plus all the world's armies be at that time? There would be no force that could stop God's will. I have my dark angels too. They tell me the Guf is all but empty, and all that is needed is for the seals to be reunited and broken, and the final trumpets will sound. Your choices are not good. What do I care about you or your companions? I am indestructible until He returns and lifts from me the binding chains of two thousand years of misery. I have learnt to gamble in my time. Your chances are poor. I will kill her first, and then him." He tapped their tombs. "If that fails, the third element will be used in conjunction with air to make the flames hotter... earth, air, fire, and water. You, Rockwell will follow the footsteps of the martyred Saint Lawrence. I was there to witness it, you know, as he was roasted alive on a grid iron by the Romans... a very unpleasant way to die." He pointed to the glowing hot brazier. "I give you thirty minutes. Give it to me and I may set them free, but that's a gamble you will have to take. We shall leave you alone, for now, for some quiet reflection." He gave a small wave and Gallo and the other men followed him out.

The glass walls had begun to steam up. Dirt had reached the level of his lower waist.

Damp … wet … and clinging.

Cloggy spats had penetrated and entered every exposed orifice. He could feel them beginning to smear into his hair, block his ears, his nostrils, the corners of his eyes, and into his mouth. It wasn't physically uncomfortable … but fear made it so.

He could make out the blurred outline of the stone coffin holding Rachael, and the trussed-up form of Rockwell further back. He prayed they were still alive. Not a sound penetrated the thickness of the glass. He knew that soon, the lack of air would be a problem, adding to what he was already facing. It seemed that whatever their fate was to be, it had been postponed. For now. *Has he told them where the Seal is being hidden?*

At that moment, he felt his insides churn in a furious fear-filled spasm.

Taphophobia wrapped itself around him. He could not imagine being buried alive. His mind, moving in slow motion, dredged up long forgotten memories.

When Joshua was seven years of age, he and two friends had entered the disused sand and gravel quarry. Not long after their games, they were sitting on a long piece of timber, throwing stones into a puddle not far off, when a section of rotten timber above them had given way, and tons of gravel and sand crashed in over them. He had been submerged, but managed to dig himself out. Being seated the furthest off, he avoided the full force and weight of it. He tried to help his friends but there was too much sand and the pile of gravel was thicker than a house. Joshua had run home, crying and screaming. But his friends died all the same.

The horror, and the shame. It was happening all over again.

He blocked the mental rerun but the fear remained. *This is it, this will be my final punishment. Please, let it be quick! God, look after Rachael and Simon.* He hung his head and gave up attempting not to swallow lumps of dirt.

Rachael, partially submerged in her black tomb, lay shivering and on the edge of unconsciousness. Her eyes were closed and she tried to keep her head above the water with what little strength she had, but her breathing had become rapid and shallow. Her heart pounded and panic overcame her. She could hear and see nothing, but knew the water had been switched off.

It is not a time for rational thought. Above her, was a stone lid, above that the cave system of Beit-Guvrin, and above that fresh clean air and a blue sky. I am being sensory deprived before I drown. Oh, Great Christ, what if they just leave me here like this?"

She spluttered out a scream.

It went unanswered

Then from somewhere, a glimmer of blue entered her mind.

Chapter 61

THE WANDERING JEW was alone, naked, with his body glistening with oils.

He raised his arms upward to form a diagonal cross with his body. The aesthetics of his perfectly proportioned muscular formations gave him pleasure. The subtle blending of tattoos etched around the countless scars, the mounds and ripples adding depths of strength were the result of work across the centuries. They could not be bettered. He gave thanks to God for his fine work.

Now the time he had waited for so long was almost upon him. No more false alarms, no more frustrations, and the never-ending curse of moving on to some new country or assuming another identity, forever cursed, persecuted, despised, and spat upon. Christ killer! He stood accused of Deicide. He had borne the burdens, and suffering had been welded into his frame. No God would make another suffer as he had done. He had seen so many terrible crimes and brutal killings across the centuries. How many times had he begged Christ for forgiveness and been refused? For too long, the levy had surely been paid in full. Mercy, and an elevation to the highest must be his.

He felt nothing for those who had been killed in the name of the AWC. They were Christ's appointed warriors.

Tears formed in his eyes, and he swept his hand into the salty trickles, to look at them suspended on the end of his finger. He had not seen tears since his early days in Judea. They were a sign of the miracles that were about to occur.

He wept for all he'd been through ... and for the release he had long waited for.

Chapter 62

THERE WAS NO time for sentiment. To ask questions would be a waste of time. He swept in, followed by an eager to please Gallo. He gestured to Gallo who went and dragged the lid off the coffin to reveal the shivering and terrified form of Rachael, resembling Millais's *Ophelia*. The water lapped a fraction below her ears. Her head from that point was the only part visible from beneath the water.

She began screaming. "Get me out of here! Please, don't make me die like this!"

He made another gesture and Gallo pulled the lid back into position, muffling her screams.

Rockwell could only watch. This was to be a deadly game.

The Grand Keeper crossed over to Joshua and peered hard into the misty glass. He nodded again to Gallo. "Twenty-five per cent flow for both."

Gallo adjusted the dial that controlled the leverage and pulled on the handle. The dirt began to drop in a small but steady stream. It piled up in a pyramid shape on Joshua's head before it collapsed and rebuilt yet again.

Joshua wriggled and struggled, but to no avail.

Next, Gallo turned the tap in exactly the same manner as he had the hopper. The water could be seen flowing into the coffin in slow trickles. Rockwell struggled, even knowing it was futile. "Let them go, you bastard. They were your staff. Have you no pity or compassion?"

"I was shown none, nor mercy in all my eternal wanderings, and I will show you none. Only what I received will you see." He turned to Gallo. "Stop the water flow and let him watch."

The lid was hauled back. Rachael was still alive, but the water level had risen up over the bottom of her chin. Another inch. and it would be in her mouth. The earth continued to drop down on Joshua.

"Think on it, Rockwell. Not long from now, both will perish in an unpleasant manner. Their deaths will be slow and agonising. Believe me, I have seen this many times. Do you want that on your conscience for the sake of a metal seal you don't even believe in? Worse still, you will then be roasted alive. By then, without doubt, you will talk. Of course, you can stop it right now. Just tell me what I want to know."

Silence.

The soft sound of water gurgling. The rumble of tumbling earth.

Rockwell's mind raced with a thousand ideas, none of which were of any use. He had reached his limitations. He'd been outplayed, outsmarted.

He lifted his head in desperation. "All right. Stop it! Switch them off. I'll tell you."

Ahasver turned to Gallo and gave a curt nod. He continued to remain silent, walking over to sit behind the altar. Rockwell could see his lips muttering, even stranger, his hands were shaking.

"Let them out, will you? You promised." Rockwell

bellowed.

"I did no such thing. I said I might. I have been thinking. It seems to be that you three have been part of this great plan. If I release you, and only if, I need the seal and I want you to witness the truth of my quest. My two-thousand-year-old endeavour would not have faced its final phase without your input. So, before you die, I want you three to witness the great power of the seals. If you doubt it, then ask yourself How I, the Eternal, the Wandering Jew have survived every known conflict, attack, war, execution, disease, pestilence, and catastrophe. Look at me." He stood and moved closer to Rockwell, and let his robe fall from him so that his defined, scarred, and tattooed body was on full view.

Rockwell gasped. Its symmetry defined any attempt at ageing, as did his face that could have been that of a young man or one in his middle years. The thought crashed through his mind. He could be crazy or, oh my God! He could be right, and all this is true. He looked around at Gallo, and he and the foot soldiers were on their knees in praise of him. *Am I going crazy? This could be true, but it can't possibly be.*

"It's not a fairy story." Ahasver had read his mind. "Where is the seal?

"If I told you, you wouldn't be able to find it. Even I, will have trouble. It's not far from here."

"You lied earlier?"

"I lied."

He picked up the discarded robe and wrapped it around his body.

"This is what I propose …"

"Till that her garments, heavy with their drink,
Pull'd the poor wretch from her melodious lay
To muddy death."

Ophelia words echoed in Rachael's mind, but could not enter her psyche. Try as she might, her spectral image had been barred. Rachael, in her watery tomb, was finding contentment and peace. She could no longer feel the coldness of the water. Warmth, relaxing and comforting, permeated her entire being, body and soul. The soft dribbles of water searching for a way into her body were purifying, cleansing her of all sins, of all the banks of filth, both physical and mental, that she had inherited since the day she had been born.

The blue light, faint, fluttering, as if uncertain of its intent, slithered through the lapping wetness of the stone tomb, and across the dormant form of its protected ward.

It was to wake her. It waited.

The stone lid began to move away from the top to allow the light to enter.

Rachael's eyes sprung open and she began to splutter. Her world was full of blue. Her mouth opened and shut. *I'm alive. What happened? Where have I been?*

Rough hands hauled her into a sitting position.

Opposite her, Josh had been released from his stand up grave. He lay sprawled on a large pile of soil, his face pressed sideways into the sandy earth.

All three remained bound.

Chapter 63

The Vatican

A WATERY SUN struggled to traverse the sky before its inevitable plunge below the horizon. He had always admired the Roman landscape, the city, the beauty and sacredness of Saint Peter's and the blessed Basilica. They were dear to his heart … a heart more open than his Cardinals wanted their holiest structure to be open to. Their conservative opposition, he knew well, but God had told him his path would not be an easy one. At fifty-seven years of age, and by Papal standards, he was too young to be in charge of the world's largest religion. He removed his scapular, the sign of his unity with Christ Jesus and the Holy Virgin, Mary. He brushed his hand through his thinning blonde Swedish hair. His selection had come as a surprise, but it had been a narrow victory … so it was rumoured. The previous incumbent, Pope Leo X, had reached the age of ninety, and had collapsed and died whilst administering Mass to the faithful in Saint Peter's Square.

The day had been one of tedium, a day that would have tested the most blessed of the saints. Pope Linus II had numerous tussles, and the latest was the contentious issues of the Sacraments being given to divorced couples, same sex couples, and women priests. His duty, he fervently believed, was to bring the church into focus with the modern world. His opponents argued that the scriptures forbade such heresies, and they were not the word of God, but of Satan.

He put that behind him. It was Thursday, and as usual, he had his weekly dinner night with his Camerlengo, Cardinal Riario, and the Papal Prefecture for Economic Affairs, Cardinal Pacca. He saw it as a welcome break from the divine duty of running a faith with multi millions of loyal adherents. The two cardinals had proven to be excellent dinner hosts, and their regular Thursday night dinner figured high on his enjoyment list.

Before leaving his quarters, he prayed in his small private chapel, rubbed his hands together, and made his way to the dining area. For his age, he had succumbed to portliness, and being of small stature, it was more evident than if he had been inches taller. Yet, his face portrayed much gentleness. For those who cared to look more closely, could be seen creases, stitched together with barbs of steel. His bishops and cardinals had soon discovered Pope Linus II had tiger's teeth. Some, to their cost, had found themselves with outlandish postings in faraway places. Now, his worldwide Encyclical, *Libero Corde et Animum*, concerning the acceptance of other faiths as a path to God, open hearts, open minds, had been roundly and frequently attacked as unheard of, unbelievable, and heretic.

No one comes to the Father but through me ...

There were moments during the heated debate when he thought a certain clutch of cardinals were beginning to regard him as the Antichrist. What nonsense!

A Swiss guard, posted at the door bearing his iconic pike, but with his modern weaponry concealed beneath the flamboyant costume, pushed the expansive double doors open. Pope Linus entered.

"My word, God be praised." His nostrils expanded at the aroma issuing from beneath the three silver domed chaffing platters. *"Aah! Pan quaglie arrosto con funghi."*

The table, set to perfection but with certain homeliness, was always a welcome sight. Cardinals Riario and Pacca rose to greet him as he lumbered in through the doors. They had learnt not to kiss his hand or kneel before him, after he told them that such performances contributed to a personality cult and unnecessary subservience. He gestured for them to be seated. They took the chairs opposite him.

"Well, my good Cardinals, it has been a trying day. Why is it that every time I attempt to bring Christ's simple message to all men through my Encyclical, those Judases, Jesuits, the right-wing bunch of die-hard, Latin obsessed priests and Cardinals attempt to block my moves. I ask that our beloved Mother Church play an important role in everyone's lives, not just to those who believe that one way is the only way…" He paused. "I've ranted enough today." He tucked the crisp white serviette behind his front collar. "And what's wrong with you two tonight? You look as if you've seen a ghost."

"Not so, Your Holiness," Riario replied. "As you said, the day has been trying with nothing resolved. I'm afraid we have more days like this to face. Let's forget it for an hour or so and enjoy our dinner. We knew you enjoyed roast quail." He looked up for the expected praise.

"*Si*, I could smell it from down the corridor. An excellent choice, and just what I need after today's nonsense."

Cardinal Pacca offered thanks for the meal about to be eaten. Riario then lifted the silver domes off each chaffing dish, followed by the side dishes. The savoury aroma glided through the ornate room. Next, he poured three ample measures of the finest Barolo wine into the large glasses.

"*Salute e felicità.*" Pope Linus raised his drink for a toast, and the two Cardinals responded. All three glasses touched.

"*Salute e felicità.*"

They proceeded to enjoy the roast birds and vegetables.

Pacca threw a concerned glance at Riario who studied his vegetables with an uncommon attentiveness. He gave a furtive look at his Holiness who had begun to carve into the small bird on his plate.

As his rule and custom, he never spoke whilst eating.

He had always said that God provided the food, and as such, one's full attention should be given to it, and once started, not a scrap should be wasted. To do so, he had said, was tantamount to saying that God's bounty lacked in some way.

For a moment, both Cardinals peered over their raised forks to watch him eat. The quail went down well. He cleared his plate of every morsel, sat back, patted his stomach, and then drank several large mouthfuls of Barolo.

"That's what I call a meal. God be praised. What's wrong with you two? You're eating like a pair of lovesick tortoises." He laughed at his own simile.

Aware of the Holy Father's disapproval of wasted food, they carried on eating without enjoyment. Their minds and thoughts were waiting for the moment the hemlock would kick in. It should happen within an hour or so. They could see perspiration forming on his forehead.

The Pope had a secret weakness. Cigarettes.

He had tried many times to give them up. To an extent, he had limited his indulgence to after-dinner occasions. He argued with himself that God wouldn't mind such a small indulgence on his part. After an excellent meal, a small brandy, and coffee, a cigarette would be allowed, as long it was only the one.

Pacca stole a glance at his watch. An hour was almost upon them, and they had a flight to catch later.

Cigarette smoke drifted around the table and the conversation had halted. Pope Linus II's complexion had developed a waxiness that hadn't been there before.

He felt his heart flutter.

"My dear Cardinals." His voice had changed to a lower pitch, and his words had a tremulous edge. "I'm not feeling too w...well. I keep getting p...pins and needles, like electric sh...shocks to my feet. Can you see me back to my room, please? And call a doctor." He coughed several times and held onto his chest. "This is painful." He began to take in huge and rapid gulps of air. "Something is... is... n...not right here. Quickly, let's go." He did not see the triumphant look that passed between the Cardinals.

They supported the Pope as they returned to his quarters.

Pope Linus staggered to the bedroom. His feet were not obeying him. Paralysis had started creeping in. The doctor was called and both Cardinals remained until he arrived. He deteriorated fast.

"How long has he been like this?'

"After his meal, he had a few drinks, lit a cigarette, and then complained of feeling ill."

"Looks like a coronary problem. The Papal ambulance is outside." The doctor clicked his fingers and the two paramedics hovering in the background hurtled into action, and inside a minute, the Pope was whisked away at high speed to Rome's Memorial Hospital.

In such events, a stream of actions are initiated, and put into place. The two Cardinals, on this occasion, would not be playing their expected roles. Should the Pope die, the Camerlengo's most important role would be to remove the Fisherman's Ring, the Pope's seal of authority, from the finger of the dead Pope, and destroy it in full view of the assembled conclave of Cardinals and Bishops. He would then be the temporary Pope until a new one is elected.

The Camerlengo didn't think that would be necessary.

Two and a half hours later, two things happened: The Holy Father, Pope Linus II, died. He did so, fully conscious, but in a paroxysm of paralysed agony. Medical teams had not yet discovered the cause of death.

'The pope is dead.' These urgent words were wired throughout the world, and every news agency worldwide interrupted their programming with the announcement of these four words. A sense of wonderment and curiosity about papal Rome reignited, as the world tuned-in to watch the calling of the Conclave of Cardinal-Electors, and waited for the installation of the successor to the See of Peter.

At the Vatican basilica, as the bell of the *Arco delle Campani* tolled the death knell, and bells all over the city peeled in sorrow at the news of the pope's death, officials of the Holy See lost their power and position. The Church, for all intents and purposes, came to a grinding halt. The See of Peter was empty. Cardinals had to be notified. Officially, the Camerlengo of the Church, the cardinal who had been nominated by the pope prior to his death, to serve the Church during the *Sede Vacante* as administrator rather than as head, assumed his temporary position over the Vatican.

Try as they might, he could not be found.

The El Al flight from Rome's Fiumicino Airport was en route to Tel Aviv's Ben Gurion Air Terminal. Jerusalem's Attorot Airport had been closed for security reasons. Passengers for Jerusalem would be bused from Tel Aviv to the city. On that flight were two cardinals, a wealthy international banker, an arms dealer, an Italian government minister, and a British Knight of the Realm, and acting senior NATO attaché.

Chapter 64

RACHAEL LOOKED LOST in a dream. The expression in her eyes was not of this world. She looked far away, somewhere, where few had been able to return from. Her near nakedness as she stood before them all did not seem to affect her. She made no effort to cover herself as water dripped from every part of her body. Joshua turned his head away, embarrassed for her.

Rockwell wasn't sure how to respond. For a fleeting moment, he realized that she was beautiful. Then, he shouted, "Give her a towel and her clothes, will you? You're not complete animals, for God's sake."

Ahasver nodded at one of his men. He found her clothes and a roll of cloth she could use as a towel. They were dropped at her feet. Ahasver pulled his hood back on, as if reluctant to be seen without it. He turned to Rockwell and Joshua. "I am glad you agreed to my proposal. I need all three of you to witness the truth of my words. Violence is inherent in all men and can be controlled; but of the will of God, men have no power whatsoever. Retrieve the seal, and you may retain it, but in doing so, you will be led to where the conjunction will occur. Once there, you will give me the seal and you will be free to leave. It will matter not, you will perish anyway. I'm certain that as archaeologists, the curiosity in your blood will compel you to stay and witness. If you refuse now, you will die right here, and your skeletons will be added to this accursed place. So, are we going to retrace your steps, Professor?"

"Unbind us first."

"No. That will only happen when we have the Seal and when we reach our destination. Are we to proceed or not?"

Rockwell looked at Joshua who nodded. He turned to Rachael. She made a brief nod … although she still wore that dreamy expression.

"Let's go."

Ahasver bowed before the altar, wrapped the six other seals in a purple cloth and placed them with loving care into a side bag he had slung around his neck.

"This way." Rockwell bent his head and began the walk towards the area from which they had first emerged. He knew that once the last step was reached, he had to count one hundred and fifty to where he concealed the artefact, and the X that marked the place. One man walked beside him and another behind. Rachael and Joshua followed close in line. Gallo, brandishing his Uzi, followed last, with Ahasver in front of him.

The climb was arduous. After their torture episode, the effort of lifting one leg up in front of another placed a heavy toll on their already tired muscles. Rockwell turned to Rachael. She looked disheveled and her hair had slicked back into a limp, non-drying rat's tail down her back.

"Are you okay?" His voice contained unfamiliar concern.

She didn't reply. She heard his words as if they were a thousand light years away. She nodded, the slight smile on her lips made her look like a Zen monk who had just experienced his first *kensho*.

"Rachael?"

"Keep moving and shut up." The guard clouted his gun into Rockwell's ribs, causing him to gasp out.

Rachael did not mind the climb at all. She felt like she was gliding, floating over each step. Fear had left her, submerged forever back in her waterlogged tomb. Just when she thought she was dying, something wonderful had happened. She could not explain it or demonstrate it … it just was … and it was with her, and would be so to her dying day.

SHE … will be with me. She loves and protects me and I am her instrument. She needs me, and I will serve her.

Rachael had not seen Rockwell conceal the Seventh Seal. But, she knew where it was.

It called to her.

She heard its blue whispering in her mind.

And she replied, *I am coming … wait for me.*

"I need to take a breather." Rockwell's chest heaved with the effort. There were still eighty steps before they reach the spot where the seal had been hidden.

"Very well, a few minutes only." Ahasver's voice bellowed across the vast space.

The troop sat down on the rocks and their flashlights danced patterns across the numerous boulders that spanned the depth below and to the side of them.

Rachael remained standing. "I'm fine." She, like Joshua and Simon, remained bound. She stood apart, aware that Rockwell and Ahasver were staring at her. Their predicament had little relevance to what she continued to experience. One she knew they would not understand. Except for Ahasver. She knew of him, his unbelievable truth, and wondered how she had ever doubted it.

For him, she felt only pity.

From the way he looked at her, she knew he sensed what was happening to her. He had understood the moment she was released from the water-filled tomb, that the very source he was attempting to reach and use for his own release had indeed been guiding her. She knew he regarded her as a threat.

They understood each other.

Turning, and in the half-light, she fixed her gaze into the darkness of his hood where she knew his eyes were located. The force that came from it stunned her.

Hate. Pure hate.

She lifted her head towards the darkness above and closed her eyes.

The blueness flickered, but the malice of the Wandering Jew billowed all around. There will be blood.

"Please resume," Ahasver snapped. "Rockwell, how much further?" His voice quivered with unconcealed excitement.

"Another eighty steps or thereabouts."

"Get going then."

They continued their ascent.

Not a word was uttered as Rockwell counted each upward step. As he neared the end, he began thinking of how to release himself and Joshua.

They had not been searched, and still possessed their concealed weapons. He just had to find a way to remove their restraints.

Five steps remaining, and Rockwell directed the flashlight onto the sidewall, hoping to see the X that marked the exact spot.

At four-thirty p.m., the diverted Jerusalem El Al flight from Rome touched down at Ben Gurion International Airport, Tel Aviv. Six serious looking men, unbeknown to most, and in whose hands much of the world's future rested, exited and made their way through customs. Their ample baggage was collected for them. Six separate limousines were waiting, and they drove off at thirty-second intervals. Forty-five minutes later, they turned into King David Street and were lining up outside the David Citadel Hotel.

A retinue of uniformed bag carriers descended on the fleet. They were expected and had between them booked the entire top floor.

Each of them experienced a flutter of nerves. Years of praying, plotting and planning had brought them to this moment in time. As instructed, they were to remain silent, and keep to their rooms until they heard from the Grand Keeper. How long that would be, they had little idea. The news from the Israeli news channels confirmed one major item. A sombre faced newscaster announced the death of the current Pope, Linus II. The announcement gave few details, apart from he had been taken suddenly ill and had died in a hospital in central Rome.

The Vatican and Rome were in an uproar amidst accusations and possible recriminations. People demanded the whole story. Almost as an adjunct, the newscaster added:

"There is increasing concern around the disappearance of two important Cardinals who have not been seen or heard of in the last twenty-four hours, Cardinals Riario and Pacca. Their whereabouts is as yet unknown. They were last known to have dined with the Holy Father.

The newscaster reminded viewers that Cardinal Riario would be acting Pope until the conclave of two hundred and twenty-five Cardinals, otherwise known as 'Princes' of the Catholic Church, elected a new Pontiff. The Camerlengo was vital for only he was authorized to destroy the Fisherman's Ring. Until it was destroyed, there could be no process nor a new gold ring made.

Riario, who had a position of considerable power in the Church, had plenty of time to reflect. He had no qualms about his momentous decision to abandon the Catholic faith, and the role he held. His new role was greater for he had helped kill the Antichrist.

Sacris Sancti Homicidium.

Riario and Pacca had discarded their vestments and were now wearing sharp designer suits, dark Ray-Bans, and had signed in under their birth names with false passports and ID.

All six men waited in silence, prayer, and meditation. It

seemed to each of them that the entire world held its breath. The seals were to be reunited, of that they were certain. The Grand Keeper had told them so.

The first step had been taken, a Pope was dead, and news around the globe also told of unprecedented and violent weather across the planet. A chain of undersea volcanoes a thousand miles northwest of New Zealand, known as the Kermadoc Arc, had *all* started erupting. Worldwide tsunamis of enormous power and destruction could follow.

But there was more to come.

NASA's findings stated that an asteroid, named WF9, half a mile wide, would miss the earth by eighteen million miles. But the Russians are saying it will collide with the earth within a month, and destroy most life on the planet.

There wasn't a man among the six Keepers who didn't believe that the End of Times had begun.

Chapter 65

THE FLASHLIGHTS LIT the stony steps and craggy walls where the Seventh Seal had been concealed. Gallo received a nod from his Master and moved forward.

"Well, where is it, Simon? You said it would be here, but we can't see it." The metallic click of the safety catch being released was loud and clear in the overbearing silence.

"It should be here. I marked the place with an X and I counted the exact number of steps. Keep shining those torches, it must be around here somewhere. It can't just have vanished."

Five powerful flashlights interplayed over the ancient wall surface in all directions. Gallo and Ahasver watched as everybody began staring and rubbing at the wall to find the elusive X.

No sign.

Rockwell looked perplexed, and Joshua's face showed his concern.

Rachael stood back, her face a blank canvas. Ahasver moved forward. In the light, he resembled a Russian Orthodox priest, but not with a message of peace. "I warned you, Professor Rockwell." His voice resonated with savage fury. "*Sacris Sancti Homicidium!* Drop her over the side." He pointed at Rachael and then down into the black abyss below.

Rough hands grabbed her and propelled her to the edge.

"Wait. You can't do this! We had an agreement!" Rockwell roared.

Joshua joined in. "No, not her. Push me instead." He moved across to stand in her place.

"Very noble, Agar, but my mind is made up. Do it now!" Ahasver pointed to the inky blackness again. Gallo moved to grab a hold of Rachael.

Before the fatal push could be made, Rachael, in a strange voice that anybody who knew her would not have recognized as her own, spoke. "If you, do you will never know where it is."

"Hold it!" Ahasver held up his arm as Rachael wavered on the edge. "Where is it? You know where it is?"

'Yes, and you will too, if you switch off your torches."

Ahasver paused. "Hold her tight, and cover those two. Now, Dr. Carver, explain. Why should I do such a thing? There's nothing you or your two other idiots can do. You stand seconds from death."

"Her voice remained at an uncanny pitch. "You will see at once where the seal is. We're in the wrong place. Professor Rockwell can't count. Turn off the lights and you will see."

Ahasver was intrigued by her lack of fear. "We'll do it. If you are playing games, it will be the last one you will ever play." He looked around. "Switch off your flashlights."

The columbarium was plunged into blackness.

The blanket of darkness lasted no longer than the briefest of seconds. Further up the steps came a discernible pulse of blue light.

"There," she said. "That's it."

Nobody spoke.

In the eerie blueness, Joshua and Rockwell looked at each other. They were speechless.

Whatever Ahasver thought, he wasn't saying. It was another confirmation that heaven held his hand. "Lead on, please. Your life, this time, is spared."

The steps looked clear in the blue light, and they left their flashlights off.

Within minutes, they were at the place. No matter how hard he looked around at the wall, Rockwell found no trace of the X he drew to mark its location. But the glow was decreasing, and the flashlights were switched back on.

"Untie him, and then you pull out the seal, Rockwell, and no tricks."

The restraints were removed, and guns covered him. Rockwell squeezed his hand into the crevice and took hold of the seal. The soft blue light flickered before it faded away.

"I have it. Shine your torch here." He held it aloft and removed it from its leather bag.

Gallo looked in awe, and Ahasver stared at it as the torch beams played across its unremarkable surface. His voice came out in a loud and reverential whisper. Tears formed in his eyes as he raised them upwards.

"How long have I waited for this? Many centuries have passed me by, and now the time is nigh. You fools cannot imagine or sense my feelings at the gravity of this moment. I wish to hold it, but I am not to touch it until we reach our destination. As I promised, Rockwell, you are to carry it. Place it in your top pocket and button it down. Leave it there and do not attempt to take it out until I tell you. Any deviation and Gallo will put a bullet through you. Now, restrain him again." His order produced an instantaneous response.

"Where are we heading for?" Joshua, soaked in sweat, asked angrily.

Before Ahasver could answer, Rachael did so. "The Mount of Olives."

Ahasver shot her a perplexed stare. "How did you know that?"

Everybody turned to stare at her.

She shrugged. "It's obvious. That's where He was last seen. Ascension has always, in legends and myths, signified divine origin. Where else could the Seven Seals be united?"

Rockwell shook his head in disbelief. He couldn't deny the empty feeling in his heart, as something he couldn't understand chewed into the boundaries of his logical consciousness, threatening to reveal the bizarre world of the subconscious … an area he had always denied. But now, it demanded release.

Chapter 66

THEY CLIMBED IN silence. When they reached the last step, the only two who had not succumbed to the muscle breaking fatigue of the steep ascent were Ahasver and Rachael. They appeared impervious to fatigue. The others were dripping in sweat, and clasped at their protesting thighs. From that high point, they then moved in a single file towards the restricted entrance. The passage became lighter as the faint shimmer of daylight grew closer.

Outside, below the access point into the caves, stood two large military style trucks, plus a 4x4 Jeep. The drivers stood around, wearing baseball caps and armed with assault rifles and side arms.

Gallo swung into action. He separated Rachael from her two colleagues and placed her in one truck, and the two men in the other. They remained bound.

Standing a short distance apart, Ahasver spent considerable time on his phone. The Keeper's worldwide network was now on its highest critical alert, as each unit contacted its allocated members and cells, in a network that encircled the globe in all directions. All that would be required would be a single text from the Grand Keeper to trigger the commencement of a global Holy holocaust. He closed the phone and stepped forward. Without emotion, he made a simple announcement.

The evil Antichrist, the Pope, is dead. Next, will be all his followers and believers. A New World Order will arise and with Christ's forgiveness and blessings, I shall rule over. With his guidance, we cannot fail Unbelievers and false religions have had their day. Now, hell and oblivion await them. For us, there can only be Paradise. We travel now to the Mount of Olives, where the unification will commence and the truth revealed."

The announcement caused a collective gasp.

He bowed his head and for the briefest moment, a look of inconceivable age passed across his face and body. He lifted both arms and his head skywards "Listen to my words. *Har Magedon,* Armageddon begins. It is upon us. We are small in number, one hundred forty-four thousand as prophesied, but with Christ's help, victory will be ours. We shall restore what is true and blessed in the eyes of Christ." His eyes swept around his small mesmerised audience, as copious streaks of sweat rolled down his ancient face. With one last roar, he yelled out, "All blessings to Cosimos Ricci who showed us how … *SACRIS SANCTI HOMICIDIUM!"*

As they journeyed to the Mount of Olives, Rockwell took stock of the situation and had to remind himself that he wasn't in the middle of some unbelievable nightmare. But it was hard to believe. Events had moved far from his perceptions of what constituted scientific enquiry and validity. That Ahasver claimed he was two thousand years old, had arranged killings and tortures, added up to nothing less than the actions of a crazed and dangerous lunatic. *How did a man like that become the head of a world-famous university?*

The Mount had now become visible. It formed part of the Judean mountains and stood beyond the Old City, dividing Jerusalem from the desert. Close by, was the ancient Garden of Gethsemane.

As they moved closer to the Garden, the weather suddenly changed. Bright sunlight gave way to an accumulation of massive dark clouds. Raindrops spattered down as loud as pebbles being rattled in a tin can, accompanied by brilliant lightning flashes and drumrolls of mighty thunder. Ahasver and his retinue remained unfazed. It was the overture to the main event.

They passed by the Basilica of Agony, the place where Christ said his last prayer. It wasn't given a second glance. The fury of the weather dispersed any straggling pilgrims and tourists. The way to the summit was clear. They reached the point where the vehicles were no longer able to pass, and Rockwell, Joshua, and Rachael, were bundled out into the lashing rain and pushed into the shelter of a few trees.

"What the hell's going to happen to us?" Joshua spat out from behind clenched teeth.

Rockwell looked at them both. "I've no idea, but I've a hunch we're going to find out real soon." He turned to Rachael, and as he did, he felt an emotion stirring within him. It was as if recent events and their now perilous predicament had brought them to the surface.

"You okay, Rachael?" It was an inadequate thing to say, but words failed him.

She lifted her head, and through the rain running down her hair and face, he detected the faintest of smiles.

"I'm fine, Simon. We will arrive there soon."

"Arrive where? Isn't this the Mount of Olives?"

"It is, and we're going all the way to the top."

He didn't know how she knew that, but asked, "Why to the top?"

"We're going to the Edicule of the Ascension. It's an octagon chapel right at the very top, built over ancient structures. It's sacred, and according to tradition, it's the exact spot from where Jesus ascended to heaven, forty days after his resurrection. In it is the Ascension Rock, where the right print of Christ's foot was enshrined. It is believed to be the last place he had touched before being taken up into heaven." She glanced up at the menacing clouds. "It's about to stop raining. Do you still have your weapons?" she whispered.

"Yes, but our Kevlar's gone. God knows what this lunatic is going to do when we get there. Tied up like this, there's little we can do."

She gave a curious expression. "I don't know what he intends, but all I can say is you need not be afraid. Trust me."

Rockwell's eyebrow lifted. "No more mumbo jumbo, please. It's enough that everybody thinks the blue light that keeps hanging around is something mystical. It's not. It's a reaction from the chemical elements in the rock and other metal components. As for an 'Ascension,' that's nothing more than a progression of pagan myths, where when a leader died, they were dragged up into another heavenly realm to meet their Gods."

Rachael said nothing.

At that moment, all three received a rough shove in their backs and they began the eight hundred-metre trek to the summit.

Unseen, Joshua struggled to free himself from the duct tape.

The Chapel of the Ascension stands centrally within the walled compound. Its ancient bricks proclaimed the location of Christ's ascension into heaven. Its soil is sacred, its purpose to proclaim in its quiet way the truth of Heaven.

Within its small, hallowed, but circular walls, a gentle arc of stone bricks arose to form an unremarkable domed roof, illuminated by two windows way up in the structure.

Upon the floor was a sunken area where allegedly, Christ's footprint can be seen, embedded until the end of time. Around this was a canopy of sweet smelling candles competing with the heady aroma of frankincense which rose from an array of gold and bronze censers. The fragrance drifted ever upward to an unseen heaven.

Six figures in fine purple robes and hoods stood inside to form a semicircle. Riario, Pacca, Woodford, Menendez, Moro, and Anderson. They have performed their tasks perfectly. Every conceivable possibility had been examined and prepared for.

This was their moment.

In a low and growling cadence, they began an old Templar war chant.

Crucem sanctam subiit,
qui infernum confregit,
accinctus est potentia,
surrexit die tertia. Alleluia.
SACRIS SANCTUM HOMICIDIUM!

He bore the holy cross
who shattered hell
He was girded with power
He rose on the third day. Alleluia!
THE SACRED ACT OF HOLY MURDER!

Approaching them from the Holy City below was the culmination of their ancient quest. Nothing less than the work of the blessed hands of John of Patmos, the inspired intentions of God Almighty that had been absent from the lives of men, causing them to lose their way and earn the wrath of God. Now, they will get what they deserved.

All six men felt galvanized as they watched the small band move closer, and with them could be seen the blessed and tall figure of the Grand Keeper, and his faithful seneschal, Gallo.

Chapter 67

THE SIX BOWED low as the Wandering Jew, Ahasver, their Grand Keeper, moved into the chapel with Gallo and his three captives. The foot soldiers remained outside. Rockwell, Joshua, and Rachael were bundled hard inside, and made to stand up against the wall directly facing Ahasver. Joshua, thankful for being placed where his hands could not be seen, continued his attempts to dislodge the tape behind his back.

The six picked up and recommenced the mournful chant. They would continue until told to stop. Ahasver remained upright and stood in a central position facing the sacred footprint. In his silence, he looked composed, perfectly still, and his eyes were closed.

With a sweeping movement of his arms, he prostrated himself flat before the sunken imprint of Christ's foot. He lay still, not moving for several minutes. He repeated the gesture and imploration twice more. Around him, the small chapel swelled with the steady cadence of the six Keepers chanting the Templar war song.

Pulsating ... Rhythmic ... Inspirational.

The Wandering Jew, as he had done many times in his long life, pleaded for redemption. He begged in a way he had never thought he would be capable of. Mixed in with the chant, the beat of his words could be heard, directed into the sunken area where the footprint was embedded.

"Have mercy upon us, O Lord, have mercy upon us.
For we have had more than enough of contempt.
Our souls have had more than their fill for we have sinned."

Joshua ignored the ritual. His hands were almost free, but not enough. He was a Guardian and Guardians had a function; to protect the Seven Seals from breakage and evil, which will elevate mankind's doom. Breakage told the Heavens that the time had arrived. No matter how seductive, how compelling the scene became, it was drenched in evil.

He looked across at Rockwell who had an expression of grim despair.

He glanced at Rachael. Her stare focused directly ahead, her face expressionless. He wasn't certain, but was that a flicker of starry blue light that passed down from her head to her toe? *What the hell's going on here?*

The chanting went on for some time and Joshua welcomed it, as his hands were now almost free from his bindings. He had to wriggle with care so as not to be seen. Finally, he freed one hand, which he kept tight behind his back.

The Grand Keeper stood straight. His eye glittering with a wild light. He addressed his Inner Circle. "You have called and they will come." He opened the chapel door. "They have heard your call. Behold." His arm pointed down the long trek that led up to the Chapel.

A blast of unprecedented lightning streaked and flashed across the darkened August sky. The thunder rolled loud but the rain had ceased. Making their way at a slow pace up the steady gradient, and illuminated by the lightning flashes, was a small procession of grey hooded figures with heads bent low, many of whom carried crosses or torches. They too were chanting the *Crucem Sanctam Subiit.* Its mournful and dark tones reverberated in harmony with the sky display that rolled across the Holy City. They were the true followers of Christ. Summoned by the Inner Circle whom they obeyed without question. Their vows were ancient and traceable back to Cosimos Ricci and way beyond.

The column made its way into the walled arena, and around the circumference of the entire structure.

Rockwell spoke. "This is crazy!"

Rachael appeared transfixed. She simply repeated, "There's nothing to be afraid of." She looked at nobody but fixed her gaze onto the sunken well where the sacred footprint was embedded. For a moment, she lifted her head with a faraway look in her eyes, and without warning or surprise to her, her restraints dropped to the floor.

She made no sound or movement. It was if she hadn't noticed, or if she had, she didn't care. She maintained her posture as if nothing had happened. None of the Keepers had seen.

Joshua's mouth dropped open in disbelief, same as Rockwell.

"This is getting beyond my comprehension. Something weird has happened to Rachael. I don't want to believe it, but it's true. Is she possessed? This is not like her. I didn't believe all this rubbish but now, I'm not sure. Not one bit of it makes an ounce of sense. What's going to happen now?"

"He'll take the Seal from you, and then I expect there'll be a firework show of some sort, and he wants us to see it. I have sworn to protect it, and keep it from being broken, and that seems like an impossible task. My arms are free now but they mustn't know. How did Rachael free herself?"

"I wish I knew, but she doesn't seem of this world right now."

The flickering light of hundreds of candles lent an eerie magnificence to the small Chapel. The Grand Keeper held his arms aloft and produced from beneath his robes an ancient scroll that he reverentially unfurled.

His voice filled the entire complex. "Warriors, I have here the testimony of Cosimos Ricci. I helped him write it. Yes, my soldiers, I was his seneschal before I initiated him step by step to make our society the wonderful instrument it is today. I have had many guises and have had to disappear many times, but I have always been with you. Know that the time has arrived as Cosimos prophesized years ago to this date, August 15, 1560. The date when the seals would come together as one. Yes, I am he who was condemned by Christ to wander the Earth until he came again. That time is about to befall us in this place and on this very spot. He will come again to rid the world of false religions and governments. We have the choice to invite worldwide destruction, or allow him to lead us with our forces poised and ready to annihilate the unbelievers and those who stand in our way ... *Sacris Sancti Homicidium!*" His ancient voice travelled across the damp air and into the hearts and minds of his devotees. His eyes blazed with fire. "He will give us this choice. I ask you now, what will it be? Cosimos has prophesized that this event would happen on this day and in this year. The six seals will soon be reunited with their lost brother, the Seventh. The Pope, the so-called Vicar of Christ, is dead, and in his place, I stand as Christ's appointed Bishop on Earth. If this is what you want, let me hear it from you."

He knew what their response would be, as he held aloft the six small seals for all to see.

There came an enormous roar from the assembly.

WE ARE UNSTOPPABLE!

The assembly began their shuffle around the sacred chapel for seven times. When that was completed, they would await the reunification. The seals will be united and once in place, they would be broken.

The Second Coming was imminent, and a New World Order would be established across the world. At the moment of breakage, the one-word code would be activated, and a global battle would commence.

The procession speeded up on each lap. Their chanting got louder, and arms began waving around in hysteria. The thunder ceased, a sign of heavenly approval as the seventh lap was completed.

The Seventh and the Seventh and the Seventh … Seven by Seven. It was all in place.

Rockwell had managed to free himself and it no longer seemed to matter who knew. He had a feeling that events were now unstoppable and somehow, he was connected to it. Between them they had two pistols. That would not be enough to stop these crazed idiots who didn't seem to care. If they had to die for their cause … then they would. He'd never been a religious person, but he saw it all in a flash. These people in their silly robes, the abandoned, soulless, desperate for salvation, having long ended their relationship with their faith, but still looking for reason and sense, unable to truly let go of the bells, smells, and the sacred chants.

Rockwell moved towards Rachael and nobody tried to stop him. There were so many people, escape would be impossible. Joshua was right behind him. Rockwell touched her shoulder.

"Are you okay, Rachael?"

She turned to face him. Her face glowed, and her clothes flickered with a blue hue.

"I am fine, Simon. Put your weapons away. She has not left me … it's him that needs to be certain. He expects an event, and there will be one." She gestured to the looming figure of Ahasver, who stood elevated on a small platform above the throng.

Rockwell followed her gesture, and saw Ahasver's gaze was fixed directly on him. *This is not looking good.*

"Joshua," Rockwell whispered with urgency. "It's time for the pistols or we are never going to escape this madhouse."

Both men reached for their guns, grateful that nobody thought of searching them. Rockwell reached out to grab Rachael.

"C'mon, Rachael. It's time we left!"

She resisted. "I said put them away. It's not time."

"What? What are you on about?"

"Wait and see."

It was then they noticed that the entire complex had fallen silent, and all eyes were fixed on them. Before they could react, rough hands had seized them and their weapons removed. All three were stood around the sacred flooring where His footprint was embedded.

The Grand Keeper spoke. "I have the six seals." He held them up. "All here, in this place, look in awe and fear for you are about to witness the end of the old order and the beginning of the new. Gallo, bring him forward. I promised you three fools that before you died you would see the extent of my powers. Take the seal from him."

Rockwell attempted to punch at Gallo's hand as it reached into his top pocket. He was prevented by a massive kick into the back of his leg that half threw him to the floor. Joshua struggled, but he couldn't break away from the three men who held him tight.

The Wandering Jew was unable to control the tremor in his hands, nor wipe away the tear that rolled copiously down his aged cheeks. Two thousand years. It had been too long. He moved them closer together.

A blue light flickered around the sacred objects.

Blueness hung from her like a graceful robe and in her head the church bells rang loud, clear, and joyful. She heard her. The Holy Mother spoke to her directly.

Ego te absolve a peccatis tuis, in nomine Patris at Filii et Spititus Sancti.

Rachael automatically made the sign of the cross. For her sins, she had been forgiven.

She opened her eyes, and lifted her arms wide. "Stop! Ahasver, stop!"

Ahasver, his face wet from tears and sweat, had no intention of stopping. "Two thousand years I have waited and now it is time. There is no stopping now. They will be united and we shall break them. Prepare!"

He joined the Seventh with the other six that had awaited their brother for so long. He displayed them dangling from his skinny arm, and began to encircle the chapel.

Rachael cried out aloud. 'Stop! You have made a dreadful mistake."

As she spoke, a blue light began to descend upon them from above. "Today is August 15th. It is the Assumption of the Blessed Mary into heaven. What you expect will not happen. She has interceded on heaven's behalf, and ours too. He will not appear!"

Joshua and Rockwell stood astonished, as did everybody. The area was now aglow with a pulsating blue colour, the same as the glow they saw from the ossuary. Now all those present saw it too. Ahasver quivered with uncertainty.

For the first time, they saw on Rachael's uplifted arms, blood emanating from the marks of the stigmata that had been embedded in both her wrists and feet.

She turned to her men. "Don't look upwards. Keep your eyes focused down. Believe me, *I KNOW!*" She reached up and pulled their heads downwards and covered them with her arms. "Only I am safe. She protects me, and I shall protect you." Without knowing why, they believed her.

A slight rustling sound filled the air before it transformed into a massive swirling wind. A fluttering noise enveloped the entire top of the mount and chapel, inside and out. It whipped and thrashed around everyone present like some crazed beast.

There was nothing to see, and the celebrants became gripped with terror. For in everyone's minds, they heard a voice, loud and clear. Ahasver covered his ears, but to no avail. The voice boomed in his head and those of his followers.

"I am the Angel Asroilu, Guardian of the Seven Seals. It is not time and they shall not be broken. Our Sacred Mother protects those here who wish the seals no harm. I was the first carrier, and I shall be the last. So, let it be."

The fluttering grew louder, but their eyes still saw nothing. The message continued.

Escape was in everyone's thoughts. But there was no escape. All the exits had ceased to exist.

"Stay with me and hold on, but don't move." Rachael bellowed her command and continued to wrap herself around the two men, who were now huddled into tight cradle postures, their heads pressed into the sandy surface.

The rumbling and fluttering grew louder, and was now accompanied by the shrieks and shouts of fear from the assembly who had nowhere to turn.

Ahasver recovered from the initial surprise and began to stand. He held the seals aloft and attempted to snap them in half. They remained firm. He hurled them to the ground, stomped and jumped on them, but nothing happened. They were enveloped in the blue light of the Holy Mother.

One by one, his Inner Circle were swept away into nothingness, as swirling blue tendrils, their vaporous fingers reaching out and clutching each of them, expunged them in a twisting white screaming plasma.

"In the name of Jesus, I am owed this!" The Grand Keeper's voice matched the intensity of the swirling torrent of fiery wind. He turned his head towards the skies. "Have pity, I beg you!"

His face registered total disbelief. Aeons of plotting and planning were collapsing all around him. "How can you ignore me? Everything I did, I did for you. I've killed many for your sake on this hellhole called Earth. Do you want more? Is that it? You want more? Then so be it!"

From beneath his robe, he produced an automatic pistol, and without taking aim, blasted off a shot at the crouching figures of Joshua, Rachael, and Rockwell.

Joshua gave a low moan and tumbled to his side. He'd taken a shoulder hit. Rockwell, without thinking, moved and covered him with his own body.

"Does that satisfy you?" Ahasver addressed the crashing volume of wind, "or must you have more?" Before he could release another shot, Asroilu's voice thundered inside his mind. There was no chance of firing another bullet. His limbs had been paralysed.

"Ahasver, listen. You will be handed over to the Angel Azrael who rules the Kingdom of Death. You're tired of this accursed Earth? Then Hell will be the abode of your warped soul forevermore. Begone!"

The seals clattered to the floor, as the Wandering Jew finally got the release he had long waited for, but not in the manner he had expected.

There would be no worldwide uprising, no message was sent, and already, a network of counter revolutionaries, troops, and police across the globe had been alerted to the threat by the Guardians. With that thought rushing through his disintegrating brain, his physical form swirled in a gavotte of pirouetting mould and decay. His crumbling flesh dissolved, and his face, a reflection of agonized horror, vanished in a whirlwind that scooped up his dust and that of all his followers, spreading them infinitely through time and space.

Only Gallo remained standing. His face wore the expression of shocked horror. He was on the verge of a mental breakdown. "Oh, Great God, what has gone wrong?" His voice came as a disjointed whisper.

"I'll tell you." Rachael faced him and raised her arms. The wounds of her stigmata remained clear for him to see. "I bleed for Him, as did his Holy Mother, with whom I've found favour. The Collyridians were not all wrong as you can see by my wounds, unlike you and your satanic master, Ahasver, or whatever you wish to call him. Thousands have died because of him, starting with Christ, whom he urged to hurry up and get on his cross. A Pope has been slaughtered but a new one will be elected, of which your New Order will never play a part. You are finished. Your Inner Circle, along with all your other fools, have been evaporated into trillions of atoms spread across the universe. Their corrupt souls will scream and fester for eternity, as will his. Your battle stations are lost and destroyed. What remains?" Rachael stared hard into his desolation. "Only you."

Joshua, clutching at his shoulder wound, looked around for Rockwell who had a look of incomprehension on his face. He shook his head at Joshua, but neither spoke.

Rachael continued, her voice as cold as ice, drove itself into Gallo's senses like a steel spike. "What is to become of you, my Lord of Mistrust and Devious Cunning? What?"

The answer came in a shaft of blue light that filled the interior once more. The shape of a woman could be seen, but her face was concealed behind a cowl softly draped across her head. She too had marks on her wrists and feet, identical to Rachael's who now knelt before her. Not a word was spoken.

Rockwell and Joshua could only gasp. Gallo had frozen to the spot. For the briefest of moments, there came another almighty rush of fluttering wings, with one tantalizing flash of gold before it stopped.

Rachael turned to her colleagues. "Cover your eyes." Her voice came full of command.

They obeyed at once, neither having a desire to look.

Asroilu, as a ghostly golden apparition, appeared, carrying an enormous heavy chain, which he placed around Gallo's neck ... causing him to sink to the ground. The chain vanished, but the weight remained.

"No! No! I beg you. Not that!"

He heard the voice in his head. *"You worshipped an evil wanderer who is lost to the universe. However, you shall replace him. For your crimes and greed, you will walk this earth for eternity, as did he. GO!"*

There was an explosion of light, followed by a massive rushing noise of wind expiring.

The Chapel of the Ascension was as it was, empty, quiet, except for the three amazed scientists.

Gallo had vanished, but where, was not known.

It was finished.

EPILOGUE

Behold I come quickly: and my reward is with me, to give every man according to his work shall be. I am Alpha and Omega, the beginning and the end, the first and the last.

Five years later...

THE PRESIDENT OF the United Nations Siberia's Frozen Tombs Program had got used to the amount of media and press releases that landed on his desk or computer. The agency used remote sensing to identify buried tombs from a culture dating back 2500 years, in a race against time, before melting permafrost ruined them. Because of this, every weirdo, alien searcher and extra-terrestrial evangelical crackpot, would forever be reporting strange sightings and close encounters. Most were rubbish. One or two were inexplicable.

It was not what the President, Professor Simon Rockwell had planned. Since the Seven Seals, his whole world had been turned inside out and upside down. He had become naked and exposed to all his human frailty. His scientific beliefs lay scattered around him, as much as the discovery of the love he had for Rachael.

That could never be. She had considered his proposal, but none could have been more surprised than herself at her rejection of it.

Joshua had vanished. He had been the first to make a major decision.

One month after the traumatic events at the Mount of Olives, none had seen or heard from him. Not a word. His wound had healed, but internally, he hurt. He told nobody. The recent events had left him shaken. What he thought as important, now no longer seemed so. The need for the Guardians had gone. The seals had vanished, and back presumably with the angels where they rightfully belonged. The entire episode had unbelievability about it.

But, he hadn't gone entirely.

In Rockwell's morning mail, he found a book that got his immediate attention. It gave him a start. He recognized the book cover photograph. Joshua Agar, now Dr. Joshua Nathaniel Agar, stared up at him. *My God, where is he?*

The book was entitled, *'Religious Miracles: Worlds Beyond Science: An investigation based on real life events.'*

Rockwell didn't have to open it to know what it would be about. He gathered from the explanatory notes that Joshua had now become a tutor at Hanazono Japanese Buddhist University, where he now headed the Department of Comparative Religious Studies. Joshua, he guessed, was still looking for answers ... and peace of mind.

He made the decision to locate and email Joshua. They both needed to talk, and there was much they should discuss. They were a pair of upended souls.

He held the book to his chest and experienced a pang of enormous sadness. He knew, because of what had happened, that he could never read it. There existed things and events he could never bring himself to speak of. He'd become detached from two close friends, his scientific firmness had all but liquefied, and the wounds had barely healed. But their testimony, Joshua's book, would remain in a privileged position in his bookcase until his dying day.

The Island of Patmos, Greece
The Convent of the Annunciation
August 15th

For a nun, uncertain of her emotions, a life of prayer seemed the right one. She listened to the bell tolling the hours of the office. Today, she knew that she would ignore them, and that as the years passed, on this special day, she would always ignore them.

She had promised herself that on this very evening, she would make every year her own obeisance.

She had every right.

The large statue of the Blessed Virgin Mary stood under its stone canopy, offering peace and gentleness to the entire world.

The nun, entering her middle years, bent low and produced her gardening trowel. With care, she scraped away the soft soil at its base, and dug deeper until she had reached her elbow's depth.

Mary smiled upon her.

She felt her warmth.

From the deep pocket of her habit, she felt its cold surface on her fingers. A small metal tablet, no bigger than a credit card was in her grasp.

For a moment, the nun held it up as an offering to the Holy Virgin.

Mary smiled upon her as a blue dazzle emitted from the tablet, surrounding her before she buried it with all the reverence she could muster.

She had sworn to return it to her. If one looked closely, the nun displayed on her wrists the signs of stigmata.

Another nun's voice called over to her.

"Sister Rachael, hurry or you're going to be late for Compline."

ABOUT THE AUTHOR

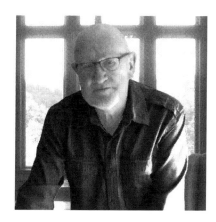

Bestselling author, Ken Fry, holds a university Master's degree in literature and has extensively travelled around the world. The places and events are reflected in his stories and most of his tales are based on his own experiences.

He was a former publisher before deciding to retire and devote his full time to writing. He lives in the UK and shares his home with 'Dickens', his Shetland Sheepdog.

Visit Ken Fry's Website:

www.booksbykenfry.com

Connect on Twitter:

@kenfry10